DISEASES AND DISORDERS OF THE HORSE

DEREK C KNOTTENBELT

BVM&S, DVM&S, FACVSc
University of Liverpool, UK

REGINALD R PASCOE

AM, BVSc, DVSc, FRCVS, FACVSc
Director
Oakey Veterinary Hospital
Oakey, Queensland, Australia

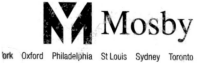

Mosby

ork   Oxford   Philadelphia   St Louis   Sydney   Toronto

MOSBY

An affiliate of Elsevier Science Limited

© 1994, Mosby–Year Book Europe Limited

ISBN 0 702 02743 X

British Library Cataloguing in Publication Data
A catalogue record for this book is available from the British Library.

Library of Congress Cataloging in Publication Data
A catalog record for this book is available from the Library of Congress.

your source for books,
journals and multimedia
in the health sciences

www.elsevierhealth.com

Contents

Preface

The contents of this book are the culmination of many contributors' efforts over many years and we would like to thank those who have offered their valuable material for our consideration, whether this was finally included in the contents or not. The book could easily have been many times its size with the inclusion of some unique and superb pictures which were sent to us from all over the world. The list of contributors is shown on page 7, but to the numerous contributors whose slides we have been unable to include (almost always only through limitations of space) we extend particular thanks. We would like to commend to the reader of this book the idea of always "having a camera handy", for without this the collection could not possibly be so complete. Photographs not only provide a colourful means of recalling interesting cases one has seen, but also act as a permanent reservoir of knowledge to which future reference can easily be made. We are dedicated to the principle of colour illustration, on the grounds that it makes subjects more interesting and easier to recall, and after all, we should be able to see what we actually see! The text is not heavily referenced but suggestions as to further reading material have been made at the end of each chapter. Most of these text books contain extensive lists of references and we see no point in repeating these.

We have tried (sometimes in vain or with limited success) to obtain material from those parts of the world where particularly poor photographic records have been kept and tried hard to obtain illustrations for diseases which are very restricted in geographical distribution or are common in some areas but rare in others. Diseases, which have been eradicated from some countries, are still very significant in others, and, while there are geographic limitations to some diseases, the modern freedom of movement of horses across the world makes it important that veterinarians recognise the major diseases of our time.

In order to structure the contents in a reasonably logical fashion a rough categorisation of the material has been followed. Included in each chapter is a text relating to the disorders and diseases of the relevant body system. The contents of the text specifically excludes extensive consideration of most aspects of treatment but some diagnostic help is proffered which might assist the clinician in both specific cases and in his/her understanding of the underlying disease processes. The chapters are designed to provide an easily assimilated, brief summary of the conditions shown in the accompanying illustrations, and is in no way a definitive treatise on each specific disorder. Thus, at the start of each system chapter, we have tried to cover the congenital and hereditary disorders, followed by the non-infectious conditions beginning with traumatic disorders, immunological/autoimmune disorders, nutritional/metabolic diseases, and then neurogenic, chemical/toxic, cardiovascular, iatrogenic/ idiopathic disorders, in roughly that order. These are then followed by a description of the infectious diseases affecting the system, beginning with the viral, bacterial and mycotic conditions and ending with the protozoal and metazoan diseases. The last section in each chapter refers to the neoplastic disorders affecting the particular body system. Where it has been possible to combine the salient features of particular sign such as nasal discharges, we have placed these together to facilitate application to particular circumstances which practicing veterinary surgeons might encounter. Suggested differential diagnoses are supplied with a number of common clinical signs to provide a broader view of the possible conditions involved. Clearly, there will be some degree of overlapping and contradictions to this scheme and, where this is so, we believe that the format we have adopted is clinically appropriate. We hope that the reader will find cross referencing a relatively easy process, particularly as we have tried to incorporate aspects of differential diagnosis into both the pictorial content and the text so that, where individual clinical signs are common to several disorders, she/he can consider the wider implications. We hope that readers will find this approach useful and will have reason to consult the book regularly. However, in a book of this size and type, it would be impossible to cross-reference every disease and every symptom of every disease. We crave the readers indulgence where there are inadequacies. Furthermore, the book is not intended to be used on its own, and we hope that it will prove to be a useful supplement to those texts which have few or no illustrations, and those which are poorly reproduced in monochrome. This book also contains some hitherto unexplored material relating in particular to the placenta and other aspects of the reproductive tract. We hope that these sections, as well as the others, will stimulate and interest the reader and thereby advance our knowledge of equine medicine. More specialised and comprehensive books in this series are (or will be) available in limited specialised fields of equine (and other) veterinary science, and we commend these to those readers wishing to expand their knowledge beyond the scope of this one. We hope that, however, this will become a standard text for initial consultation.

Acknowledgements

There have been many supporting roles in the preparation of this text book. We would both like, firstly to acknowledge the patience and understanding of Joy and Morna, our wives, who have soldiered on without us! The burden on us has been considerable but on them it must have been even greater!

Our gratitude is, particularly, extended to those mentioned below for their contributions and or comments and help, lesser or greater numerically - all appreciated, absolutely!

Professor G.P.Carlson, University of California, Davis, USA

Dr John Cox, University of Liverpool, England

Dr Hugh Cran, Nakuru, Kenya

Dr Joe Fraser, University of Edinburgh, Scotland

Professor James Duncan, University of Glasgow, Scotland

Professor Barrie Edwards, University of Liverpool, England

Dr Rod Else, University of Edinburgh, Scotland

Dr Ursula Foggarty, Irish Equine Centre, Ireland

Professor Murray Fowler, University of California, Davis, USA

Dr Christine Gibbs, University of Bristol, England

Professor John Hughes, University of California, Davis, USA

Professor Leo Jeffcott, Cambridge University, England

Professor Don Kelly, University of Liverpool, England

Dr Karen Long, University of Edinburgh, Scotland

Dr Sandy Love, University of Glasgow, Scotland

Dr Pat McCue, University of Davis, California, USA

Dr R. A. McKenzie, Queensland, Australia

Mr James McLaughlin, Veterinary Research Laboratory, Dublin, Ireland

Professor Stephen May, Royal Veterinary College, London, England

Dr Andy Mathews, Kilmarnock, Scotland

Dr Joe Mayhew, Animal Health Trust, Newmarket, England

Dr Richard Miller, Brisbane, Australia

Dr David Pascoe, Oakey, Australia

Dr John Pascoe, University of Davis, California, USA

Dr Christopher Pollitt, University of Queensland, Australia

Mr Chris Proudman, University of Liverpool, England

Professor M. Rodriguez, Falcultad de Veterinaria, Madrid, Spain

Dr Alan Rowlands, University of Edinburgh, Scotland

Professor Dr.M. S. Saleh University of Giza, Egypt

Professor Danny Scott, Cornell University, USA

Dr Marianne Sloet von Oldruitenborg Osterbaan, University of Utrecht, Netherlands

Dr Tony Stannard, University of California, Davis, USA

Professor John Stick, Michigan State University, USA

Dr Susan Stover, University of California, Davis, USA

Professor Mike Studdert, University of Melbourne, Australia

Professor Ed Usenik, University of Zimbabwe, Harare, Zimbabwe

Dr James Vasey, Shepparton, Australia

Dr T.E. Walton, United States Department of Agriculture, Laramie, Wyoming, USA

Dr Katherine Whitwell, Animal Health Trust, Newmarket, UK

Dr Lesley Young, University of Edinburgh, Scotland

Dr W.R. Allen, Cambridge, England

Professor F.W.G. Hill, University of Zimbabwe, Harare, Zimbabwe

Editor, Veterinary Record

This book is dedicated firstly to Joy and to Morna, our wives, and then to the horse, a beautiful and noble animal, which provides us with so much enjoyment and intellectual challenge.

1. Conditions of the alimentary tract

Including the mouth, oesophagus, stomach, small intestine, caecum, large colon, small colon, rectum and anus.

Part 1: The Mouth

Disorders of the mouth form an important group of conditions in the horse and, while in most cases deviations from normal can be seen directly, some are more subtle and require diagnostic aids.

Developmental Disorders

Congenital or hereditary conditions of the soft tissues of the mouth are rarely encountered in the horse and are apparent at an early stage in the life of the animal. However, **hard palate clefts** occur relatively often as a developmental abnormality (**1**). The degree to which these are heritable is not well defined. The extent of the cleft may be considerable and they are often complicated by concurrent clefts of the soft palate (*see* **185**) and a relatively high proportion of foals with a cleft palate have other developmental abnormalities, including cardiovascular defects and bone and joint abnormalities. There is a relatively high incidence of epiglottic entrapment (**Plate 5m**, page 113) in foals with a cleft in either hard or soft palate, or both. Foals in which a significant hard palate cleft occurs may show dramatic nasal regurgitation of milk during nursing (**2**). In some cases, particularly those with relatively small clefts or clefts in the soft palate, nasal return of milk becomes obvious only after feeding (**Plate 6n**, page 122) and may be relatively minor in amount. Small clefts may not always be easily visible or produce significant

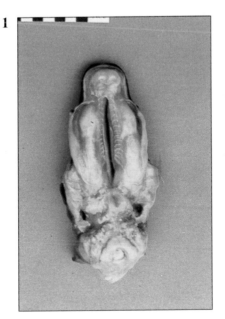

1 Cleft hard palate.

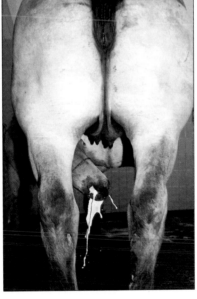

2 Cleft hard palate.
Note: Profuse nasal return of milk during nursing.
Differential Diagnosis:
i) Cleft or hypoplastic soft palate
ii) Sub-epiglottic cyst
iii) Neurological dysphagia

nasal return of food and, occasionally, some are only detected after some years, when nasal reflux of grass and more solid food material, may be present. Lesser clefts may be encountered and result in correspondingly less obvious clinical abnormality such as a mild nasal discharge with flecks of food material. Consequent rhinitis and nasal discharges may not be immediately identifiable as resulting from a cleft palate. Occasionally the cleft is sufficiently small to produce no detectable evidence and these are sometimes identified incidentally during clinical or post mortem examinations. Large palatal defects in young foals have profound effects including failure to ingest adequate amounts of colostrum, starvation and inhalation pneumonia. While the presence of clefts of the hard (or soft) palate may pass unnoticed for some years affected horses almost invariably finally succumb to inhalation pneumonia (*see* **210**).

Gross deviations of the skull, known as '**Squiffy Mouth**' or '**Wry Nose**' may be present from birth (**3**) and most result in severe malocclusion of the incisor teeth (**4**). The defect is possibly due to pressure and malpositioning during gestation. The consequences upon the well being of the foal depend largely on the extent of the distortion and whether any occlusion occurs. While most are able to suckle effectively, some cannot. Severe malformations will preclude effective grazing and such animals, which survive to adulthood, are commonly stunted and remain a permanent management problem. Probably the commonest congenital defect involving the maxilla and/or mandible is **inferior brachygnathia** (**Parrot Mouth** or **Undershot Jaw**) (**5**).

This is thought to be an inherited disorder. In the milder cases, the full extent of the discrepancy between the upper and lower jaw length, in which the upper jaw is relatively longer than the lower, may not be obvious at birth, becoming more apparent as the permanent incisors erupt and grow into their normal occlusal positions. The failure of significant occlusion results in an increasing overgrowth of the upper incisors (**6**) ('**Rabbit Toothed**') and impingement of the mandibular teeth into the soft tissues of the hard palate. Individuals with lesser degrees of inferior brachygnathia may be less affected but the lingual edges of the lower incisors may become sharp and lacerate the gums and hard palate. More commonly the lower incisors tend to prolong the line of the lower jaw and the labial margins of the upper incisors become long and sharp (**6**) and may lacerate the lower lip. Simultaneously there is usually a discrepancy in the length of the lower molar arcade and a rostral hook will often develop on the first upper cheek teeth (**7**) with an equivalent caudal hook on the last lower cheek teeth. Interestingly, foals affected by inferior brachygnathia at birth may also have concurrent ruptured common extensor tendons (*see* **437**), poorly developed pectoral muscles and/or goitre (*see* **357**). The relationship between these conditions is not clear.

Superior brachygnathia (**Monkey, Sow** or **Hogg Mouth**) is more rarely encountered (**8**). Associated with it are projections (hooks) on the rostral edge of the first lower cheek teeth and the caudal edge of the last upper cheek teeth.

Even extensive overgrowth of either superior or inferior brachygnathism, where little or no effective

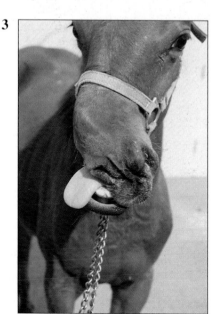

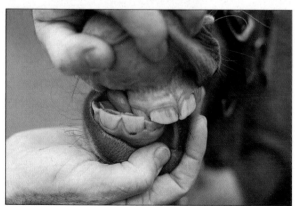

3 Wry nose (Squiffy face).
Differential Diagnosis:
i) Fracture of premaxilla

4 Occlusal malformation in a foal affected by Wry nose.

occlusion is present, appears to cause little hindrance to prehension in many cases, with the cosmetic and aesthetic effects being of concern in the early years of life. Effects upon growth and condition are therefore unusual, provided that suitable forage is available. Short grazing however, makes prehension very unrewarding for the horse, and weight loss and poor growth are to be expected. Clearly, once the overgrowth becomes severe, difficulties with prehension are more likely. Current opinion indicates that both inferior and superior brachygnathism are a result of defects in the mandible and not the premaxilla.

'**Shear mouth**' arises when there is a discrepancy in the width of the upper and lower jaws. In the normal horse the upper jaw is wider than the lower and where this discrepancy is exaggerated, even slightly, there is an excessive angulation of the table surfaces of the cheek teeth. The buccal margins of the upper cheek teeth and the lingual margins of the lower become excessively long and often very sharp (**9**). Although this disorder may be encountered in young horses as a result of developmental differences between the jaws, it is more often the preserve of older animals where irregularities of wear and 'normal' age-changes in the shape of the lower jaw, result in an increasing size discrepancy. The possible secondary consequences of this change include a marked reduction in the movement of the temporo-mandibular joints and the development of osteoarthritis. A primary joint disorder including degenerative joint disease or fractures/dislocations of the mandible, resulting in limitations of joint movement, might also be expected to cause shear mouth as a consequence of poor lateral movement of the jaw over a prolonged period of time.

5
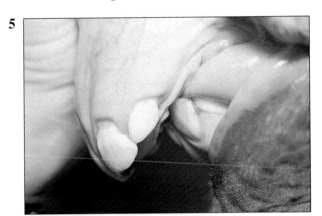

6
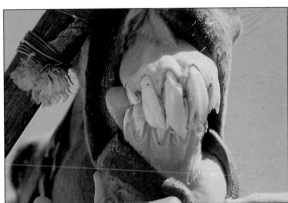

7
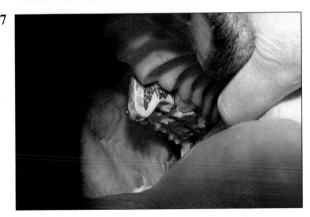

8
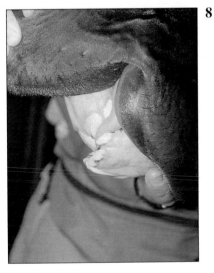

5 Inferior brachygnathism (Parrot mouth).

6 Inferior brachygnathism (Parrot mouth).

Note: Overgrowth of upper incisors in a 14 year old gelding. The lower incisors were extremely sharp and impinged upon the hard palate causing difficulty with mastication. The horse showed little difficulty with prehension, however.

7 Inferior brachygnathism (Parrot mouth)—Dental hook.
Note: Hook on first upper cheek tooth. There was a corresponding hook on the last lower cheek tooth.

8 Superior brachygnathism (Sow mouth, Hog mouth).

Defects of the teeth relating either to genesis or eruption are relatively common. **Oligodontia** (absence of teeth) is a developmental disorder when one or more teeth are absent through failure of genesis. The incisors are the most commonly affected in this way **(10)** but the molars may also be affected. In the latter cases the most common missing tooth is the first molar (fourth cheek tooth) **(11)** which should erupt at around one year of age. Examination of the molar arcade is often very difficult and lateral and oblique radiographic projections are often necessary for their identification (*see* **11**). It is often helpful to compare similar normal radiographic views **(12)** with the suspected abnormal. In the case of the incisors, true oligodontia is reflected in an absence of both temporary and permanent teeth, this being consistent with a complete absence of the dental germ cells. Although the absence of teeth may be a true developmental defect, most frequently missing and malerupted teeth are due to previous traumatic damage to the dental germ buds or to systemic infections involving these during their maturation. The consequent maleruption of teeth may cause a significant deformity of the incisor dental arcades in particular **(13)**.

Supernumerary incisors and **molars (polyodontia)** are not uncommon and develop as a result of multiple dental stalks from a single germ bud of a permanent tooth. In some cases there may be a complete double row of incisors but more often one or two extra teeth will be present. This polyodontia (dental duplication) may be restricted to one or more teeth, and affects incisors **(14)** more often than premolar or molar teeth. Due to lack of wear by an opposing tooth, the extra tooth usually becomes elongated and may ultimately cause soft tissue injury to the opposing palate or tongue.

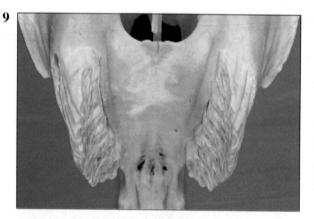

9 Severe parvinathism (Shear mouth).
Note: Inability to masticate effectively caused weight loss. Concurrent severe degenerative joint disease of both temporo-mandibular joints.

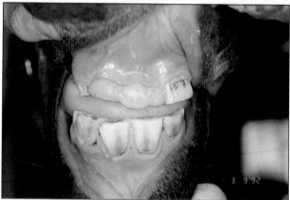

10 Oligodontia (incisor).
Note: Both temporary and permanent central and right lateral incisors absent.

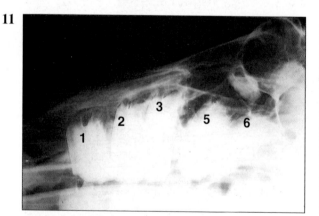

11 Oligodontia (molar).
Note: Lateral radiograph of the head of a 6 year old Arabian gelding with a missing first molar. No dental surgery had ever been performed.

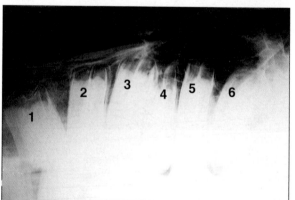

12 Normal lateral (30°) oblique radiograph (of the maxillary arcade).
Note: Roots of the maxillary teeth and their relationship to the sinuses.

Supernumerary molar teeth occasionally occur. Their position in the dental arcade is irregular but they are found caudal to the third molar tooth in jaws which are longer than normal. Less often they are located either lingual or buccal to a normal molar and may in the latter case show obvious facial swelling. They often have a draining sinus onto the side of the face or into the maxillary sinus (*see* **19**).

The '**wolf teeth**' are the vestigial first upper permanent premolar and while many horses have these some do not. In some cases their presence is blamed for a number of behavioural problems including head shaking, failure to respond to the bit and bit resentment. A wolf tooth is located just rostral to the first upper cheek tooth and may be in close apposition to this or may be somewhat removed from it. It is believed that the latter state is the more significant with respect to abnormalities. They should not be confused with the normal canine teeth which occur in many (but not all) male horses and are located in the interdental space of both upper and lower jaw. Incomplete removal of the wolf teeth may result in persistent pain and fragments of enamel or root may be present. More usually, provided that the remains of the tooth are not exposed, there is little pathological effect.

Persistent temporary dentition may be accompanied by obvious or, occasionally, mild dental deviations of the permanent tooth and most often affects the incisor arcade (**15**). Retained temporary incisors are usually firmly embedded in the gums and the permanent tooth usually erupts behind it rather than under it and so fails to occlude the blood supply to the temporary tooth or to push it out. They are however, ordinarily loose and easily removed. Total retention of the temporary molars is much less common. In some cases, the temporary tooth creates a dental cap on the permanent tooth which may be so persistent as to make their identification difficult. However, as the first cheek teeth are most commonly affected, it is usually possible to see the cap on the erupted permanent tooth (**16**). **Persistent, temporary premolar caps** overlying the erupting permanent teeth may occasionally cause oral discomfort and masticatory problems. In the event that these caps rotate there may be associated cheek swelling and in this case the displaced temporary cap will be easily visible. Under such circumstances more significant abnormalities of mastication may be present with quidding (spitting out of partially chewed food material) and reluctance to eat. Most of these caps will resolve spontaneously but some will require removal.

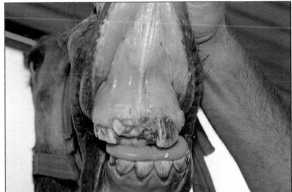

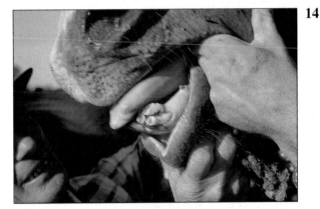

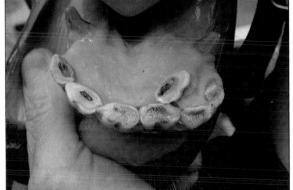

13 Maleruption (right central incisor).
Note: Developed after the temporary tooth had been damaged and extracted.

14 Polyodontia.
Note: An extra corner incisor developed at 5 years of age and remained for the rest of the horse's life. Picture taken at 12 years of age. The extra tooth is visible lateral to the normal one and had a tubular form.

15 Maleruption (lingual) (permanent corner incisor).
Note: Permanent tooth erupted inside the temporary tooth resulting in persistence of the temporary corner incisor.

Local trauma to dental germinal cells or to an erupting tooth, such as might accompany mandibular or maxillary fractures (*see* **25**), or orthodontic surgery to repair such fractures may result in significant deformities of location and consequent discrepancies of wear. The extent of the damage to the dental germinal cells and erupting teeth may be minimal but create a significant defect of either formation or eruption. The third upper cheek tooth, being the last to erupt, is most likely to suffer from defects of eruption with gross deformity of the face over the site (**17**). Radiographic examination and comparison with the normal arcade anatomy (*see* **12**) shows a variety of deformities ranging from complete absence of the tooth to an obvious tooth growing in an abnormal direction or position. Sometimes however, definite dental structure cannot be identified in a mass of abnormal tissue (**18**).

Maleruption of the molar teeth may, on occasion, only become apparent in later life, and most often affects the eruption of the fourth upper permanent premolar (third, upper cheek tooth) which is the last cheek tooth to erupt and may be identified at ages of 4 years and over. Abnormalities of dental eruption may present with maxillary (**19**), or nasal (*see* **17**) swelling associated with abnormal positioning or abnormal eruption of the permanent premolar and molar teeth. The last premolar would be most likely to suffer from defects of eruption (*see* **19**) created by a lack of space and wedging out of

16

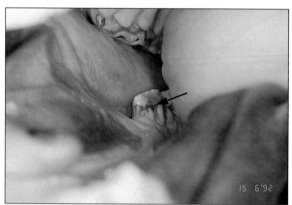

16 Premolar cap.
Note: Cap firmly attached to the erupting crown of the first permanent cheek tooth (arrow) in a 3 year old thoroughbred showing difficulty with mastication. The cap was fairly easily dislodged and no harmful effect was present.

17

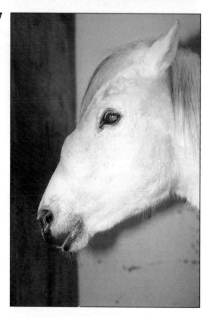

18

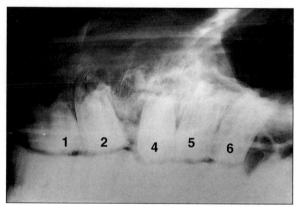

17 Maleruption (third upper cheek tooth).
Note: Facial deformity first appeared at 5 years of age and gradually became more severe. The swelling was not hot or painful and a slight catarrhal nasal discharge was present.

18 Maleruption (third upper cheek tooth) (Lateral radiograph of maxillary teeth and sinuses).
Note: Same horse as described in 17. Last permanent premolar is malerupted and diffuse dental tissue is present in its place. Deformity of the nasal and maxillary bones has been created by the expanding dental tissue.

the permanent tooth (**20**). Inability to erupt effectively results in considerable growth pressure within the associated rostral maxillary sinus. A discharging tract or enlarged sinus with a nasal discharge in a young horse should alert the clinician to the possibility of maleruption.

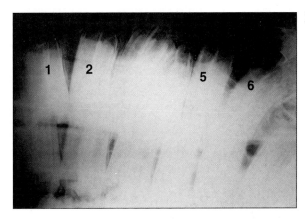

19 Maleruption of the second permanent cheek tooth (third premolar) resulted in the appearance of a discharging sinus tract which lead directly to a mass of dental tissue and a horizontally aligned molar tooth.

20 Lateral radiograph of the maxillary arcade of a 3 year old hunter gelding, showing impaction of the third and fourth cheek teeth leading to maleruption.

Obvious tooth structures or tooth-like material, identifiable radiologically and pathologically, may occur at remote sites from the normal location of teeth. The presence of a **dentigerous cyst (temporal odontoma)** in a two-year-old (or older) horse, is frequently indicated by a discharging sinus which is characteristically, but not exclusively, located mid-way-up the anterior margin of the pinna (**21**) with a cystic or firm swelling at some point below this. Most often the cysts are situated against, or on, the petrous portion of the temporal bone of the skull, but may sometimes be located on the forehead or in the frontal or maxillary sinuses. Carefully positioned radiographic projections can confirm the presence of an aberrant tooth-like structure (**22**) which is either firmly attached to the cranium, or loosely enclosed in a cystic structure and may in either case be surrounded by a collar of bone forming an apparent alveolus. The cyst-like structures may contain no obvious dental tissue or remnants and may then be described as a **conchal cyst**. These may be radiographically unconvincing, but consist of a cystic structure with a smooth lining and an associated chronic discharging sinus. Dental remnants may be identifiable in other sites including the maxillary sinuses.

21

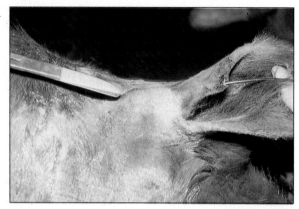

22

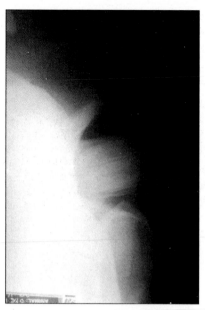

21 A discharging sinus had been present on the anterior margin of the pinna (probe inserted) for two years. The tract lead to an obvious solid non-painful mass just rostral to the base of the ear. This is the typical clinical appearance of a dentigerous cyst.

22 Oblique radiograph of the temporal region of the same horse as described in 21. An obvious tooth-like structure with an associated 'alveolus' is present and is typical of many cases of dentigerous cysts. In the absence of obvious tooth-like material contrast radiography will identify a distinct (or occasionally) a poorly defined cystic structure at this or a neighbouring site.

Non-Infectious Disorders

Swellings of the horizontal ramus of the mandible (**chronic ossifying alveolar periostitis, pseudo-odontoma**) are often encountered in young horses around the time of the eruption of the associated cheek teeth, and are probably due to alveolar periostitis around fluid-filled, active, dental sacs. In a few cases they may be associated with dental overcrowding and horizontally aligned unerupted teeth. Although the apparent deformity of the mandibular bone may be obvious (**23**), radiographs of the area will demonstrate the presence, in young horses, of a normal dental sac, without any evidence of periapical inflammation or infection. Usually the extent of the defect improves somewhat with age, but persistence of some thickening and deformity is to be expected. Such swellings are totally benign and, in spite of apparently severe cosmetic changes they are of little or no clinical significance and are in any case untreatable.

'**Lampas**' or inflammation/edema of the mucosa of the hard palate (**24**) has historically been regarded as a recognisable clinical disorder warranting treatment. However, edema of the hard palate commonly occurs in young 'teething' horses and is of no clinical significance. Pathological 'lampas' was previously recognised as significant when swelling was sufficient to result in the mucosa of the hard palate being below the level of the incisor occlusal margin. It is now accepted that the condition is a normal physiological response to feeding and may become more prominent during the eruption of the permanent incisor and permanent premolar teeth. It is of little or no clinical significance and certainly does not warrant any treatment save ensuring that the diet is acceptable and causes no further irritation. The disorder is occasionally reported to occur in older horses when irritant substances/foods are ingested.

One of the commonest oral injuries sustained by horses is **fracture of the premaxilla** or **mandible**. The fractures may involve the whole premaxilla (**25**), but quite frequently only one or more of the incisor teeth are distracted, and broken back from the alveolus. In the former cases the effect on dental eruption is likely to be minimal but the consequences of the fracture, if left, are likely to be serious with little or no incisor occlusion possible after healing. The latter cases have more serious effects on eruption and less long term serious effects on occlusion, although an individual tooth may be severely displaced or even fall out.

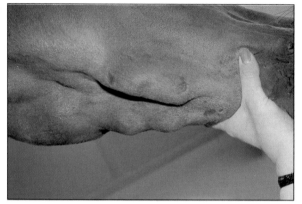

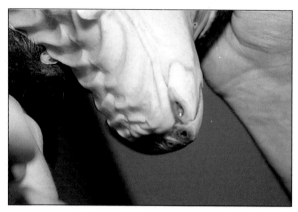

23 Benign dental lumps on the mandible of a 5 year old mare. The lumps were cold, non-painful and remained in this form for the rest of the animals life.

24 Edema of the hard palate (Lampas) noted incidentally in an otherwise normal horse. Historically this extent of hard palate swelling would have been regarded as clinically significant, warranting treatment, as the mucosa was below the incisor occlusal margin. The condition is benign and of no clinical importance.

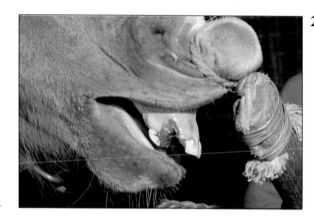

25 Fracture of the premaxilla as a result of a wire injury.

The wear patterns of the incisor and molar teeth may be due to traumatic displacement, pathological softening of enamel or, more often, are a reflection of the type of diet available and/or abnormal occlusal movements of the dental arcades against each other. Almost every normal horse, at some stage of its life, develops **sharp enamel points** along the lingual edges of the lower arcades and the buccal edges of the upper arcades. These enamel edges frequently result in buccal (or lingual, where the edges are sharp on the lower teeth) erosions and ulceration, salivation and even a reluctance to eat. As the lower jaw and the cheek teeth themselves are narrower than the upper, the buccal margin of the upper teeth is most often affected and it is therefore more common to encounter buccal ulceration.

Painful or physical reasons for alteration of normal occlusal movements including oral ulceration, dental pain and/or abscesses, temporomandibular arthropathy, fractures of the mandible or soft tissue lesions, result in corresponding **variations of the wear pattern** of the incisor or molar teeth. Disorders inducing significant changes in the physical shape of the teeth (*see* **9**) have, of necessity, to be long-standing with the normal rate of wear of the cheek teeth being only approximately 3–5 mm per year. **Fractures of the maxilla** (*see* **25**) or temporo mandibular joint pain may ultimately induce severely abnormal incisor and/or molar wear patterns. Once present, the function of the jaw may be permanently abnormal but in some cases the occlusion will gradually return to normal, once the instigating factors have been corrected. Abnormal wear patterns involving the cheek teeth may have marked clinical consequences. While many such cases arise from painful focuses in the masticatory structures including the temporomandibular joints, the masseter muscles and the nerves supplying them and, of course, the teeth themselves, others arise from defects of tooth structure or from the ingestion of abrasive substances. Localised differences in the density of the occlusal surfaces of the molar teeth may also have marked effects upon the occlusal efficiency and the development of abnormal wear patterns. Alternate hard and soft areas in the structure of the cheek teeth or, more commonly, stereotyped chewing behaviour, may result in the development of '**Wave Mouth**' in which either a series of waves develops on the occlusal surface **(26)** or individual teeth wear faster or slower than their neighbours giving a much coarser irregularity of occlusal surfaces **(27)**. In other cases, there may be one (or more) tooth which, often for inexplicable reasons, wears excessively. This results in gross variations in the height of the teeth ('**Step Mouth**') **(27)** and necessarily limits the occlusal efficiency. The full extent of the condition may only be apparent from lateral radiographs when gross variations in height and pyramid deformities of the crowns of the molar teeth may be present. While the loss of lateral grinding movement of the molars will initially induce sharp buccal margins on the upper teeth this may progress, given suitable restrictive movement, into a severe and debilitating **parvinathism** ('**Shear**' / '**Scissor Mouth**') (*see* **9**) in which lateral movement, which is essential for normal chewing, is prevented. These unfortunate horses are often noted to have an abnormally narrow lower jaw but, while under these circumstances it is regarded as a developmental deformity, the same dental deformity may develop as a consequence of a sensitive molar tooth (or teeth) in the opposite arcade or from pain associated with the temporomandibular joints. This results in the upper molars becoming bevelled from the inside outwards with the lower molars worn in the opposite fashion. This deformity prevents further lateral movement of the teeth and seriously interferes with mastication. It represents one of the most serious deformities of the horse's mouth and carries a poor or hopeless prognosis.

In areas where horses have, of necessity, to eat and chew large amounts of sharp sand or other abrasive substances the occlusal surface of the cheek teeth may become completely smooth and therefore ineffective as grinders of food. Failure to masticate efficiently results initially in difficulty with swallowing and slow eating.

26

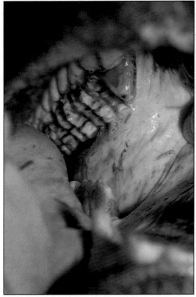

27

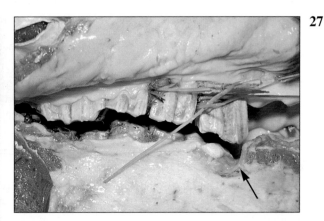

26 Stereotyped chewing behaviour was thought to be the cause of this Wave mouth.
Note: The rostral hook on the first cheek tooth was present without any inferior brachygnathism. Prominent latero-medial ridging of the occlusal surfaces.

27 Step mouth. Post mortem specimen of an aged horses mouth showing loss of one upper and one lower cheek tooth with severe occlusal irregularities including overgrowth of the first upper tooth and marked irregularity of the wear.
Note: Coarse straw wedged between the upper teeth and lower gingival damage associated with the grossly overgrown first upper cheek tooth (arrow).

Latterly, weight loss, as a result of ineffective digestion, is commonly present. Under similar circumstances, because these horses are usually grazing very short pasture or having to find food in soil or sand the incisors may become severely worn down ('**Sand Mouth**') (*see* **30**). Very old horses commonly have smooth occlusal surface even when they have no history of abrasive diets. In some cases the table of the molar teeth is completely smooth and concave and has almost no enamel ridges. This severely limits the effective mastication of fibrous food and has debilitating effects. Individuals with occlusal difficulties of all types which result in poor mastication exhibit an inordinately high long-fibre content of feces.

As a result of dental pain, or inefficient mastication, or as a consequence of some neurological deficits of sensation within the oral cavity, food material may become impacted between the cheek and the cheek teeth. In some cases this might pass unnoticed but in others an obvious lump may be visible.

Overgrown cheek teeth may arise from the absence of the opposite occlusal tooth. Such defects may follow either from normal old age shedding, or from failure of normal eruption or, more often, from surgical extraction of one or more of the cheek teeth. Molar teeth with no occlusal pressure are likely to grow faster than normal teeth and in addition have no occlusal abrasion. The resultant loss of normal control of dental growth creates abnormal wear patterns which are usually visible as gross overgrowth (**28**). Pyramidal peaks on the tooth opposite the gap are common where the gap created by a missing cheek tooth is narrowed by angulation of the adjacent teeth but leaving a relatively small area of non-occlusion. Many of these deformities are directly visible but radiography may be required to accurately identify the site, etiology and extent of the defect. Normal shedding of molar teeth usually begins when the horse is over 25–30 years of age and the first molar tooth,

being the oldest, would be expected to be lost first. Under these circumstances the scope for subsequent overgrowth in the opposite occlusal teeth is minimal and dental hooks, overgrowths or pyramids are usually of marginal significance. The loss of any of the cheek teeth except the first and last, leaves a gap in the dental arcade which may narrow significantly (and sometimes completely) with time as the adjacent teeth angle inwards. However, where the first or the last tooth is lost from an arcade the consequences are usually more obvious (*see* **28**). Dramatic overgrowth of the opposite occlusal tooth develops at about 3–4 mm per year, in the absence of any corrective measures. Where narrowing of the gap occurs the extent of regrowth is limited and the angulation of the adjacent molars results in a typical pyramidal pattern of overgrowth. Although these defects may be less in size than the more dramatic overgrowth encountered in either the first or the last tooth the secondary consequences may be more significant and arise more quickly. Thus, limited overgrowth may result in gross discomfort and inability to chew effectively within months of the onset. Alternatively overgrowth may continue unabated for years before any clinical effects may become apparent. Overgrowth impinges upon the opposing gingiva causing ulceration, necrosis and possibly infection of the ulcerated area.

While severe incisor wear is sometimes encountered where grazing is short and large amounts of sand or other abrasive substances are ingested, the wear pattern of the incisors, in particular, may be influenced by behavioural factors. 'Crib-biting' is a common, unpleasant habitual vice (neurosis) developed by horses (*see* **718**) showing a characteristic wear pattern on the rostral margin of the upper incisor teeth which is variable in extent according to the severity and duration of the vice, and to some extent upon the structural character of the teeth. The earliest indications of the vice may be gained from close examination of the rostral

28

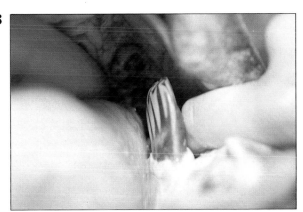

28 Severe overgrowth of the first lower cheek tooth arising as a result of dental extraction of the opposite upper tooth. The surgery had been performed some 8 years previously and the overgrowth was approximately 25mm.

margin of the upper central incisors where a worn edge will be detected (**29**). The persistence and severity of the effort involved in cribbing is often enough, even in young horses to cause severe wear of the central incisors, often down to gingival level (**30**). Horses showing this abnormality should always be regarded with suspicion and examination of the neck may detect the characteristic hypertrophy of the *sternocephalicus* muscle or the presence of rub marks on either side of the throat, indicating the prior use of a cribbing strap.

Habitual grinding of the teeth on metal rails or concrete walls results in wear patterns involving, usually, the corner and lateral incisors. The pattern is usually such that it is hard to visualise any normal behaviour pattern which could produce them. Usually only one side is affected (**31**).

Dental tartar commonly accumulates on any, or all, of the teeth and is most obvious on the lower canine (**32**). It is unusual for this to cause any significant gingival inflammation and/or alveolar infection. Extensive accumulations of tartar on the cheek teeth may be an indication of underlying systemic disease or dietary conditions but is commonly an incidental observation in healthy (particularly, old) horses. Chronic gingival inflammation caused by dental calculus or other irritants may give rise to a **benign inflammatory hyperplasia (epulis)** of the gum (*see* **32**). Again, the most obvious site for this is the buccal margin of the canine teeth but it may equally develop at any other site along the tooth-gum margin. It seldom reaches significant size although localised cheek swelling may be detected in severe cases. The subsequent development

29

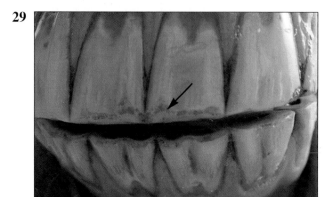

29 Mild (early) 'crib biter'.
Note: Prominent wear on the rostral margin of the upper central incisors (arrow).

30

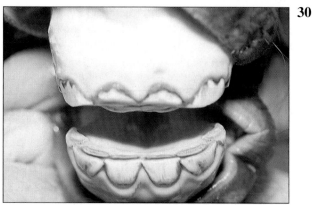

30 Severe 'crib biter'. The teeth are temporary incisors and the foal had apparently learned the habit from its dam, starting at an early age and was not resolved.
Note: Wear of central upper incisors almost down to gingival margin. A similar appearance to this occurs in horses grazing for long periods over sandy soil.

31

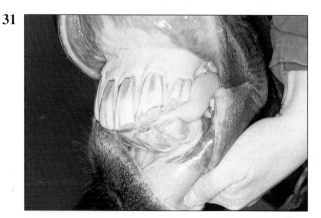

31 Wall raker. This horse spent considerable periods of time grinding his upper lateral and corner incisors along a concrete door post, creating this defect. No other abnormality was found.

32

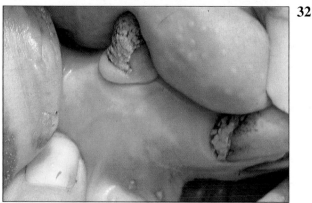

32 Dental tartar and gum hyperplasia (epulis).

of neoplastic tissue, usually fibroma or fibrosarcoma but occasionally squamous cell (or undifferentiated) carcinoma, at these sites suggests that the inflammatory reaction may have longer term significance.

Long-standing **defects of molar occlusion** resulting from **degenerative temporomandibular joint disorders**, have severe consequences upon the horse's ability to wear the occlusal surfaces in a coordinated fashion. Once a significant defect of occlusion has developed it may be impossible for normal masticatory movements to take place. Under these circumstances extensive overgrowth (*see* **9**) or bizarre dental deformities may be encountered. This may, itself induce secondary temporomandibular arthropathy as the animal attempts to chew with the sides of the molar teeth. It is, in most cases impossible to identify whether the occlusal problem arose first and caused secondary joint degeneration, or whether the occlusal deformity is the result of abnormal jaw movement created by joint inflammation and degeneration.

One of the commonest important dental disorders is **alveolar periostitis**. Most cases are the result of food material and infection gaining access to the dental alveolus. The incisors are much less often affected than the molar teeth. Horses in which the molar teeth are separated from each other by a gap and those in which gum recession and/or inflammation/infection of the periodontal tissues develops, have a high incidence of alveolar periostitis (**33**). Food of poor quality may be a predisposing factor (*see* **27**) and, indeed, cases are not restricted to the older horse, with some cases being encountered within the first few years of life. Gingival and alveolar infection results in progressive loosening of the dental ligaments, gum recession and penetration of infection (*see* **33**) with increasing scope for food material impaction. Localised periodontal disease (alveolar periostitis) may result in localised abscesses within or adjacent to the affected alveolus (**34**). This may have secondary effects particularly where the affected tooth is situated within one or other part of the maxillary sinuses. Secondary **infective sinusitis** (*see* **38**) or focal abscessation onto the face or into the nasal cavity are common effects of periodontal disease (*see* **19**). Loosening of the cheek teeth may also be the consequence of degenerative disorders of the alveolar ligaments such as occur in nutritionally deprived horses or in those ingesting relatively large amounts of phosphate in their diet (*see* **356**). Horses affected by pituitary adenoma (*see* **362**) commonly suffer from degenerative changes within the dental alveoli and consequent loosening of teeth. Old horses have a natural slowly progressive loosening of the teeth which ultimately results in shedding but the process of natural shedding is seldom accompanied by prolonged or serious alveolar infection.

33

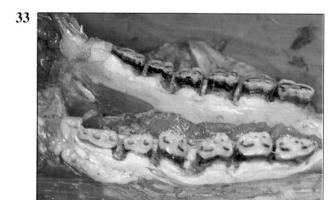

33 Severe periodontal disease resulting in gum recession, loosening of the mandibular cheek teeth and alveolar infection. Both upper and lower arcades were affected similarly and the alveolar infection in the former had extended into the maxillary sinuses creating extensive bone necrosis and a foetid odour was associated with a bilateral purulent nasal discharge.

34

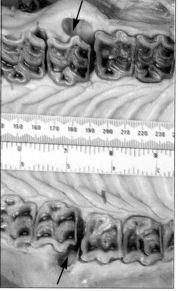

34 Localised periodontal disease resulting in focal gum recession and abscessation (arrows).

Dental caries is a localised, progressively destructive, decay of the teeth which originates in the enamel. Dental decay in the horse is not common although, where it exists, the consequences may be severe. **Incisor caries (35)** is particularly unusual and may be secondary to defects of enamel or to fluorosis or other defects of dental structure. In some cases it arises from previous trauma including cracks or abnormal wear patterns. Where caries develop in the temporary teeth, infection of, or damage to, the underlying germinal cells of the permanent teeth may result in a complete absence or deformity of the permanent structure. **Caries in the cheek teeth** is much more commonly encountered, but is, initially, much less obvious, with the long term secondary consequences of discharging sinus tracts or maxillary sinus infections being, usually, the major presenting signs. Infection within the pulp cavity of the molar teeth may arise from cement hypoplasia of the maxillary teeth, and caries arising from the fermentation and decay of food material impacted within a patent infundibulum **(36)**. The infundibulum is normally filled with cement, and when this is either not present, or is defective, or is eroded, food material may be forced into the cavity under occlusal pressure. The decay of this material produces organic acids and provides an ideal environment for bacterial multiplication. As the upper cheek teeth have prominent infundibuli these are most often affected by such necrosis. The defective infundibulum is often very small and difficult or impossible to visualise directly, but persistent pressure of food material and secondary infection results in severe apical infection and **alveolar periostitis** (*see* **40**). Horses with **secondary sinusitis** as a result of dental disease often have a characteristic unilateral purulent nasal discharge (**Plate 7b**, page 143) and a fetid odour on the breath.

Fractures or splitting of the enamel layers from the sides of the cheek teeth may be encountered. The two deep and prominent infundibular cavities of the upper cheek teeth provide a potential line of weakness in the sagittal plane along which fractures may occur **(37)**. Sagittal or other fractures of the lower teeth are much less common, as they have no infundibular cavities and are in any case much narrower and denser than the corresponding upper teeth.

The second and third cheek teeth in the lower jaw and the third and fourth in the upper jaw are the most frequently diseased teeth in the horse. As the first maxillary molar (fourth cheek tooth) is the oldest tooth in the mature horse, this is probably, overall, the most often diseased. The relative positions of the upper teeth in relation to the rostral and caudal maxillary sinuses and their respective drainage pathways, result in the characteristic clinical features of dental infections or defects of eruption/locality in the upper arcade. The rostral root of the third upper cheek tooth and the two

35

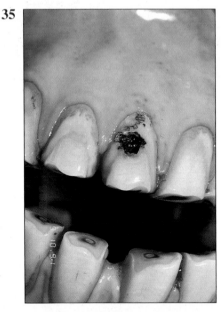

35 Dental caries in the central incisor of an aged mare. No alveolar infection was present and the mare was not apparently affected with either pain or discomfort.

36

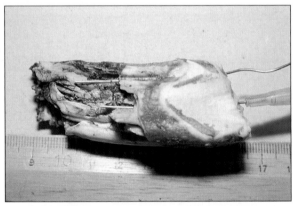

36 This third upper cheek tooth was removed from a thoroughbred gelding which was suffering from secondary sinusitis of the rostral maxillary sinus. A fetid odour and a unilateral, scanty, purulent nasal discharge was present. After removal of the tooth it was possible to pass probes up two infundibuli and into the obviously decaying roots of the tooth which contained obvious rotting food material. Cement hypoplasia was thought to be responsible for a weak and easily decayed infundibulum.

more rostral premolars usually have roots which are not related directly to the sinuses, and infections in these induce focal facial swellings and discharging sinus tracts at the appropriate site (*see* **19**). More unusually these drain into the nasal cavity, producing a purulent, unilateral nasal discharge (**Plate 7b**, page 143) and a characteristic fetid breath without any apparent deformity of the face. Where the caudal root of the third upper cheek tooth (fourth premolar) or any of the upper molars are involved, sinusitis will generally develop. The rostral and caudal maxillary sinuses drain independently into the nasal cavity by separate drainage ostia. The bony barrier separating the caudal and rostral sinuses is seldom disrupted except by trauma or persistent sinus infection and a common drainage channel is only then available. Most often the rostral sinus becomes infected and while drainage into the nasal cavity continues, appearing as a unilateral nasal discharge, distortion of the face just above the rostral

half of the facial crest, will gradually develop (*see* **232**). Enlargement of the caudal maxillary sinus is usually less obvious as the drainage is more efficient and less liable to occlusion as a result of localised inflammation or physical obstruction from purulent material. Radiographic examination of horses with purulent material in the sinuses as a result of periapical (or other dental or localised) conditions shows the presence of an obvious air-fluid interface (**38**). In almost every case of sinusitis with underlying dental disease there is an offensive necrotic odour on the breath, which will be restricted to the affected nostril. Trephination of the offending sinus invariably releases a quantity of purulent material (**39**). Such trephination also permits a detailed endoscopic examination of the contents of the sinus and the roots of the associated teeth. This diagnostic technique provides very useful information and is simply performed in the standing horse under local analgesia. Long-standing apical infection in the more

37

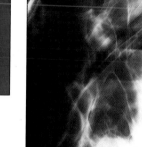

37 Sagittal fracture of the fourth upper cheek tooth (first molar).
Note: split joining the two infundibuli.

38 Standing lateral radiograph of the maxillary area of a horse affected with secondary maxillary sinusitis. The fourth upper cheek tooth removed from this horse is shown in **37**.
Note: Fluid level (air-fluid interface) in caudal maxillary sinus (Arrow).

38

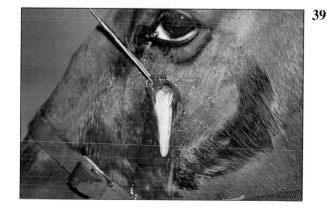

39

39 Trephination of the caudal maxillary sinus of the horse shown in **38**, released purulent material, and was associated with secondary sinusitis resulting from a fractured upper fourth cheek tooth.

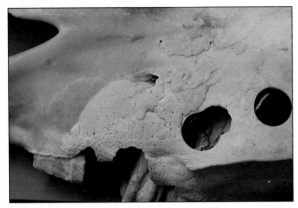

40 Marked new bone formation and remodelling of the maxilla was a direct consequence of a persistent infection of the alveolus and root of the second cheek tooth.

rostral teeth may result in moderate or severe bone erosion and the laying down of soft, diffuse new-bone around the area (**40**).

Lower arcade defects induce less extensive secondary effects and those involving even the most caudal teeth produce firm circumscribed swellings, usually on the ventro-lateral aspect of the mandible which may, or may not, be associated with an innocuous-looking, discharging sinus tract (**41**). The amount of discharge is often deceptively small. Radiography with a probe inserted into the sinus tract will usually enable accurate identification of the diseased tooth (**42**). Usually there is some degree of radiolucency around the offending root and variable degrees of rarefaction of the root itself (*see* **42**). In spite of the rather benign appearance, these tracts seldom, if ever, heal without attention to the underlying problem.

Where the alveolus and the periodontal tissues are affected by dystrophic bone disease (such as osteodystrophia fibrosa or '**Bran Disease**') there may be gross irregularities and consequent distortion of the face and dental arcades (*see* **355, 356**) which may result in significant abnormality of the occlusal surfaces such as have already been described. Horses affected with nutritional secondary hyperparathyroidism following persistent ingestion of large amounts of high phosphate, low calcium diets over many months show gross, usually symmetrical, enlargement or thickening of the facial flat bones (*see* **355**). The substitution of the thin, facial bone plates by very thickened masses of fibro-cartilaginous tissue has a significant effect upon the

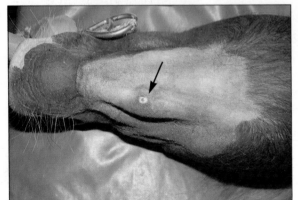

41 Firm, non-painful, swelling and an innocuous-looking sinus tract in the mandible over the root of the second cheek tooth (arrow), of a nine-year-old mare. The sinus had been present for several years and while the discharge was scant the bony swelling became progressively larger. No apparent pain or discomfort during mastication was present.

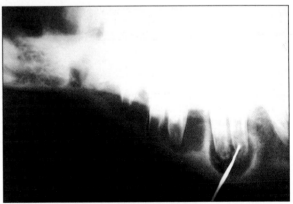

42 Oblique radiograph of the mandible of a horse suffering from a chronic swelling and discharging sinus tract over the root of the third lower cheek tooth. A probe has been inserted into the tract.
Note: Area of lucency with sclerotic margin indicating osteolysis and lytic roots of the tooth typical of apical abscessation.

position of the molar teeth in particular and the strength of the alveolar attachments (*see* **356**).

Oral ulceration and/or diffuse inflammation (**stomatitis**) may arise from ingestion of caustic or irritant chemicals, such as organophosphate anthelmintics. Diffuse, multiple oral ulceration occurs occasionally after, or during, medication with non-steroidal anti-inflammatory drugs. More focal inflammatory lesions may also arise from coarse or sharp food materials such as plant awns (**43**). The ulcerations and erosions which are seen in these disorders may appear to be similar but recognition of the underlying cause is very important when considering the treatment and prognosis.

Traumatic lesions involving the tongue (44) occur relatively commonly in the horse. The blood supply to the tongue and the buccal mucosa is good and rapid healing is usual with these, and other oral lesions. Although the trauma may be extensive, the function of the tongue may still be adequate after the wounds have healed (**45**). Excessive tension on the tongue during examination may induce severe tearing of the frenulum or, sometimes, even fracture of the hyoid bone. In the former case healing is usually rapid and complete with minimal scarring and disability although some tongue flaccidity is commonly present for months. In the latter there may be moderate or severe, transient or permanent, neurological damage as a result of traumatic disruption of the cranial nerves within the guttural pouch. In both cases, loss of tongue tone and dysphagia might be encountered, particularly if there are concurrent neurological deficits.

43

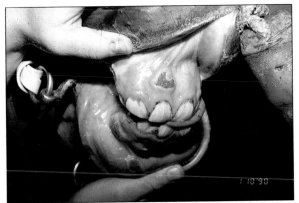

44

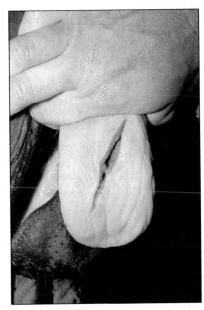

43 Focal area of ulceration in the upper lip of a horse ingesting irritant plant awns. There were several such lesions in the buccal cavity and on the lower lip. Biopsy of the lesion revealed numerous spicules of plant material embedded in the lesion.
Note: Well defined ulcerated area with thickened margin.

44 Tongue laceration. The lesion had virtually healed by 7 days and during this time the horse appeared little affected.

45

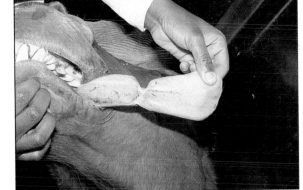

45 Some 5 years previously this horse had been restrained by the application of a tongue twitch. In spite of the severe constriction the tongue was mobile and showed no atrophy of the distal portion. The horse showed no apparent ill-effect.

An unusual inflammatory response to oral insults is the production of **hyperkeratinized oral mucosa (46)**. The changes are usually most prominent in the sub lingual tissue but the reasons for it are not clear. Once the insults are removed and the mouth is allowed to heal, the abnormal mucosa is gradually replaced and returns to normal. Horses so affected should be carefully examined to ascertain the cause of the chronic repeated or persistent oral inflammation.

Glossal weakness in neonatal foals is characterised by a protruding tongue which, either cannot be withdrawn into the mouth or has a noticeably poor withdrawal tone when pulled gently. Affected foals are often dysphagic with a poor suckling ability. Although the condition is usually temporary and mild, severely affected foals may become weak. The disorder is possibly related to the delayed maturation of the trigeminal nerve. Inhalation pneumonia is a possible sequel. **Tongue sucking** (*see* **720**) is a well recognised behavioural problem of adult horses and usually occurs without concurrent dysphagia in spite of the tongue having an apparently flaccid character. No overt neurological or physical disorder can usually be established and the condition is usually without serious clinical significance. Racing horses frequently protrude the tongue during and after racing and this is probably due to the presence of the bit and is, again, usually of no importance. **Tongue flaccidity** is a cardinal sign of **Botulism** (*see* **735**). The disorder has few other pathognomonic signs and horses of all ages suffering from an apparent tongue paralysis should be carefully assessed for this possibility. Failure to recognise the earliest signs makes treatment almost impossible.

The position and function of the tongue may reflect abnormalities of function and/or local damage or disease. **Fracture/dislocation of the mandible** and/or **fracture of the stylohyoid bone** usually manifest as a dropped jaw with dysfunction of the tongue, and abnormalities of mastication and deglutition. Where the condition has been present for a considerable time there may be obvious concurrent **masseter atrophy** (*see* **687**) which in these cases is usually bilateral.

Damage to the cranial nerves within the guttural pouch as a result of fracture of the stylohyoid bone presents a complex series of neurological deficits including **Horner's Syndrome** (*see* **695** *et seq.*).

Neurological deficits associated with cranial nerves IX, X, and XII, such as might occur centrally in **equine protozoal myeloencephalitis** (*see* **737** *et seq.*), or peripherally in **guttural pouch mycosis** (*see* **251**), or with localised neurological damage following trauma, usually result in an inability to move the tongue and jaw effectively. Partially masticated food material accumulates between the teeth and the cheeks and there may be a loss of oral sensation if the sensory functions of the trigeminal nerve (cranial nerve V) are also impaired. Horses lacking in oral co-ordination and/or sensation frequently bite their cheeks and the tongue along its buccal margin. Minor lacerations in this area are more usually due to sharp enamel points on the lingual margins of the lower cheek teeth or the buccal margins of the upper teeth. **Bilateral trigeminal neuritis** of central origin with loss of motor function results in an inability to close the mouth effectively, and the tongue is seen protruding from the mouth (*see* **686**). Other muscles innervated by the trigeminal nerve, including the *Temporalis* m. and the distal portion of the *Digastricus* m. undergo rapid atrophy. Additional signs which may accompany damage to the trigeminal nerve include enophthalmos and a slight but obvious drooping of the upper eyelid on the affected side(s). **Unilateral atrophy of the masseter muscle** mass occurs when unilateral neuritis or damage to the peripheral course of the trigeminal nerve has been sustained or subsequent to local myopathies affecting specific muscle masses. Unilateral neuropathies involving the motor innervation of the tongue may be detected by careful palpation of the musculature of the body of the tongue. Unilateral atrophy of the affected side may be detectable. **Equine protozoal myeloencephalitis** (*see* **737**) and *polyneuritis*

46

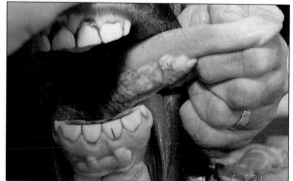

46 Chronic oral irritation accompanied by repeated episodes of salivation and dysphagia had been present in this case. Marked hyperkeratosis of the sublingual mucosa and the buccal surface of the lower lip became thickened and hyperkeratotic. A change in diet resulted in a gradual improvement until no abnormality could be found after 6 months.

equi (**cauda equina neuritis**) (*see* **711**) are also, on occasion, responsible for unilateral trigeminal neuropathies which are manifest by unilateral atrophy of these muscles.

Masseter myopathy associated, equivocally, with selenium and vitamin E deficiency, is encountered in stabled horses, maintained under poor management. It is characterised by severe swelling of the masseter muscles (*see* **469**). There is marked local pain and resistance when the jaws are opened, and affected horses are understandably anorectic. A marked resistance to jaw movement is also a prominent feature of **Tetanus** (*see* **731**), but in all cases of this condition there are other signs which are usually more prominent.

Bullous pemphigoid, which is probably associated with an immunological disorder is very rare but may

result in severe ulcerative glossitis and stomatitis.

The buccal mucosa may be a significant and important indicator of the circulatory status of the horse and may, furthermore, show significant changes in colour and appearance in many other disease conditions. **Petechial hemorrhages** are seen in conditions of vasculitis including purpura hemorrhagica (*see* **296**) and in bleeding diatheses. Icterus (yellowing) (**Plate 8f**, page 179) may be present in hepatic or hemolytic disorders such as **neonatal isoerythrolysis** (*see* **312**). Pallor (**Plate 8e**, page 179) may be present in disorders involving blood loss. There are many disorders which are reflected in the character and colour of the oral mucosa and it therefore acts as an important diagnostic aid in the investigation of a wide variety of disorders involving other systems.

Infectious Disorders

Viral (vesicular) stomatitis occurs rarely and there are usually large numbers of ulcers and vesicles over the oral mucosa, although in many cases, these are limited to the dorsum of the tongue and the lips (**47**). The udder of mares and the prepuce of males are often involved. Clinically the disease is usually transient and the salivation and anorexia are quickly resolved over a day or two. The condition may be confused primarily with the appearance of stomatitis which is caused by irritant chemicals.

Botulism (*see* **735**), **encephalomyelitides** (including the Togaviral encephalitides (*see* **724**), **heavy metal poisoning** (such as **lead** and **mercury**), **Yellow Star Thistle poisoning** (**nigropallidal encephalomalacia**)

(*see* **716**) and **leukoencephalomalacia** (**Mouldy Corn Poisoning / aflatoxicosis**) (*see* **717**) may all have marked effects upon the function of the tongue and the ability of the affected horse to prehend and masticate effectively. Most of these are characterised by a flaccid paralysis of the tongue with saliva accumulations and overflow.

The larval stages of ***Gasterophilus* spp. flies** migrate through and within the tissues of the tongue, gingivae and dental alveoli, where they cause significant inflammation of the margin of the gums and the formation of characteristic circular raised ulcer like lesions on the lips (**48**), tongue, palate and buccal mucosa. Similar lesions may also be caused by focal irritations from sharp grass awns.

47

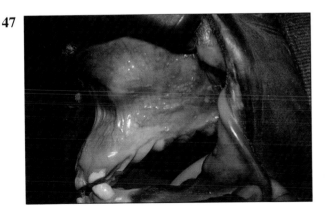

47 Viral (vesicular) stomatitis.
Note: Numerous small blister like vesicles over lips and gums. The dorsum of the tongue was equally affected but other areas of the mouth were apparently unaffected.

48

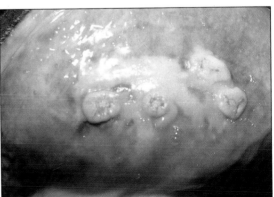

48 Typical lesions on the mucosa of the upper lip caused by the larval stages of *Gastrophilus intestinalis* (Bot fly).

Neoplastic Disorders

Neoplastic lesions of the mouth and associated structures are rare. **Squamous cell carcinoma** is the most prevalent true neoplastic lesion of the oral cavity of the horse and affects either the tongue (**49**) or the buccal mucosa. In some cases the lesion is large, resulting in facial deformity. The tumour may infiltrate the cheek and ulcerate onto the side of the face (**50**). A similar ulcerative appearance may be seen with fibrosarcomas involving the cheek. Involvement of local lymph nodes in horses affected with either squamous cell carcinoma or fibrosarcoma is uncommon but the parotid lymph node is usually hyperplastic if not infiltrated with neoplastic tissue. Metastases are not usually encountered from these tumours originating at this site.

Adamantinomas in the mouth may represent a development of benign or malignant epulis rather than a primary disorder. Most occur in the incisor region of the mandible and are highly infiltrative, rapidly involving the underlying bone of the mandible (**51**). Teeth included in the proliferating mass may become loose or displaced. Most occur in mature horses without sex or breed predilection. A congenital ameloblastoma which may include teeth and tooth like material is exceptional.

Ossifying fibromas are occasionally encountered in the mandible of young horses (**Plate 8a**, page 178) and although these are unsightly they are often slow growing or static. They are sometimes associated with defects of dental eruption or trauma. Occlusal radiographic examination usually establishes the true character of the mass.

The skin in the immediate area around the mouth is liable to the development of **sarcoid tumours** with the verrucose form (*see* **524**) being the most common type encountered in this site. As is the case with sarcoids at other locations they may take on a more fibroblastic appearance (*see* **527**) following surgical or other trauma.

49
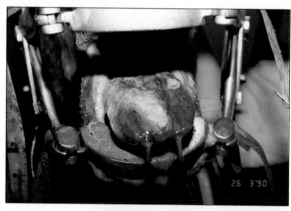

50
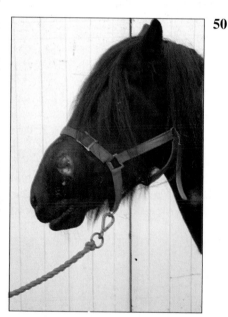

51
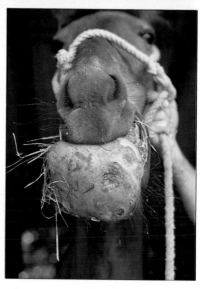

49 Squamous cell carcinoma of the tongue.

50 Squamous cell carcinoma of the buccal mucosa ulcerated onto the surface of the face in this 13 year old pony. The tumour had also invaded the nasal cavity but no metastases were found.

51 Adamantinoma (ameloblastoma) of the lower jaw.

Part 2: The Salivary Glands and Ducts

Developmental Disorders

Congenital salivary mucoceles resulting from defects in the salivary duct or the integrity of the gland may reach considerable size **(52)**. A more frequent cause of saliva-filled cystic structures is trauma to the associated duct(s) or to the glands themselves. Needle aspiration from these structures produces a viscid, saliva-like substance which may be slightly blood tinged when of recent origin. These cysts are commonly noted to vary in size from day to day but ultimately they become large pendulous bags of skin (*see* **52**) which fill with saliva at irregular intervals.

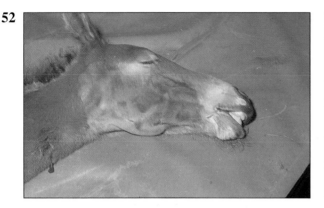

52 Salivary mucocele in a young foal. The lesion in this case was present from birth and fluctuated in size from day to day. Aspiration revealed a fluid with all the characteristics of saliva. The lesion is clinically indistinguishable from acquired salivary cysts.

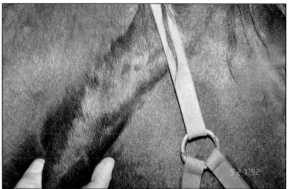

53 Parotitis (Idiopathic sialadenitis). The gross enlargement of the parotid salivary glands shown here was bilaterally symmetrical and appeared within 2 hours of being turned out in nine out of ten ponies. The condition resolved in all the affected horses within 4 hours of being stabled again. The condition recurred over the following 6 weeks each time the animals were turned into the field.

Non-Infectious Disorders

Significant pathological disorders of the salivary glands of the horse are not often recognised. **Ptyalism** as a result of oral irritation is seen in normal horses under a variety of circumstances such as excitement, oral irritation and when coarse food is fed. Horses which mouth persistently on the bit may produce large amounts of foamy saliva at the mouth. This is seldom of any clinical importance. Occasionally profuse salivation is seen in horses fed on preserved grass products and this has been attributed to the fungus *Rhizoctonia leguminicola*. The extreme salivation which is seen under these conditions is particularly severe immediately after feeding and usually ceases after withdrawal of the offending foodstuff. A similar profuse ptyalism may accompany the migration of larvae of *Gastrophilus* spp.

through the tissues of the mouth and oesophagus. Parasympathetic stimulation induces a profuse but short lived salivation, while parasympatholytic drugs and plants such as *Belladona atropina* reduce the extent of salivation and produce a dryer than normal mouth. Cases of **Grass Sickness** (*see* **129** *et seq.*) and any alteration in the function of the cervical sympathetic trunk (such as might occur in Horner's Syndrome) might also influence the function of the salivary glands. Foals (and occasionally adult horses) which have gastric ulceration (*see* **93**) often salivate significantly (*see* **92**).

Idiopathic sialadenitis is encountered relatively commonly in grazing horses in particular, and occurs either sporadically or in outbreaks; indicating the possibility of infectious aetiology or hypersensitivity conditions. Affected horses show a bilaterally symmetrical enlargement of either the parotid (**53**) or the submandibular (**54**) salivary glands. In some cases all the glands may be involved. The non-painful, firm, glandular swelling, which often develops within a few hours of being turned-out into the pasture and which may reach alarming proportions, resolves equally quickly when the affected horse is brought back into a stable. It is likely from the speed of the reaction and its repeatable course from day to day that the disorder represents a hypersensitivity disorder rather than an infection. Epidemics amongst grazing horses are suggestive of either a plant poisoning or an infectious aetiology. Salivation is not a prominent feature and this further suggests that it arises from direct inflammation of the gland rather than as a result of oral irritation. Salivation may also be present in horses with stomatitis or traumatic injuries but this is most often accompanied by malodorous breath, sanguineous saliva and/or a swollen tongue.

Obstructive disorders of the salivary ducts are usually restricted to the superficial (Stenson's Duct) and intra-glandular portions of the parotid duct. Obstructions are most often due to **sialoliths** lodged within the common duct, often in the more distal portion where it passes along the anterior border of the masseter muscle (**55**). Sialoliths are usually spherical or oval and consist of calcium carbonate (**56**) deposited around a nidus created by a foreign body or inflammatory cells originating in the gland or duct. Their size is very variable with some weighing up to 0.5 kg and others being pea-sized. The actual size may, or may not, relate to the extent

of the obstruction. Thus, some very small calculi may cause more severe obstructions than the obvious larger ones and this may be more a reflection of the speed of onset of the obstruction and the rate of development of the calculus. Continuous enlargement of sialoliths occurs over some years, as more and more mineral content is laid down. Most long-standing cases are those in which the obstruction is partial and saliva continues to pass around the mass. In these circumstances the secondary effects upon the gland are minimal. However, where there is abrupt and complete obstruction a dramatic and painful enlargement of the associated gland is usually induced. Occasionally there may be localised obstructions within the substance of the gland itself. Such cases show varying degrees of localised swelling and pain and radiographic or ultrasonographic examination may be required to identify these. Obstructions sufficiently severe to cause rupture of the duct or traumatic disruption of the associated gland result in the release of saliva into the adjacent tissue. **Salivary mucoceles** develop progressively as the saliva is produced and creates a cystic structure in the throat region (*see* **52**). The size and content of the cyst-like structure will be noted to vary in relation to feeding patterns and the speed of development largely depends upon the extent of the rupture and whether any saliva can pass the site of obstruction. Sometimes a defect develops in the overlying skin and the continuous salivary secretion into the lesion prevents healing, often never resolving naturally. Chronic small, or large, discharging sinuses or large areas of ulcerated glandular tissue (**57**) result.

54

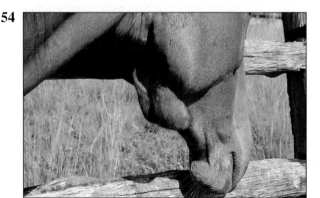

55

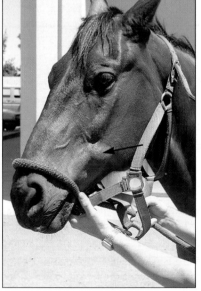

54 Idiopathic sialadenitis (Bilateral inflammation of the submandibular salivary glands). The condition persisted for some weeks and only gradually resolved. No obstruction was present in either of the ducts.

55 Parotid salivary duct calculus. The calculus can be seen in the parotid salivary duct (Stenson's Duct) on the anterior edge of the masseter muscle (arrow). The swelling was very hard, non-painful and developed over some months without any apparent clinical effect.

56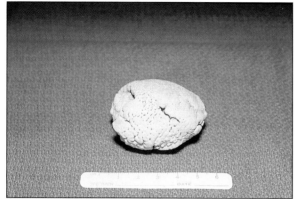

57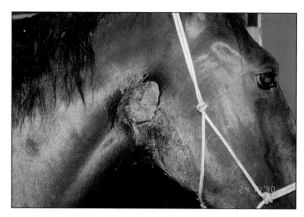

56 Salivary calculus removed surgically from the parotid duct of the horse described in **55**. No recurrence occurred and healing was uneventful.

57 Acute obstruction of a major branch of the parotid duct by a calcium carbonate calculus (which was identified by radiography and ultrasonography) resulted in a gross, painful and hot swelling of the parotid salivary gland. The swelling burst onto the surface of the skin discharging a quantity of blood stained saliva. The lesion failed to heal, becoming progressively larger and discharging saliva over 8 months without any sign of healing.

Infectious Disorders

Sialadenitis, an active inflammation of the salivary glands, seldom occurs as a primary disorder. This is usually a diagnosis made after histopathological examination of affected glands. Conditions in which sialadenitis is a feature include **Rabies** (*see* **721**), **equine herpes virus-1** and **4** (*see* **211**) and some bacterial conditions such as *Streptococcus equi* **infection** (*see* **226**). The presence of abnormal amounts of saliva should be differentiated from an inability to swallow normal amounts, such as might occur where a pharyngeal foreign body or intraluminal oesophageal obstruction (**Choke**) are present (*see* **64**). Conditions which result in dysphagia and/or pharyngeal paralysis such as **Grass Sickness**, **lead poisoning**, **Rabies**, **African Horse Sickness** and several others, may show significant overt salivation and pooling of saliva in the mouth and pharynx. The extent of salivation in many of these cases may be marked and attempts at swallowing may be accompanied by profuse nasal reflux of saliva and food material (**Plate 6o, Plate 6r**, page 123).

Neoplastic Disorders

Neoplastic disorders of the salivary glands are effectively restricted to **melanoma** and **melanosarcoma** in grey horses (**58**). The often gross enlargement in the parotid area of grey horses suffering from melanoma masses is sometimes due to the presence of the tumour masses in the adjacent lymph nodes but tumours in lymphoid tissue within the salivary glands may reach massive proportions. The existence of these lesions in the salivary glands and adjacent structures may or may not be accompanied by the presence of tumours elsewhere (*see* **813**). Detailed endoscopic examination of the guttural pouches may identify the presence of small or large foci of pigmented tissue in many grey horses and these are probably hamartoma (abnormal accumulations of normal tissue components) (*see* **274**) and are probably not neoplastic. However, in some cases obviously more aggressive melanotic foci may be present (*see* **275**) and these are likely to be neoplastic lesions. Extension from the dorso-lateral wall of the guttural pouch, which is a predilection site for the development of melanoma masses, is relatively rapid in many cases. On some occasions melanomas are not present in any other detectable site and the extent of changes within the guttural pouches may be a useful guide to the existence of lesions elsewhere. The character of the solid tumours is clinically usually simply assessed. Needle aspirates from the mass contain black cells which are very

characteristic. Surgical biopsy is not necessary and indeed may be contraindicated.

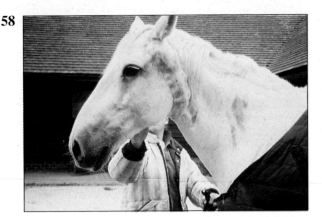

58 Melanosarcoma in the parotid salivary gland of a 12 year old grey mare. The lesion had become progressively larger over some years and endoscopic examination of the guttural pouches showed the presence of large numbers of aggressive looking melanotic lesions. The right side was not affected, although the guttural pouch contained several focal melanotic patches and 2 larger spherical melanotic masses.

Part 3: The Esophagus

Developmental Disorders

A number of clinically important developmental anomalies of the esophagus have been recognised including atresia, fistulation, diverticula, cysts and strictures. **Congenital intramural cysts** are usually located in the proximal third of the cervical esophagus **(59)**. The clinical signs associated with these include dysphagia and regurgitation. They are assumed to be embryonic remnants of bronchogenic cysts and are usually soft and fluctuant (fluid filled). While most affected foals are not unduly distressed by their presence, weight loss and inhalation pneumonia are serious complications. Naso gastric intubation may prove difficult with marked resistance at the site. Contrast radiography (particularly with the aid of fluoroscopy) reveals a filling defect of the esophagus proximal to the cyst itself, which in most cases, effectively acts as a partial or complete, intermittent or permanent, obstruction.

Localised or generalised **esophageal dilatation** or laxity in the cervical and/or the thoracic esophagus occur occasionally and in spite of marked local changes the defects may only become apparent when dysphagia and inhalation pneumonia are presented. Generally these disorders only become apparent when the affected foal begins to eat significant amounts of solid food from ground level. The normal nursing foal may be regarded as being posturally fed in its early life, with liquid feed

passing into the cervical esophagus easily (provided that bolus formation and deglutition are normal). The formation and swallowing of normal boluses of food material, whether this be milk in the young foal, or solid food, is dependent upon efficient, coordinated neuromuscular function of the tongue, mouth, pharynx and the intrinsic neural control of the esophagus. Horses with developmental defects of neurological or physical function of the cricopharyngeal structures at the cranial end of the esophagus may have significant difficulty in swallowing. **Crico-pharyngeal laxity** may be recognised endoscopically when the apparently flaccid esophageal opening may be readily seen above the apex of the arytenoid cartilages **(60)**. This condition is erroneously called an achalasia, but this is a misnomer as the esophageal opening is flaccid and not firmly closed.

The definitive diagnosis of neurologically related esophageal dilatations, whether related to sphincter control at either end of the organ, or to its intrinsic motility, is difficult, and relies heavily upon endoscopic and static or dynamic contrast radiographic studies. Diffuse, often extensive, **dilatation (mega-esophagus)** arising from generalised neuromuscular dysfunction, primarily affects the proximal (striated muscle) portion and contrast radiographic studies (using double, positive and negative, contrast) will usually identify a well

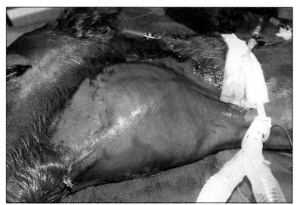

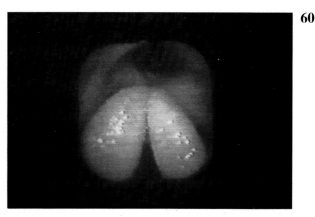

59 Esophageal cyst.
Differential Diagnosis:
i)   Esophageal abscess
ii) Esophageal diverticulum
iii) Salivary mucocele

60 Cricopharyngeal laxity.
Note: Open, apparently flaccid esophageal opening above arytenoids.

defined narrowing at the cardia (**61**) situated caudal to the base of the heart. Post mortem examination of the dilated esophagus will confirm the flaccid, thin nature of the proximal dilated portion. The appearance of the disorder is suggestive of neurological deficits within the intrinsic nerve plexuses controlling esophageal contraction and co-ordination. However, there is usually no pathological evidence of this or of an achalasia or spasm of the cardia. The length of esophagus affected may be relatively short and in some cases it may merely involve limited areas of muscular wall. In other cases the effect may be diffuse and affect much larger (or even the entire) length of the esophagus (**62**). Again, contrast radiographic studies (both static and dynamic) can be used to define the extent of the dysfunction. Where greater lengths of esophagus are involved (**62**) contrast medium, whether as a swallow or a meal, will be seen to remain in the esophagus for an abnormally long time. These are, fortunately, rare disorders of limited clinical importance and carry a poor or hopeless prognosis, although individual animals may be capable of reasonable growth and function with suitable nursing and feeding regimens.

Congenital strictures are usually annular in character and most are located in the proximal third of the cervical esophagus (**63**). They vary widely in their character and consequent clinical effects. Thin superficial strictures (webs), involving the mucosa and sub-mucosa only, may be more common than is realised. Most, though not all, are probably disrupted, in early life, by natural bouginage (dilatation) with increasingly firm food and these present no detectable clinical abnormality. Thicker mucosal strictures, and those

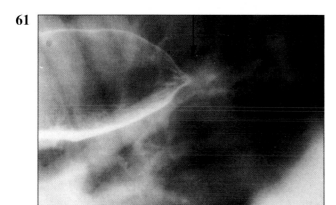

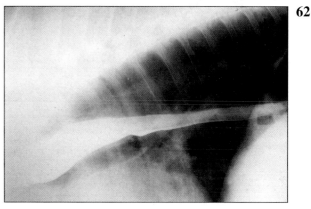

61 Megaesophagus.
Note: Four-month-old foal demonstrating use of double contrast esophagram. Arrow at the level of the diaphragm.

62 Esophageal dilatation (megaesophagus) (contrast study).

involving the deeper layers of the esophagus, are potentially more serious and may not resolve spontaneously with increasing dietary-fibre intake. Strictures of congenital origin resulting in a functional obstruction of the lumen of the esophagus are usually partial, allowing liquid feed to pass without hindrance but, as soon as the foal starts to ingest fibrous food, clinical evidence of obstruction may be seen. Affected foals are often presented with a history of **recurrent 'choke'** (*see* **64**) and while these may resolve spontaneously, more often they become increasingly severe. On occasions, the accumulation of food proximal to a stricture (whether due to a congenital or acquired obstruction) may be visible and palpable (**65**). The presence of a stricture may be confirmed by contrast-meal radiography. Dynamic studies with contrast fluoroscopy will reveal a significant retention of food at the site with variable proximal dilatation. Negative contrast (using air) may also be used effectively in identifying the width and firmness of the stricture itself (**63**). Endoscopic examination provides an ideal means of assessing the extent and character of the stricture from the lumen. In many cases however, the foal is presented with considerable esophageal accumulation of food and saliva and this may have to be resolved first. Congenital strictures should be differentiated from those which arise as a result of esophageal trauma and the clinical signs are initially indistinguishable from those of intraluminal esophageal obstruction ('choke') due to food impaction or foreign bodies. Esophageal strictures may be found in horses of any age. The prognosis for foals affected with developmental strictures is largely dependent upon the extent to which the stricture can be dilated naturally. Surgical corrections are difficult and carry a very guarded prognosis.

A developmental hypertrophy of the esophageal musculature (particularly that of the distal third) results in an unusual form of functional esophageal stricture. Clinical signs of esophageal obstruction typically develop only once the foal starts to ingest solid food. Endoscopically the esophagus looks normal but passage of a nasogastric tube is very difficult. Barium meal radiography is required to establish the diagnosis. The prognosis for these foals is hopeless.

63
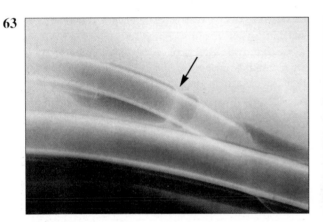

64
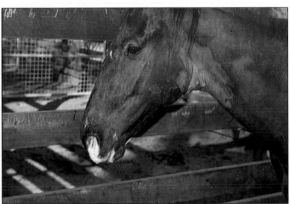

63 Esophageal Stricture.
Note: Negative contrast radiograph of the proximal cervical esophagus. An endotracheal tube was inserted into the esophagus and the cuff was inflated. Arrow points to the stricture, which only just allowed the 12 mm tube to pass.

64 (Intraluminal) esophageal obstruction (choke).
Note: Food and saliva at nostrils and mouth.

Non-Infectious Disorders

Note: Even gross esophageal disorders such as strictures, ulceration or diverticula are often impossible to visualise endoscopically without persistent insufflation. Examination is usually best performed during the withdrawal of the endoscope, while maintaining insufflation pressure. Contrast radiographic studies using positive or negative contrast (or both) may also be applicable in the investigation of acquired esophageal disorders.

Intraluminal obstruction ('choke') is probably the commonest disorder involving the esophagus of the horse. The most common causes of obstruction are the ingestion of food of abnormal consistency, and foreign bodies. In the United States of America and most other countries the majority of choke cases are due to corn-cobs and other foreign bodies. Around 95% of cases in the United Kingdom are direct consequences of the ingestion of dried (or partially soaked) sugar beet pulp. Even small amounts of dry feed such as (dry) sugar beet or cubed/pelleted feed, may cause intraluminal obstruction. Greedy feeders, horses which are poorly fed at irregular intervals, and those with dental disease, are particularly liable to the condition. Also, Shetland ponies, in which the esophagus is thought to be narrower than in other breeds, appear particularly prone to the disorder. Medication by bolus (particularly in Shetland ponies) has historically, been a frequent cause of complete obstruction. The signs, which have a characteristically acute onset, include marked discomfort/pain with repeated swallowing attempts accompanied by arching of the neck and squealing. Pain appears to be most severe with foreign body obstruction as opposed to the more diffuse impactive condition caused by dry feeds. Profuse salivation and the nasal regurgitation of saliva mixed with food particles (**64**) is usually present, particularly after swallowing attempts. Rarely, some blood may be present in the regurgitated food and saliva. The esophagus may be visibly distended (**65**) or the obstruction may be palpable. Long-standing cases may have an unpleasant, fetid breath. In spite of the dramatic appearance it is remarkable how well horses tolerate the condition. The proximal extent of the obstruction can be located by passage of a naso gastric tube or by endoscopy (**66**), or by contrast radiography. None of these would, however, necessarily, define either the type of material responsible, or the site, or the full extent of the obstruction. Some horses affected by complete intraluminal obstruction continue to eat, particularly where the obstruction is situated in the thoracic or distal cervical esophagus. The character of the endoscopically visible obstruction (**66**) may, therefore, be very different from the inciting cause. In some cases the obstruction

65

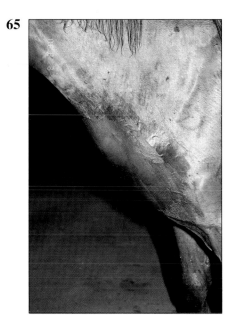

66

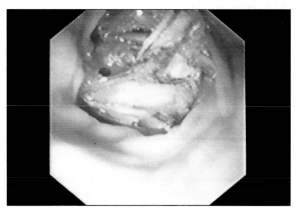

65 (Intraluminal) esophageal obstruction (choke). **Note:** Visible distension of the esophagus at thoracic inlet. The horse continued to eat hay and straw for some hours after eating a feed of dry sugar beet pulp.

66 (Intraluminal) esophageal obstruction (choke). **Note:** Endoscopic view of proximal end of esophageal obstruction (same horse as **65**). The presence of straw was not indicative of the inciting cause which was found to be sugar beet pulp.

is, at first, incomplete and results in proximal dilatation of the esophagus which, sometimes over considerable periods of time, becomes complete with the proximal accumulation of fluid, saliva and food material. Repeated refluxing of this liquid-based material as a result of muscular contractions of the esophagus results in marked nasal regurgitation of non-acidic material which is salivary in appearance, but which may not contain any obvious food material. Sometimes, particularly in those animals with continued access to food, the esophagus may become filled with food material up to the pharynx. In these cases, and more rarely in the milder forms of choke, food material and saliva may be inhaled into the trachea (**Plate 4 l**, page 104). Fortunately, this is seldom significant, although, in prolonged or neglected cases, inhalation pneumonia may develop and be of life-threatening severity (**210**). This complication seems particularly common in foals affected by esophageal obstruction, regardless of the cause, with some of these cases developing severe aspiration pneumonia within hours of onset. Although the clinical signs of choke are dramatic, diffuse obstruction, such as that commonly caused by sugar beet impaction, is seldom immediately life-threatening and mucosal damage is usually minimal or non-existent. Obstructions due to firm foreign bodies such as corn cobs, rough straw, wood shavings, potatoes, apples, carrots etc. are, however, potentially more serious. These obstructions may be partial or complete, and the firm nature of most such objects, results in significant local spasm of the esophagus around the foreign body. Variable degrees of **mucosal ulceration** develop. Limited depth (mucosal), longitudinal or linear ulceration is relatively common and may take the form of a single broad ulcer (**67**) or multiple, finer, short, linear lesions. These shallow, mucosal ulcers have little long-term consequence and heal rapidly. **Circum-ferential ulceration** involving the mucosa only, or the mucosa and the superficial muscular layers, or more severe lesions affecting the deeper layers of the wall of the esophagus (**68**), may be visualised endoscopically, and occurs particularly with rough or sharp foreign bodies. Whilst, in most cases, the area of ulceration is more diffuse, bolus medications and dry corn cobs, in particular, seem to result in a sharply demarcated circumferential ulceration (**69**). The circumferential nature of these lesions makes their long-term consequences more serious than the longitudinal ulcers. **Fibrous (scar tissue) strictures** commonly develop some days or weeks later (*see* **71,72**). Their depth and density is variable, and depend upon the depth of the original ulcer and the extent to which stricture development can be prevented or controlled by natural healing processes or through therapeutic measures. **Acquired strictures** may be sufficiently severe to cause repeated episodes of choke which are usually progressive in severity, following an insidious onset. Sometimes there is no previous history of choke, with the first episode being severe. The site of the stricture may be evident if it is located in the cervical esophagus, as even small amounts of food result in an obvious proximal filling defect (**70**) cranial to the site. Endoscopically the severity of the stricture may be marked (**71**). Post mortem examination of the esophagus of horses suffering from tight, full-thickness-stricture development, confirms their depth and extent and reveals the proximal dilatation associated with repeated and persistent choke (**72**). It is entirely

67

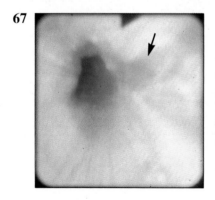

67 (Intraluminal) esophageal obstruction (choke) (After treatment).
Note: (Linear) esophageal erosion (arrow) which resulted from long-standing esophageal obstruction.

68

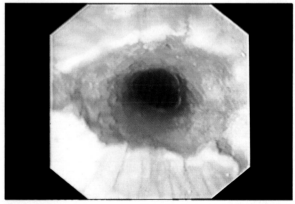

68 (Severe) circumferential ulceration (proximal cervical region).
Note: Due to intraluminal obstruction with a corn-cob.

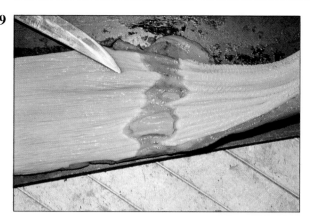

69 (Well defined) circumferential ulceration (mucosa and submucosa).
Note: Following obstruction by bolus medicant (Shetland pony).

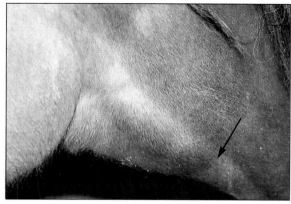

70 Esophageal stricture.
Note: Recurrent choking episodes of increasing severity and duration with an obvious swelling having a sharp cut-off point (arrow).

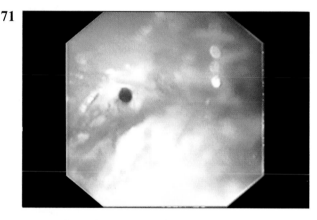

71 Esophageal stricture (endoscopic view).
Note: Same horse as **68** and **70** (3 weeks later). Proximal dilatation of esophagus (also insufflated) with very small (1 cm diameter) lumen to stricture.

72 Esophageal stricture (post mortem specimen).
Note: Same horse as **68** and **71**. Obvious full-thickness scarring and contraction with proximal distention of esophagus (left).

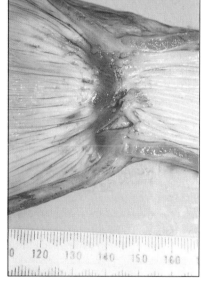

understandable that natural bouginage would not easily result in any improvement in such a case, and that continuing contraction of the fibrous tissue stricture would result in recurrent or persistent obstruction. Natural bouginage and attempts to dilate the stricture surgically would, likely, be unrewarding, if not entirely impossible. Most full thickness circumferential ulcerations and the consequent strictures are, therefore, extremely serious and frequently carry a hopeless prognosis, requiring surgical resection, which itself may result in a further stricture. Early diagnosis and aggressive treatment is essential if even mild scar tissue strictures are to be treated effectively. The full length of the esophagus of all horses which have suffered from any 'choke' due to a sharp foreign body should, therefore, be carefully examined endoscopically.

Esophageal ulceration and inflammation involving greater or lesser lengths of the organ which are more severe at the proximal end are characteristic of the ingestion of irritant chemicals such as phenylbutazone, organophosphates or some poisonous plants (including the hepatotoxic plants of the *Crotalaria* spp.). The latter cause well-recognised hepatic and esophageal diseases, such as **Chillagoe Horse Disease** in Australia, and **'dunsiekte'** in South Africa. In these, esophageal ulceration is particularly severe at the proximal end (**73**)

73

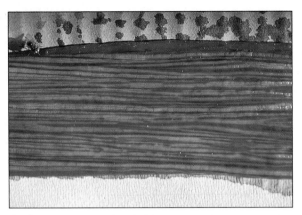

74

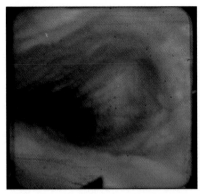

74 (Pulsion-type) Esophageal diverticulum (Endoscopic view).

73 Esophageal ulceration (Chillagoe Horse Disease / *Crotalaria aridicola* poisoning).
Note: Proximal esophagus. Signs of hepato-encephalopathy were also present.

in contrast to the similar ulcerative esophagitis encountered at the distal end as a result of gastro-esophageal reflux such as occurs in **Grass Sickness** (*see* **133**), in particular. Diagnosis depends upon the use of an endoscope and critical assessment of the extent of the inflammation /ulceration and in most of these conditions the esophageal lesions are only a relatively minor sign accompanying obvious cranial and/or hepatic signs.

Numerous, small, **focal** and sometimes very deep, **ulcerative esophageal lesions** may be caused by the ingestion of irritant drugs or caustic chemicals and, while most are of no clinical significance, loss of the protective mucosa may have serious immediate and long-term consequences including infection and local abscess. Cases of Grass Sickness (*see* **129** *et seq.*) sometimes show extensive diffuse, linear esophageal ulceration which is particularly severe in the distal third (*see* **133**). This is probably due to repeated or persistent, acidic, gastro-esophageal reflux and is likely to be exacerbated by the paralysis of the esophagus which is a feature of the disorder (*see* **132**).

Mucosal necrosis, **perforation of the esophagus**, or other localised, non-circumferential esophageal lesions, resulting possibly from foreign body damage, may result in the formation of an **esophageal diverticulum**. Acquired diverticula of the esophagus are usually of little consequence if the neck of the diverticulum is wide, such as sometimes occurs following surgical esophagotomy or the spontaneous healing of esophageal wounds. These are described as traction diverticula, and probably arise as a result of peri-esophageal scarring and subsequent scar contraction. Some of these develop without any apparent instigating factor. They may be encountered anywhere along the length of the esophagus, and may be a result of a longitudinal developmental defect in the integrity of the muscular layers, particularly in the distal, smooth-muscle portion of the organ. The diagnosis of such diverticula may be frustrating. Clinical signs of recurrent choke may be seen, although this is an irregular occurrence. Naso gastric intubation is sometimes easy, suggesting that there is no obstructive lesion, while at other times the procedure may be difficult or even impossible. Endoscopic examination will usually identify the site and extent of the lesion. **Spherical (pulsion) diverticula (74)** arising from focal muscular or mucosal damage are potentially more serious, and present with progressive (variable) swellings in the cervical esophagus (**75**). As the neck of the diverticulum is narrow, these are more prone to impaction with food material and consequent perforation than traction diverticula. Secondary effects include local occlusion of the jugular vein (*see* **75**) and **fistulation** (*see* **77**). In both types of diverticulum clinical evidence of 'choke' may be present and both may sometimes be seen to enlarge, momentarily, when the animal swallows. Combinations of ultrasound, endoscopy and contrast radiography may confirm the diagnosis.

Fistulae which may discharge saliva and food material during swallowing are effectively restricted to the cervical esophagus. Most are sequels to internal ulceration, mural or peri-esophageal abscesses or necrosis, they may also arise from traumatic rupture of the esophagus (**76**). Where this occurs in the cervical region the lesion is usually obvious, although the defect in the esophageal wall may appear to be small the consequences are greater, as the food within the esophagus is under considerable pressure. Subcutaneous contamination with food and saliva is usually extensive **(76)** but in some cases may be minimal. Where the fistula develops from lesions within the esophageal wall (*see* **75**) (such as a diverticulum) fistulation is usually preceded by local abscess formation in the esophageal wall and subsequent rupture onto the skin surface, with minimal subcutaneous involvement **(77)**. In either case the persistent food and saliva contamination prevent healing of the defect. The smooth fistula can be visualised endoscopically **(78)** or radiographically using positive contrast methods **(79)**.

Acquired failure of the neurological function of the esophagus is a characteristic sign of **Grass Sickness (equine dysautonomia)** and results in the development of esophageal flaccidity with the accumulation of food material at the thoracic inlet. The flaccidity of the wall of the esophagus may be demonstrated effectively with contrast radiographic studies when contrast will be seen to pool at the thoracic inlet and remain there almost indefinitely (*see* **132**). The esophageal mucosa characteristically shows longitudinal ulceration particularly in the distal third which is possibly due to reflux esophagitis (*see* **133**).

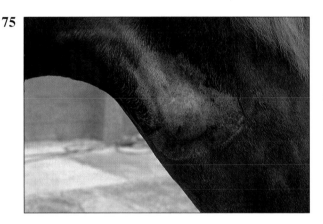

75 Intramural esophageal abscess.
Note: Confirmed by ultrasonography. Due to brush bristle. Obstruction to flow of jugular vein (not thrombosed).
Differential Diagnosis:
i) Impacted focal diverticulum
ii) Esophageal stricture
iii) Neoplasia

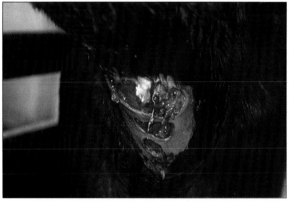

76 Traumatic esophageal rupture.
Note: Extensive necrosis and subcutaneous contamination following kick to ventral neck. Defect in esophagus was less than 1 cm diameter in post mortem specimen.

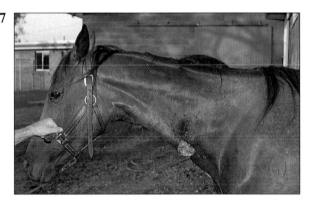

77 Esophageal fistula.
Note: Developed subsequent to an intramural abscess. The horse was not distressed although food and water issued from the fistula during swallowing. Weight loss was present.

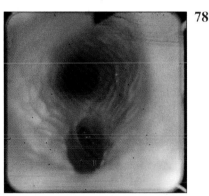

78 Esophageal fistula (endoscopic appearance).

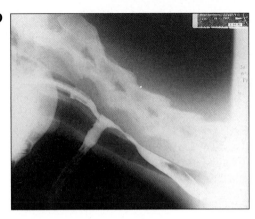

79 Esophageal fistula (contrast esophagram taken during swallowing).

Infectious Disorders

Clostridial infection of the pharynx and esophagus is sometimes encountered following the use of long-term, in-dwelling, nasogastric and feeding tubes and is characterised by the development of extensive local myonecrosis and infiltration of the pharyngeal tissues with gas (**80**). Depending upon its severity and proximity to the pharynx, severe limitations to swallowing and, often life-threatening, pharyngeal swelling (**80**) may accompany this condition. It is unlikely that even severe focal abscessation and swelling in the cervical region would be sufficiently severe to affect tracheal patency.

Single intramural esophageal abscesses are unusual but are associated with foreign bodies such as brush bristles or twigs. These present as focal solid or fluctuating swellings in the wall and may be sufficiently large to cause jugular obstruction (*see* **75**). Other effects are usually minimal. They are difficult to differentiate clinically from a diverticulum or a mural neoplasia and the use of ultrasonography and endoscopy is essential.

Traumatic rupture of the cervical esophagus may follow from kicks and other trauma to the neck. Some cases are the result of injudicious passage of a naso-gastric tube, particularly during investigation of choke and diverticula. Ruptures of the cervical esophagus are characterised by extensive subcutaneous contamination and infection (*see* **76**), but seldom cause any

immediately-life-threatening danger. Boluses of food passing down the esophagus are normally under considerable pressure and even small defects of the wall result in extensive local contamination and an acute suppurative inflammation of the adjacent subcutaneous tissues. **Bacterial contamination with anaerobic organisms** is usual and, where this occurs in the cervical esophagus, the tissues surrounding the esophagus become emphysematous, hot and very painful. Radiographic examination can be used to detect the presence of gas and extensive soft tissue swelling (**81**). A similar appearance may be found in cases of severe **oropharyngeal necrosis**, usually arising from long-term nasogastric intubation (*see* **80**). Extension of the bacterial contamination is usually towards the thorax and ultimately a severe mediastinitis develops with a fatal outcome. Ruptures of the esophagus may appear, visually, to be relatively minor when viewed endoscopically (or at post mortem examination) but the consequences of such rupture within the thorax are particularly serious, with extensive thoracic (mediastinal) contamination with food and saliva. Animals so affected are often presented *in extremis*, or may die suddenly after a short, fulminating and progressive pleuritis and mediastinitis which are complicated still further by infection with clostridial and other gas-forming bacteria.

80

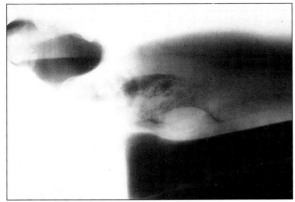

81

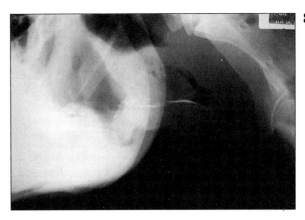

80 Esophageal necrosis.
Note: A long-term, in-dwelling, nasogastric (feeding) tube resulted in necrosis and clostridial infection (gas in peri-esophageal tissue). A large abscess developed at the site.

81 Esophageal Rupture with Infection (*Clostridia* spp) (positive contrast barium swallow esophagram).
Note: Acute suppurative inflammation of the subcutaneous tissue with extensive peripharyngeal gas production following rupture of the esophagus. Note narrowing of pharynx and upward displacement of the guttural pouches which lead to respiratory obstruction.

Neoplastic Disorders

Intra-mural space-occupying lesions of neoplastic nature are very rare but may be sufficiently large to affect food transit. Lesions of sufficient size to obstruct the esophagus in the cervical region would be expected to be palpable but may not affect the endoscopic appearance of the mucosa except in the case of squamous cell carcinoma. Masses within the thorax such as lymphosarcoma may be sufficiently large to result in an extra-luminal esophageal obstruction with proximal dilatation and present the characteristic signs of recurrent choke. Several episodes of obstruction without any endoscopic lesion should alert the clinician to this possibility. The clinical effects on the esophagus are usually of relatively minor importance in these cases.

Part 4: The Gastro-Intestinal Tract

In common with other systems the clinical manifestations of gastro-intestinal disease in the horse are somewhat limited with many possible etiological factors. Individual diseases or disorders often show only subtle variations in the basic clinical appearance. Specific diagnosis often, however, relies upon the application of further diagnostic tests including rectal examination, the examination of abdominal fluid, fecal and hematological analyses, and a number of more specialised tests. Furthermore, the critical examination of cardio-vascular and respiratory status is of vital importance in assessing the severity of abdominal diseases and disorders. Probably the single most important clinical sign associated with gastro-intestinal disorders is **colic** which is the clinical manifestation of abdominal pain. While most cases of colic can be attributed to gastro-intestinal disease, it is important to realise that abdominal pain not related to gastro-intestinal disorders may induce very similar clinical signs. Therefore, conditions of abdominal organs other than the gastro-intestinal tract, including the urinary, genital, hepatic, pancreatic and other peritoneal organs, may exhibit the same signs and may, therefore, require to be considered when investigating horses with colic signs. Horses showing colic as a result of abdominal pain exhibit a variety of clinical signs in combination. The general signs include flank watching (**Plate 1a**, page 44), restless pacing, wandering and pawing the ground (**Plate 1b**, page 44), stretching (**Plate 1c**, page 44), repeated attempts to lie down (**Plate 1d**, page 44), recumbency (*see* **Plate 1a**) associated with groaning or grunting and rolling which may be mild or violent (**Plate 1e**, page 45). The severity of pain in cases of colic may also be assessed by the type and extent of sweating (**Plate 1f**, page 45) and from the cardiovascular and respiratory status. Cold extremities, a clammy wet skin, and cyanotic mucous membranes (**Plate 8b**, page 178) are normally indicative of shock, and are signs of very serious or catastrophic disorders. Occasionally horses showing colic may adopt a 'dog-sitting' posture associated with anterior abdominal pain or catastrophes such as gastric rupture, or diaphragmatic hernia. The presence of acidic green fluid at the nose (**Plate 1g**, page 45) is suggestive of serious gastric distention with impending gastric rupture or may follow gastric rupture. The presence of significant volumes of gastric fluid (**Plate 1h**, page 45) detected by the passage of a nasogastric tube is a most important clinical sign, and its character and pH may be helpful in identifying the site of gastro-intestinal obstructions.

The amount and consistency of the feces and the frequency with which these are passed represent the other easily assessed clinical indicator of gastro-intestinal function. Reductions in the volume of feces passed may reflect a reduced intake or some hindrance to the passage of food material through the tract. Failure of efficient mastication produces feces which have an inordinately high long-fibre content but although the character of the fibres may be abnormal, this seldom results in any significant changes in overall consistency of the feces. The consistency of the feces in the horse usually reflects the motility and absorptive capacity of the large bowel. Even severe, diffuse, small bowel disease often has surprisingly little effect upon the ability of the large bowel to produce feces of normal consistency. **Diarrhea** (*see* **134**) is, therefore, generally a sign of colonic disease, although its presence would not preclude the presence of concurrent small intestinal pathology. Complete absence or marked reductions in the frequency of defecation would normally be associated with obstructive disorders of the tract and these may arise as a result of physical obstruction or physiological obstruction resulting from motility dysfunctions.

For all practical purposes physical obstruction of the bowel may be divided into:

i)   **simple obstruction** (those lesions which obstruct the lumen but, initially, do not interfere with intestinal blood supply),

ii) **strangulating obstruction** (in which the blood vessels are compromised, as well as the lumen of the bowel), and

iii) **non-strangulating infarction** (in which blood supply is occluded without the intestinal lumen being obstructed).

Horses affected by intraluminal obstructions are usually in good metabolic order (at least in the early stages). Those with non-strangulating, vascular compromise and the strangulating disorders usually show dramatic and rapidly progressive cardio-vascular effects associated with endotoxemia and shock. The efficiency of blood perfusion in cases of gastro-intestinal colic appears to be one of the most vital factors in the pathophysiology of the colic complex. Impaired neurological control of intestinal motility usually results in a reduced gut motility. The secretory and absorptive functions are typically maintained and under these conditions the proximal (secretory) organs (stomach and small bowel to the level of the distal jejunum) continue to fill, while in the ileum, large colon and cecum the sustained absorptive functions continue to render the contents progressively more desiccated. This type of disorder would result in a physiological obstruction to bowel function and would fall into the non-strangulating category of colic disorders.

The colour and content of free **peritoneal fluid** is an important diagnostic aid in the investigation of colic and other abdominal disorders. **Normal peritoneal fluid** is straw coloured and is usually present in limited volumes such that it may be difficult to obtain a sample (**Plate 2a**, page 46). **Ascites** (accumulation of serous fluid in the peritoneum) is usually evidence of circulatory, hepatic or hypoproteinemic disorders. The fluid is usually clear, watery, of low specific gravity, and only very faintly colored (**Plate 2b**, page 46). A cloudy or milky appearance may rarely be the result of **chylous leakage** from lymphatic vessels but is most often indicative of an **increased cell content** (**Plate 2c**, page 46). The cells which are present may reflect the pathological process which is present and range from abnormal (neoplastic) cells in proliferative conditions to inflammatory cells in peritonitis. The proportion of red cells in the peritoneal fluid (hematocrit) is of major importance as most peritoneal fluid is obtained by aspiration. Peritoneal fluid having the same hematocrit as a simultaneous jugular (venous) sample suggests that a peritoneal vein or artery has been entered. **Truly bloody peritoneal fluid** is indicative of intraperitoneal bleeding, such as might occur in horses suffering from verminous arteritis (*see* **145**) or rupture of the middle uterine artery at foaling (*see* **776**). In these cases the hematocrit of the fluid obtained is usually slightly higher or lower than circulating blood (depending upon the duration and extent of the bleeding and its consequences upon circulating volume). Horses suffering from **strangulating lesions** of the intestine frequently have blood-stained peritoneal fluid (**Plate 2d**, page 46) having a low packed-cell volume and an elevated protein content. The red cells contained in the fluid may sediment leaving a clear supernatant. There are, however, two major occasions when strangulating lesions may not alter the peritoneal fluid. These are **hernias** (diaphragmatic or other), when the strangulated loops are within the thorax (or elsewhere), and **intussusceptions** when the obstructed venous drainage is enclosed within the intussuscipiens (the enclosing portion of the intussusception). Peritoneal fluid with a turbid appearance, which may be slightly red or orange in colour (**Plate 2e**, page 47), is usually indicative of a high cell content and may be associated with **peritonitis** (either localised or generalised). In these cases the protein content of the fluid is also markedly raised and close examination of the cells will usually identify active and degenerate neutrophils. A dark, very concentrated, blood-like peritoneal fluid (**Plate 2f**, page 47), with a packed cell volume (hematocrit) significantly greater than that of circulating blood, is indicative of **splenic aspiration**; a finding which may, in certain circumstances, be of significance. Very large volumes of brown/red peritoneal fluid with a high cell content (including abdominal cells) are usually a result of abdominal neoplasia such as mesothelioma (**Plate 1h**, page 45, *see* **177**). The presence of abnormal cells in the peritoneum is suggestive of neoplasia and identification of the cell types is an important diagnostic aid. An abdominal paracentesis which produces a fluid which is contaminated with **food material** (**Plate 2g**, page 47) may arise from inadvertent puncture of an abdominal viscus (usually the cecum or ventral colon), or when an abdominal viscus has ruptured (usually the stomach, cecum or colon). The latter are invariably associated with severe, rapidly deteriorating colic with dramatic cardiovascular compromise.

Developmental Disorders

Congenital disorders involving the stomach are very unusual with **pyloric stenosis** being the most prevalent disorder. Affected foals usually show post-prandial bruxism (grinding of the teeth) and varying degrees of abdominal pain and colic and may regurgitate milk after nursing. Some cases are evident at a very young age but others may appear to develop when solid food is ingested at several weeks of age. There is considerable doubt as to whether the disorder is of congenital origin at all, being possibly an acquired stenosis secondary to gastro-duodenal ulceration or chronic gastritis due to other reasons.

Congenital atresia (absence of a normal opening or patent lumen) or restrictive narrowing of the intestine are rare abnormalities of development. As would be expected the intestine proximal to the obstruction is distended (sometimes greatly) while the distal portion is empty (**82**). Complete obstruction, for whatever reason, results in the distal portion being completely empty and a foal affected in this way would have no meconium in the rectum at birth. Foals with complete atresia, or any other total obstruction, are usually weak at birth and suffer from non-strangulating, unremitting colic within hours of birth. The more proximal the obstruction the

Plate 1

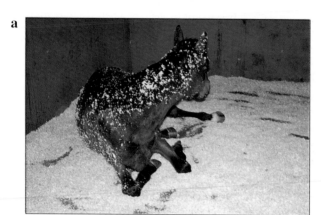

a Recumbency and flank watching.

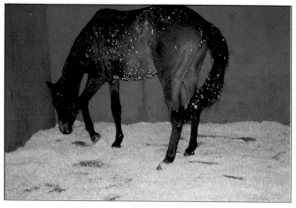

b Pawing.

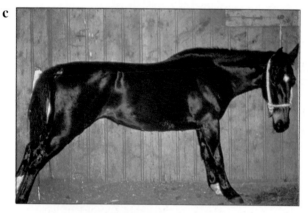

c Stretching.
Differential Diagnosis:
i) Peritonitis
ii) Cystic/urethral calculi/inflammation

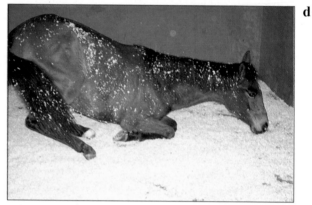

d Repeated attempts to lie down.

Plate 1

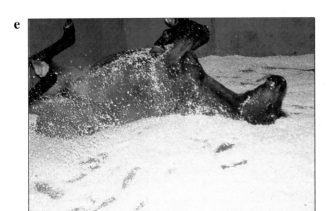

e Rolling.

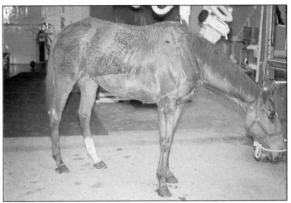

f Generalised (or patchy) sweating.

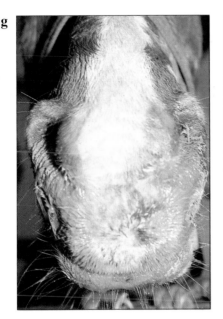

g Spontaneous gastric reflux.
Differential Diagnosis:
i)   Primary gastric distension (food material, water, Grass sickness)
ii) Secondary gastric distension (gastric outflow impairment, intestinal obstruction)
iii) Choke (esophageal obstruction)
iv) Chillagoe horse disease

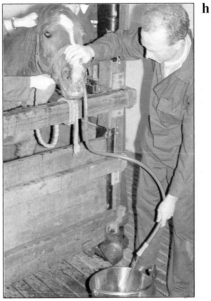

h Gastric reflux (relief by naso-gastric tube).

Plate 2

a

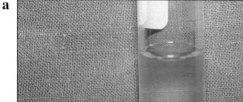

a Normal peritoneal fluid.
Note: Usually in small amounts only. Clear, straw-coloured, almost acellular with a low protein content.

b

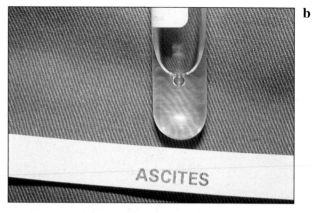

b Clear peritoneal fluid (Ascites).
Note: Clear, very pale (almost water clear in some cases) with a low protein concentration. Usually present in large amounts.
Differential Diagnosis:
i)   Starvation / hypoproteinemia
ii) Chronic hepatic failure (cirrhosis)
iii) Congestive heart failure

c

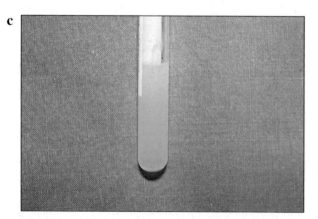

c Cloudy peritoneal fluid.
Note: Diffuse cloudy/turbulent appearance.
Differential Diagnosis:
i)   Peritonitis (raised cell content and protein concentration)
ii) Chylous peritonitis (leakage from mesenteric lacteals or lymphatic ducts)
iii) Abdominal neoplasia
iv) Biliary Obstruction (including cholangiocellular carcinoma)

d

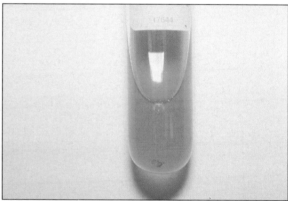

d Blood-stained peritoneal fluid.
Note: Clear fluid in greater than normal amount and containing obvious sedimenting red cells.
Differential Diagnosis:
i)   Abdominal hemorrhage (neoplasia, trauma)
ii) Puncture of minor blood vessels during paracentesis (low protein content of fluid)
iii) Strangulating intestinal lesion (high protein content and elevated white cell count)

Plate 2

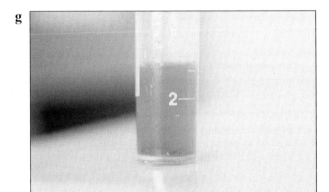

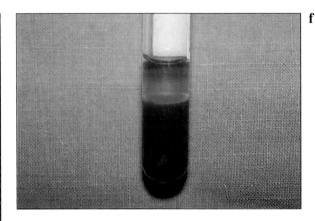

e Cloudy, blood-stained peritoneal fluid.
Note: Densely turbid and obviously hemorrhagic.
Differential Diagnosis:
i)   Peritonitis
ii) Abdominal abscess
iii) Abdominal neoplasia
iv) Parasite-induced focal infarction

f Hemorrhagic peritoneal fluid (splenic sample).
Note: High packed-cell-volume with small buffy coat (as shown) indicates splenic sample, hematocrit value similar to jugular sample indicates blood vessel sample.

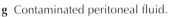

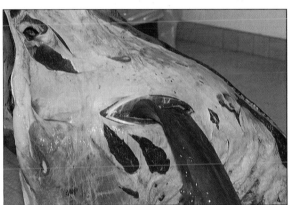

g Contaminated peritoneal fluid.
Note: Obvious brown-green colour and sediment of food/plant material.
Differential Diagnosis:
i)   Penetration of viscus (low volume, no leucocytes)
ii) Rupture of abdominal viscus (high protein content, high leucocyte count, erythrocytes)

h Brown peritoneal fluid (in large amounts).

Differential Diagnosis:
i)   Abdominal neoplasia (mesothelioma, hemangiosarcoma)

82

83

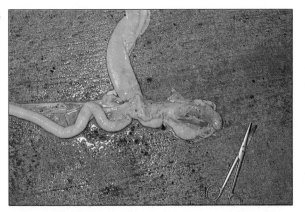

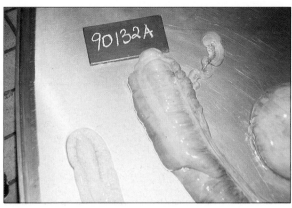

82 Atresia of jejunum.
Note: Post mortem specimen obtained from a day-old foal showing severe colic and marked cardiac abnormalities. Proximal jejunum filled/distended and distal narrow, empty segment.

83 Atresia of large colon.
Note: Right ventral colon ends in a blind sac and more distal segments are empty and poorly developed. Foal showed severe non-responsive, progressive colic starting 4 hours after birth.

more rapid will be the onset of the clinical signs. **Atresia of the colon** usually occurs in the region of the pelvic flexure, that is between the left ventral and left dorsal colon (**83**), but may affect any site in the large or small colon. Failure of continuity of the large colon results in the early development of severe, unremitting and persistent colic associated with abdominal distension and tympany. It is one of the recognised intestinal abnormalities encountered in the '**Lethal-White Syndrome**' encountered in foals of Ovaro-Paint breeding (*see* **87**). **Atresia ani** is less common in the equine than in other farm animals and may be associated concurrently with defects of the urogenital tract. In some cases, where the deficit is more anterior the terminal rectum will be completely empty but in others the rectum may be full, terminating blindly some distance from the anus. Clinically these defects may be recognised as partial or complete absence of anal structures. Straining, attempts at defecation and complete absence of any feces or detectable meconium staining are the major presenting signs and, ultimately there is extensive accumulation of food material and gas in the terminal large and small colon. In some cases the condition is complicated by the development of megacolon (**84**) which sometimes terminates in rupture. Other, often multiple, congenital abnormalities, such as cardiac defects, cleft palates and eye and joint defects, are often found in foals affected with this type of disorder.

Meckel's Diverticulum, which is formed from the persistent remnants of the vitelline (omphalomesenteric) duct, is also a possible causes of colic deriving from developmental defects. Although in many cases it never causes any problem, most affected horses are adult. The structure, whose lumen is continuous with that of the ileum, usually takes the form of a finger like projection extending from the anti-mesenteric border of the ileum (**85**). Severe, strangulating colic as a result of this developmental defect is sometimes encountered in adult (often old) horses and the extent of the strangulated intestine is almost infinitely variable. Furthermore, impaction of the diverticulum with food material may result in recurrent non-strangulating colic. Rupture of the impacted and distended organ may cause fatal peritonitis.

Persistent mesodiverticular bands, which are also possibly related to the vestigial vitelline artery, have also resulted in strangulating and non-strangulating obstructions of the small intestine. These present as small bands extending from the mesentery onto the anti-mesenteric border of the intestine. The band forms a potential cavity or hiatus (**86**) into which small intestine may pass. Once entrapped through the space, strangulating and obstructive colic may develop at any stage and the extent of the entrapped bowel may be limited, or may include considerable lengths of jejunum.

Foals born to matings of Ovaro-Paint horses which have white hair, pink skin and blue eyes (**Lethal-White Syndrome**) frequently suffer from developmental **ileo-colonic aganglionosis** in which there is a profound absence of intrinsic myenteric plexus in the ileum and colon. Affected foals are usually normal immediately after birth but develop severe, unremitting colic within 12 hours (**87**). These foals invariably die. At post mortem examination the characteristic signs of ileus will be noted. These include distension of the stomach and

84

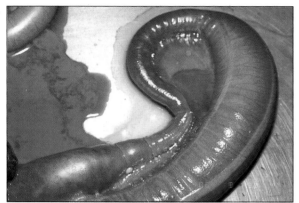

84 Megacolon.
Differential Diagnosis:
i)   Atresia of a distal segment of large or small colon
ii) Atresia ani
iii) Meconium impaction

85

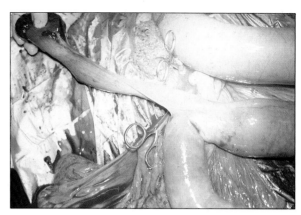

85 Meckel's Diverticulum (at proximal ileum).
Note: Strangulated distal end of diverticulum which contained impacted food material and had been responsible for obstruction of jejunum and ileum.

86

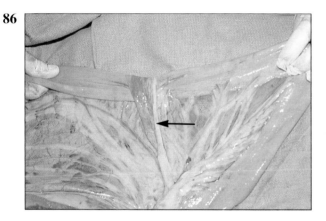

86 Mesodiverticular band (arrow).

87

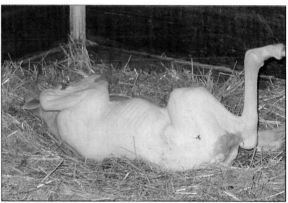

87 Lethal-White foal (Ovaro-Paint breed).
Note: Atresia coli and ileus due to intestinal aganglionosis were present. Severe non responsive colic developed within two hours of birth. Concurrent cardiac septal defect and cleft hard palate.

small intestine with secretions and milk and an empty or partially empty large colon. No physical obstruction needs to be present, although, in some cases, complex developmental abnormalities, including atresia of one or more sections of the intestine (*see* **83**), may be present.

Herniation of bowel through the umbilicus subsequent to traumatic rupture or excessive tension on the umbilical cord at birth is occasionally encountered and may be associated with both natural and assisted deliveries. The extent to which this can be classed as a developmental problem is variable. Some foals may have particularly tough cords and natural separation may then be inhibited. However, most are considered to be of traumatic origin relating to excessive tension or to abnormal parturient behaviour by the mare, or both.

Congenital diaphragmatic hernias may be extensive and result in major interference at a very early age (or even *in utero*) and are possible causes of colic in young foals. Lesions which are presumed to be congenital defects in the diaphragm are sometimes found incidentally at post mortem examination of adult horses. Occasionally, however, they become clinically significant when loops of jejunum pass into the thorax and then may result in dangerous strangulating colic. By contrast new-born colt foals often have significant lengths of small bowel herniated through the **inguinal canal** and lying within the enlarged scrotum (**88**). Lesser or greater lengths of intestine appear to have considerable freedom to move in and out of the inguinal canal and the condition usually resolves spontaneously

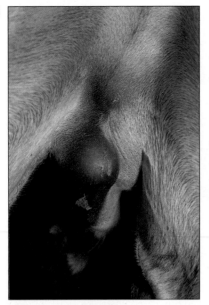

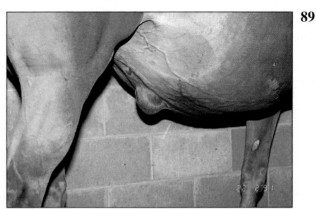

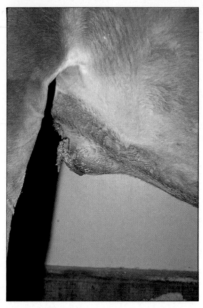

88 Scrotal hernia (left side).

89 Umbilical hernia.

90 Enterocutaneous fistula (at the site of umbilical hernia).

over the first few weeks of life. In older, entire horses variable lengths of intestine may be incarcerated within the inguinal canal. This is usually regarded as a consequence of increased intra-abdominal pressure which distorts the inguinal ring allowing herniation of a short loop of small intestine. There is little evidence to support the theory that the acquired condition in stallions is a result either of damage to the internal inguinal ring or the presence of an abnormally wide inguinal ring. Severe strangulating colic may result with gross asymmetrical enlargement of the scrotum associated with edema and swelling of the ipsilateral testicle. Open castration of horses affected by inguinal hernias or those with an abnormally wide inguinal canal may result in serious herniation of variable lengths of small intestine (*see* **837**).

Developmental **umbilical hernia** is very commonly encountered in foals and most commonly in filly foals. Small or large hernias generally appear as soft, fluctuant,

reducible swellings in the umbilical region (**89**). In most cases the defect is of little immediate importance but they may, at any stage of the animals life, be a source of bowel incarceration. Significantly, severe colic may arise in some cases when only a small portion of the bowel wall is pinched into the hernial ring. In these cases there is little or no immediate obstruction to the passage of food material and little impairment of circulation to the intestine as a whole. Commonly, however, the hernial sac contains abdominal fat and may remain benign with no long term harmful effect. Where bowel is entrapped within the hernial sac local swelling, edema and pain are usually present with other signs of acute intestinal obstruction. **Entero-cutaneous fistulation** at the site of an umbilical hernia (**90**) is one possible consequence which can develop. Almost all future performance horses are currently subjected to surgical repair of umbilical hernias for cosmetic reasons and in order to prevent future complications.

Non-Infectious Disorders

Weak, abnormal and some normal foals which receive little or no colostrum within the first few hours of birth suffer from a variety of secondary effects consequent upon a deficient immune status, and may be presented with **retention of the meconium**. These foals strain heavily, with a dorsally flexed back and elevated tail **(91)**, in contrast to the ventro-flexed back crouching posture adopted by foals with the **ruptured bladder syndrome** (*see* **328**). Hard, pelleted meconium may be passed in small amounts but, without the laxative effects of colostrum, progressive small colon impaction develops. This may be sufficient to result in the gross accumulation of feces and gas in the rectum and small colon which may be identifiable radiographically. Severely affected foals often show signs of colic with rolling, repeated lying down and the adoption of abnormal postures, particularly relating to head and neck position. Eventually rupture of the grossly distended viscus may occur, although this is very uncommon. Many foals presented with clinically-significant retention of meconium are found to be cases of failed passive transfer, having received little or no colostrum. Meconium retention/impaction is therefore, perhaps, best regarded as an immunological disorder. In rare cases it may be a secondary effect of a developmental megacolon (*see* **84**) or to other abnormalities of bowel function.

Gastric and gastro-duodenal ulceration occur frequently in very young foals, particularly when subjected to stressful circumstances and/or non-steroidal anti-inflammatory drugs such as phenylbutazone. Even those foals subjected to relatively minor stresses, such as transportation or minor surgery, are prone to the disorder. It may develop in individual foals which have no apparent stress or other inciting cause. Affected foals often exhibit salivation which, with persistent grinding of the teeth (bruxism), results in a foamy salivation **(92)**. Affected foals spend long periods in dorsal recumbency with their legs extended. They are depressed and frequently show interrupted nursing patterns and, sometimes, overt post-prandial colic. Although up to 50% of all foals show endoscopic evidence of moderate, or even severe, ulceration of the glandular mucosa of the stomach **(93)**, many show no clinical evidence of the disorder. There is also little apparent correlation between the extent of ulceration and the severity of the presenting clinical signs with some foals being mildly affected but showing marked clinical signs. Most gastric ulcers in young foals, are located in the glandular portion of the stomach, but some do occur in the squamous (esophageal) portion. The former lesions are generally regarded as those of greatest importance in the foal. Ulceration of the pyloric and duodenal areas is likely to result in gastric emptying defects. The clinical signs are most

91

![Meconium impaction in a foal showing dorsi-flexion of the back and elevated tail]

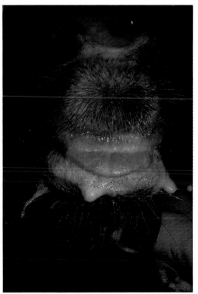

92

91 Meconium impaction.
Note: Dorsi-flexion of the back and tail elevated during straining.
Differential Diagnosis:
i)   Ruptured bladder syndrome
ii) Atresia ani
iii) Atresia coli

92 Gastric ulceration syndrome.
Note: Foamy salivation as a result of persistent bruxism (grinding of teeth).

93

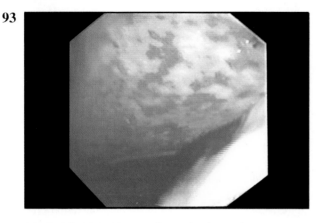

93 Gastric ulceration syndrome (endoscopic appearance of gastric ulcers in glandular portion of stomach).

94

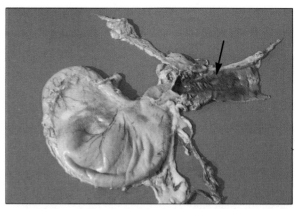

94 Duodenal ulceration.
Note: Severe duodenal bleeding and perforation (arrow). Extensive inflammation around pylorus and proximal duodenum.

95

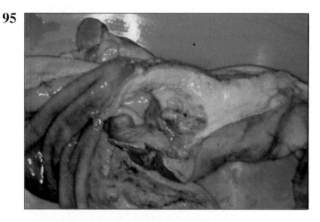

95 Chronic pyloric ulceration.
Note: Extensive scarring and thickening responsible for persistent gastric emptying problem causing recurrent post-prandial colic and terminal severe gastric distension.

96

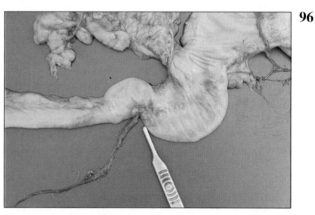

96 Duodenal stricture.
Note: Chronic flaccid distension of stomach and proximal duodenum due to chronic emptying disorder. Site presumed to be an old ulcer lesion with adhesion.

prominent in these cases, presumably due to the reflux duodenitis which is usually present. Extensive and/ or deep ulceration of the stomach or duodenum are sometimes associated with enteric hemorrhage and, while in most cases diarrhea is the most significant clinical sign, melena (passage of dark coloured, tarry feces with a high content of partly digested blood) or frank hemorrhage may be seen. **Duodenal ulceration (94)** is generally regarded as being of the greatest significance with the secondary effects being particularly serious. Secondary gastric ulcerations are frequently associated with duodenal lesions and, under these circumstances, are probably a result of duodenal reflux, which, in turn, results in gastro-esophageal reflux with marked salivation and bruxism. Hemorrhage is often

severe in the case of duodenal ulceration and perforation of the duodenum and catastrophic peritonitis may also be encountered. The presence of a duodenal ulcer frequently induces marked local inflammation and swelling as well as fibrosis in longer standing cases **(95)**. These, either independently or in combination, have been associated with the development of duodenal strictures **(96)**, when gastric emptying may be severely impaired and with adhesions between the stomach and other abdominal organs. Clinical signs of acute colic related to gastric distension are typically present. Perforation of gastric or, more commonly, duodenal ulcers results in a severe, often overwhelming generalised fibrinous peritonitis.

Gastric ulceration in horses over 3 – 4 months of age has been shown to occur frequently and again is most often encountered in stressed horses. Horses in training seem particularly prone to ulceration whilst pasture-rested animals and brood mares are probably less affected. In contrast to the foal, gastric ulceration in the adult horse occurs predominately along the *margo plicatus* (junction of squamous and glandular portions), where lesions may be extensive and coalescent (**97**) or focal (**98**). The later are usually deeper and elicit a more profound local inflammatory response than the former, and are particularly associated with prolonged oral, or parenteral, administration of non-steroidal anti-inflammatory drugs. In adult horses lesions involving the glandular portion or the duodenum are rare but again, animals receiving prolonged high doses of phenylbutazone may suffer from severe peptic ulceration. The clinical features of gastric ulceration syndrome are characteristically vague, and may be limited to a poor or intermittent appetite and mild post-prandial abdominal discomfort. More severely affected cases sometimes show more overt signs including recurrent colic. Affected horses usually show an initial enthusiasm for food but reluctance to eat more than the first few mouthfuls. Salivation and bruxism are seldom seen. Significant bleeding may occur in the adult syndrome but may only be detectable by gastric lavage/aspiration. Melena or more rarely, dark (changed), tarry blood passed with feces is an important sign of the more severe forms of the condition in both adult horses and foals. Chronic blood loss may be sufficient to induce detectable anemia but severe anemia is unlikely to develop from this alone. Perforation of ulcers is most unusual in the adult horse. Diagnosis of gastric ulceration in both young and adult horses is largely reliant upon gastroscopy and this necessarily limits the number of cases in which the condition can be diagnosed definitively. Supportive evidence for its existence can be gained from the effects of specific anti-ulcer therapy including the use of H_2-receptor-blocking drugs.

Diffuse erosions of the gastric mucosa, accompanied by severe generalised inflammation and variable hemorrhage are characteristic of the caustic epithelial necrosis caused by **arsenic compounds**, **blister beetle toxicity** and by other irritant chemicals (including organophosphate anthelmintics). A similar syndrome may also be associated with salmonellosis, colitis and a number of other systemic disorders. Clinical signs of extreme pain and depression with dramatic generalised organ failure and circulatory collapse are typical with the extent of the signs largely dependent upon the extent of the damage, and the specific toxicity of the inciting cause. The pathological changes encountered in the stomach from large doses of arsenic compounds are repeated throughout the gastro-intestinal tract and the clinical signs are associated with massive caustic burning of the intestinal mucosa. The entire tract is intensely hyperemic and massive fluid loss occurs.

97

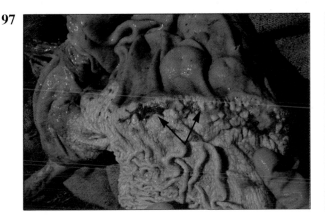

97 Gastric ulceration.
Note: Coalescent ulceration of the *margo plicatus* in an adult horse (arrows).

98

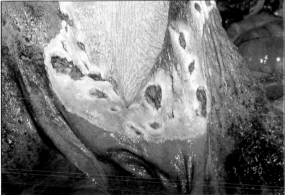

98 Focal gastric ulceration.
Note: Deep ulcers in squamous mucosa of stomach with prominent ridges. Typical of ulceration caused by non-steroidal anti-inflammatory therapy.

Acute gastric distension, from whatever cause, is one of the most painful and dangerous conditions of the horse and affected horses show prominent signs of colic with characteristically elevated heart and respiratory rates. The anatomical location of the stomach means that even severe distension is unlikely to produce any abdominal enlargement although splenic displacement may be discernible during rectal examination. Elevations of heart and respiratory rates with splenic displacement should alert the clinician to this possibility. Horses, after racing or other heavy exercise, occasionally engorge sufficient amounts of cold water to create a painful and dangerous gastric distension. It is possibly the result of a pyloric spasm which prevents onward progression of gastric contents. A diagnosis can easily be reached in these cases with the aid of a naso-gastric tube, when a large volume of clear fluid will be refluxed. Relief is invariably immediate and complete.

Gastric distension arising primarily from solid food material (**grain overload**) or secondarily to disorders of gastric motility/emptying is a serious and difficult disorder to diagnose definitively. Engorgement with, or accumulation of, fibrous food or dry food which expands within the stomach are the commonest causes of primary gastric impaction (**99**). A chronic form of gastric distension is also recognised in which there is a progressive accumulation of fibrous food material in the stomach and while this becomes larger and firmer, more liquid material may pass over it and into the duodenum. Feces continue to be passed in small amounts and the horse develops a pot-bellied appearance which is not due to fluid accumulation within the peritoneal cavity. This form is likely to be a result of failure of the intrinsic gastric motility and while starvation may eventually result in some resolution, the condition recurs once feeding starts again. A secondary somewhat similar gastric impactive syndrome may be the result of *Senecio* spp plant poisoning, but a more major symptom of this is chronic hepatic failure (*see* **167**). Horses with the more common acute impactive gastric distension syndromes are presented with mild or moderate, progressive colic. They are often severely acidotic and may progress to hypovolemic shock. Naso-gastric intubation is usually unrewarding. Diagnosis is often difficult and may only be possible with gastroscopy or at laparotomy. Chronic and recurrent gastric distension arising secondarily to pyloric obstructions are rare but heavy accumulations of parasites such as *Gastrophilus* spp larvae (Bots) (*see* **153**) may induce sufficient gastritis and pyloric swelling to cause recurrent gastric distension.

Gastric distension arising specifically from primary gastric disorders may be confirmed by the presence of large volumes of fluid having a very low pH. Distension of the stomach arising secondarily to intestinal obstructions, however, characteristically shows elevation of the pH of gastric contents due to reflux of strongly alkaline duodenal secretions. The pH is, however, seldom actually alkaline. Physical and functional obstructive disorders of the small (and to a lesser extent the large) intestine are common causes of gastric distension. Under these circumstances there may be

99

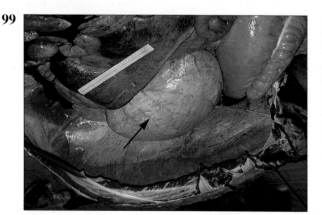

99 Gastric impaction (distension).
Note: Grossly enlarged stomach, (arrow) which contained dense impacted food material. Due to long-standing motility disorder. Similar gross appearance in all cases of gastric impaction but contents and etiology vary.

100

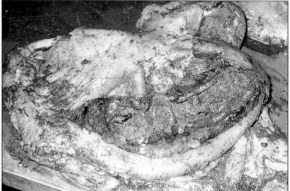

100 Gastric rupture.
Note: Due, in this case, to primary food impaction. Typical site of rupture along greater curvature.
Differential Diagnosis:
i) Grass sickness
ii) Intestinal obstruction
iii) Pyloric obstruction (neoplastic/inflammatory)
iv) Perforated gastric ulcer

spontaneous reflux of gastric fluid (**Plate 1g**, page 45) and large amounts of gastric reflux can usually be released by the passage of a nasogastric tube (**Plate 1h**, page 45). The clinical signs are otherwise similar to gastric distension due to other causes.

Gastric rupture usually occurs along the greater curvature of the stomach (**100**) and is commonly associated with neglected or untreated cases of excessive gastric distension. It is also a frequent complication of **Grass Sickness** (*see* **129** *et seq.*). Grain overload may also result in rupture but in these cases slow progressive hydration and swelling of the contents is responsible. Imminent rupture is accompanied by a dramatic rise in heart rate and sometimes an acidic, green, nasal reflux will be seen, although the latter is usually in small amount (**Plate 6q**, page 123). Rupture is associated with an apparently dramatic cessation of pain and a further small amount of reflux, often containing some blood, may occur spontaneously. Metabolically, the patient is obviously in very poor condition with deteriorating cardiovascular parameters and the rapid development of endotoxic and hypovolemic shock. Abdominal paracentesis of such a case will reveal contaminated brown or reddish fluid (**Plate 2g**, page 47) which contains a high cell content and a sediment of food particles. This latter effect is dependent upon the duration and extent of the abdominal contamination but, as gastric rupture usually occurs as a result of excessive pressure within the organ, most cases show extensive and severe abdominal contamination (*see* **109**). Rectal examination of horses affected by gastric (or other viscus) rupture has a very characteristic granular, gritty feel, often with an inordinate freedom of movement.

Significant gastric distension may, also, be due to the accumulation of gas/air in horses affected by the neurosis, **windsucking (aerophagia)** (*see* **718**), although in these the stomach is usually chronically distended and non-painful. Horses subject to this vice are often not hungry in spite of poor condition and show no other evidence of disease. They seldom show colic as a result of gastric distension but gross swallowing of air may result in clinically significant, recurrent, and occasionally acutely painful distension in the more distal alimentary tract.

A wide variety of intestinal obstructive and vascular disorders are diagnosed in horses and while many are of interest and occur commonly it is not within the scope of this book to provide a definitive description of them all.

Simple non-strangulating obstructive lesions arise in all segments of the intestinal tract as a result of intraluminal obstructions, or pressure from outside the bowel itself, or from lesions within the bowel wall. Vascular compromise is not usually prominent in most of these cases. Initially the mucosal barrier remains effective and affected horses are usually therefore in good metabolic condition, at least in the early stages. Obstructions within the small intestine are probably less frequent than those of the large bowel, due to the fluidity of the contents, although the ileum may become severely impacted. The severity of the clinical signs and their rate of progression depend largely upon the location of the obstruction, with more proximal obstructions being more acute and more severe. However, even very distal obstructions, such as those occurring at the ileum, may induce a rapidly deteriorating and acutely painful colic. Obstructions may be partial, allowing some food material (particularly the wetter and smaller particulate matter) to pass into the distal segments of the intestine.

Ileal impaction (**101**) is an infrequent cause of moderate or severe colic. Gross distension of the proximal small intestine and, ultimately, the stomach, with gas or fluid is usually encountered. Many cases have no apparent etiology but ileal hypertrophy (*see* **113**) or inflammatory swelling of the ileo-cecal opening are possible predisposing causes. Affected horses have frequently had a change of diet in the immediate past. The ingestion of poor quality forage, or inadequate mastication of coarse fibrous foods, or water deprivation may be important factors in the disorder. Large accumulations of tapeworms (*Anoplocephala* spp), at or near the ileo-cecal opening, may cause sufficient inflammation to result in narrowing and may be partially responsible for some cases of ileal impaction, particularly when this is accompanied by one or more of the other predisposing factors. Recent anthelmintic treatment in young horses carrying heavy burdens of ascarids (*Parascaris equorum*) may result in knots of dead worms obstructing the ileum. Rectal examination may identify a solid, distended ileum with proximal gas-distension of jejunum but more often there is little palpable evidence of the condition. The cecum and large colon are usually empty and few feces are passed.

Intussusception of a length of small intestine and its associated mesentery (**102**) most commonly involves the more distal jejunum or the ileum, and is most often encountered in young horses. A history of diarrhea may be present, particularly in foals. Parasitism may be an instigating factor (*see* **142**). Intussusception of the jejunum into itself, or into the ileum or cecum, results in few changes in the peritoneal fluid as the length of damaged bowel (intussusceptum) is firmly enclosed in the distal segment (intussuscipiens). However, the

101

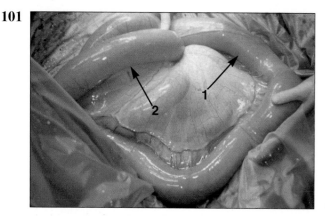

101 Ileal impaction.
Note: Ileum (arrow 1) is solid and slightly distended while proximal loops of jejunum are gas filled and grossly distended (arrow 2).

102

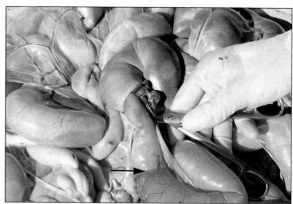

102 Ileo-ileal intussusception.
Note: Intussusception has been partially reduced to illustrate the sharply defined zone of vascular compromise of the intussusceptum (arrow). Compromised intussuscipiens and proximal jejunal distension.

103

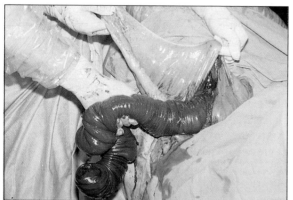

103 Ileo-(and jejuno) cecal intussusception.
Note: Severely compromised ileum and jejunum within cecum.

104

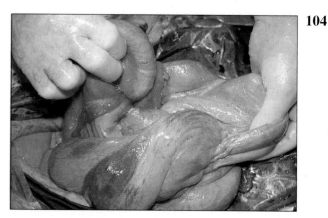

104 Ceco-cecal intussusception.
Note: Apex of cecum inverted into the body. Patchy areas of compromised cecal wall.

proximal small intestine rapidly becomes significantly distended and gastric distension with its attendant dangers may also develop. In some cases the obstruction created by an intussusception (particularly ileo-ileal intussusceptions) may not be complete with limited amounts of food material able to pass the site and, under these conditions, the severity of the clinical signs may be less. Intussusception of the ileum (and variable lengths of jejunum) into the cecum (**103**) is potentially very dangerous as the ileum has a particularly poor collateral circulation. There is little or no alteration in the peritoneal fluid in these cases, so that diagnosis may be difficult and is often dependent on rectal examination or laparotomy. The detection, *per rectum*, of distended small intestine and a large, sausage-shaped, solid object within the cecum is usually pathognomonic. Ileo-cecal

intussusceptions usually induce a complete obstruction and the clinical features are correspondingly more severe than the partial obstructions often found in ileo-ileal or jejuno-ileal intussusceptions.

Ceco-cecal intussusception (104) probably arises from impaired, or altered, motility of the organ and in these cases the degree of circulatory compromise is much less than in the small intestine, as there is little strangulation and vascular impairment. Also, there is insignificant hindrance to the passage of food material into the large colon and, although affected horses are anorexic and have mild, recurrent or persistent colic, feces of normal consistency usually continue to be passed. These may, however, contain evidence of intestinal bleeding. The clinical signs of colic in these animals are therefore less severe and slower in progression, but the long-term consequences are no less dangerous. Rectal examination is often unremarkable but the presence of melena (dark tarry feces containing changed blood) may be a significant finding for this and other types of intussusception.

Strangulating obstructions of the bowel form an extremely important group of disorders in the horse and occur when the intestinal blood supply and the lumen of the bowel are obstructed. Strangulating lesions are much more common in the small intestine than in other segments of the gut. The extent and significance of these disorders depend largely on the degree of vascular compromise, but most of them are life-threatening. The affected portion of the intestine is often devitalised rapidly. Initially, the venous drainage of the affected portion is impaired and localised swelling and edema cause progressively more severe arterial obstruction. Ischemia of the gut then results in localised spasm of the affected length and there is a consequent accumulation of gas and fluid proximal to the obstruction. Dangerous gastric distension is a common sequel which develops rapidly. Gross, intraluminal distension of the bowel results in further ischemia and disruption of the protective mucosal layers. Loss of protein-rich fluid into the lumen and passage of endotoxins into the peritoneal fluid and blood stream occur early. The systemic consequences of these changes are profound. Hypovolemic and endotoxic shock accompanied by electrolyte and acid-base deviations occur and are responsible for the continuing metabolic collapse of the patient. Vascular compromise and capillary necrosis result in the loss of high-protein fluid containing both red and white cells into the abdomen. Peritoneal fluid is usually blood stained (**Plate 2d**, page 46) and has a high protein concentration and raised total leucocyte count .

Typically, affected horses have an acute onset of severe and unrelenting, non-drug-responsive abdominal pain. Where the lesion occurs in the proximal segments of the small intestine, progression is particularly rapid and is usually accompanied by gastric distension resulting from reflux of alkaline intestinal fluid into the stomach (**Plate 1h**, page 45). Lesions occurring further down the small intestine have a somewhat slower course but all have a characteristically rapid progression over 1–12 hours. The extent of pain shown by these cases finally becomes less severe due to devitalisation of the distended and damaged intestine. Critical clinical assessment confirms that the apparent improvement is not a result of resolution of the underlying problem, and that cardiovascular compromise and terminal shock are imminent. Most affected horses will die within 24–36 hours unless treated effectively.

Strangulating lesions caused by entrapment through a natural body opening or acquired hernia or through internal openings, or as a result of fibrous mesenteric bands or from strangulating pedunculated lipomas, cause a complete luminal obstruction and result in considerable vascular compromise. The location of the proximal and distal viable or undamaged segments of the intestine is of paramount importance and in these cases this is usually evident as a sharp demarcation in the bowel wall (**105**).

Entrapment of lengths of small intestine through internal or external hernias are relatively common. In entire stallions (and rarely in geldings) loops of small intestine may become incarcerated in the inguinal canal or scrotum (**106**). The disorder is common and of relatively minor significance in the neonatal foal (*see* **88**). In some foals, and in adult horses, the disorder is however extremely serious. Umbilical hernias also provide a possible site of intestinal strangulating

105

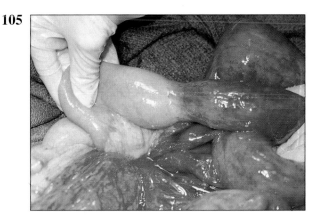

106

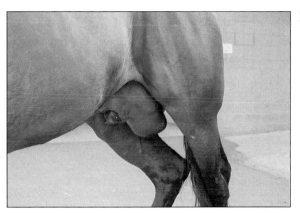

105 Strangulating lesion (of small intestine).
Note: Sharply demarcated division between compromised and 'normal' bowel. Due to strangulating mesenteric herniation.

106 Scrotal hernia.

obstruction (*see* **89, 90**). Entrapment of jejunum and/or ileum through naturally occurring internal anatomical openings, such as the epiploic foramen, occurs relatively frequently and the incidence of this particular disorder increases with age as the foramen increases in size in older horses. Rectal examination of horses suffering from epiploic foramen entrapment is often somewhat disappointing but it is the ileum and terminal portions of the jejunum, which are usually involved early in the disorder. Tension applied to the ventral tenial band of the cecum *per rectum* will often elicit a sharp pain response in these cases.

Acquired (or developmental defects) in the diaphragm or mesentery may also be responsible for the development of strangulating lesions. In the acquired defects, such as mesenteric tears or rents, incarceration probably occurs at the time of the damage to the mesentery. Most of these probably arise from physical tearing during falls, or from blows, but many have no such history. Mesodiverticular bands (*see* **86**) and pedunculated lipomas, which arise from the mesentery or from the serosal surface of the small intestine, are common causes of incarceration and strangulation of small intestine or small colon. **Lipomas** of significant size are most often encountered in horses over the age of 15 years, but while many horses have large and/or numerous lipomas without any untoward effect, some small and relatively innocuous-looking masses have serious consequences. Younger horses may also be affected. The most dangerous forms of lipoma are those with long pedicles (**107**) and while in some cases this may cause extreme and complete strangulation of small intestine (**108**) or small colon, others may have a lesser effect from tension within the pedicle. The latter are more commonly associated with large lipoma masses with relatively long pedicles. The body condition of the horse is not reliably related to the presence of lipomas with some horses in moderate body condition having large masses while some inordinately fat horses may have no, or a few, small lipomas.

Rotation of segments of jejunum or ileum through more than 180°, along the long axis of the mesenteric attachment (**volvulus**) initially results in impairment of blood supply and, later, obstruction of the lumen of the affected portion. These lesions often occur secondarily to some other obstructive or incarcerative condition such as **Meckel's Diverticulum** (*see* **85**), **adhesions** (*see* **111, 112**), **infarctions** or **mesenteric rents**. Continued twisting of the affected loop results in progressive vascular compromise and luminal obstruction. The loop becomes devitalised, while the segments proximal to the obstruction become filled with gas and fluid. Where the affected loop of jejunum or ileum becomes knotted rather than merely twisted upon itself, the term *volvulus nodosus* is applied. These strangulating obstructive lesions are easily recognised (**109**) but it is difficult to understand how they are formed. It is presumed that the underlying cause is basically a defect of motility. The clinical features are typical of severe and complete strangulating obstruction with proximal distension and distal emptying of the bowel. Peritoneal fluid is usually indicative of strangulation lesions (**Plate 2d**, page 46). Again, there is a considerable risk of gastric distension and consequent gastric rupture.

Rotation of the mesenteric root about its axis results in a severe vascular obstruction to the entire small intestine (**110**). The progression of colic signs is rapid and relentless. This stage is often followed by a period when less pain will be shown but the astute clinician will recognise that this is due to devitalisation and impending death. Gross abdominal distension may not, however, be a major feature of the disorder, although in some cases this may be present. Rectal examination is usually diagnostic, and will at least

107

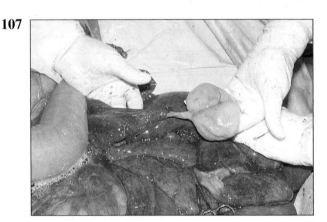

107 Pedunculated lipoma.

108

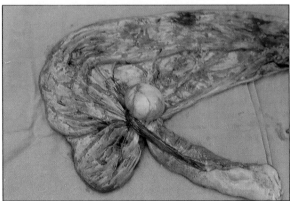

108 Strangulating pedunculated lipoma.

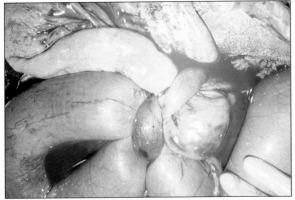

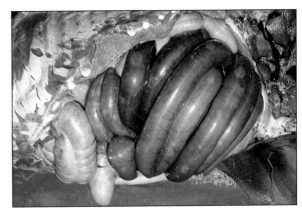

109 *Volvulus nodosus* of jejunum.
Note: Severe peritoneal contamination due to gastric rupture.

110 Torsion of the mesentery (360°).
Note: Entire length of small intestine severely compromised. Gas-filled loops lying next to each other.

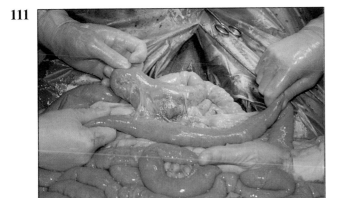

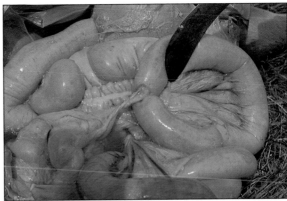

111 Fibrinous adhesions (between segments of jejunum.
Note: Probably occurred as a result of vascular compromise or peritonitis.

112 Adhesion (at site of infarction lesion).
Note: Resulted in non-strangulating obstruction.

identify that a large number of loops of small intestine are grossly dilated, tense and, in the early stages, painful to the touch. In this condition the loops of distended jejunum will be felt lying next to each other as can be demonstrated clearly at post mortem examination (**110**).

Non-strangulating obstructions of the small intestine (or other segments of the intestinal tract) may arise from alterations in the ability of the gut to move naturally and to propel ingesta distally. One of the commonest causes of this type of obstruction is the development of adhesions between adjacent loops of jejunum (**111**). These loops frequently become adherent to each other in response to peritonitis and/or areas of infarction (ischemia or necrosis) within the bowel wall (*see* **144**). Adhesions between different sections of the intestine or between the intestine and other abdominal organs, including the spleen and the parietal peritoneum, are common sequels to peritonitis or surgical interference, particularly where vascular compromise is present. The organisation of these may lead to the development of non-elastic scar tissue bands (**112**) which may create partial or complete, non-strangulating obstructions in any segment of the tract although the small intestine appears to be most commonly involved. While, there may be no obstruction to the passage of food in the early stages, the impaired mobility and motility of the affected loops result in either a physical obstruction through narrowing or kinking (*see* **111**) or to a functional obstruction with little or no ability to propel food onward (*see* **112**). Post prandial colic caused by intermittent partial obstruction of the jejunum and/or ileum is a common feature of developing or mature adhesions. One of the more serious consequences of these adhesions, which may become densely fibrosed as scarring matures within them, is their liability to cause strangulating obstructions. Even relatively harmless-looking adhesions may have a dramatic effect upon the motility of a segment of bowel and, although this may be very restricted in extent, it may act as a complete obstruction to the onward passage of ingesta. Most cases affected by this type of disorder have a history of recurrent episodes of drug-responsive, mild or moderate, colic with a single, more acute, persistent episode, with signs typical of intraluminal small intestinal obstruction. It is unusual to find signs of active peritonitis. The diagnosis of these lesions is usually only made at laparotomy but indications of the type of lesion may be deduced from an accurate history and a careful clinical assessment using all the available aids.

Persistent or long-standing partial obstruction of the ileum, either as a result of motility abnormalities or more usually as a result of **ileo-cecal stenosis** of inflammatory, neoplastic or neurogenic origin, or ileo-ileal intussusception (*see* **102**), or parasitic lesions (*see* **152**), frequently results in considerable hypertrophy of the ileal musculature (**113**). While in most cases the extent of this muscular thickening is limited to the ileum itself, considerable secondary hypertrophy may be found in the distal segments of the jejunum extending a considerable distance proximally. The presence of such a finding should alert the clinician to the possibility of chronic ileal, or ileo-cecal obstructions.

Torsion of the cecum alone (**114**) is much less common than small intestinal torsion and entrapments; most being related to large colon torsion. As there is a poor collateral blood supply, vascular compromise occurs rapidly. The amount of distension of the organ may be limited. Peritoneal fluid usually provides evidence of a strangulating obstruction but fecal output may be little affected. Rectal examination is often disappointing but a distended cecum with an edematous wall may be identifiable.

Large colon displacements occur relatively commonly and the more severe torsions of the organ represents an extreme emergency, being probably the most serious of all the colic disorders of the horse. The relatively mobile anatomical character of the large colon and its relatively high gas content make a wide range of displacements possible. In some cases displacement has no compromising effect upon the blood supply in the early stages but the size and weight of the organ, especially when filled to capacity, makes some compromise inevitable in almost all cases. Any impairment of the motility and/or the ability of gas to escape down the tract will result in a rapid gaseous distension.

One of the commonest non-strangulating disorders of the large colon, encountered primarily in large framed adult horses, is **left dorsal displacement of the colon** (**115**). In this disorder, the left colon becomes entrapped in the nephrosplenic space. While, in most cases, there is little vascular compromise, the progressive accumulation of food material in the right ventral colon, and progressive gas accumulation in the entrapped distal left colon, result in continuous, though (in most cases) mild colic. Fecal output is reduced. Rectal examination can be diagnostic, when converging tenial bands can be easily identified and the displaced colon is obviously in

113

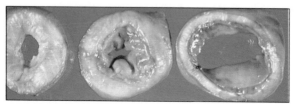

113 Ileal hypertrophy.
Note: Distal ileum on left. Centre section from mid-ileum and right from the end of the ileal fold.
Note: Progressive increase in muscular layer.

Differential Diagnosis:
i) Ileo-cecal obstruction eg *Anoplocephala* spp tapeworms
ii) Ileo-cecal intussusception

114

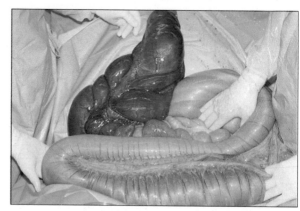

114 Cecal torsion.
Note: Severely compromised cecal apex and body with normal large colon.

the nephrosplenic space. The spleen may be displaced medially and in some cases may not be palpable. Few cases show gross distension of the abdomen but cecal tympany is common and gastric distension may be present. There may be some degree of vascular compromise at the site of the entrapment with the more distal portion (the pelvic flexure) becoming edematous (*see* **115**).

Right dorsal displacement of the large colon presents with similar, but somewhat more severe clinical signs, and again rectal examination is diagnostic in most cases when the displaced right dorsal colon can be identified by its tenia running across the caudal abdomen just forward of the pelvic brim. As is often the case with large bowel torsion the extent of compromise is very variable and there may be gross gaseous distension without much vascular compromise.

Strangulating displacements (torsion) of the large bowel are variable in their extent and effect upon the horse. The degree of rotation and consequent vascular and luminal obstruction largely dictates the rate of onset and progression and the severity of the clinical signs. Thus, minor rotations (of less than 90°), may present with no apparent vascular obstruction, and relatively minor luminal interference. Such displacements are best regarded as physiological and probably occur frequently. Rotations of between 90° and 180° cause increased, but often insignificant, luminal obstruction. Under these conditions it may be impossible to identify the disorder except by careful examination of the position and appearance of the colon at laparotomy. Torsion of 180° to 270° will obstruct the lumen and impair blood supply (and venous drainage, in particular), while degrees of rotation greater than this probably represent the most rapidly progressive and dangerous forms of colic. The latter cases are extremely serious, and there is a dramatic build up of gas within the large colon and the cecum, sufficient to result in an obvious bloating of the abdomen (**116**). Rectal examination of horses suffering from serious degrees of large colon torsion is often impossible due to the massive gaseous distension. A tense, gas-filled viscus occluding the pelvic inlet is strongly suggestive of colonic torsion, but the metabolic effects may make further exploration unnecessary. Torsion of the large colon usually occurs in a clockwise direction, when viewed from the back of the standing horse, and are most often centred around the right colon just forward of the cecum (**117**). Some involve the origin of the large colon and some even include the cecum. Vascular compromise is always severe, with gross edema and congestion of the colon and its mesenteric vasculature (**118**). Black or dark-purple mucosa, identified during surgery in cases of large colon torsion, and very low mucosal pH are grave prognostic signs. The dramatic progression of these cases is a result of a combination of serious endotoxic shock arising from massively compromised mucosal layers of the colon, and to gross distension and consequent circulatory compromise. Rupture of the grossly distended large colon (or the cecum) represents the ultimate progression of the disorder, but most cases die before this can occur.

Pelvic flexure impaction by dry fibrous ingesta (**119**) is a common cause of persistent, mild or moderate colic. Occasional cases may be more severely affected, particularly where there is gaseous distension of the colon and cecum proximal to the obstruction. The disorder sometimes follows ingestion of coarse, indigestible foods, poor mastication or reduced water intake (or combinations of these), but some cases apparently occur without any obvious etiological factor. As the site of the obstruction is a considerable distance from the small intestine and the obstruction is, at least initially, only partial, the onset of colic is slow and the degree of pain is limited. Most cases have a marked reduction in fecal output over the previous two days.

115

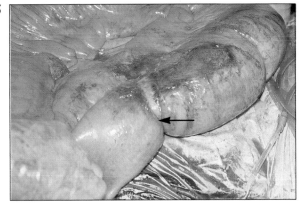

115 Left dorsal displacement (nephrosplenic ligament entrapment).
Note: Sharp demarcation at site of entrapment (arrow) in left colon with minimal vascular compromise.

116

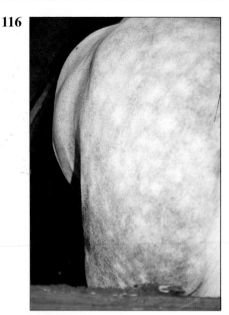

117

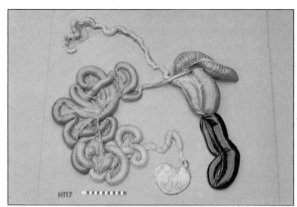

116 Bloated horse.
Note: Rectal examination was impossible due to gas filled large colon obstructing pelvic inlet.
Differential Diagnosis:
i) Large bowel torsion
ii) Simple obstruction of transverse or small colon
iii) Left dorsal displacement
iv) Right dorsal displacement
v) Fermentative colic

117 Large colon torsion (450°) (in newborn foal).
Note: Typical site in proximal segment of right colon, just anterior to caecum. Clockwise rotation (when viewed from behind the standing horse). Severe compromise of distal large colon and gas distention of cecum and small intestine. The condition is unusual in neonatal foals but this is a particularly good illustration of the problem.

118

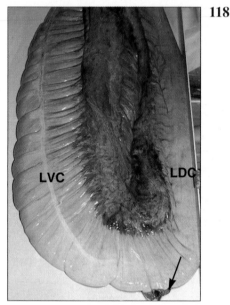

118 Large colon torsion (270°).
Note: Compromised and edematous wall of left ventral (LVC) (sacculated) and left dorsal (LDC) colon wall and mesocolon. Colon has been drained of contents at pelvic flexure (site visible at arrow). These would usually be grossly distended and the sacculations would not be visible.

Only occasional, very long-standing cases have significant small intestinal or gastric distension. Rectal examination is always characteristic, with significant impaction resulting in the displacement of the pelvic flexure into the pelvic inlet and being palpable as a firm doughy mass. The extent of the impaction may be severe in some cases but seldom, even then, warrant surgical interference.

The persistent ingestion of large volumes of sand (**sand colic**) occurs where grazing conditions are short and the consumption of sand is unavoidable, although in some individuals it may be indicative of dietary inadequacies or idiosyncratic behaviour patterns.

Mineral deficiencies are often blamed for capricious appetites but there is little evidence to support most such claims. Occasional horses persist with the eating of sand and soil in spite of the availability of adequate forage. Moderate persistent colic with an insidious onset is characteristic but some horses may show more acute colic signs. The presence of sand in the feces is usually of diagnostic help, and can be demonstrated by suspending a quantity of feces in water, when the sand will form an obvious sediment. In some cases, however, the feces may contain no detectable sand particles and in others the presence of sand may be incidental. The apex of the cecum may contain heavy accumulations of

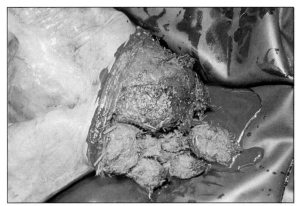

119 Pelvic flexure impaction.
Note: Firm, dry food material with mucus covering (indicative of prolonged stasis).
Differential Diagnosis:
i) Fecalith/Foreign body impaction
ii) Grass Sickness

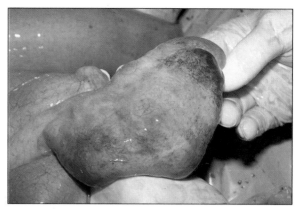

120 Sand colic.
Note: Diffuse inflammation of cecal apex. Very obvious sand/grit palpable through wall. Feces contained large volumes of sand. Concurrent diffuse inflammation of small colon was present.

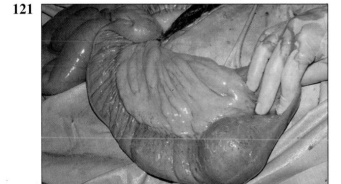

121 Enterolith (in small colon).
Note: Smooth, regular outline. Proximal slight distension (gas able to pass).

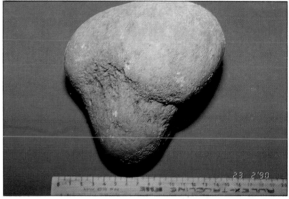

122 Enterolith.
Note: Smooth, solid stone-like nature. No facets, so probably single.

sand and this causes localised, acute inflammation of the cecal wall **(120)**. Considerable lengths of large and/or small colon may be involved in intraluminal obstructions due to larger amounts of sand. The mucosal surface of the affected bowel is also usually, acutely inflamed and the motility of the affected portions is often first increased and then reduced. Fecal output is commonly normal in the early stages but becomes reduced and may ultimately cease altogether.

Ingestion of foreign bodies such as nylon carpeting or fibres from nylon-belt fences also affects the patency and progressive motility of the large and small colon in particular and may lead to obstruction. There are few pathognomonic features of these forms of colic but an accurate history may assist.

Concretions of fecal material known as **fecaliths** (a hard mass of inspissated feces) or **enteroliths** (intestinal calculi formed of layers surrounding a nucleus of some hard indigestible substance swallowed) may be found in the small colon of horses. They are associated with the development of small colon obstructions. Foreign bodies such as baler twine, rubber or nylon string/fibres are often responsible for the original accumulation with fecal material accumulating around the object to form large obstructing masses. They are usually formed in the large colon and most often result in simple luminal obstruction within the transverse or small colon **(121)**. The more solid, rock-like concretions (enteroliths) **(122)** are usually composed of ammonium and magnesium phosphate complexes and, although they are smoother,

123

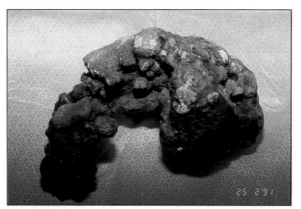

123 Enterolith.
Note: Found incidentally in left ventral colon. Curved shape and 'cast' of sacculations indicating prolonged location.

124

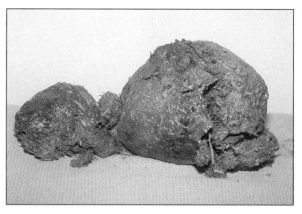

124 Fecalith.
Note: Relatively uniform shape and obvious fecal nature. Very hard and difficult to break up.

they may also cause intraluminal obstructions in the large and small colon. These are much slower to develop than fecaliths (*see* **124**) and may be found incidentally in any part of the large colon. Objects of significant size, found in the small colon, are usually causes of obstruction. The shape and location of the developing mass largely dictates the associated clinical signs. Thus, roughened and irregular enteroliths occurring in the cecum or large colon (**123**) may have little or no pathological effect or may produce mild, recurrent episodes of colic associated with local bowel-wall irritation. The commoner larger, smoother, enteroliths (*see* **122**) and fecaliths (**124**) characteristically cause obstructions in the narrower portions of the large bowel including the pelvic flexure, transverse colon and small colon. Rarely, enteroliths may be multiple, smooth and conforming, and these are often more tetrahedral in shape than spherical. Some masses of limited size may be passed normally in the feces. Obstructions caused by enteroliths or fecaliths may be complete, when acute clinical signs associated with the gross proximal accumulation of gas and ingesta may be seen but are more usually incomplete. In the latter cases the clinical signs are similar to those of impactions at the relevant anatomical sites. Intermittent impactions may be associated with slow and intermittent movement of the object through the colon. Rough objects located within the cecum or large colon (*see* **123**) may not, however, have any obstructive effects but may cause quite extensive intermittent (and sometimes persistent) inflammation of these organs and each episode might be accompanied by significant colic symptoms. Rectal examination may or may not detect the presence of these objects depending on their location and weight.

A variety of intramural lesions such as abscesses, neoplasia and intramural hematomas may also result in significant non-strangulating colic. Intramural (usually abscessed lymphatic tissue) or mesenteric **abscesses**, resulting from systemic spread from respiratory infections, are relatively common. Most are due to *Streptococcus equi*, *Streptococcus zooepidemicus*, *Rhodococcus equi* (*see* **225**) and *Corynebacterium pseudotuberculosis*. Although few cause any significant bowel disorders, some result in intermittent, recurrent colic associated with chronic weight loss. The commonest obstructive condition caused by these lesions are adhesions between loops of bowel or between bowel and other peritoneal organs. **Cecal abscess**es may reach considerable size and involve extensive portions of the jejunum and ileum (**125**) and other abdominal structures. There is little known about their pathogenesis, but they are most often centred around the ileo-cecal or ceco-colic openings. The clinical signs are insidious in onset and only when peritonitis and/or bowel obstruction occur are acute signs of colic presented.

Submucosal hematomas occur in the wall of the small colon and exert the same effect as other obstructions. They are often large and result in partial or complete luminal obstruction. Chronic ulceration of the small colon at the site of the hematoma, iatrogenic damage following rectal examination and other as yet unidentified factors, may be responsible for their development. The pain associated with this obstruction is usually inordinately severe when compared to that due to other forms of small colon obstruction and this is possibly due to the tension created by the swollen mass on the visceral peritoneum.

Prolapse of the rectum is usually the consequence of persistent, intense tenesmus (straining) and it may, therefore, be a sequel to intestinal disorders (diarrhea, constipation, enteritis, parasitism or other factors which result in local inflammation), or urinary or genital tract disorders in which straining is a prominent feature. Horses which ingest man-made, fibrous material such as carpeting, nylon twine or fibre-glass, may develop a severe and protracted proctitis which is sufficient to result in rectal prolapse. **Rectal prolapse** should be differentiated from intussusception of the small colon and several different forms of the disorder are recognisable. **Mucosal prolapse** alone has a characteristic appearance and represents the simplest form. These vary from mild partial or intermittent prolapses, to severe, complete prolapses with extensive mucosal edema **(126)**. Necrosis drying and laceration of the prolapsed mucosa is a frequent complication of prolonged or neglected cases. In this type there is usually no serious compromise of the underlying rectal wall. The more severe, **complete prolapse** with invagination of the colon **(127)** may be complicated by intussusception of the peritoneal rectum or colon through the anus. Under these circumstances the rectum (and if involved, the colon) rapidly becomes compromised and extensive necrosis of varying lengths is a common complication. Severe prolapse of the colon may accompany parturition in old mares in particular. Differentiation of small colon intussusception and rectal prolapse can be made by detailed examination of the mucosal reflection at the anal ring. In the former case a probe (finger) can be inserted a considerable distance between the anus and the prolapsed organ whereas in the latter, the reflection occurs at the anal ring or just inside it. A probe (finger) cannot be inserted beyond this reflection.

125
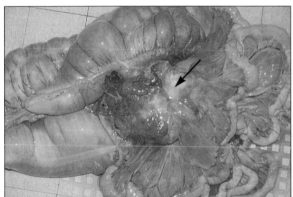

126
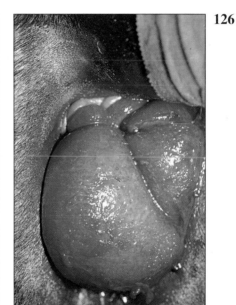

127
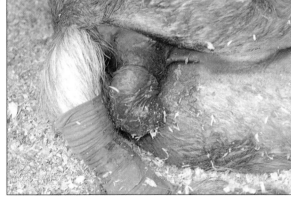

125 Cecal abscess.
Note: Large abscess (arrow) centred on ileo-cecal region and involved ileum, cecum and the ceco-colic opening. *Streptococcus equi* isolated.

126 Rectal mucosal prolapse (eversion).
Note: Drying and edema of exposed mucosa.

127 Rectal Prolapse (with small colon eversion).
Note: Compromised (cyanotic) prolapse.

Rectal tears are a relatively common occurrence and while most are certainly iatrogenic, being consequent upon rectal examination, some occur spontaneously. Nervous and young horses are more often affected, possibly as a result of the difficulties these create with respect to rectal examination. The most common initial presenting sign of damage is the presence of fresh blood on the rectal sleeve of the operator or fresh blood in the feces of spontaneous cases. However caused, most tears are located in the dorsal rectal wall and are classified according to their depth into four grades. The extent of the damage varies from mucosal tears only (Grade I), to complete disruption of the wall **(128)** (Grade IV) with consequent contamination of the surrounding tissues. Where the tear occurs in the retroperitoneal part of the rectum the consequences are likely to be somewhat less severe than those occurring in the more anterior portions. In the former cases the consequences include peritoneal abscessation or generalised intrapelvic infection. In the latter, peritoneal contamination usually occurs particularly rapidly and these cases carry a grave prognosis even when identified early. Affected horses usually strain heavily within a few minutes (or hours) of the initial incident. Peritoneal contamination (as evidenced by rising neutrophil counts in peritoneal fluid) or gross peritoneal contamination **(Plate 2g**, page 47) results in peritonitis and abdominal guarding (indicative of parietal pain). Sweating and colic developing within a few hours of rectal examination, should alert the clinician to the possibility of rectal tears, even if blood was not seen on the sleeve at the time of the examination. Diagnosis of rectal tears should be made with the aid of careful rectal examination and endoscopy, accurate location and characterisation of the tear will enable the clinician to make the appropriate therapeutic decisions. Blood on a sleeve following rectal examination should never be ignored.

Impaired gastric and/or intestinal motility may arise from **paralytic ileus** following gross, persistent distension of the small intestine in particular, or from excessive handling of bowel during surgery, or from a number of specific disorders of motility including **Grass Sickness (equine dysautonomia)**. The clinical signs associated with all forms of paralytic ileus are largely similar with gross accumulation of ingesta and secretions in the stomach and jejunum. The consequent pain is usually obvious.

Cases of **Grass Sickness** are presently largely restricted to limited areas of Europe and more specifically to the United Kingdom. While most cases are encountered in grazing horses under 10 years of age, in spring or early autumn, rare cases occur in older horses, stabled horses and during the winter months. The etiology of the disease is unknown, but epidemiological evidence suggests that a toxic principle primarily affecting autonomic function of the distal jejunum and ileum (amongst other effects) is involved, and is probably pasture-related. Cases are encountered more commonly when warm wet weather has prevailed over a few days, and both outbreaks involving several horses, and single sporadic cases, are recognised. Specific fields seem to be particularly associated with Grass Sickness, but many cases occur in isolated places without any apparent reason and sometimes when pasture has had no previous horse contact. The disease has a wide range of clinical manifestations which are largely dependent upon the speed of onset and the extent of the characteristic alimentary paralysis. In **peracute Grass Sickness** the stomach and small bowel are worst affected, and these horses show dramatic and rapidly deteriorating physiological status with severe colic. Spontaneous nasal regurgitation of greenish, acidic fluid **(Plate 1g**, page 45) is common and indicative of dramatic, dangerous gastric distension and impending gastric rupture. Patchy sweating **(129)** and triceps fasciculations are regular signs. Horses affected with the peracute form invariably die within 24–48 hours of onset, in spite of the best nursing efforts. Perhaps the most important means of prolonging the life of the unfortunate horse until a

128

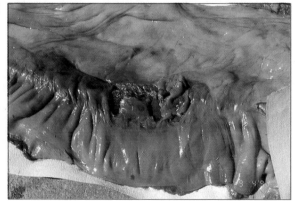

128 Rectal tear.
Note: Typical site in dorsal wall, full thickness tear, resulted in fulminating peritonitis and colic with sweating and straining two hours after rectal examination. Extensive damage to mesorectum.

specific diagnosis can be established, is gastric intubation and balanced, parenteral fluid administration. The signs characteristic of **acute Grass Sickness** are attributable to affects on both the stomach and duodenum, as well as to some, less obvious, signs of colonic and ileal hypomotility. In these cases continued secretion into the stomach, duodenum and jejunum and concurrent progressive desiccation of digested food material in the more distal parts of the alimentary tract occurs and these result in the onset of mild or more severe colic. The effects on the colon may pass unnoticed with death usually intervening after 36–96 hours. The **chronic form** of the disorder appears to exert more effect upon the ileum, cecum and colon, than on the stomach and proximal, secretory parts of the small intestine. Progressive desiccation of the contents of the hypomotile colon results in dramatically reduced fecal output and hard, black, pelleted feces are characteristic

(130). These are often covered with a slimy mucus, indicative of prolonged small colon transfer time. Although colonic hypomotility is the usual finding, occasional cases of Grass Sickness develop profuse diarrhea – presumably as a result of the deranged motility. Paralysis of the esophagus and consequent dysphagia (**Plate 6r**, page 123) are also common features. Dysphagia and dramatic weight loss result in a boarded, tucked-up abdomen **(131)**. The speed of development of this typical appearance, in horses living in areas where the disease is endemic, is almost pathognomonic for Grass Sickness. A dry, dark greenish accumulation is often encountered in the nostrils of chronic Grass Sickness cases (**Plate 6p**, page 123). Positive contrast esophageal radiography may be used to demonstrate the flaccid paralysis of the esophagus with pooling of contrast medium at the thoracic inlet **(132)**. Many, but by no means all, affected horses show superficial, mucosal,

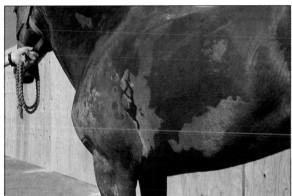

129 Grass sickness
Note: Patchy sweating. Triceps fasciculations were obvious.

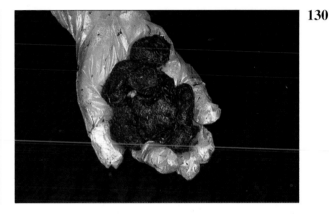

130 Grass sickness (chronic form).
Note: Dry, black, hard, pelleted feces, often with mucus covering.

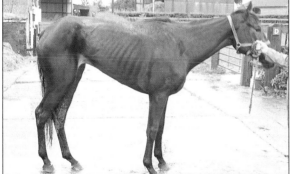

131 Grass sickness (chronic form).
Note: Severe, 'tucked-up' ('herring-gutted') appearance.

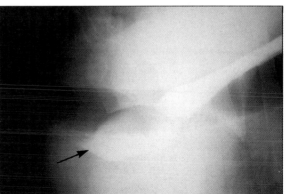

132 Grass Sickness (Chronic Form) (Barium contrast lateral thoracic radiograph).
Note: Esophageal paralysis. Pooling of contrast at thoracic inlet (arrow) and distention of thoracic esophagus.

linear esophageal ulceration which is sometimes demonstrable endoscopically (**133**). This probably arises from persistent gastro-esophageal reflux and profound esophageal paralysis which are characteristic of the disorder. The more chronic cases often survive for weeks or (occasionally) months but almost all eventually succumb. All forms of the disorder are, at present, best regarded as fatal, and therefore early recognition and prompt euthanasia are important. Post mortem examination in the acute cases, reveals the grossly distended stomach which contains a greenish mucoid fluid, while the contents of the cecum and colon, in cases surviving for more than 48 hours and in a few of the more acute cases, will be desiccated and scanty. For a disease which is so highly fatal both the clinical and post mortem signs are somewhat disappointing and laparotomy or post mortem examination is usually required to eliminate the other possible causes of gastric distension or fecal volume reduction (or both). A definitive antemortem diagnosis is currently based on histopathological examination of the intrinsic myenteric plexus in the ileum, while post mortem diagnosis can be made with certainty from examination of the mesenteric autonomic ganglia. The finding at laparotomy of a markedly reduced or an obvious hyper-motility (without any apparent co-ordination of movement of the bowel) in an animal without any other apparent cause for this, should be treated as suspicious in areas where the disease is known to exist.

Impairment of the absorption of food from the intestine may be associated with degenerative conditions of the small bowel or lymphatic obstructions. Inflammatory bowel disorders include diffuse alimentary lymphosarcoma (*see* **155**), tuberculosis (*see* **141**), histoplasmosis, and granulomatous/eosinophilic enteritis complex. These disorders form a complex of conditions in which impaired intestinal absorption is the major presenting sign (Malabsorption Syndrome) The clinical signs are inseparable and diagnosis relies heavily upon the use of a barrage of investigative procedures including absorption tests, motility studies and biopsy. Affected horses frequently have chronic intractable diarrhea (**134**), mild anemia (**Plate 8d**, page 178) and often show ventral and dependent edema (*see* **161**) associated additionally with impaired protein metabolism and protein-losing enteropathy. All these disorders carry a guarded or poor prognosis. It is important to differentiate the cases with a poor outlook from those conditions with similar general clinical signs, but which are resolvable, such as heavy parasitic infestation, dental disease and diet-related digestive disturbances.

133

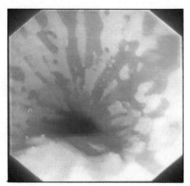

133 Grass sickness (chronic form) (endoscopic view).
Note: Extensive, linear and coalescent, mucosal esophageal ulceration and gastro-esophageal reflux of bile-like liquid.
Differential Diagnosis:
i)   Chillagoe horse disease
ii) Irritant ingestion

134

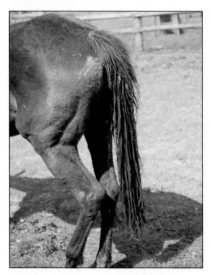

134 Granulomatous (eosinophilic) enteritis (chronic diarrhea).
Differential Diagnosis:
i)   Parasitism (particularly Cyathostomiasis)
ii)   Intestinal lymphosarcoma/adenocarcinoma
iii) Grass Sickness
iv)   Tuberculosis
v)   Malabsorbtion/maldigestion syndromes
vi)   Salmonellosis
vii) Dental disorders
viii) Hepatic failure
ix)   Granulomatous enteritis

Infectious Disorders

Infections with enteric pathogens are relatively uncommon in horses when compared to other species of large animals. However, several viral and bacterial infections are significant causes of disease.

Virus Diseases: Rotavirus diarrhea is probably the commonest cause of infectious enteritis in foals. While most affected horses are less than 6 months old, it is likely that the virus affects all ages of horse, exerting more or less effect depending upon its virulence and the immune status of the host. Adult horses are usually solidly immune following previous challenge but foals, particularly those stressed by environmental or other factors are susceptible. A profuse, watery diarrhea is typically present **(135)** and affected foals are mildly febrile and anorectic. However, many cases show only limited, transient diarrhea without any other systemic effects. The disease is more severe in foals receiving heavy challenges of virulent strains of the virus. A presumptive diagnosis can usually be made on clinical and epidemiological features but specific identification of the virus particles by ELISA (enzyme-linked immunosorbent assay) or electron microscopy are definitive means of diagnosis. A few foals show a persistence of diarrhea and chronic ill-thrift following the disease, possibly due to more severe and persistent changes in the mucosal structure of the intestine.

Bacterial Diseases: Bacterial enteritis in foals is usually the result of Gram-negative pathogens such as *Escherichia coli* and *Salmonella* spp. Very young foals,

or those suffering from stress, or those affected by immunocompromising disorders (including failure of passive transfer of colostrally derived antibodies), are most likely to suffer from bacterial enteritis. The infections are usually septicemic and this group of organisms is responsible for most cases of the **neonatal septicemia syndrome** in which clinical signs of enteritis may or may not be prominent. In most cases the origin of the infection is likely to have been the alimentary tract or the umbilicus. Septicemic foals are dull, febrile and anorectic. Diarrhea, which often contains blood and/or shreds of mucous membrane, may be seen **(136)**.

Adult carriers of ***Salmonella*** spp. organisms may develop a fulminating and highly fatal diarrhea syndrome shortly after they are subjected to stress. Even short transportation or apparently minor surgical procedures may be sufficient to allow the organisms to multiply and invade the mucosa of the large intestine with serious consequences including profuse, dark diarrhea **(137)**, often containing shreds of mucosa and blood, dullness, and in many cases, rapid death. The **Colitis-X Syndrome** may be associated with a peracute, fulminant salmonellosis or clostridiosis and in some cases diarrhea may not have time to develop before death intervenes although cases surviving for more than 24 hours usually have a profuse, fetid and hemorrhagic diarrhea. Affected horses are often collapsed, showing signs of severe endotoxemia, metabolic derangement and shock. Some cases are possibly associated with the

135

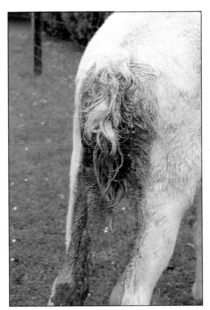

136

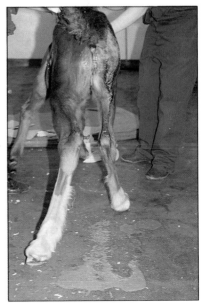

135 Rotavirus diarrhea.
Differential Diagnosis:
i)   Enteric bacterial infection
ii) Faunation (Foal-heat) diarrhea
iii) *Rhodococcus equi* (intestinal form)
iv) Parasitism (*Strongyloides westeri*, cyathostomiasis)
v)   Digestive disorders (lactase deficiency)
vi) Villous atrophy (following previous or concurrent enteric infection)

136 Salmonellosis.
Note: Febrile, profuse diarrhea, often with blood and shreds of mucosa, and systemic illness. This 5-day-old foal did not receive any colostrum.

137

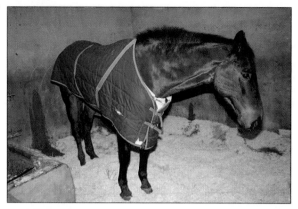

137 Acute salmonellosis (post surgical).
Note: Profuse dark diarrhea over wall of stable. Diarrhea contained blood and shreds of intestinal mucosa. Very low circulating white cell count, fever and severe depression.

138

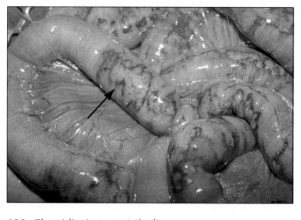

138 Clostridiosis (acute) (foal).
Note: Well defined patches of compromised small-intestinal wall (arrow). Extension to serosal surface and peritoneum. Ileus (generalised intestinal stasis) was present and resulted in gastric distension and nasal reflex.

139

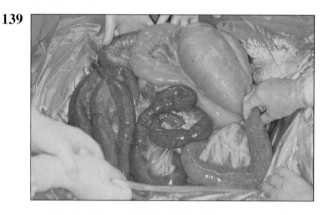

139 Proximal (anterior) enteritis (duodenitis/jejunitis) syndrome.
Note: Extensive severe inflammation of jejunum which is not distended. Proximal distension (portion held) and normal large colon. Severe gastric distension was present and spontaneous nasal regurgitaion of gastric (gastro-duodenal) fluid (**Plate 1g**, page 45) was present.

administration of certain antibiotics and some non-steroidal, anti-inflammatory drugs, but other cases have no such history, apparently developing spontaneously. At post mortem examination the wall of the large colon and/or the cecum are grossly edematous, and the mucosa has a characteristic, necrotic, brown-red appearance.

Clostridial infections within the gut may cause severe enteritis in both adults and foals. In the foal a fetid, bloody diarrhea with colic and rapid death are characteristic. Clinically the condition closely resembles the Colitis-X syndrome of older horses. At post mortem examination extensive, severe inflammatory changes are present in the small and large intestine (**138**). Gross distension of the jejunum is usually found and this is responsible for gastro-duodenal reflux. In adult horses, however, two syndromes are recognised. The first is the **proximal (anterior) enteritis(duodenitis/jejunitis) syndrome** in which proliferation of clostridial organisms occurs in the proximal segments of the small intestine. Affected horses are presented with symptoms attributable to a severe, simple, non-strangulating obstruction of the small intestine. Pain is often moderate to severe and progresses rapidly to depression. Extreme, often violent, colic results from ileus due to inflammation of the duodenum or proximal small intestinal segments and the consequent gastric distension. Acute inflammation, which can be recognised by extensive, diffuse, intestinal inflammation (**139**) or more limited areas of serosal hemorrhage (**140**) in affected length(s) of small intestine, results in edema and a firm, obstructive swelling of the bowel wall. The extent of the visibly affected small intestine is often limited and may even be restricted to a few serosal hemorrhages over short segments. The clinical signs are attributable to peracute, proximal small-bowel obstruction and endotoxemia. There is voluminous gastric reflux (often spontaneous) of alkaline or slightly acid fluid (**Plate 1h**, page 45), and progressive and rapid hemoconcentration. Gastric fluid is replaced extremely rapidly after removal. Confirmation of the involvement of *Clostridia* spp bacteria may be obtained from gastric fluid or from intestinal contents.

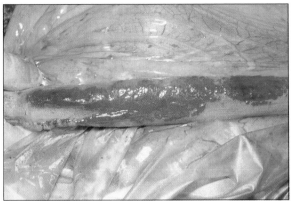

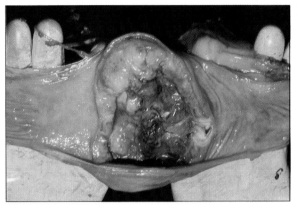

140 Anterior (proximal) enteritis (jejunitis) syndrome. **Note:** Very limited area of distal jejunum and proximal ileum affected. Horse showed moderate pain and repeated nasogastric reflux.

141 Intestinal tuberculosis. **Note:** Granulomatous lesion in wall of ileum associated with recurrent mild colic episodes and recurrent fever over some months.

Streptococcus equi (*see* **231**), *Rhodococcus equi* (*see* **225**) and a number of other bacteria, including *Mycobacteria* spp and a number of Gram-negative organisms, are occasionally responsible for a variety of clinical syndromes in which bowel obstructions or diarrhea or digestive disturbances occur. **Granulomatous enteritis** has been reported in horses between 1 and 5 years of age, in several parts of the world including the United States of America, Canada, South Africa and Australia. Chronic, progressive weight loss, poor appetite, diarrhea (*see* **134**) and intermittent colic are present. Recurrent episodes of pyrexia and dependent edema are reported. The clinical syndrome is not distinctive, but rectal examination reveals enlargement of the mesenteric lymph nodes and palpable thickening, with some obvious masses, in the wall of the small (and large) intestine. In some cases the focal, larger, lesions may cause partial obstructions of the lumen of the intestine, and these often exhibit intermittent and recurrent colic. Both diffuse and focal granulomatous lesions (**141**) may be found at post mortem examination and cultures from these may contain acid-fast organisms. Concurrently, lesions may be present in the lungs and other organs and may be associated with the **generalised granulomatous disease of horses**.

Bacterial abscesses involving the cecum (*see* **125**) are relatively common and may arise from foreign body penetration of the cecal wall or from other focal lesions which become infected. They are usually very large and may involve adjacent structures including the ileum and the origin of the right ventral colon. They result in vague persistent colic signs and weight loss but seldom cause diarrhea.

The development of normal microflora in the large bowel of foals occurring, usually, at about 7 – 14 days of age, is probably responsible for the development of profuse, watery but transient diarrhea. This normally coincides with the post-partum estrus (foal heat) in the dam, but there is little evidence to support the theory that the milk of the dam changes sufficiently to result in diarrhea. Affected foals are usually systemically normal, being bright and apparently unaffected by the diarrhea. Spontaneous resolution usually follows, although occasional foals may develop persistent diarrhea. It is likely that these are due either to digestive deficiencies or superimposed viral or bacterial infections resulting in long term damage to the mucosal lining of the large colon.

Parasitic diseases: Strongyloidosis (due to *Strongyloides westeri*) affects foals less than 2 months old inducing a persistent yellowish, milky diarrhea and weight loss. However, even extremely heavy infestations often show no detectable pathological effect. The adult worms are slim, up to 1 cm in length, and characteristically lie in close contact with the wall of the small intestine. Spontaneous resolution usually follows and few foals over the age of 4 months will harbour significant numbers of the parasites. The role of *Strongyloides westeri* in the incidence of neonatal diarrhea is uncertain.

Parascaris equorum, the equine ascarid, has a well defined hepato-tracheal migration route. The adult worms which are usually found in the distal jejunum and ileum, are often very large and may occur in large numbers (**142**). There is a true, age-related resistance which is acquired at about 6 months of age and is frequently accompanied by a dramatic expulsion of the

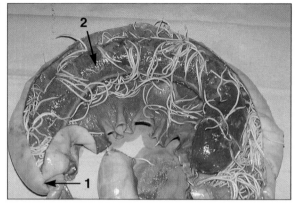

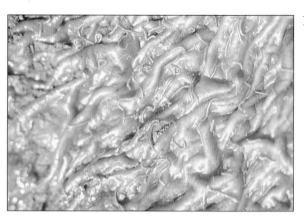

142 Ascaridiasis (*Parascaris equorum*).
Note: Ileo-ileal intussusception (arrow 1)with severe compromise of intussusceptum (arrow 2). Heavy ascarid burden.

143 Strongylosis (mixed large and small strongyles).
Note: Large numbers of pinkish and beige parasites on surface of mucosa.

adult worms from the gut, the worms often appearing in the feces in considerable numbers. Adult horses are not usually infested unless there is concurrent immune suppression, such as occurs in Cushing's Disease associated with pituitary adenomas (*see* **362**). If present in large numbers they may have limiting effects on growth and vitality with poorly grown, pot-bellied and poor-coated foals. Diarrhea is unusual. Acute ileal obstruction or ileo-ileal intussusception (*see* **142**) may be encountered, particularly after a significant number of mature worms are ejected simultaneously (either through natural resistance or anthelmintic therapy). Lumenal obstruction by live adherent ascarids is unusual. The migratory pathway involves the liver and lungs and conducting airways. Clinical signs of migration are usually limited to coughing and a muco-purulent nasal discharge, but hepatic scarring (*see* **172**) and small, focal hemorrhages and lymphocytic nodules in the lungs may be seen at post mortem examination.

Perhaps the commonest group of parasites affecting the horse are the **Strongyles**, which may be divided on clinical and morphological grounds into two groups. Over 40 different species have been identified with parasitic disease world-wide. The **large strongyles** include the *Strongylus spp.* and the adult stages of these worms are to be found in the large colon where they are readily visible as relatively stout, reddish-grey or pink worms, some 3 – 7 cms in length (**143**). They are firmly attached to the mucosa by elaborate mouthparts, and feed on blood or plasma and on the intestinal contents. Most of these parasites have tortuous and prolonged migratory patterns within the body. The migration pathway of the larvae largely dictates the pathological effects of a particular species, for the adult worms are probably of relatively lesser pathological importance.

The pathological significance of large burdens of adult worms should not, however, be under emphasised. Weight loss, anemia and chronic diarrhea (*see* **134**) are also encountered in heavily parasitised animals. The somatic-migrating, larval stages of the large strongyles are frequent causes of thromboembolic colic. Non-strangulating infarction conditions of the intestine occur relatively commonly and, although most of these are considered to be related to the migration of *Strongyle spp.* larvae, and more particularly to the migratory habits of *Strongylus vulgaris*, others have no obvious cause. Infarction of variable lengths of intestine occurs in the absence of any strangulating lesions and these are probably best classified as thromboembolic causes of colic. Almost every horse suffers at some point from strongyle infestation and the life cycle of *S. vulgaris*, in particular, involves a migration through the walls of the mesenteric (and other) arteries. Localised damage to end-arteries within the wall of the intestine may result in a well defined, often circular, patch of damage to the mucosa and wall of the intestine (**144**). The subsequent leakage of bacteria and possibly food material through the defect is one of the commonest causes of diffuse peritonitis and is associated with cloudy red or orange peritoneal fluid (**Plate 2e**, page 47). The presence of migrating larvae in the intima of the arterial walls results in more or less local inflammatory response and vascular luminal compromise. The most obvious lesions occur at the root of the **cranial mesenteric artery** as an area of **arteritis** (**145**). At post mortem examination it is often possible to identify larvae within the roughened, granulating lesions within the artery. It is easy to imagine emboli from this tissue and/or larvae themselves flowing down the major arteries. The extent of the consequences of this migration are considerable, with lesions ranging from

144

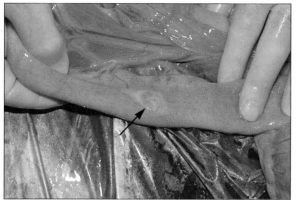

144 Strongylosis (focal infarction in jejunum) (arrow).
Note: Peritoneal fluid cloudy and reddish (**Plate 2e**, page 47).

145

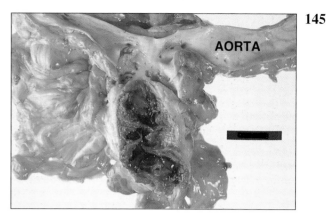

145 Verminous anterior mesenteric arteritis.
Note: In a 6 month old foal. Distention and thickening of cranial mesenteric artery with hemorrhagic thickening of the vessel wall. Parasitic larvae were visible embedded in the wall.

146

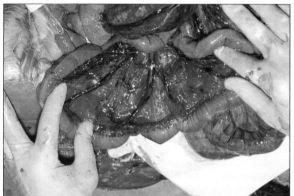

146 Parasitic infarction (of major mesenteric artery).
Note: Extensive infarction and consequent necrosis, no lumenal distension.

147

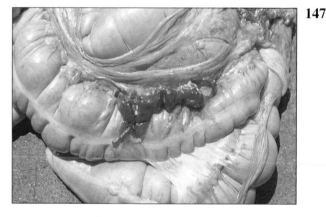

147 Parasitic infarction (of minor artery in wall of right dorsal colon).
Note: Lesion was due to *Strongylus edentatus*.

acute occlusion of major mesenteric vessels, resulting in gross infarction of large areas of jejunum (**146**), or lesser obstructions resulting in smaller, well defined areas of infarction. Occlusion of end-arteries in the cecum and/or large colon, results in well defined infarctive lesions (**147**) which almost always have serious consequences. In all cases where focal infarctions occur there is a high tendency for adhesions to develop between the infarcted area and adjacent structures. However, some localised lesions will have almost no clinical effect where collateral circulation overcomes limited vascular compromise. Ileal or ceco-colic vessel infarction may also cause a variety of lesions according to the location of the obstruction, but the extent is necessarily greater in these areas due to the poor collateral circulation. In the latter cases the migration of *S. edentatus* is often implicated (*see* **147**). The most severely affected areas are therefore those with the worst collateral circulation and those at the most distal points of the circulation such as the apex of the cecum and pelvic flexure. The clinical features of these disorders therefore range from catastrophic infarction to minor, transient colic signs or even no clinically detectable disorder. The more major lesions involving end-arteries have, however, serious effects on motility and integrity of the affected portion. A diagnosis of verminous arteritis is usually based upon the identification of a thickened root of the cranial mesenteric artery, or very occasionally the finding of a large arterial aneurysm at this site. It is important to realise that the migration stages of these parasites are of major importance and during this stage fecal worm eggs may not be present at all.

Many apparently normal horses show obvious discrete focal lesions in the terminal jejunum and the ileum as a result of hemorrhagic infarcts, probably caused by migrating *Strongylus vulgaris* larvae which exert local effects only and in most cases have no clinical effects. The condition, which is usually identified incidentally, is known as ***hemomelasma ilei*** (**148**) . Long-standing lesions become darker and more focal, often appearing as black dots or nodules in the wall of the ileum and are obvious from the serosal surface. Their importance lies only in the fact that they indicate prior parasitic infestation.

The **small strongyles**, or *Cyathostome* spp. which form a complex sub-family of the *Strongylus* spp. inhabit the large colon and cecum, are much smaller in size than the large strongyles, being between 0.5 and 1 cm long, and thread like (*see* **143**). Cyathostomes generally restrict their developmental stages to the wall of the large colon and cecum and do not migrate extensively. The pathological effects of the cyathostome group are often dramatic but individual animals may be heavily parasitised without showing any evidence of clinical disease. The ability of the larvae to delay their development within the intestinal wall (hypobiosis) makes it possible for synchronous emergence of large numbers of fourth/fifth stage larvae to occur. It is probably this which results in the extensive edema and inflammation of the large colon which is characteristic of **cyathostomiasis**. Vast numbers of maturing larvae may appear in the feces as writhing masses of fine pale pink or cream thread-like worms, coincident with the emergence of the larvae from the wall of the colon. As the life cycle of almost all the species of cyathostome is restricted to the large colon, the effects upon absorption and fecal consistency are often considerable. Accordingly, profuse diarrhea (*see* **134**) and weight loss are prominent signs of infestation. Severely affected horses may develop obvious dependent edema as a result of serious protein-losing enteropathy and, although appetite is often ravenous, some affected horses become inappetant. Large numbers of parasites (including the large strongyles) may, furthermore, have serious competitive demands upon the available food material. Detailed post mortem examination of the mucosal surface of heavily infested large colon shows the presence of varying stages of the maturing larvae in the mucosa (**149**) and adult worms closely attached to the surface with the larger, more mature larval and adult stages most prominent. This condition is now regarded as a major cause of debilitating and performance limiting disease.

A chronic and debilitating diarrheic disorder which is characterised by the pathological findings of diffuse eosinophilic infiltration of both the large and small colon may be related in some cases to this condition. A diagnosis of cyathostomiasis may be particularly difficult to confirm as the clinical features are largely non-specific and the presence of large numbers of worm eggs in the feces may not necessarily be related to pathological numbers of the worms. The absence of worm eggs in the feces may likewise not be a reliable indicator of the absence of the parasites. The effect of larvicidal anthelmintics may, however, be supportive in the diagnosis in some cases but again, the conclusions are often unreliable when there is chronic and extensive long-term damage to the intestinal wall and its function.

148

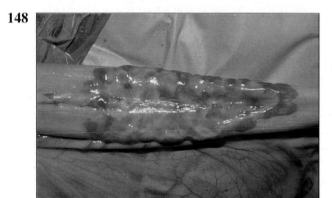

148 *Hemomelasma ilei.*
Note: Found incidentally at laparotomy.

149

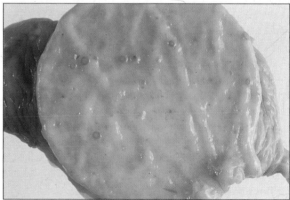

149 Cyathostomiasis.
Note: Sudden onset of acute diarrhea, anorexia and low grade colic occurred in spring. Mucosal thickening of cecum due to congestion and edema. Small (1–3 mm) discrete pink lesions enclose visible cyathostome larvae.

Cyathostomes are known to develop resistance to some anthelmintic drugs, and benzimidazoles in particular and regular worming with agents which have no certain effect upon migrating larvae, may not neccesarily preclude a diagnosis.

Oxyuriasis due to *Oxyuris equi*, which occurs in many parts of the world, causes an acute, often severe, peri-anal irritation which is associated with the egg laying habits of the worm. Affected horses will often rub the tail-head against solid objects causing breakage of hair and thickening of the tail head skin. Significant, acute, self-inflicted skin trauma with large inflammatory lesions on the perineal skin (**150**) are often encountered. Adult females may be up to 10 cm in length, white or cream in colour and have a characteristic tapered appearance. Large numbers of the parasites may be present in the feces of affected horses but in spite of this there are few pathological effects apart from the irritation.

The nematode species *Habronema* and *Draschia* are closely related and are transmitted between horses by flies of the *Musca* and *Stomoxys* species. While the most common clinical manifestations of **habronemiasis** are the cutaneous (*see* **584**) and ocular (*see* **649**) forms the presence of the parasite in the stomach may induce significant superficial gastric irritation or abscessation (**151**). In the case of *Draschia* spp. eosinophilic submucosal granulomas may develop in the wall of the stomach. These may coalesce and form solid fibrous, nodular lesions up to 5 – 7 cm in diameter. In most cases, however, no clinical disease results, but obstructions of the pylorus due to diffuse fibrosis have been encountered and in rare cases the lesions may abscess (*see* **151**) and result in chronic and recurrent gastric-related colic. In some cases long-standing infestation with *Habronema* or *Draschia* spp. parasites has been implicated in the development of gastric squamous cell carcinoma (*see* **154**).

The significance of ***Anoplocephala spp.* tapeworms** in the region of the ileo-cecal opening is disputed but it is likely that they are of importance in relation to ileal or cecal causes of colic. *Anoplocephala perfoliata* is the commonest tapeworm in horses, and is usually found in the distal ileum, cecum and proximal large colon. *Anoplocephala magna* is much larger and less common, and this species is restricted to the small intestine and has correspondingly less pathological effect. While adult tapeworms evenly distributed about the cecum may appear to cause few pathological effects, the area of attachment of each adult parasite is often acutely inflamed and ulcerated. Large numbers of worms congregating in the area of the ileo-cecal and ceco-colic openings (**152**) may cause localised inflammation, ulceration and edema of the openings themselves. Indeed, this finding is encountered at post mortem examination in many parasitised horses, most of which have not shown overt signs of colic or any other symptom. Significant hypertrophy of the ileo-ceco-colic region has, however, been attributed to high numbers of these parasites and prolonged partial obstruction to the ingress of food material from the ileum. This may result in significant muscular hypertrophy of the distal segments of the ileum (*see* **113**) which may extend, secondarily, to

150

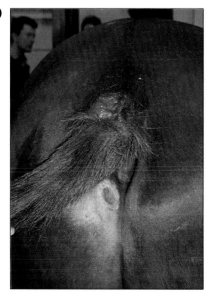

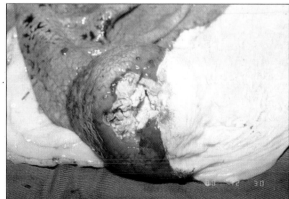

151

150 Oxyuriasis (*Oxyuris equi*).
Note: Lesions on perianal skin and base of tail caused by self-inflicted trauma.
Differential Diagnosis:
i)   Pediculosis (louse infestation)
ii) Culicoides hypersensitivity (Sweet itch)
iii) Chorioptic mange

151 Gastric habronemiasis (abscess lesion).

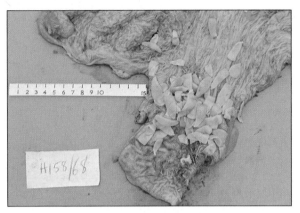

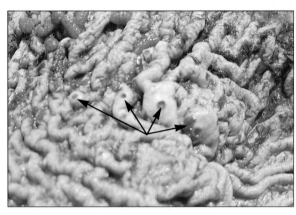

152 Cestodiasis (*Anoplocephala perfoliata*).
Note: Removal of the parasites revealed extensive mucosal ulceration and edema in the underlying cecal mucosa. The sample was obtained from a horse which suffered from a ceco-cecal intussusception (See **104**) and ileal hypertrophy (See **113**).

153 *Gastrophilus intestinalis* (Bots).
Note: Reddish larvae and discrete areas of inflammation, swelling and ulceration associated with previous attachment sites (arrows).

significant lengths of the distal jejunum. It is clear, however that ileal hypertrophy of this type is also encountered in the absence of tapeworm infestation. Ileo-ileal (*see* **102**), ileo-cecal (*see* **103**), ceco-cecal (*see* **104**) and ceco-colic intussusceptions have been found in association with large numbers of *Anoplocephala* spp. tapeworms but an etiological relationship has not yet been definitely established.

The larvae of ***Gastrophilus spp*** (**Bots**), which occur all over the world, hatch on the skin of horses in summer, from eggs laid by the adult female fly on the hair of the legs, face and mane. They migrate through the tissues of the mouth (*see* **48**) and esophagus to the stomach where they attach to the wall (**153**). A high proportion of horses are infested by the parasite at some time. Although large numbers may be present and they have been blamed for some cases of pyloric obstruction, more usually, they appear to induce no detectable clinical effect. Examination of the gastric mucosa shows, however, that there is a significant focal inflammatory response and ulceration at the site of attachment (*see* **153**).

Neoplastic Disorders

Squamous cell carcinoma of the stomach which characteristically affects the squamous (esophageal) area adjacent to the cardia (**154**) is one of the commonest neoplastic lesions of the gastro-intestinal tract and is certainly the commonest gastric neoplasm. Most are invasive with adhesions extending from the greater curvature of the stomach to the diaphragm and/or liver. They may reach considerable size and have an ulcerative, invasive and proliferative appearance. They are often ulcerated and secondarily infected. In these circumstances their surface may have a greyish-white and hemorrhagic appearance. Metastatic spread from this site occurs frequently with miliary secondary tumours in the lungs and occasionally elsewhere. Their development is possibly associated with parasitic conditions of the stomach such as habronemiasis (*see*

151) or infestation with *Gastrophilus* spp. (*see* **153**). Horses affected with gastric squamous cell carcinoma almost always lose weight dramatically and have a capricious appetite. Recurrent, episodic pyrexia is commonly encountered. Significant amounts of blood are lost into the lumen of the stomach and melena may be seen. Gastric contents obtained by nasogastric intubation might also show significant hemorrhage. Anemia and intermittency of appetite often associated with post-prandial colic are the most common clinical manifestations of the disorder. Pyloric stenosis as a result of neoplastic (or inflammatory) changes may cause recurrent gastric accumulations with repeated requirement for decompression. Endoscopy and cytological examination of peritoneal fluid obtained by abdominocentesis are most useful aids to the diagnosis

154

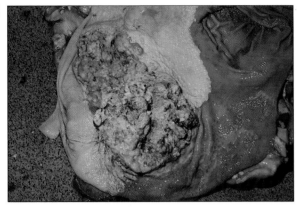

154 Gastric squamous cell carcinoma.
Note: Typical, proliferative, ulcerative lesion. The lesion extended through the gastric wall into the peritoneum and liver. Secondary (metastatic) lesions were found in the lungs.

155

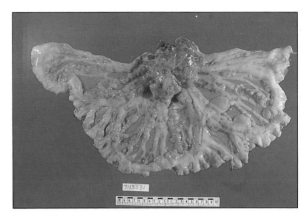

155 Diffuse intestinal lymphosarcoma.
Note: Diffuse thickened small intestine and lymphatic infiltration. Patient suffered from progressive weight loss, recurrent fever, hypercalcemia and chronic intractable diarrhea which was due probably to serious motility disturbances.

156

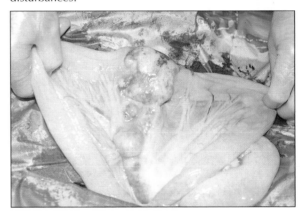

156 Focal intestinal lymphosarcoma.
Note: Extension of tumour masses up mesenteric lymphatic vessels. Mesenteric lymph nodes at root of mesentery were markedly enlarged but no other organ was involved.

of this disease. Squamous cell carcinoma of the anal ring typically only occurs when the perineal skin is depigmented and is in any case a rare neoplasm.

Alimentary tract manifestations of **lymphosarcoma** are relatively frequent neoplastic lesions of the horse. While in many cases the affected animals are in the older age groups, horses as young as 2 years of age may be affected. Both diffuse and localised lymphosarcoma lesions occur in the intestine and the clinical manifestations are therefore varied. The **diffuse form of lymphosarcoma** usually involves the small intestine (**155**), although the stomach and colon may be affected. The more unusual, **focal lymphosarcoma (156)** is commoner in older horses, and may present with recurrent colic and/or an acute abdominal crisis resulting from mechanical obstruction of the lumen of the intestine. General signs of weight loss, inappetence and ventral edema are found in all forms. In cases of diffuse lymphosarcoma involving the colon, diarrhea is a regular sign (*see* **134**), but in other forms it is not common. In both forms the tumour generally extends into the mesenteric lymph nodes which may be palpably enlarged at rectal examination. Affected horses are often anemic (**Plate 8d**, page 178) and, in common with other forms of lymphosarcoma (and other internal neoplasia), are sometimes reported to have periodic 'unexplained' febrile episodes lasting up to several days at a time. Examination of abdominal fluid obtained by paracentesis will often reveal neoplastic cells in both forms of the disorder. A definitive diagnosis may be difficult to reach without surgery but intestinal absorption tests (using glucose or xylose), elevations in serum calcium and changes in blood protein distribution may be helpful. Laparotomy or post mortem examination of horses affected by the diffuse form shows either a generalised thickening of the wall of the affected lengths of intestine with gross extension along mesenteric lymphatic vessels (*see* **155**) or focal dense lobulated lesions (*see* **156**). In the focal form, lesions tend to be well defined solid, often multiple and affect

157

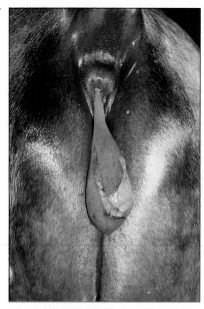

157 Rectal polyp.
Differential Diagnosis:
i) Rectal prolapse
ii) Prolapsed intussusception

only a limited length of bowel but obvious mesenteric spread towards the mesenteric lymph nodes is common (*see* **156**). Cases of intestinal lymphosarcoma may be affected by other forms of this neoplasm including the mediastinal (*see* **323**), multicentric and cutaneous forms (*see* **591**).

Pedunculated, **rectal polyps** develop slowly from the wall of the terminal rectum (**157**) or the immediate anal area and are dramatic in appearance but of little clinical significance. They are usually small but can reach considerable size and occasionally bleed quite heavily. They are totally benign.

Further reading

Problems in Equine Medicine
Brown, C.M. (1989) Lea & Febiger, Philadelphia, USA
Current Therapy in Equine Medicine (2)
Ed Robinson, N.E. (1987), W B Saunders, Philadelphia, USA
Current Therapy in Equine Medicine (3)
Ed Robinson, N.E. (1992), W B Saunders, Philadelphia, USA
Equine Clinical Neonatology
Koterba, A.M., Drummond, W.H., and Kosch, P.C. (1990) Lea & Febiger, Philadelphia, USA
The Equine Acute Abdomen
White, N.A. (1990) Lea & Febiger, Philadelphia, USA
Veterinary Parasitology
Urquart, G.M., Armour, J., Duncan, J.L., Dunn, A.M. and Jennings, F.W. (1987) Longman, Scientific and Technical, Harlow, UK

Equine Colic Research (Proceedings of the Second Symposium at the University of Georgia)
Ed Moore, J.N., White, N.A. and Becht, J.L. (1986) Veterinary Learning Systems, New Jersey, USA
Equine Colic Research (Proceedings of the Third Symposium at the University of Georgia)
Ed Moore, J.N., White, N.A. and Becht, J.L. (1993) Veterinary Learning Systems, New Jersey, USA
Manual of Equine Practice
Rose, R.J., and Hodgson, D.R. (1993) WB Saunders, Philadelphia
Equine Parasites
Jacobs. G. (1986) Baillière Tindall, U.K.

2. Conditions of the liver, peritoneum, and pancreas

Developmental Disorders

There are no clinically significant common congenital hepatic, pancreatic or peritoneal abnormalities of the horse, although very rarely porto-caval shunts have been described which induce neurological signs, typical of hepatic failure, when dietary protein levels are increased after weaning.

Part 1: The Liver

Non-Infectious Disorders

The wide range of disorders of the liver reflects the diversity of its metabolic functions and the clinical signs of hepatic failure may, in turn, reflect the loss of one or more of these. Specific disorders therefore tend to produce a diversity of non-specific clinical signs, reflecting the severity of hepatocellular damage and the effect which this has on the metabolic, catabolic, anabolic, detoxification and synthetic functions of the organ. Mild hepatocyte damage, for example, might be insufficient to produce any detectable clinical abnormality, with the only evidence for its existence being found in analysis of blood samples. The liver has a large functional reserve, and overt clinical signs associated with hepatic dysfunction may only become apparent when more than 70 – 75% of hepatic tissue is non-functional. In some cases however, specific metabolic processes are deranged and this results in conspicuous clinical signs which may not immediately be attributable to the liver. Clinical signs associated with hepatic disease tend, therefore, to be vague and may even pass unnoticed in many cases. When signs of hepatic failure become obvious damage is usually severe, whether this is of chronic or acute onset. Evidence of hepatic failure may be found in failure of detoxification of absorbed toxins, metabolites and chemicals, and/or in disorders of metabolism, and/or impaired anabolic and synthetic functions.

Hepatic disease in the horse is a relatively common occurrence, but only those with either biliary obstruction or extensive hepatic parenchymal disease (or both) will exhibit easily identifiable signs of hepatic failure. The onset of clinical signs is invariably acute, even though the damage might have been long-standing and even mild, acute insults sustained weeks, months or years previously may become significant at a later stage. The organ does however, have some regenerative capacity and may regain some, if not all of its complex functions even after severe acute insults. Acute hepatic damage therefore provides the clinician with therapeutic opportunities while chronic severe changes are usually frustratingly unmanageable.

Overt **icterus** (jaundice) **(158, Plate 8f**, page 179) may be particularly difficult to assess accurately in the horse, not only because of the inherently high blood concentrations of natural, harmless, carotenes in some grazing horses, but also because starved horses may be icteroid (seemingly jaundiced) in the absence of any hepatic pathology. Starvation for as short a period as 24 hours, whether through non-availability of food or through inappetence, results in significant increases in blood bilirubin concentration which appears as icteric pigmentation of the mucous membranes. Furthermore, icterus is, itself, not necessarily always a result of hepatic disorder, but may reflect either an excess of demand upon the mechanisms for breakdown of hemoglobin-derived metabolites or interference in the mechanisms of excretion of conjugated bilirubin via the biliary tract (*see* **169**). As a rule, however, icterus in the horse is intense in acute hepatic failure and less obvious in chronic failure. Most non-hepatic icterus is a result of excessive red cell destruction, such as occurs in **equine neonatal isoerythrolysis syndrome** (*see* **312**) and **equine Babesiosis** (*see* **319**), or is due to extensive biliary tract obstruction. The latter may occur within the

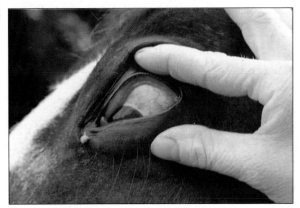

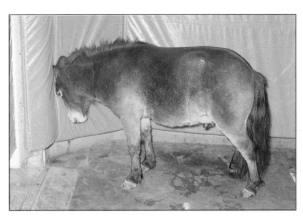

158 Icterus (jaundice) of the sclera.
Differential Diagnosis:
i)   Internal bleeding
ii) Intravascular hemolysis eg neonatal isoerythrolysis, Babesiosis
iii) Acute (or chronic) hepatic failure
iv) Biliary obstruction (cholelithiasis, neoplasia)
v)   Starvation
vi) Equine infectious anaemia

159 Hepatoencephalopathy (head pressing).

liver itself, when there is intra-hepatic inflammation and swelling, when there are physical obstructions due to fibrosis or neoplasia, and when there are obstructive hepatic or biliary calculi. **Abdominal neoplasia** also results in some cases of obstructive jaundice, particularly where the primary lesion is in the pancreas or where there is extensive peritoneal involvement in the anterior abdomen, such as might occur in gastric squamous cell carcinoma (*see* **154**). The establishment of the cause of icterus is obviously important and biochemical analysis of the proportions of conjugated and non-conjugated bilirubin in circulating blood may be required to accurately identify the type of icterus which is present and thereby provide indications as to its origin.

The most obvious clinical signs of **acute or chronic hepatic failure** usually involve the central nervous system or the skin. Affected horses show depression (*see* **161**), repeated yawning, head pressing (**159**), un-controllable circling, compulsive walking/pacing (**160**), convulsions and coma. The earliest signs of ataxia and yawning may easily be missed. These central nervous signs are probably a result of hepato-encephalopathy due to high circulating concentrations of ammonia and other metabolites (including organic acids), which reflects a failure of the detoxification functions of the organ. These compounds produce nervous signs through their effect upon nervous tissue and neural junctions. Some of the signs may also be attributable to hypoglycemia which reflects the failure of anabolic and catabolic functions.

Horses lacking the normal detoxification capacity as a result of either acute but more commonly, chronic

hepatic failure frequently become excessively sensitive to ultraviolet light. **Photodynamic agents** are derived endogenously as a result of metabolic processes (particularly in the intestine), or from ingested chemicals, including phenothiazine, and some plants, including *Hypericum peroratum* (St John's Wort) (**Plate 3a**, page 84), *Polygonum fagopyrum* (Buckwheat) and *Lolium perenne* (Perennial ryegrass). Failure to detoxify a number of photodynamic agents including phylloerythrin (a product of bacterial degradation of the plant pigment chlorophyll) results in accumulation in the circulation. In normal animals any absorbed photodynamic agents are removed from the portal circulation and excreted in bile, precluding the general distribution of the agents to the skin and other organs. Photodynamic compounds circulated in the skin are activated by ultraviolet radiation in sunlight causing massive release of inflammatory mediators. The consequent tissue damage is usually restricted to white areas of the skin (*see* **502**). It is not always only the obvious areas of unpigmented skin which become affected, but the restriction to white skin is almost pathognomonic for **photosensitisation**. A number of other chemicals such as phenothiazine may have strong photodynamic effects. Occasionally, very pale-skinned horses may suffer from sunburn, without any underlying organic disease and in the absence of any ingested photodynamic agent. In these cases it is unlikely that the inflamed areas will include the distal limbs which are often severely affected in photosensitised horses. An unusual form of photosensitisation which occurs under

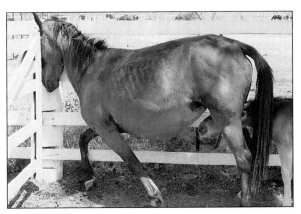

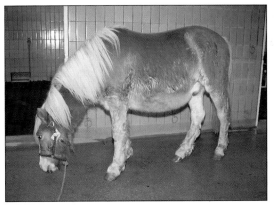

160 Hepatoencephalopathy (compulsive walking/circling).
Note: Ascites (distended, pot-bellied abdomen), poor body condition.

161 Hepatic failure (ventral edema and depression).
Differential Diagnosis:
i)   Hypoproteinemia (starvation, hepatic failure, malabsorption, protein losing enteropathy/nephropathy)
ii) Vasculitis
iii) Congestive (right-sided) heart failure
iii) Local circulatory disorders (eg thoracic neoplasia)
iv) Pleuritis
v)   Hyperlipaemia
vi) Lymphosarcoma
vii) Renal Failure

the same conditions as the more common dermatosis, involves the development of an **immune-mediated (photoactivated) vasculitis** (*see* **297**). In these, the lesions remain confined to non-pigmented areas of the lower extremities. Severe edema, erythema and crusting occurs with punctate foci of hemorrhage, and, significantly, the lesions are painful rather than pruritic. All horses showing photosensitisation and/or sunburn should be thoroughly screened for all these possibilities. Photosensitisation may, as can be appreciated, be of non-hepatic origin and in some cases may be a curiosity but may also be a sign of serious hepatic disease or serious poisoning, or both.

Failure of the anabolic functions of the liver is reflected in a depression of glucose and albumin synthesis. While the reduced blood glucose shows few specific signs, reductions in circulating albumin have profound effects with distinctive clinical signs. Significant hypoalbuminemia results in peripheral and ventral edema (**161**) and chronic weight loss. Gross abnormalities of albumin synthesis and increased portal pressure, arising as a result of hepatic fibrosis, often result in the accumulation of large volumes of clear, watery, fluid with a low specific gravity, low protein content and negligible cell count, within the abdomen (ascites) (*see* **Plate 2b**, page 46). Horses with significant ascites have a pot-bellied appearance (*see* **160**) and it may be possible to percuss a fluid thrill across the abdomen. Animals suffering from terminal hepatic

failure may show obvious intravascular hemolysis with prominent hemoglobinuria (*see* **471**). The reasons for this development are not clear.

The liver is also responsible for the synthesis of a wide range of important metabolic proteins including clotting factors, amino acids and other nutrients required for red cell and hemoglobin production. **Hepatic failure** then results in a number of related clinical signs, including hemorrhagic diatheses, and anemia (**Plate 8d**, page 178). Although overt spontaneous hemorrhage is not a common sign associated with hepatic failure, bleeding into the intestine or into the major conducting airways and prolonged or excessive bleeding from wounds may be encountered.

A number of other signs are also commonly associated with hepatic failure, including **laminitis** (*see* **409**), **colic** and **generalised or focal pruritus**.

The diagnosis of **acute or chronic hepatic failure** in the horse is largely based upon the detection of the characteristic, but non-specific, signs and confirmation usually relies heavily upon laboratory studies involving concentrations of enzymes and plasma proteins. The release of enzymes into the circulating blood from damaged hepatocytes is an index of the extent of the cell damage although the magnitude of the enzyme concentration increase does not always correlate closely with the degree of hepatic dysfunction. The extent to which hepatic function is impaired by disease processes can be separately assessed by testing the function of the organ. Bile acid concentration in the plasma and the ability of the liver to excrete an exogenously administered substance, such as bromosulphothalein (sulfobromophthalein) (BSP) provide a useful index of function. The serum concentration of ammonia is also an index of the functional ability of the liver. Liver biopsy, which is a relatively safe and simple procedure, provides definitive histological evidence of the type and extent of the pathological process. As almost all the significant hepatic disorders occurring in the horse are diffuse, biopsy is a most useful aid to their diagnosis. Although chronic hepatic failure may be accompanied by blood clotting disorders the procedure is seldom accompanied by dangerous blood loss. The prior administration of normal plasma is usually sufficient to render the procedure totally safe. In some cases the liver is particularly small and percutaneous biopsy may be difficult or impossible without additional ultra-sonographic or laparoscopic guidance. Some of the more common means of assessment of liver pathology are shown in Table 1. The table is by no means definitive and the clinician should seek suitable combinations of specific and non-specific indices which may, together with the clinical features, be used to confirm a presumptive diagnosis of acute or chronic, diffuse or focal hepatic failure.

Table: Hepatic 1. Some of the more commonly employed aids to the diagnosis of **hepatic disease** in the horse.

	RELATIVE VALUE OF TEST (and comments)		
	acute diffuse hepatic failure	chronic diffuse hepatic failure	focal hepatic /biliary disease
ULTRASONOGRAPHY	LITTLE VALUE	USEFUL	VERY USEFUL
LIVER BIOPSY	USEFUL	ESSENTIAL	ONLY IF ULTRASOUND GUIDANCE AVAILABLE
BSP[1] CLEARANCE/ RETENTION	SHOULD NOT BE USED	USEFUL	ONLY USEFUL IF MAJOR OBSTRUCTIVE DISORDER
BILE ACIDS	LITTLE USE	VERY USEFUL	NO VALUE (unless major obstructive disorder)
ASPARTATE AMINOTRANSFERASE (AST)	VERY USEFUL (elevated)	USEFUL (marginal elevation may be present)	NO VALUE (possible increase)
γ-GLUTAMYL TRANSFERASE (GGT, γGT)	VERY USEFUL (marginal increase initially)	VERY USEFUL (Significant increase)	NO VALUE
LACTATE DEHYDROGENASE[2] (LDH$_5$)	VERY USEFUL (specialised laboratory)	VERY USEFUL (specialised laboratory)	NO VALUE
SORBITOL DEHYDROGENASE (SDH)	VERY USEFUL (labile enzyme)	LITTLE VALUE	NO VALUE

[1] Bromosulphothalein Clearance/Retention Test
[2] Lactate dehydrogenase isoenzyme-5 (also found in skeletal muscle)

Acute hepatic disease may be more common than is appreciated but mild cases may pass unnoticed due to the large functional reserve of the organ. A relatively well recognised form of acute hepatic failure known as **Theiler's Disease** occurs in adult horses. Individuals may be affected but outbreaks involving several horses may also be encountered. Outbreaks of Theiler's Disease occur relatively frequently in the autumn months in the north western states of the United States of America. Many parts of the world have no reported cases. A number of cases have been associated with the prior administration of serum or other biological products and a virus etiology has been suggested in view of some extensive outbreaks amongst horses in close contact. Several other possible causes have been suggested including mycotoxins, alkaloid toxicity and others. The clinical signs, which generally have a peracute onset, do not differ significantly from the general signs of acute or chronic hepatic failure. The course of the disease is usually about five days with most cases either dying of hepatic failure or gradually recovering over seven to ten days although commonly recovery may be protracted and incomplete. Mild forms of the disease are also recognised, presenting with a vague malaise accompanied by elevated serum hepatic enzyme concentrations. Post mortem examination of affected horses shows the liver to be pale and enlarged with rounded edges (**162**). The cut surface shows diffuse mottling giving a characteristic nutmeg-like appearance (**163**).

Hyperlipemia is one of the commonest forms of acute hepatic failure and is most frequently encountered in overweight ponies in which a dramatic reduction in dietary carbohydrate intake has recently occurred, either as a result of starvation or appetite suppression. Affected ponies (or, more rarely, horses or donkeys) are often pregnant or lactating, and although most cases occur in overweight animals, body condition may be normal, or even poor. Affected animals typically show depression and weakness (*see* **161**), ataxia, muscle fasciculations and often have a greyish white coating on the tongue (**164**). Concurrent myopathy affecting the skeletal muscles and particularly the masseter masses are commonly encountered. Icterus is not usually a prominent sign but individual cases may be obviously icteric. Blood samples are usually noticeably lipemic and it is often helpful to compare the plasma with that of a normal horse (**165**). The extent of the hyperlipemia is not necessarily proportional to the severity of the clinical syndrome. There may be an intercurrent azotemia and an insulin-resistant hyperglycemia. Secondary laminitis (*see* **409**) is a common complication. Mortality is usually very high in spite of even the most aggressive treatment. At post mortem examination the liver is large, friable, pale-yellow in colour and markedly fatty (**166**). Pieces of affected liver will float in 10% formal saline.

Chronic hepatic failure is a particularly common clinical entity and is usually a sequel to repeated toxic insults. The most common cause for chronic failure is poisoning with plant-derived pyrrolazidine alkaloids, such as are found in *Senecio* spp. (**Plate 3b**, page 84), *Crotalaria* spp. (**Plate 3c**, page 84), *Lantana camara* (**Plate 3d**, page 84), *Echium plantagineum* (Patterson's Curse) (**Plate 3e**, page 84) and others. Most countries in the world have at least one plant which is capable of inducing chronic liver failure and the local dangerous plants are usually widely appreciated amongst stock owners. The plants are, however,

162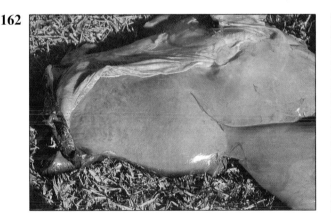

163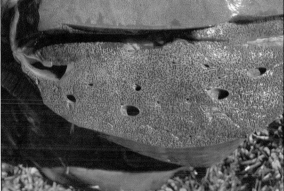

162 Theiler's disease (acute hepatic failure).
Note: Generally pale liver with swollen rounded edges.

163 Theiler's disease (liver, cut surface).
Note: Characteristic nutmeg appearance.
Differential Diagnosis:
i) Right-sided heart failure
ii) Cholelithiasis (*see* **169**)

Plate 3

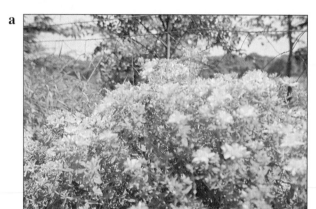

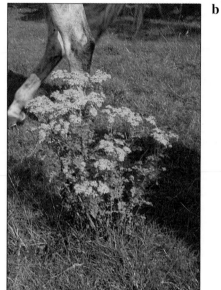

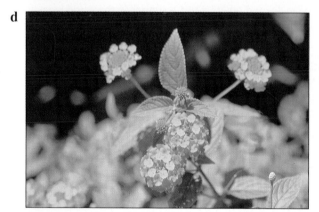

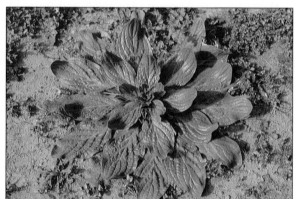

a *Hypericum peroratum* (St John's Wort).

b *Senecio jacobea* (Ragwort).

c *Crotalaria crispata.*

d *Lantana camara* (Marmalade Bush, Cherry Pie).

e *Echium plantagineum* (Patterson's Curse).

164

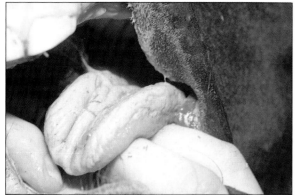

165

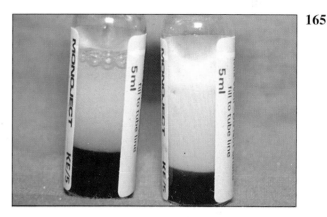

164 Hyperlipemia (hyperlipidemia) (white, 'furry' tongue).
Differential Diagnosis:
i) Terminal renal failure

165 Hyperlipemia (plasma, compared to normal horse on left).

166

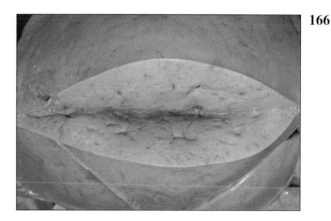

166 Hyperlipemia (liver, cut surface).
Note: Pale, waxy appearance. Liver grossly enlarged with rounded edges and a piece floated in 10% formol saline.

not usually palatable to grazing horses and ingestion directly from the pasture is not common except where no other food is available. However, the dried or wilted plants appear to be undetectable when they are included in preserved fodder such as hay or silage. Although there are sensitive detection methods available for the chemical agents in blood, long-term, low-level poisoning usually passes unnoticed. Ultimately, however, the damage is sufficient to result in the acute onset of clinical signs which are typical of hepatic failure. **Photosensitive dermatosis** (*see* **502**) is often the first reported sign in these cases. It is unusual for the clinical signs to develop slowly but chronic weight loss with ventral edema (*see* **160**) and soft "cow-pat" feces may be present in the early stages, and may be indicative of sub-clinical hepatic disease.

In **chronic hepatic failure** a small, densely fibrotic liver is usually found (**167**). The cut surface is usually dark, dense and fibrous with prominent biliary tracts (**168**). The carcase of horses dying from chronic hepatic failure is not often obviously icteric except when secondary bile duct obstruction, either within or outside the liver, has occurred. Generalised edema of the subcutaneous tissues, fluid accumulations in the body cavities and poor body condition are usually presented.

Secondary hepatic failure arises in cases of toxemia, septicemia and other apparently unrelated disorders, as a direct result of hepatocyte insult and impairment of one or more of the functions of the organ. **Right-side heart failure, aflatoxicosis, leukoencephalomalacia (Mouldy Corn Poisoning)** (*see* **717**), **duodenal ulceration in foals** (*see* **94**) and several other disorders may progress to hepatic failure. Several **heavy metals** such as **lead, arsenic and mercury** also have hepatic related effects although in most of these the hepatic effects are overshadowed by more obvious signs of the poisonings.

Biliary obstruction may occur in horses over 9 years of age, as a result either of the development of calculi within a bile duct (**169**) or from cholangiohepatitis and results in mild, or sometimes more severe, recurrent colic, with a course lasting up to several years. **Calculi** may be lodged in the common bile duct or the more minor ducts and, in the latter case, there may be almost

167

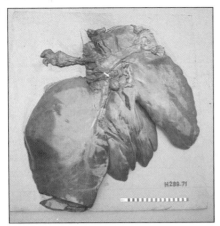

168

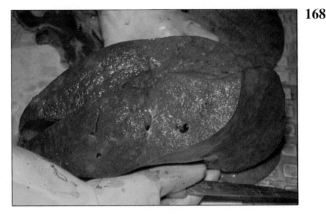

168 Chronic hepatic failure (fibrosis, cut surface).
Note: Dense fibrous appearance (difficult to cut), prominent biliary tracts. Liver taken from horse shown in **159**.

167 Chronic hepatic failure (cirrhosis/fibrosis).
Note: Small, dense lobes with bile duct stasis. Due to chronic ingestion of *Senecio jacobea*.

169

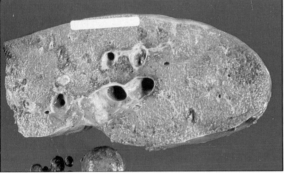

170

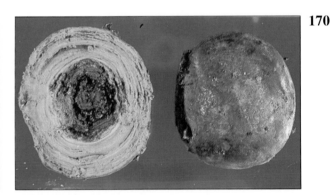

169 Cholelithiasis.
Note Extensive biliary fibrosis resulting from chronic obstruction of major bile duct.

170 Cholelithiasis.
Note: Bile stone in section showing laminated appearance due to deposition of bile salts and smooth, mottled, marble-like patterning on outer surface.

no helpful pathognomonic clinical signs apart from recurrent colic. Intermittent fever and marked icterus which may vary in severity are sometimes present, particularly when the obstructive lesion is situated in more distal parts of the biliary tract. Complete obstructions of the common bile duct will, of course, result in severe icterus and persistent colic which can become extreme. Usually animals affected in this way have a history of previous milder episodes, but it is possible to encounter the disorder without such a history. Signs of hepato-encephalopathy are less common than in chronic or acute hepatocellular disorders, particularly with choledocholithiasis (calculi lodged in common bile duct), but dementia and dullness may form part of the clinical syndrome in some cases. Peritoneal fluid is sometimes increased in amount and has an orange-yellow colour and may contain a few cells indicative of active inflammation, particularly if bile ducts are disrupted. Ultrasonographic examination may be most useful in identifying the dilated bile duct and the choleliths within them. Larger calculi may be more significant and ultrasonography may demonstrate the obstructed bile duct. Biliary calculi, which may also be found incidentally at post mortem examination, vary in size from 2 – 12 mm diameter. Their slow development within the biliary tract is emphasised by their laminated appearance in cross section (**170**).

Foals affected by the **gastro-duodenal ulceration syndrome** (*see* **94**) may suffer from a severe and life threatening bile duct obstruction. The clinical signs include marked icterus but clinically other signs may be more obvious.

Infectious Disorders

Virus/Bacterial Diseases: The central role which the liver plays in the metabolic and circulatory functions provides opportunities for systemic virus and bacterial infectious processes to affect the organ. While any viremic or bacteremic condition provides maximal opportunity for the sequestration of organisms into the liver it is remarkable that it is so seldom affected by infectious diseases of this type. It is possible that the functional reserve makes the clinical effects of hepatocyte damage minimal and that such processes are sub-clinical in nature. Infectious diseases of the liver are virtually restricted to the foal and include infection with **equine herpes virus type-1 (EHV-1)** or *Bacillus pilliformis* (**Tyzzer's Disease**). Foals infected with equine herpes virus-1, *in utero* may be born with severe hepatic necrosis, showing rapid onset of clinical signs attributable to acute, terminal hepatic failure, including progressive weakness, convulsions, collapse and death, but without marked jaundice. Necrosis of bowel and myocardium are also often present in these foals and the hepatic failure may be overlooked. Usually, however, such foals are born dead or are aborted in a non-viable state (*see* **212**).

Tyzzer's Disease is a well recognised clinical entity caused by *Bacillus pilliformis*. The disease is an acute or peracute, highly fatal, septicemic hepatitis occurring in foals between 1 and 6 weeks of age. Death is often the first sign of the disorder, but cases surviving for over 24 hours are severely depressed, intensely icteric and often show nervous signs attributable to advanced hepatic failure. Post mortem examination of affected foals reveals a severely swollen, pulpy and necrotic liver which on cut-section shows little or no recognisable architecture **(171)**. Diagnosis may rely on histopathology, when the large bacteria can be identified in the liver substance, and on bacterial culture.

Focal, well circumscribed **abscesses in the substance of the liver** are relatively commonly found at post mortem examination as an incidental finding **(172)**. While most are old and no specific organism can be identified, they are usually regarded as the product of septicemic dissemination. Organisms which have been blamed include *Streptococcus equi*, *Staphylococcus aureus*, and *Rhodococcus equi*. **Scars** or **"milk spots"** on the liver capsule (*see* **172**) are frequently found in normal horses and while the larger of these may reflect normal pigmentary changes in the capsule (*see* **172**), others may be scars associated with the hepato-pulmonary migration of *Parascaris equorum*. Even extensive numbers of these lesions appear to cause no detectable harm.

Parasitic Diseases: Considerable numbers of **large cysts** associated with *Echinococcus granulosis* var *equinus* may occur in the peritoneal cavity and particularly on the liver capsule **(173)**. The parasite is a relatively common finding in parts of the world where horses co-exist with infected dogs. Although the appearance may be dramatic they are probably of little clinical significance. The parasite is probably host specific for the horse and has no known zoonotic importance.

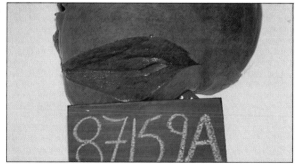

171 Tyzzer's disease.
Note: Specimen obtained 10 minutes after death. Loss of normal hepatic architecture. Liver was diffusely 'mushy' in consistency.

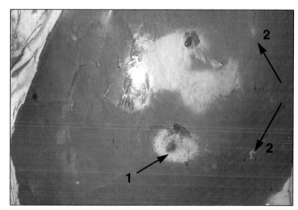

172 Focal hepatic abscess (arrow-1) and (small) 'Milk Spots' in capsule (arrow-2).
Note: Extensive pale area on capsule usually regarded as normal finding.

173

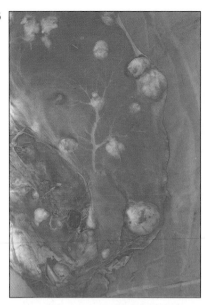

173 Hydatidosis (*Echinococcus granulosis* var *equinus*).
Note: Multiple cyst like lesions containing proscolices in a clear fluid attached to liver capsule. No hepatic involvement. Lesions were also present in lungs (detected radiographically and endoscopically).

174

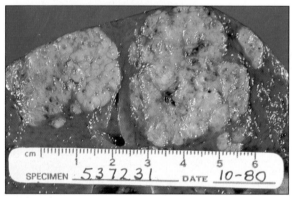

174 Hepatic carcinoma (primary).

175

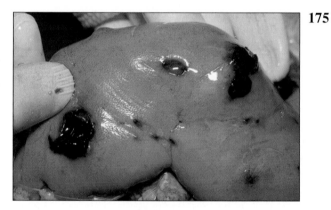

175 Secondary (metastatic) hemangiosarcoma.
Note: Pale liver associated with chronic, severe anemia. Lesions contain amorphous hemorrhagic material.

Neoplastic Disorders

Neoplastic lesions involving the liver substance may be primary or secondary to malignant neoplasia elsewhere. All such disorders of the liver are, fortunately, rare. **Cholangiocellular carcinoma** is the only primary neoplasm likely to be encountered in the horse and affects older horses exclusively. The clinical signs are those associated with biliary obstruction and extensive hepatocellular destruction (**174**). Peritoneal fluid is of an orange-red, turbid nature (**Plate 2c and 2f**, page 46) and abnormal cells can be identified easily, although the specific origin of these is almost always impossible to identify in the living horse. The advent of sophisticated ultrasonographic techniques may assist the diagnosis.

Horses affected by **hepatic lymphosarcoma** show varying degrees of abdominal distension due to lymphatic and hepatic obstruction with elevation of portal pressure. The peritoneal fluid tends to be clear or cloudy (**Plate 2c**, page 46) but is seldom hemorrhagic. Abnormal lymphocytes can usually be identified in this fluid.

The commonest neoplastic changes involving the liver are **secondary metastases** from malignancies elsewhere. Secondary tumours occurring in the liver substance are usually blood born but local trans-peritoneal metastasis, such as occurs with **gastric squamous cell carcinoma** (*see* **154**), is possible. Secondary tumours of all types are usually multiple, arising from hematogenous spread from a primary lesion elsewhere. Gastric squamous cell carcinoma (*see* **154**) occurs relatively frequently and often involves local direct, and hematogenous, spread to the liver. **Secondary hemangiosarcoma** lesions in the liver are soft or spongy, poorly defined and contain dark hemorrhagic amorphous tumour tissue (**175**).

Part 2: The Peritoneum and Pancreas

Infectious Disorders

The horse has long been considered, perhaps unjusti-fiably, to be particularly prone to **peritonitis**, especially following laparotomy. However, peritonitis may arise spontaneously and is always potentially extremely serious. **Focal peritonitis** (*see* **144**) or **diffuse fibrinous peritonitis** (*see* **176**) are relatively common and where the inflammation extends to the parietal peritoneum affected horses show a characteristic reluctance to move, stretching (**Plate 1c**, page 44), a tense 'boarded' abdomen and pain and resentment on abdominal palpation. **Spontaneous or iatrogenic rupture of the intestine or stomach** generally result in a **catastrophic diffuse peritonitis** (*see* **109**) which may be detected by abdominocentesis (**Plate 2g**, page 47) and by rectal examination when a granular, gritty feeling is detected, with an impression of abnormal freedom of movement within the abdominal cavity. Usually, in catastrophic cases the extent of peritonitis is masked by overwhelming endotoxic shock. Rectal examination of infected or long standing cases of peritonitis give an impression of lack of abdominal mobility, probably due to the extensive adhesions which develop between the loops of small intestine (**176**) and extensive binding-down of the large colon to the abdominal wall.

Abscesses within the peritoneal cavity may affect both the liver and other abdominal organs and are usually a sequel to either bacteremic conditions, such as **disseminated (Bastard) Strangles** (*Streptococcus equi* septicemia) and **tuberculosis**, or **penetrating wounds from the abdominal wall or from penetrations of the gut**, such as occurs after **cecal perforations** and **rectal tears**, or from surgical interferences such as **castration**. Most abdominal abscesses remain discrete and may reach considerable size (*see* **125**). The clinical signs of peritoneal abscesses are usually vague and ill-defined. They may be detected by rectal examination and they frequently involve the cecal head (*see* **125**) and/or the spleen. A detectable lack of mobility of a normally mobile organ within the peritoneal cavity may indicate the presence of adhesions between it and other organs or to the parietal peritoneum and, in some cases, this arises from abscesses in the wall of the intestine, the cecum or other abdominal organs. Rupture of peritoneal abscesses causes either a focal or diffuse peritonitis and

176

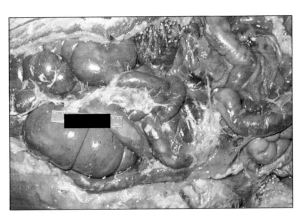

176 Diffuse fibrinous peritonitis.

unless intestinal contents are involved the former are more common.

Both **acute and chronic pancreatitis** have been encountered in the horse. **Acute pancreatic failure** causes a fulminating and rapidly progressive shock and endotoxemia with severe colic, gastric distension (*see* **Plate 1h**) and cardiovascular compromise. These signs are also encountered in cases of anterior enteritis (*see* **139,140**) and, indeed the two conditions may be inter-related or co-exist making specific diagnosis even more difficult. Voluminous gastric reflux (**Plate 1h**, page 45) is usually obtained. Peritoneal fluid is darkly hemorrhagic, brown coloured and flocculent, and may be seen to contain large and small globules of free fat. Fortunately the disorder is rare but may be under diagnosed as it is most difficult to confirm before death

and the signs are not specific. At post mortem examination, the pancreas is diffusely "mushy" with a dark and often gaseous texture. *Clostridia* spp. bacteria may be identifiable.

Chronic pancreatic failure results in exocrine pancreatic insufficiency. Affected horses suffer from weight loss and maldigestion but these aspects are masked by the particular characteristics of the horses digestive tract. Acute or sub-acute episodes accompanied by peritonitis, colic and laminitis may be superimposed upon the chronically failing pancreas. Post mortem examination shows the pancreas to be severely atrophied. Both acute and chronic pancreatic disease are fortunately extremely rare, and there are few helpful clinical features; most cases are diagnosed at laparotomy or, more often, at post mortem examination.

Neoplastic Disorders

Primary (or secondary) pancreatic neoplasia is very rarely encountered in the horse. The clinical effects include non-specific signs of weight loss, diarrhea, icterus and fever.

Mesothelioma involving the peritoneal cavity (and occasionally the pleural cavity) is more common and is associated, usually, with the development of massive

numbers of discrete lesions on the parietal and visceral peritoneal (and pleural) surfaces (**177**). Clinically, affected horses show a progressive anemia and massive peritoneal effusion of a brown pigmented fluid (**Plate 2h**, page 47) in which abnormal mesothelial cells can be identified. Involvement of the liver substance is not usual, however.

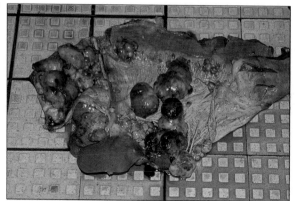

177 Mesothelioma (peritoneal).
Note: Extensive peritoneal fluid (**Plate 2h**, page 47), no hepatic involvement. Further secondary lesions in pleural and pericardial cavities.

Further reading

Problems in Equine Medicine
Brown, C.M. (1989) Lea & Febiger, Philadelphia, USA
Current Therapy in Equine Medicine (1)
Ed Robinson, N.E. (1987), W B Saunders, Philadelphia, USA
Current Therapy in Equine Medicine (2)
Ed Robinson, N.E. (1992), W B Saunders, Philadelphia, USA

Manual of Equine Practice
Rose, R.J., and Hodgson, D.R. (1993)
WB Saunders, Philadelphia
Equine Clinical Neonatology
Koterba, A.M., Drummond, W.H., and Kosch, P.C. (1990) Lea & Febiger, Philadelphia, USA

3. Conditions of the respiratory tract

Developmental Disorders

Foals born with mild **deviations of the nose (178)** seldom show any significant effects on breathing, but where the extent of the deviation is severe, there may be marked unilateral (or occasionally bilateral) respiratory obstruction and obvious prehension and mastication difficulties (*see* **3,4**). Air flow through the nostrils will then be markedly asymmetric. Gross distortions of the nares and/or the rostral structures of the nasal cavity occur occasionally as developmental abnormalities. While most are minor and of cosmetic significance some are much more severe and liable to induce life-threatening respiratory difficulties.

Hypoplasia of the nasal turbinate bones is occasionally seen during routine endoscopy and although in some cases it is profound in extent the effect upon the animal is minimal.

Congenital persistence of thyroglossal remnants is usually presented as a **sub-epiglottic cyst (Plate 5h,** page 112) and is occasionally encountered in new born foals. The presence of the cyst at this site may have little effect upon the well-being of the animal and may be detected incidentally at any age during endoscopic examination of the pharynx. In foals, the major presenting signs are coughing (a result of inhalation of food material), inspiratory dyspnea (from obstruction of the *aditus laryngis*), a nasal discharge which commonly contains milk or other food particles, and inhalation pneumonia. Affected foals may be reported to collapse dramatically when attempting to suckle. The cysts may be relatively small in the early years of life but commonly enlarge slowly with time and therefore a progressively deteriorating respiratory noise with exercise limitations develops. Epiglottic cysts are quite frequently detected at a later age, during investigation of respiratory noises or poor performance. Often, they are only detected when horses are required to perform. While some cases show no clinical effect, passing unnoticed for years, others may cough or may even be markedly dyspneic at rest. The cyst may be sufficiently large as to almost occlude the pharynx, although most lie beneath the epiglottis being spherical and between 1 and 5 cm in diameter **(Plate 5h,** page 112). They usually contain a thick viscid mucus. Cysts located in the sub-epiglottic tissue may not always be visible while the epiglottis is in its natural position relative to the soft palate, being located under the rostral palatine border. Swallowing will, in these cases, usually reveal the cystic structure which may in some cases, be flaccid and appear only momentarily from beneath the epiglottis. Concurrent epiglottic entrapment in the redundant folds of mucosa surrounding the cyst is often found with this form **(Plate 5i,** page 113). Sub-epiglottic cysts in adult horses may produce signs of dysphagia and nasal discharge but contrary to those occurring in foals they seldom produce inhalation (aspiration) pneumonia. Horses in which the epiglottis is very prominent and apparently upright, giving the impression of being tightly held by the rostral border of the soft palate **(Plate 5j,** page 113), may be so because of an epiglottic cyst under the soft palate. In most such cases, however, no cyst can be identified and radiographic examination will usually confirm or deny their existence. Where no cyst is present the position of the larynx relative to the soft palate is regarded as a normal variant.

Pharyngeal cysts may be located in the mucosa of the dorsal naso-pharynx and these tend to be larger **(179)**. Such a cyst is not directly visible endoscopically, but symmetric or asymmetric dorsal pharyngeal compression, which is not attributable to guttural pouch enlargement, is visible and lateral radiographs of the pharynx confirm their presence. Concurrent developmental defects of the epiglottis are sometimes present and these influence the clinical effects and endoscopic and radiographic appearance. Repeated dorsal displacement of the soft palate may be present **(Plate 5a,** page 111), possibly as a result of inadequate free rostral length **(Plate 5k,** page 113) or inadequate stiffness of the epiglottis **(Plate 5l,** page 113).

Epidermal inclusion cysts (atheroma) are characteristically located in the caudo-dorsal area of the nasal diverticulum (false nostril) **(180)**. These spherical structures are usually unilateral and 2 – 5 cm in diameter, but in unusual circumstances may be bilateral and much larger. They are only of cosmetic significance. The cysts are soft, fluctuant and non-painful but may also have a firm texture giving the impression, on palpation, of a solid mass. They may be moveable in the surrounding tissue or relatively fixed, and contain a sterile, grey, creamy, odourless, thick material.

Congenital disorders of the nasal cavities and paranasal sinuses are very rare. However, unilocular or, more usually multilocular, fluid-filled **maxillary cysts** may be encountered within the paranasal sinuses in

178

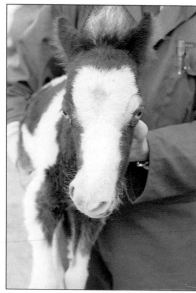

179

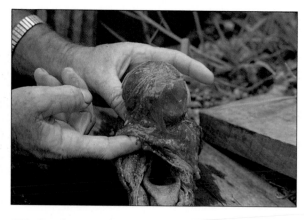

178 Developmental nasal deviation (mild) ('Squiffy/Wry nose').

179 Pharyngeal cyst.
Note: Large cystic structure in dorsal pharyngeal wall. Responsible for respiratory noise and dorsal pharyngeal compression in a 3-year-old Thoroughbred presented for investigation of poor performance. The cyst was not visible endoscopically, but could be identified on lateral radiographs.

180

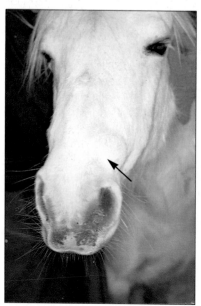

181

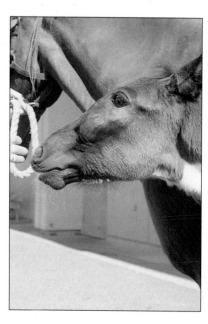

180 Nasal atheroma (dermal inclusion cyst) (arrow).

181 Maxillary sinus cyst (Developmental)
Note: Progressive maxillary distortion and increasing dyspnea - emergency tracheostomy tube inserted.

young foals (**181**). The caudal compartment of the maxillary sinus is most often affected but the cysts may extend from here into the frontal sinus. They are possibly related to the germ buds of the permanent cheek teeth, although most affected foals show no developmental dental defect in later life. Congenital cysts are obvious at birth or develop in the first few weeks of life. Very large cysts have a significant effect upon the nasal cavity and facial appearance (*see* **181**). Progressive enlargement results in a worsening obstruction of the nasal cavity and displacement of the nasal septum (**182**) which can be identified by ventro-dorsal radiographs. Distortion of the maxilla and the nasal cavity, with bony resorption and dental defects, may result (*see* **182**). The clinical effects are largely dependent upon the extent of dental and nasal distortion. Where the erupting premolar teeth are grossly displaced by progressive bone resorption, foals may show difficulty with mastication; food material accumulating in the sides of the mouth. There may also be some loss of solid food from the mouth (quidding) but there is usually no difficulty with suckling, except where the hard palate is also distorted (**182**). They often have a marked effect on respiratory function when the

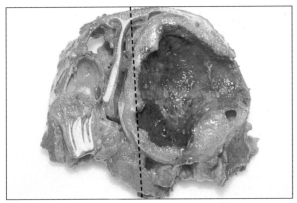

182 Maxillary sinus cyst (Developmental).
Note: Same case as 181. Single fluid filled cavity with spongy mucosal lining. Severe occlusion of ipsilateral nostril and deviation of nasal septum to occlude contralateral nostril. The mid-line is shown by the dotted line.

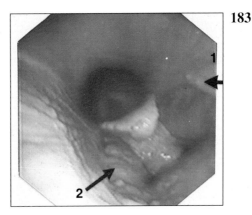

183 Aplasia of soft palate (Complete).
Note: Remnants of palatal shelves (arrow 1) and prominent sublingual lymphoid hyperplasia (arrow 2). Mare presented at 4 years of age with dysphagia and severe proximal tracheal contamination (**Plate 4m**, page104).

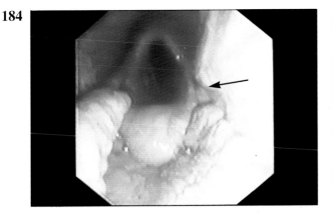

184 Unilateral hypoplasia of soft palate.
Note: Single (left) palatal shelf absent (arrow). Dorsal displacement of 'normal' palatal shelf above epiglottis

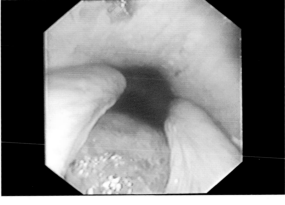

185 Cleft soft palate.
Note: Both palatal shelves present but no fusion. Food material in oropharynx and nasopharynx.

distortion of the nasal cavity is sufficient to result in occlusion of both nasal cavities (**182**). While most of these cysts have a thick spongy epithelial lining others have a thinner mucosal lining (**182**). In both types, incomplete plates of bone are often present. The cyst itself is usually filled with a sterile, turbid, yellowish fluid with little or no odour. Radiographically, fluid filled structures, with multiple air-fluid interfaces, soft tissue mineralisation and gross deviations of the nasal septum are characteristic. Dental distortions and nasal cavity occlusion may be evident endoscopically. Very similar structures occur in horses over 9 years of age (*see* **267, 268**). There is little evidence to suggest that the latter are developmental cysts which have lain dormant, and they may be more related to ethmoidal hematomas (*see* **259 et seq.**) which are encountered relatively frequently in adult horses.

The **congenital absence of an effective naso-maxillary opening** creates a discrete single-structured secretory cyst within the affected maxillary sinus, and lined by the normal sinus mucous membrane, known as a **mucocele**. In these cases, the contents of the cyst are thick and mucoid but, in contrast to the sinus cysts and infected sinuses, are usually clear and sterile. They may be difficult to differentiate from maxillary cysts but, radiographically, gas-fluid interfaces are not usually present. Facial deformity is often marked and, as most occur in the rostral maxillary sinus, facial swelling over the third and fourth cheek teeth in foals up to 6 months of age is suggestive of the presence of a mucocele.

Hypoplasia and clefts of the soft palate are relatively frequent congenital defects of the horse. The defect may be hereditary in some cases. The extent of the deficit in the soft palate may be marked where there

186

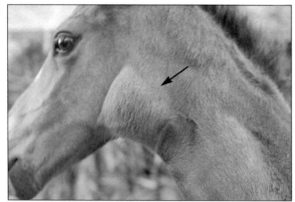

187

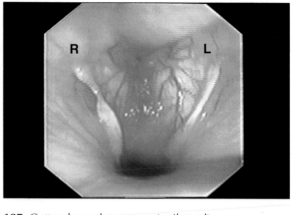

186 Guttural pouch tympany.
Note: Obvious swelling (tympanitic) below tendon of *Sternocephalicus* muscle (arrow).
Differential Diagnosis:
i) Guttural pouch empyema
ii) Strangles
iii) Esophageal cyst
iv) Salivary mucocele

187 Guttural pouch tympany (unilateral).
Note: Curled ostium of right auditive (eustachian) tube. This failed to open effectively during low pressure phase of swallowing. Left side normal.

is a **uniform hypoplasia of the whole soft palate (183)**. Lesser clefts involving **unilateral hypoplasia** of a single palatal shelf only **(184)**, or the **failure of fusion of the soft palate** in the mid-line with normal palatal shelves (**true cleft**) may be encountered **(185)**. The failure of fusion of the soft palate represents a significantly different developmental problem from unilateral or bilateral hypoplasia. In the former, which arise as a result of failure of developmental fusion (which normally starts at the rostral end of the palatal shelf), concurrent clefts of the hard palate are often encountered (*see* **1**). In the latter, which is less usual, there is clearly no opportunity for fusion to occur at all. The two disorders, therefore, represent different embryological abnormalities. Typically, clefts of the soft palate alone or hypoplasia of one (or both) palatal shelf(ves) induce post-prandial, nasal regurgitation of food/milk in the same way as clefts of the hard palate (*see* **2**), but there is usually less nasal regurgitation during the actual process of suckling. Although serious or extensive soft palate cleft or hypoplasia may be directly visible from the mouth, in the absence of intercurrent clefts of the hard palate, oral inspection may not reveal the extent of the lesion and endoscopic examination is usually essential. Intercurrent epiglottic entrapment is frequently present. Affected foals usually fail to thrive or succumb to inhalation pneumonia at an early age. However, in spite of severe tracheal contamination (**Plate 4m**, page 104), some cases survive reasonably well into adult life, showing little or no hindrance to growth or maturity for many years.

Ultimately, however, aspiration pneumonia develops, and a normal life-span is not to be expected.

Guttural pouch tympany is a common, possibly developmental, disorder involving usually one (but occasionally both) of the openings (ostia) and/or the pharyngeal component of the auditive tube in the nasopharynx. The condition occurs predominately in young Thoroughbred foals, with a preponderance of females being affected. One (or both) ostium(ia) appears to become an effective 'one-way' valve, allowing air to pass into, but not out of, the guttural pouch (diverticulum of the auditive tube). The defect in function may be a result of inflammatory changes in the mucosa of the opening, but excessive tissue/mucosal bulk in the auditive tube or around the ostium, may be responsible. Many cases, however, show no detectable physical abnormality or any evidence of inflammation, suggesting that the problem is functional rather than anatomical. Clinically, within the first few weeks of life (but occasionally up to one year of age) affected foals develop a prominent, non-painful, non-elastic, tympanitic distension in the parotid region **(186)**. The extent of the swelling may be variable, and, while it is more usual for the condition to affect one side only, both sides of the pharynx may be swollen. The swelling from the affected side in unilateral cases often results in a bulging of the (normal) contralateral side and in some cases, the pharyngeal deformity so created results in an effective occlusion of the unaffected ostium and auditive tube, resulting in a secondary tympany. The extent of unilateral swelling may be such that a bilateral condition

188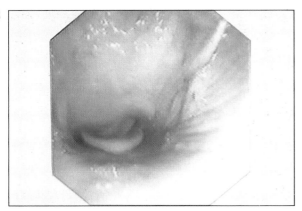

189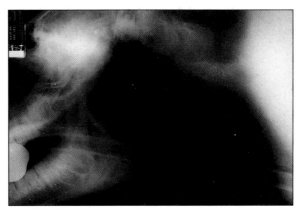

188 Guttural pouch tympany (dorsal pharyngeal compression).
Note: Collapse of pharyngeal vault onto larynx causing distortion of arytenoids and occlusion of *aditus laryngis*.
Differential Diagnosis:
i) Guttural pouch empyema
ii) Pharyngeal paralysis (bilateral)
iii) Hemorrhage in guttural pouch
iv) Pharyngeal abscess/necrosis
v) Dorsal pharyngeal cyst
vi) Strangles

189 Guttural pouch tympany (bilateral) (lateral radiograph).
Note: Grossly enlarged, air-filled, guttural pouches extending to fourth cervical vertebra. Marked dorsal pharyngeal compression - Note: relationship of roof of pharynx to endotracheal tube.

is suspected. The swelling is generally somewhat more ventral than might be expected because of the overlying *sternocephalicus* tendon (*see* **186**). Dynamic endoscopic examination of the pharynx during deglutition in these foals suggests that neurological dysfunction may be involved, with the ostium only opening during the high pressure phase of swallowing. The free border of the ostia are often slightly curled in these cases (**187**), and noticeably fail to open effectively during the low pressure (second) phase of swallowing, as the larynx is lowered. Stertorous (noisy) breathing and possibly dysphagia with nasal regurgitation of food, as a result of dorsal pharyngeal compression or distortion may be evident (**188**), particularly if the neck is flexed. Suckling foals may have considerable difficulty feeding from the mare and sometimes adopt bizarre feeding positions in an attempt to limit the pharyngeal distortion and allow normal swallowing. The full extent of the problem can be clearly identified and differentiated from other causes of parotid swelling and pharyngeal compression by lateral radiographs. The gas-filled, grossly distended pouch(es) will be clearly seen beyond the normal limit at the second cervical vertebra (axis). In severely affected foals, the affected pouch may extend to the level of the fourth cervical vertebra or even lower (**189**). In the absence of intercurrent infection or fluid accumulation, no air-fluid interface or solid content will be detectable. Endoscopically, the lining of the pouch is generally diffusely inflamed and the pouch is obviously

distended, although introduction of the endoscope results in instantaneous collapse of the swelling. Relief of one side without simultaneous resolution on the other is indicative of bilateral tympany.

The Thoroughbred has been shown to be prone to what is believed to be a developmental **epiglottic hypoplasia** which may be diagnosed where the epiglottis appears, endoscopically, to be visibly short (**Plate 5k**, page 113), or when it appears to be flaccid (**Plate 5l**, page 113) regardless of the length (which may be normal or, in some cases, greater than normal). Lateral radiographs of the pharynx will also identify the shortened epiglottic cartilage which can usually be measured accurately, making allowances for magnification. The normal epiglottic length is 8 – 9 cm and an abnormal shortening is usually associated with a length of less than 7 cm. These animals appear to be particularly liable to epiglottic entrapment (**Plate 5m; Plate 5n**, page 113) and dorsal displacement of the soft palate (laryngopalatal dislocation) (**Plate 5a**, page 111). There are few significant primary effects from epiglottic hypoplasia itself, with most of the secondary consequences affecting performance through airway distortions and displacements. Dysphagia and a marked tendency to mouth breathing may be encountered, but both of these are likely to be secondary to displacement of the soft palate, and failure to close the nasopharynx effectively during deglutition. Diagnosis of the disorder is not always easy and there is some doubt as to whether the condition exists at all. Dynamic, endoscopic airway studies performed during treadmill work are often necessary to confirm the effects of the hypoplasia.

Abnormalities of the shape of the thyroid cartilage, arising secondarily to a developmental abnormality of the fourth branchial arch, have been blamed for the development of the severe forms of **rostral displacement of the palatopharyngeal arch**. The condition is important with respect to abnormal respiratory noises and poor exercise tolerance and it is easily recognised endoscopically **(Plate 5d**, page 111). Most cases are only detected when extra exercise-demands are placed upon them, and they can not open the *aditus laryngis* to allow an increased air supply. Affected horses show a severe limitation to exercise with harsh rasping inspiratory (and often expiratory) sounds which are localised around the larynx.

Miniature horses and pony breeds, including the Shetland, are prone to developmental malformation of the trachea known as **'Scabbard Trachea'** or 'collapsed trachea'. The latter name possibly gives the wrong impression of the congenital disorder in which the trachea is flattened ventro-dorsally **(190)** or, more rarely, laterally. Limited lengths of the trachea are affected but longer lengths are sometimes involved. The passage of a food bolus through the esophagus can be appreciated during tracheal endoscopy due to the flaccid dorsal ligament which replaces part of the normally solid cartilaginous ring. Some cases are found to have intact tracheal rings with a marked flattening and sharp angles at each side (*see* **190**). While it is almost certainly a developmental abnormality, it is usually found incidentally during endoscopic examination (or post mortem examination) of mature ponies. It appears to cause little or no detectable effect upon respiratory function, perhaps because of the limited exercise demand on most of these animals. Some cases do, however, show a harsh grating respiratory noise on both inspiration and expiration, which is exacerbated on exertion, and a few may cough. Extreme respiratory embarrassment may be encountered, particularly where intercurrent respiratory disease, with airway inflammation and edema, is present. The **acquired (trauma-induced) form of tracheal collapse** is, however, often accompanied by paroxysmal, harsh coughing and obvious inspiratory and expiratory noises and is, naturally, not restricted to the pony breeds.

Spiral deformity of the trachea is a developmental abnormality, also primarily affecting the miniature breeds, in which the tracheal rings take on a spiral contour **(191)**. This is usually more prominent in the proximal cervical trachea. Again there are seldom any clinical effects, being found incidentally during respiratory tract endoscopy or post mortem examination.

190

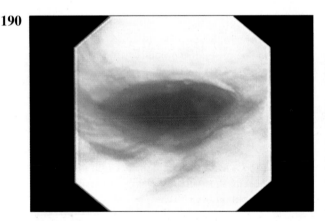

190 Scabbard trachea.

191

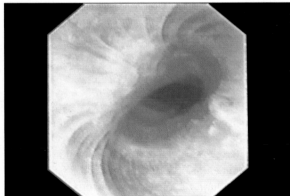

191 Spiral trachea.

Non-Infectious Disorders

Foreign bodies lodged in the nasal cavity are unusual in the horse, and result in a unilateral nasal discharge of acute onset, often with small amounts of fresh blood **(Plate 7f, page 144)**. Affected horses show considerable discomfort, being head-shy and snorting a great deal. Sneezing is unusual in the horse under any circumstances. Untreated cases may result in local abscesses or the development of mineralised concretions within the nasal cavity and a foul-smelling breath from the affected nostril.

Thorny twigs, brush bristles, and other sharp objects lodging in the pharynx are possibly more common than foreign bodies within the nasal cavity. They usually result in an acute-onset dysphagia and more or less respiratory obstruction. The clinical signs will, however, depend largely upon the type of foreign body involved. Large solid objects such as pieces of apple would be expected to have marked effects upon respiration, particularly on inspiration and the effects are consequently dramatic and of peracute onset. In most cases these are transient with the object dislodging spontaneously and resolution is immediate and complete. In some cases, however, the object appears to be firmly lodged and a life threatening respiratory obstruction may be presented. Short, thorny twigs are a relatively common **foreign body in the pharynx** of horses **(192)** and are most often derived from hay; normal horses seldom voluntarily eat woody or thorny vegetation. Horses which, however, habitually chew wooden fences and doors are also liable to pharyngeal obstructions as a result of pieces of wood. Sharp, small foreign-bodies present little immediate threat to life and do not often cause respiratory embarrassment. However, an acute onset of severe and distressing difficulties with swallowing are frequently presented. The affected horse presents with nasal regurgitation of food material and saliva **(Plate 6o, page 123)** and attempts to drink are accompanied by nasal regurgitation, squealing and arching of the neck. Occasionally unilateral (or in some cases bilateral) epistaxis is present **(Plate 7f, page 144)**.

Tracheal foreign bodies are unusual but are sometimes surprisingly large. The inhalation of small grass seeds and particles of dust and grass is common when horses are exercised hard under appropriate conditions. These seldom cause any marked effect and coughing is usually sufficient to dislodge the foreign matter. A residual tracheitis may be present for a day or two thereafter. Plant twigs represent a relatively common tracheal foreign body **(193)** and are often responsible for an acute onset of a severe and frequently paroxysmal coughing. Tracheal hemorrhage is usual and there is often some inflammation and reflex spasm of the airway **(193)**. Where plant twigs are inhaled into the bronchial tree their location may be very difficult and only painstaking endoscopy will establish the site and character of the object. It is sometimes possible to trace the hemorrhage but inflammation is extensive. Foreign bodies of this type and size which are not retrieved become firmly lodged within the airway and create a persistent site of irritation, inflammation and abscess formation.

Traumatic lesions involving the facial bones result in almost infinitely variable distortions of the shape of the

192

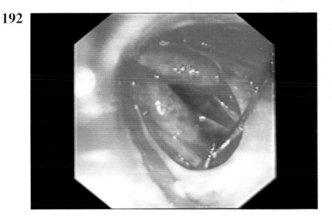

193

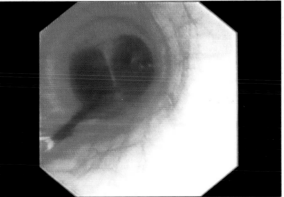

192 Pharyngeal foreign body.
Note: Dorsal displacement of soft palate unable to correct. Marked inflammation and hemorrhage. Unilateral epistaxis was present.

193 Tracheal foreign body.
Note: Acute inflammation of carina and reflex spasm of bronchi.

head, often as a consequence of depression fractures of the facial, frontal, nasal and maxillary bones. The extent of the fractures can be defined by careful lateral and appropriate oblique radiographs. Evidence for caudal maxillary (and frontal) sinus involvement can be obtained from endoscopic examination of the common drainage pathway of these sinuses in the caudal nasal cavity (**194**). Facial trauma may also impair the drainage from the maxillary and/or frontal sinuses. Injuries involving the sinuses or the nasal turbinate bones are usually accompanied by slight, moderate (**Plate 7f**, page 144) or heavy bleeding (**Plate 7i**, page 145) from the ipsilateral nostril. The immediate consequences of such injuries are related primarily to the bleeding and to any consequent nasal edema and swelling. Sufficient damage to result in an effective occlusion of both nostrils is, fortunately very rare, even in cases with gross facial damage. Even considerable nasal bleeding seldom seems to result in marked distress, although affected animals will understandably resent handling of the face. Physically and radiographically, such cases may present with bizarre anatomy which may appear to be dramatic but the external deformity might represent a relatively minor part of the consequences of such trauma. Relatively minor trauma to the facial bones (*see* **665**) commonly results in damage to, or disruption of, the bony portion of the nasolacrimal duct which may be occluded, resulting in epiphora, or may be totally disrupted (*see* **666**), in which case epiphora may not be a prominent sign. Consequent sinus empyema (**195**), involving either of the maxillary sinuses and/or the frontal sinuses, represents a serious complication of failure of drainage and infection following traumatic injuries to the face. In most cases involving nasal cavity or sinus trauma, therefore, the secondary effects may be far more serious than the obvious facial deformity which is, itself, only of cosmetic significance.

Most traumatic episodes involving the nasal cavity result in severe hemorrhage from disruption of nasal turbinate bones (**Plate 7i**, page 145). Significant epistaxis is usually obvious but only more severe trauma will cause extensive turbinate damage. However, iatrogenic damage from misdirected nasogastric tubes may cause severe hemorrhage within the ipsilateral nostril (**Plate 7i**, page 145). Usually this follows introduction of the nasogastric tube into the middle, rather than the ventral, meatus of the nose, and the damage typically involves the ethmoturbinate region.

The identification of the source of **epistaxis** in the horse is clinically very important. Unilateral hemorrhages may be associated with small (**Plate 7g**, page 144) or larger (**Plate 7h**, page 145), venous bleeding within the ipsilateral nasal cavity or from the ipsilateral guttural pouch. Bilateral epistaxis however, may be a result of simultaneous damage causing bleeding in both nasal cavities (**Plate 6f**, page 121) or to hemorrhagic disorders (**Plate 6g**, page 121) or to arterial (**Plate 6h**, page 121) or venous (**Plate 6i**, page 121) (**Plate 6j**, page 121) hemorrhage from structures caudal to the nasopharynx. Heavy (particularly arterial) bleeding from one guttural pouch or from one nasal cavity may also produce bilateral epistaxis (**Plate 6h**, page 121).

Traumatic damage to the respiratory tract caudal to the nasal cavity is rarely encountered but foreign bodies lodged within the pharynx (*see* **192**) may cause serious, protracted and sometimes permanent damage to the laryngeal cartilages, in particular, including **chondritis of the arytenoid corniculate process (Plate 5q; Plate 5r**, page 114). While some cases have definite or implied histories of pharyngeal foreign bodies, many cases of **corniculate chondritis** do not. Severe chondritis of one or both cartilages is encountered relatively frequently in young Thoroughbred horses, in particular, perhaps as a secondary consequence of respiratory tract infections. In most cases both arytenoid cartilages are affected (**Plate 5s**, page 115), although the extent of involvement of the two may be markedly different with one severely and the other relatively mildly affected (**Plate 5r**, page 115). There may be obvious granulation tissue projecting into the airway

194

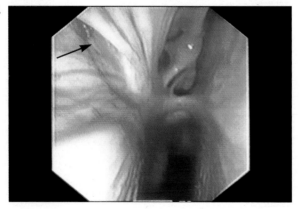

194 Facial trauma (hemorrhage from maxillary sinus)(arrow).
Differential Diagnosis:
i)   Maxillary sinus cyst
ii) Hemorrhagic diatheses
iii) Sinus aspergillosis

195

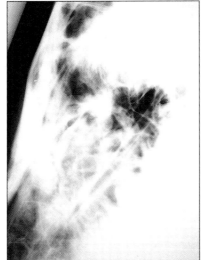

196

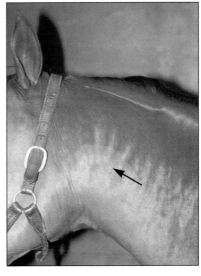

195 Facial trauma (fracture nasal/maxillary and frontal bones).
Note: Maxillary sinus empyema (loss of air content of maxillary sinuses).

196 Ruptured trachea.
Note: Subcutaneous emphysema (and edema) of neck (note: hand imprint (arrow)) due to traumatic dislocation of crico-tracheal ligament.
Differential Diagnosis:
i) Clostridial myositis
ii) Pharyngeal necrosis
iii) Retro-pharyngeal abscess
iv) Anthrax

from the mucosa overlying the corniculate process (**Plate 5r**, page 115). The central portion of the arytenoid cartilage may become necrotic and cavitated, and sinus tracts open from the granuloma and adjacent tissue into the airway. Some pharyngeal and perilaryngeal abscesses arise directly from corniculate chondritis. A significant loss of effective abduction arises from concurrent involvement of the adjacent abductor muscles and the crico-arytenoid articulation on one (**Plate 5q**, page 114), or both sides (**Plate 5s**, page 115), and from the marked thickening of the cartilage and overlying mucosa (**Plate 5s**, page 115). This results in the appearance of a flaccid *aditus laryngis* with collapse of one or both arytenoids into the airway. On some occasions the *aditus laryngis* may be reduced to a mere slit (**Plate 5s**, page 115) with neither abduction nor adduction ability. There are consequently severe limitation upon respiratory function. The clinical effects of the disorder are, therefore, usually related to the acute onset of respiratory obstruction. However, in some cases, it may be insidious in onset, progressing slowly over some weeks. In these cases corniculate chondritis is discovered while investigating poor performance and/or abnormal inspiratory noises. Individuals with less demand upon airway efficiency may show no overt signs until pharyngeal abscesses develop. Cases in which there is extensive cartilage destruction develop severe and life-

threatening respiratory obstruction (**Plate 6m**, page 122), with obvious inspiratory and, to a somewhat lesser extent, expiratory dyspnea at rest. Horses affected by right sided laryngeal neuropathy/paralysis (**Plate 5cc**, page 117) should be examined particularly carefully for evidence of chondritis, which may be primarily responsible for the paralysis, although most of these are caused by irritant extra vascular injection in the right jugular groove.

Occasionally, **damage to pharyngeal structures** results from foreign bodies or from iatrogenic injury during laryngeal surgery, with the epiglottis being most often affected (**Plate 5g**, page 112). An appropriate history is usually available to establish the cause and the long-term clinical consequences are usually minimal, in spite of the obvious physical deformity. There may be a tendency to dorsal displacement of the soft palate (**Plate 5a**, page 111) in cases in which the epiglottis is grossly distorted.

Severe (or occasionally minor), blunt trauma to the ventral neck may cause **tracheal fracture** or **avulsion of the tracheo-laryngeal junction**. Disruption of the tracheal mucosa sufficiently to allow air-leakage into the surrounding tissues may be present. **Tracheostomy** is also commonly responsible for the development of secondary **subcutaneous emphysema**, and although the defect in the mucosa of the trachea may be very small e.g. following trans-tracheal aspiration, significant air

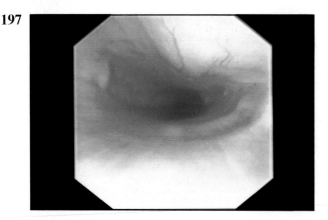

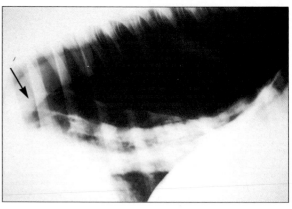

197 Tracheal collapse.
Note: Collapse of limited length of trachea (3 rings), occlusion of nostrils caused collapse to become very obvious.
Differential Diagnosis:
i) Scabbard trachea
ii) Hypoplasia of tracheal rings (food bolus can be seen passing along esophagus and compressing the prominent dorsal tracheal ligament)
iii) Esophageal foreign body
iv) Space occupying mass (particularly if at thoracic inlet)

198 Pneumothorax.
Note: Obvious loss of radiodensity in caudo-dorsal thorax with increased density ventrally and prominent aorta (arrow).

accumulation may also occur. Large amounts of air will result in subcutaneous emphysema **(196)** which can readily be identified as a non-painful crackling under the skin. In spite of considerable air accumulations and local edema, affected horses often show little or no discomfort and there is, at least initially, little systemic response. Extra-lumenal gas in the pharyngeal and cervical tissue is often radiographically obvious in such cases. Small amounts of leaked air migrate distally until, in some cases, a pneumomediastinum is induced, which is much more serious. Complicating infection of the original wound or of the emphysematous tissues (particularly where this is due to gas-producing bacteria such as *Clostridia* spp.) results in a similar appearance, but the difference is clinically obvious, with severe inflammation, pain and reluctance to swallow or bend the neck. Bacterial infection of this type may also be introduced during the use of in-dwelling nasogastric tubes which traumatise the dorsal pharyngeal wall (*see* **80**). Where infection exists, the extent of subcutaneous emphysema is much less and the horse is plainly seriously ill.

The insertion of emergency, or permanent, tracheostomy tubes or traumatic injuries to the trachea are common causes for the development of localised granulation tissue within the trachea. This occurs more particularly when the cartilage rings of the trachea are damaged during the procedure with the resulting tissue

being usually classified as a **chondroma**, but which may only consist of granulation tissue. The healing of tracheostomy wound sites is often accompanied by distortions of the tracheal rings beneath the mucosa, but it is unlikely that these would be responsible for significant impairment of air flow except where consequent tracheal stenosis or collapse develops, following cartilage damage and/or necrosis. Horses with severe inspiratory obstructions within the nasal cavity or pharynx may become affected by spontaneous tracheal collapse due to the high negative pressure of inspiration. In the early stages of this type of disorder the mucosa of the trachea may be visibly loose and edematous **(197)**.

Traumatic injuries involving the chest and its contents are surprisingly unusual, in spite of the apparent superficial severity of some of the injuries. Wounds penetrating the thoracic wall almost always result in **pneumothorax** and subsequent infection of the pleural cavity. However, in some cases pneumothorax may arise from traumatic tearing of the visceral pleura with ingress of air into one or both pleural spaces **(198)**. Pneumothorax may occasionally also arise spontaneously in foals suffering from fetal atelectasis or failure of normal lung inflation at birth. In these foals the visceral pleura is not invariably disrupted initially, and air may accumulate in small or large, subpleural **(199)** or intrapulmonary bullae.

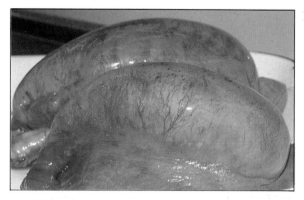

199

199 Subpleural bullae.
Note: Newborn foal presented with severe dyspnea. Primary atelectasis (anectasis, non-expansion of lungs after birth) affected most of lung tissue.

All horses affected by pneumothorax (or more rarely by hemothorax) show moderate to severe dyspnea with an increased abdominal component. Percussion of the chest will establish an abnormal resonance and auscultation will reveal an absence of audible lung sounds over the affected areas. In the event that hemothorax is present the ventral percussible border of the lung is often elevated above the normal level which lies on a line joining the *tuba coxae* (external angle of the ilium) and the point of the elbow.

Multiple, smaller bullae in the lungs are a rare complication of long-standing allergic (or other) respiratory disease and are most often associated with **chronic allergic small airway disease (chronic obstructive pulmonary disease, 'Heaves', COPD)** (*see* **204** *et seq.*) or other disorders resulting in loss of pulmonary compliance (elasticity). Radiographic and ultrasonographic examinations and pleurocentesis are often helpful in the investigation of pneumothorax and accumulations of fluid within the chest.

Racing horses of all breeds are particularly prone to pulmonary bleeding following heavy exercise. Whilst it is probably normal for horses to show some **exercise-induced pulmonary hemorrhage** following extremes of exercise, occasional cases are more severely affected, and some may even die as a result. Young horses in their first year of training are particularly prone to this type of pulmonary bleeding. However, it seldom becomes significant and, indeed, may only be detectable by careful laboratory examination of tracheal aspirates. The etiology of the disorder is equivocal, but spontaneous physical disruption of lung tissue is one of the possible factors in the pathogenesis. Furthermore, the condition is more common, in all its forms, in horses suffering from other lung or airway pathology, and in particular, those suffering from either chronic small airway disease (chronic obstructive pulmonary disease / allergic lung disease / allergic bronchitis) (*see* **204** *et seq.*) or from **idiopathic laryngeal neuropathy (Plate 5u** *et seq.*, page 115). The

combination of physical disruption of areas of lung where movement is greatest, and a concurrent loss of elasticity, as a result of other pulmonary pathology, seems to be the most likely etiopathogenesis. The relationship between exercise-induced pulmonary hemorrhage and chronic airway disorders is reasonably well established, but it is also clear that not all horses affected with one condition will inevitably suffer from the other. Characteristically, severely affected horses show moderate or severe post-exercise, bilateral epistaxis. In most such horses the bleeding is bright red (**Plate 6h**, page 121) and evident within 30 minutes of exercise. In rare extreme cases, horses may die either during or immediately after racing with extreme arterial-like epistaxis and cyanosis. The horse may pull up suddenly and large amounts of fresh, bright-red, blood are evident immediately. The chest and neck of the horse (as well as the rider) may be spattered with blood on completion of the race. Some affected horses show poor performance throughout the race, while others may 'tail-off' dramatically while others may 'pull-up'. Affected horses are often described by the rider as having "gurgled, "swallowed" or "choked-up". There are, however, other possible causes of this type of report from riders including dorsal displacement of the soft palate (**Plate 5a**, page 111) and epiglottic entrapment (**Plate 5m**, page 113). Milder degrees of exercised-induced pulmonary hemorrhage are commonly detected, endoscopically, in apparently normal racing and other performance horses, without any detectable clinical effect. Endoscopic examination of acute 'lung-bleeders' usually shows moderate to severe intra-tracheal bleeding, which may be seen to originate from one (**Plate 4f**, page 103) or both lungs. In milder cases bilateral epistaxis is often detected and will, most often, be posturally related (**Plate 6i**, page 121) or, alternatively, may be inapparent, with no overt epistaxis. The nasal evidence of pulmonary bleeding may only become apparent some 24 hours after racing, and under these circumstances, blood may be found in or around water buckets or on-floor feeding troughs. The posture related

Plate 4

Note: Tracheal fluids accumulate at thoracic inlet i.e. at most dependent point of trachea. Clearance from this site is reliant upon coughing, mucociliary escalator, postural drainage and inspissation.

a
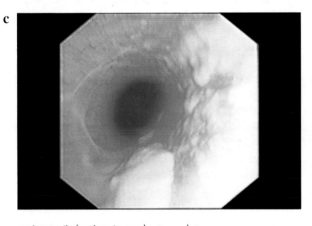

b
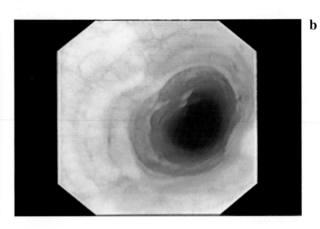

a Acute (infectious) tracheitis.
Differential Diagnosis:
i)   Acute viral rhinotracheitis (equine herpes virus, equine influenza)
ii)   Acute irritation (smoke etc)

b Acute purulent exudate.
Differential Diagnosis:
i)   Bacterial (*Streptococcus* spp) secondary infection (following virus)
ii)   *Rhodococcus equi* infection

c
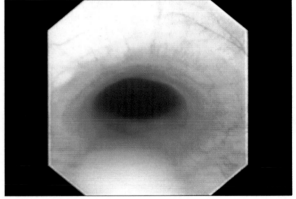

d

c Acute (infectious) purulent exudate.
Differential Diagnosis:
i)   Strangles (*Streptococcus equi*)
ii)   False Strangles (*Streptococcus zooepidemicus*)
iii)   *Rhodococcus equi* infection (pulmonary form)
iv)   Inhalation pneumonia
v)   Pleuritis/bronchopneumonia
vi)   Iatrogenic (following McKay-Marks Operation)

d Catarrhal exudate.
Differential Diagnosis:
i)   (Chronic) small airway disease
ii)   Chronic tracheal irritation (smoke, noxious gas)

Plate 4

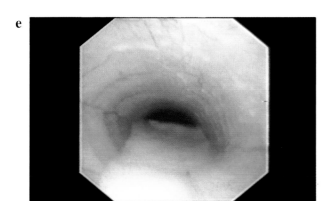

e Muco-purulent exudate.
Differential Diagnosis:
i)   (Chronic) small airway disease
ii) Pulmonary edema
iii) African horse sickness
iv) Congestive heart failure

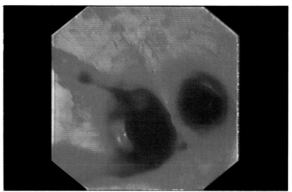

f Acute (fresh) tracheal (bronchial) hemorrhage.
Differential Diagnosis:
i)   Exercise induced pulmonary hemorrhage (<12 hours post exercise)
ii) Pulmonary arterial rupture

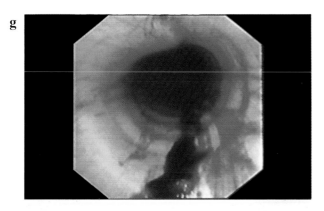

g Tracheal hemorrhage (static, dark).
Differential Diagnosis:
i)   Exercise induced pulmonary hemorrhage (24–36 hours)

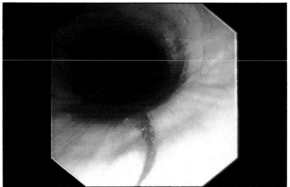

h Tracheal hemorrhage (serosanguineous, scanty, dark).
Differential Diagnosis:
i)   Exercise induced pulmonary hemorrhage (36–72 hours)
ii) Clotting disorders

i (Scanty) serosanguineous tracheal fluid.
Differential Diagnosis:
i)   Exercise induced pulmonary hemorrhage (72–144 hours)
ii) Pulmonary neoplasia
iii) Hemorrhagic diatheses (purpura hemorrhagica, thrombocytopenic purpura, clotting disorders)

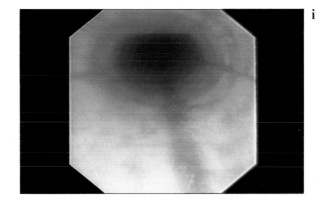

Plate 4

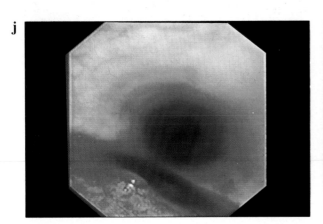

j (Profuse) serosanguineous tracheal fluid.
Differential Diagnosis:
i) Pulmonary/tracheal neoplasia
ii) Exercise induced pulmonary hemorrhage with (chronic) small airway disease
iii) Warfarin poisoning

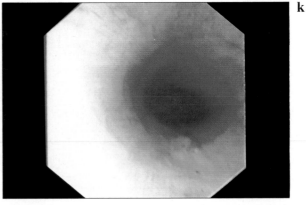

k Foreign material (scanty).
Differential Diagnosis:
i) Normal after heavy exercise in dusty or other environment
ii) Mild dysphagia (eg pharyngeal foreign body)

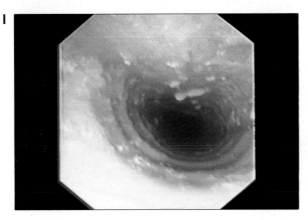

l Tracheal food-contamination.
Differential Diagnosis:
i)   Dysphagia (neurological or physical)
ii) Choke
iii) Cleft soft palate
iv) Pharyngeal foreign body
v)   Laryngeal prosthesis surgery

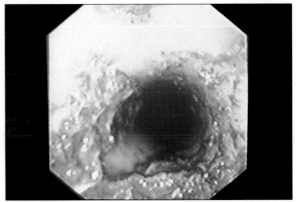

m Severe tracheal food-contamination.
Differential Diagnosis:
i) Cleft (or hypoplastic/aplastic) soft palate
ii) Chronic dysphagia (neurological or physical)

200

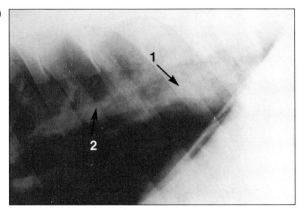

201

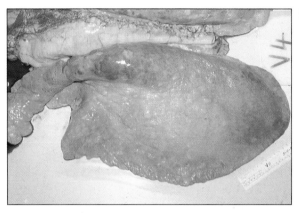

200 Exercise induced pulmonary hemorrhage (radiograph).
Note: Characteristic radiodensity in phrenico-diaphragmatic angle (arrow 1) with single prominent bronchial density (arrow 2).

201 Exercise induced pulmonary hemorrhage.
Note: Intrapulmonary blood in dorsal and caudo-dorsal lung regions.

epistaxis in these cases is usually bilateral, and is most often dark in colour (**Plate 6i**, page 121) reflecting the longer time taken to reach the external nares. Endoscopic examination shows hemorrhage of varying extent ranging from dark pools of stagnant blood (**Plate 4g**, page 103) to thin, almost inapparent 'lines' of dark blood (**Plate 4h**, page 103) or blood-stained mucus along the floor of the trachea (**Plate 4i**, page 103). Horses with intercurrent mucus hypersecretion usually show accumulated pools of blood-stained fluid in the trachea, particularly at the thoracic inlet (**Plate 4j**, page 104) which is the most dependent segment of the trachea. Small or larger amounts of dark blood in the pharynx is strongly suggestive of bleeding from lower down the airway (**Plate 5b**, page 111). In the milder cases, blood is usually only endoscopically apparent in the first 4 – 6 hours after exercise, but tracheal aspirations contain macrophages with hemosiderin deposits which can be detected by suitable staining methods. The interpretation of such a small amount of blood should be made carefully, in view of the frequency with which it is found in 'normal' animals performing up to expectation. Epistaxis might, equally, originate in sites rostral to the trachea and in particular from within the nasal cavity or may be associated with hemorrhagic diatheses. Radiographic changes in the more severe cases of exercise-induced pulmonary hemorrhage, are usually detectable between 1 and 7 – 10 days (or more) and, characteristically, present a diffuse opacity in the phrenico-diaphragmatic angle of the caudo-dorsal lobes of the lung (**200**). The age of the bleeding can be roughly assessed by the radiographic density of these areas, with marked radiodensity (*see* **200**) being indicative of a fresh hemorrhage (24 – 36 hours old), while progressively reducing density indicates correspondingly older lesions.

The post mortem examination of the lungs of horses suffering from moderate, or severe, exercise-induced pulmonary hemorrhage show obvious dark, hemorrhagic areas in the phrenico-diaphragmatic angle, in particular (**201**). The distribution of the bleeding is entirely consistent with the endoscopic findings and radiographic changes.

Extensive chest trauma, which does not always (or even generally) have obvious external evidence, may also result in serious pulmonary bleeding which is often sufficient to be fatal. Affected animals may present with a similar clinical syndrome although the history will usually be different and, furthermore, hemorrhage into the pleural cavity is also commonly present. This may be detected by an obvious elevation of the percussible ventral border of the lung and confirmed by pleuro-centesis when pure blood will be present in considerable amounts. Post mortem examination of such cases, however, shows distinct differences from the appearance of exercise-induced pulmonary hemorrhage with massive, diffuse bleeding in areas not normally associated with the non-traumatic disorder (**202**).

The horse is liable to the development of **amyloidosis**, in which glycoproteins are deposited in various organs. The nostrils, nasal cavity, nasal septum, conchae and, more rarely, the guttural pouches, pharynx and skin, are the usual sites for this deposition. The disorder occurs in animals with continued immune stimulation of the reticulo-endothelial system; the liver producing abnormal proteins. Horses which are being (or have been) used for the production of hyperimmune serum are probably most frequently affected. In rare cases, neoplasia or other chronic inflammatory disease may be an instigating factor. A sero-purulent nasal discharge (**Plate 7c**, page 143), which may occasionally

202

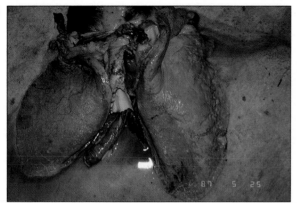

203

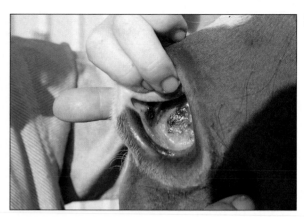

202 Traumatic intrapulmonary hemorrhage.
Note: Yearling ran into fence at full speed and died almost immediately with severe epistaxis.
Note: Generalised hemorrhage through left lung and medial part of right lung.
Differential Diagnosis:
i) Exercise induced pulmonary hemorrhage

203 Nasal amyloidosis.
Note: Minor trauma induced persistent hemorrhage from the site.

include flecks of blood or more overt hemorrhage (**Plate 7e**, page 144)**,** abnormal respiratory noises, recurrent mild epistaxis (**Plate 7g**, page 144) from one (or both) nostrils, poor exercise tolerance and weight loss are associated with the disorder. The clinical syndrome presented will depend upon the nature of the underlying disease process and the extent to which the deposition of amyloid proteins are confined to the nasal cavity, but impaired function of major organs including the liver, kidneys and heart, are to be expected. The nasal lesions are characteristically raised, firm, plaque-like areas of discoloured mucous membrane (**203**). These plaques are notoriously easy to traumatise and profuse bleeding may result from relatively minor interference such as palpation or nasogastric intubation. In some cases the lesions are not directly visible at all, and the first evidence of a problem is when relatively trivial interference results in unexpectedly severe nasal bleeding. Sometimes there are no apparent lesions in the nasal cavity and such cases are a considerable diagnostic challenge.

Acute allergic airway disease is less common than the chronic form and cases show a sudden onset of severe inspiratory and, occasionally, expiratory dyspnea associated with laryngospasm and/or tracheo-bronchial spasm and edema. Respiratory function may be sufficiently impaired to be life-threatening with obvious cyanosis, 'air hunger' with flaring nostrils (**Plate 6m**, page 122) and distress. Auscultation of the thorax usually detects wheezing and whistling sounds associated with high air speeds and narrow airways (*see* **207**). Crackling and fluid sounds are evidence of

emphysema and/or pulmonary edema, both of which are commonly encountered under these circumstances.

Small airway disease (chronic obstructive pulmonary disease/COPD/Heaves/allergic airway disease/allergic bronchitis) is one of the most common respiratory disorders of the horse in temperate areas of the world, and occurs particularly where horses are stabled for long periods and fed and bedded on preserved cereal and/or grass products. The probable etiology of the disorder is repeated mucosal allergic challenge in the conducting airways. Various specific etiological factors have been identified with more or less certainty, but most opinion attributes the development of the syndrome to hypersensitivity (or allergy) to inhaled environmental contaminants, including fungal spores, plant pollens and possibly other protein materials. A history of a preceding respiratory viral or bacterial infection is often reported, giving the mistaken impression of a persistence (or recurrence) of the infection. The exercise tolerance of affected horses is frequently adversely affected, with a significant number being presented, initially, for investigation of poor or inadequate athletic performance. Cases generally have an abnormally high resting respiratory rate, often with more or less flaring of the nostrils. A chronic, harsh, non-productive cough, which is usually worse when the animal is stabled, is characteristic. Without treatment, the severity of the cough often increases over weeks or months, sometimes with episodes of a more acute syndrome superimposed from time to time. Severely affected horses lose weight dramatically and the increased expiratory effort commonly results in marked hypertrophy of the muscles of the caudo-ventral thorax producing the so-called 'heave line' (**204**). In the severe cases, an obvious, extra, expiratory 'push' from the abdominal and thoracic muscles is present, possibly with an associated grunt. A slight or sometimes more profuse, bilateral, postural, catarrhal nasal discharge is usually present (**Plate 6b**, page 120). Endoscopic examination of the respiratory tract shows poor mucus clearance from the trachea with varying accumulations of muco-pus at the thoracic inlet in particular. In most cases this is grey and catarrhal in character (**Plate 4d**, page 102) but, particularly in the more acute cases, the accumulation of muco-pus in the trachea is sufficient to almost occlude the airway and breathing movement results in a 'tidal wave' of fluid (**Plate 4e**, page 103) and even in foam-formation. Where secondary infection is present the accumulation may be more purulent in character (**Plate 4b**, page 102; **Plate 6c**, page 120). Tracheal aspirate or broncho-alveolar lavage, in such cases, reveals inflammatory cells in proportion to the severity of the underlying disease and this provides an effective quantitative measure of the severity of the underlying pathology. Comparison of tracheal bifurcation (carina) appearance between the normal, unaffected horse (**205**) and that of diseased horses, shows the latter to have an obvious, edematous, thickening of the tracheal and bronchial mucosa, and a more or less obvious rounding and thickening of the carina. The extent of these changes is roughly proportional to the extent of the allergic response with milder cases showing a moderately narrowed airway and a thickened carina (**206**) and severe cases having an obviously very narrowed airway with a markedly thickened and rounded carina (**207**). The changes present at the carina are reflected throughout the tracheo-bronchial tree. Radiographic examination of the chest has been used to assess the extent of the pulmonary changes but it is limited by the technical difficulties and pathological changes can easily be confused with the normal changes in bronchial pattern associated with advancing age. Lateral, inspiratory radiographs of the caudo-dorsal lung fields may, however, show a mixed pattern of radio-density throughout the lung fields and prominent bronchial patterning with obvious 'tram-lining' and 'dough-nut' lesions, indicative of thickened conducting airways. In some cases pulmonary hypertension will also be detected on the radiographs. While extensive efforts have been devoted to the interpretation of thoracic radiographs in horses affected by small airway disease, they are perhaps best limited to differentiation of this from other, more focal, disorders. The application of cytological techniques, lung biopsy and measurements of intra-pleural pressure and other dynamic airway studies are likely to be more useful in confirming the existence of the disease. Supportive evidence of small airway disease can also be obtained from blood gas analysis.

Nasal edema is unusual in the horse but may be very significant, resulting in severe nasal obstruction. As the normal horse cannot breath via the oral cavity, this may be life-threatening. The commonest causes of nasal edema are circulatory disorders of the head, including bilateral jugular thrombosis (*see* **291, 292, 293**), congestive heart failure (**Plate 6l**, page 122) and disorders associated with vasculitis (*see* **293**). Postural, passive congestion of the head is sometimes severe enough to cause nasal edema (**Plate 6g**, page 121) and is a possible complication of neck injuries. Significant nasal edema is also commonly encountered following prolonged general anesthesia in dorsal recumbency, and while other factors relating to circulatory efficiency may be involved, the postural effects are probably the most significant. A severe life-threatening nasal edema is also occasionally encountered as an undesirable side-effect of certain drugs, and particularly quinidine sulphate, and as a result of some hypersensitivity/allergic disorders related to anaphylaxis. Localised anaphylactoid reactions such as those associated with snake envenomation may cause extreme swelling and nasal obstruction (**208**). In all these conditions endoscopic examination shows marked narrowing of the nasal cavity with extensive edema and congestion of the mucosa.

Neuropathy of the recurrent laryngeal nerve affecting most frequently, but not exclusively, the left nerve, is a very common disorder which may affect all types of horse. Young horses, between 2 and 6 years of age, and horses over 16 hands in height, are, however, most often affected. Certain breeds, including the Hannovarian, Shire, Irish Draught, Dutch Warmblood and other large breeds, appear to be particularly liable to severe forms of the condition which apparently develops spontaneously. The Thoroughbred, Standard-bred and Quarter Horse breeds are also affected commonly with a range of mild to severe forms of the disorder with up to 80% of Thoroughbred horses possibly affected to some extent. The majority of these have mild degrees of the condition in which little or no clinical effect is detectable. Animals affected by the spontaneous or **idiopathic form of left recurrent laryngeal neuropathy** are often noted to have a narrow intermandibular space. In normal large horses greater than a four- or five-finger-width is usual, whilst affected horses often have widths of less than three fingers. Most horses with significant laryngeal neuropathy are presented for investigation of inspiratory noises and/or

204

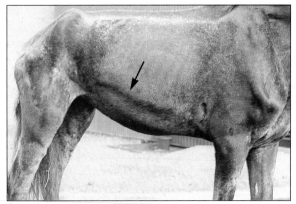

204 (Chronic) small airway disease (chronic obstructive pulmonary disease, COPD, 'Heaves', allergic lung disease).
Note: Weight loss, prominent muscular hypertrophy along caudo ventral thorax ('Heave line') (arrow).

205

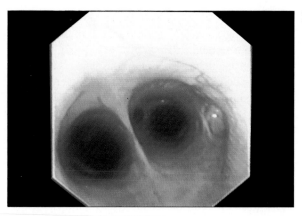

205 Normal tracheal carina.
Note: Sharp 'keel-like' central division at tracheal bifurcation.

206

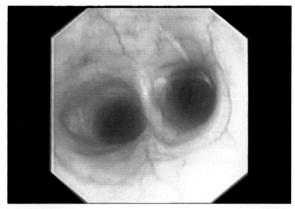

206 Chronic small airway disease (chronic obstructive pulmonary disease, COPD, 'Heaves', allergic lung disease) (mild).
Note: Thickened carina and narrowed bronchial diameter (compare to normal in **205**).

207

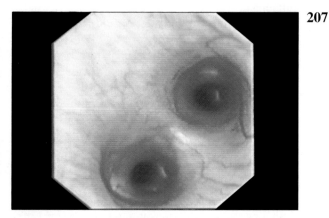

207 Chronic small airway disease (chronic obstructive pulmonary disease, COPD, 'Heaves', allergic lung disease).
Note: Very thickened edematous carina and marked narrowing of bronchial diameter (compare to normal in **205**).

poor exercise tolerance. While it is to be expected that exercise limitations will be present in the advanced cases, milder degrees produce correspondingly less clinical effect. However, even mild cases commonly show various levels of inspiratory dyspnea known as '**roaring**'. The paralysis is usually only left-sided, and may be partial (in which there is some abduction movement of the arytenoid), or complete, (in which no abduction is visible). In the normal larynx (**Plate 5t**, page 115) the movement of the left and right arytenoids is symmetrical and their apices are positioned in the 12 o'clock position. The left and right arytenoids, vocal folds and aryteno-epiglottic folds, furthermore, look alike, and all their movements are in

synchrony. Quivering of the arytenoid which results in similar fine movements of the aryteno-epiglottic and vocal folds, and loss of left-right laryngeal synchrony in relation to arytenoid movement, are regarded as the mildest forms (Grades I and II) of the disorder. An apparently normal, or near normal, full abduction of the arytenoid is present, particularly after swallowing or during exercise, or when the nostrils are occluded for a few moments, but there is almost always some asymmetry of appearance or function. The arytenoid is usually fairly stable in these and it seldom obstructs the airway until extremes of exercise are undertaken. In the more severe cases an apparently 'weaker-looking' arytenoid can be recognised on the affected

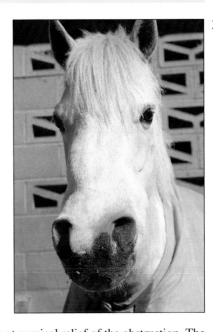

208 Nasal edema.
Differential Diagnosis:
i)   Anaphylactoid reactions (Snake/spider bite)
ii) Disseminated intravascular coagulopathy
iii) Local circulatory obstructions
iv) Congestive heart failure
v) Postural edema (neck injury etc)
vi) Disseminated intravascular coagulopathy

(usually the left) side and the apex of the arytenoid cartilage will appear to be set lower than the unaffected side, giving an impression of a rotation away from the twelve o'clock position (Grade III) (**Plate 5u**, page 115). Abduction movement is still present in the affected arytenoid but is limited in extent and response to exercise. Progressively more severe neuropathy results in a progressive displacement of the arytenoid apices towards the affected side (Grade IV) (**Plate 5v**, page 116). Where the condition is severe (Grade V) (**Plate 5w**, page 116) there is no abduction of the arytenoid and extreme asymmetry is obvious, particularly when the unaffected arytenoid is fully abducted (**Plate 5w**, page 116). There is little or no stability of the paralysed cartilage, and it may 'flop' across the airway (**Plate 5x**, page 116). When such animals are exercised, the airway may become almost totally occluded as the arytenoid is drawn into the *aditus laryngis* by the high negative pressure within the trachea. This results in a flaccidity and stretching of the aryteno-epiglottic fold which becomes increasingly apparent (**Plate 5x**, page 116). Such cases are usually severely handicapped by even minimal exercise and make a loud inspiratory noise. This is particularly obvious during canter or galloping work and is coordinated with the stride being audible when the front feet are off the ground (i.e during inspiration). Less affected horses, during dynamic endoscopy at exercise, show a marked asymmetry of the laryngeal opening but less intrusion of the left arytenoid into the airway with correspondingly less noise and less limitation on exercise capacity. Comparative endoscopic examination of the larynx, at rest and at exercise, is particularly useful in establishing the extent of the dysfunction and whether any prior attempts have been made at surgical relief of the obstruction. The 'Slap Test', which tests the integrity of the thoraco-vagal reflex by observing (or palpating) contralateral laryngeal adduction and abduction in response to a 'slap' applied to the thoracic wall, may also be used to demonstrate the malfunctioning of the affected side. The atrophy of the *cricoarytenoideus dorsalis* muscle may be suggested by palpation of the muscular process of the arytenoid on the affected side which becomes characteristically prominent (**209**). Right-side (**Plate 5cc**, page 117) and bilateral paralysis are sometimes encountered but the etiology of these are usually better defined. Extravascular injection of irritant drugs in the jugular groove, guttural pouch mycosis (*see* **252**), poisoning by *Swainsonia spp* plants, heavy metals or organophosphates, bacterial or other toxemia and thiamine deficiency (bracken poisoning) have all been implicated in individual cases of laryngeal paralysis. Horses recovering from the Australian form of Stringhalt (*see* **708**) are frequently left with a severe right laryngeal neuropathy which may not be clinically obvious, initially, due to their inability to move fast. One of the most common causes of right sided and bilateral paralysis is the presence of arytenoid chondritis (**Plate 5r; Plate 5s**, page 115) with secondary extension of the inflammation and degeneration into the abductor muscles. In these cases the primary problem is likely a myopathy and muscle atrophy is therefore less obvious than in those cases in which denervation atrophy is effectively present. Post mortem dissections of the larynx of idiopathic laryngeal neuropathy cases confirm the presence of marked atrophy of the *cricoarytenoideus dorsalis muscle* on the affected side and prominence of the ipsilateral muscular process (**209**).

209

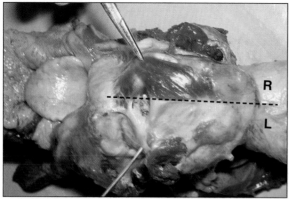

209 Idiopathic laryngeal neuropathy (ILN) (roaring, laryngeal hemiplegia, laryngeal paralysis).
Note: Marked atrophy of *cricoarytenoideus dorsalis* muscle on left side and prominent muscular process of left arytenoid cartilage (the pointers locate the muscular processes).

Horses which have been subjected to surgery to relieve the noise and performance-limiting signs, present characteristic endoscopic features. The recognition of these is important. **Lateral ventriculectomy (Hobday's Operation)**, in which the lateral laryngeal ventricles are surgically ablated has been used for many years to reduce the respiratory noise. Endoscopic examination will readily detect the absence of one or both laryngeal ventricles (**Plate 5y**, page 116). A **prosthetic ligature (McKay-Mark's Operation)** is currently widely used to stabilise and abduct the affected arytenoid cartilage. This operation has considerable advantages in reducing the noise and also stabilising the arytenoid and thereby preventing inspiratory occlusion of the airway. Horses which have been subjected to this procedure show a stabilised (immobile) arytenoid which, in the resting horse, is ideally slightly abducted from the normal neutral position (**Plate 5z**, page 117). During exercise, only the unaffected cartilage will be seen to move, the fixed cartilage remaining in the same relative position throughout (**Plate 5aa**, page 117). At certain stages of performance the larynx will regain some semblance of symmetry. The insertion of a prosthetic ligament prevents any adduction and therefore precludes closure of the *aditus laryngis* during swallowing. Thus, horses in which the arytenoid is fixed in a markedly abducted position lose their ability to protect the airway during swallowing and consequently food material can, sometimes, be seen in the airway (**Plate 4l**, page 104). Some cases cough persistently following the surgery and this is sometimes explained by food inhalation or chondroma formation at the site of the suture. Some cases which prove refractory to treatment by the milder surgical interferences are subjected to **sub-total arytenoidectomy** and the endoscopic appearance of these is very obvious (**Plate 5bb**, page 117).

Histopathological examination of the affected recurrent laryngeal nerve may identify the progressive loss of distal myelinated nerve fibres. This may result from physical factors such as excessive stretching, such as might occur in a jumping horse, or even from persistent trauma from pulsations in the aorta, around which the left recurrent laryngeal nerve passes. The term idiopathic laryngeal neuropathy (ILN) is applied to these cases and the onset is generally insidious, with a progressive deterioration over months or years, in some cases a static non-progressive stage is reached which is not always the most extreme form. Although in most cases of left laryngeal neuropathy, and some cases of right sided paralysis, the etiology is unknown, any damage to the recurrent laryngeal nerves will have the same effect.

Abnormal, persistent **dorsal displacement of the soft palate (Plate 5a**, page 111) occurs during exercise (and occasionally at other times) in Thoroughbred and Quarter horses, in particular. The normally air-tight seal between the caudal free border of the soft palate and the epiglottis is broken and the horse may then breath through the mouth. This is virtually impossible, and, indeed, is strongly resisted, in normal horses, even in the face of severe and life-threatening nasal obstructions. The displacement has a profound effect upon respiratory function, with narrowing of the nasopharynx and consequent air turbulence. In most cases the disorder is intermittent or occasional, but some horses are said to be persistently and severely handicapped by it. Where the dislocation occurs during fast work the performance of the horse may be momentarily affected by a sudden, transient asphyxia. Under these circumstances, the horse shows a characteristic 'gurgling' sound and an abrupt loss of pace. A number of possible predisposing factors have been identified such as retraction of the tongue, swallowing, opening of the mouth at full pace, flexion of the neck or inflammatory disorders of the pharynx including pharyngeal lymphoid hyperplasia (*see* **213**).

Plate 5

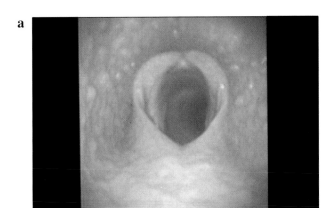

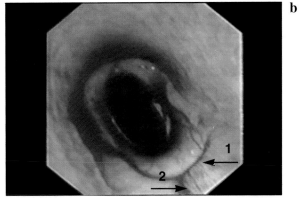

a Dorsal displacement of soft palate.
Note: Epiglottis not visible. Mild pharyngeal lymphoid hyperplasia present in this case.

b Soft palate resection surgery.
Note: Excessive resection of free border of soft palate (arrow 1) resulted in permanent displacement of epiglottis relative to soft palate.
Note: Evidence of hemorrhage (exercise induced pulmonary hemorrhage) on free margin of soft palate (arrow 2) and left laryngeal paralysis (asymmetry).

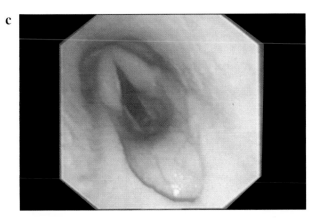

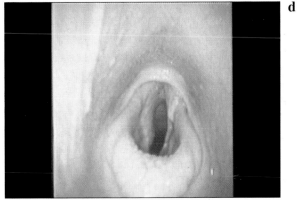

c Soft palate resection surgery.
Note: Wedge excision excessive and resulted in persistent dislocation of soft palate.
Note: Soft palate passing around apex of arytenoids. Should not be confused with epiglottic entrapment (See **Plate 5m**, page 113).

d Rostral displacement of palatopharyngeal arch (dorsal laryngopalatal dislocation).
Note: Epiglottis visible but apices of arytenoids hidden behind palatopharyngeal arch. Arytenoid abduction impossible.

Plate 5

e

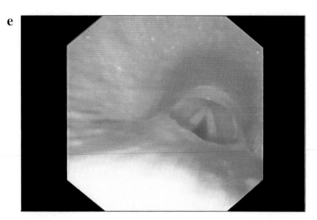

e Complete dislocation of soft palate.
Note: Epiglottis and apices of arytenoids hidden and circular soft palate shape is obvious. Little impairment of arytenoid function. Only occurs momentarily in most cases. This is quite frequently encountered in sedated horses after endoscopy and can be easily differentiated from the serious rostral displacement of the palatopharyngeal arch by allowing a single swallow.

f

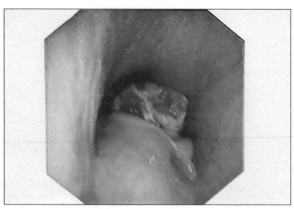

f Pharyngeal neoplasia (primary lymphosarcoma).
Note: Causing persistent dorsal dislocation of the soft palate. Horse presented for investigation of progressive, deteriorating dysphagia. Defect in soft palate margin probably incidental or secondary to persistent displacement and difficulty with deglutition.

g

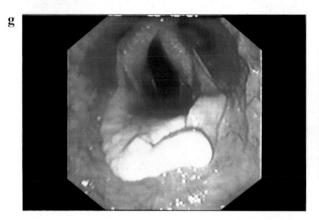

g Traumatic epiglottic deformity.
Note: Followed surgical relief of epiglottic entrapment using a hooked bistoury. No apparent effect on the horse; found incidentally.

h

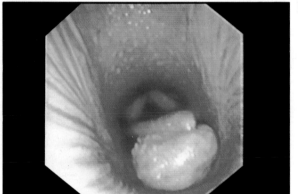

h Sub-epiglottic cyst.
Note: Animal presented as 4-year-old for investigation of abnormal respiratory noise at exercise and poor athletic performance.

Plate 5

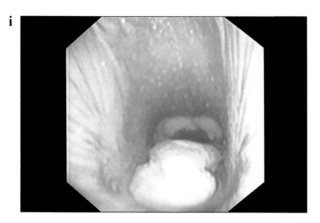

i Sub-epiglottic cyst complicated by concurrent epiglottic entrapment.
Note: The epiglottic entrapment was intermittent and the cyst was not always visible (sometimes being located under the free border of the soft palate).

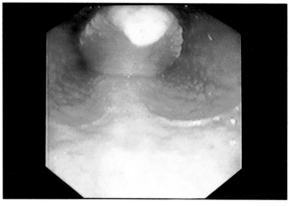

j Upright epiglottis.
Note: Usually regarded as a normal variant but may be associated with sub-epiglottic cysts located under the soft palate.

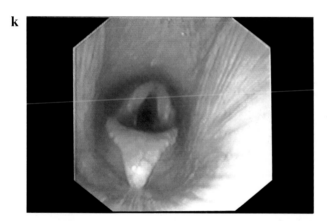

k Epiglottic hypoplasia.
Note: Epiglottic length measured from lateral radiograph (with allowances for magnification) was 5.8 cm. Recurrent dorsal displacement of the soft palate and epiglottic entrapment were noted.

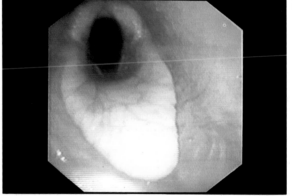

l Epiglottic hypoplasia.
Note: Length normal but epiglottis flaccid and recurrent dorsal displacement of soft palate noted.

m Epiglottic entrapment.
Note: Shape of epiglottis present but loss of detailed structure (blood vessels and crenated free margin). Caudal margin of entrapping membrane is visible (arrow) and only a small part of the epiglottic body is apparent. (Compare with dorsal displacement of soft palate **Plate 5a**, page 111).

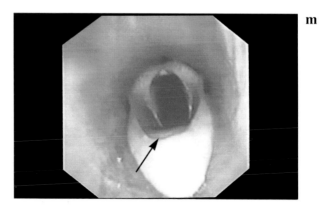

Plate 5

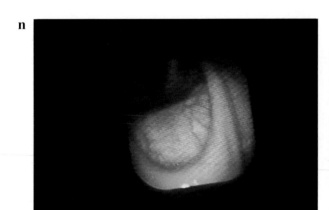

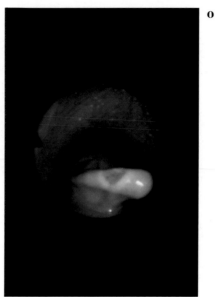

n Epiglottic entrapment.
Note: Intermittent/incomplete form. Epiglottis became entrapped and peeled out frequently and particularly associated with swallowing.

o Epiglottic entrapment (chronic).
Note: Ulcerative lesion on glossoepiglottic fold entrapped over epiglottis. Crenated border of epiglottis not visible.

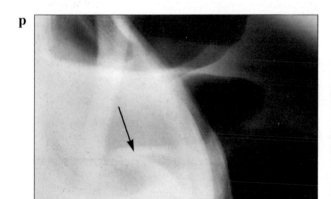

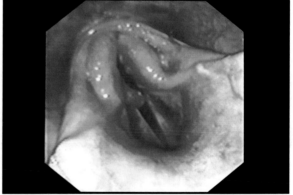

p Epiglottic entrapment (radiographic appearance).
Note: Prominent epiglottis (arrow) with thick margin held away from soft palate.

q Arytenoid (corniculate) chondritis (bilateral).
Note: Enlarged and edematous arytenoid cartilages. Prominent axial displacement of left arytenoid and impaired abductor function (paralysis) and partial rostral displacement of palatopharyngeal arch which are typical. Narrowing of *rima glottidis.*
Differential Diagnosis:
i)   Laryngeal hemiplegia (idiopathic and neurological forms)
ii) Laryngeal neoplasia
iii) Laryngeal polyps
iv) Laryngeal granuloma
v)   Laryngeal cartilage hypertrophic ossification

Plate 5

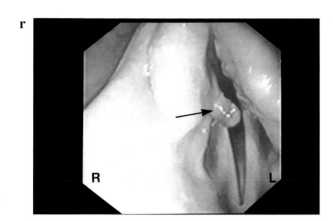

r Arytenoid (corniculate) chondritis (bilateral, asymmetric).
Note: Ulcerative lesions on medial margin of left cartilage and granuloma (associated with discharging tract) in corniculate process of right cartilage (arrow).

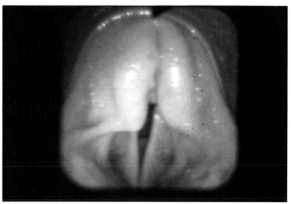

s Arytenoid (corniculate) chondritis (bilateral).
Note: Prominent right side arytenoid abduction disability. Thickened cartilages and edematous overlying mucosa. Perilaryngeal abscessation was present.

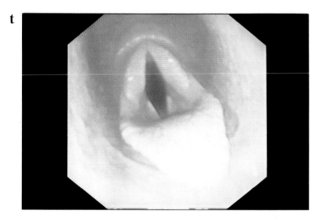

t Normal (symmetrical) larynx (resting horse).
Note: Photograph taken mid-inspiration.

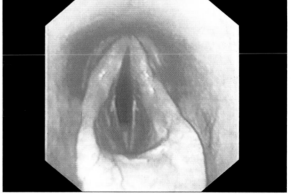

u Idiopathic laryngeal neuropathy (ILN) (Grade III).
Note: Some abduction was present but obvious asymmetry developed during exercise. Slap test positive (normal) both sides. Photograph taken mid-inspiration.

Plate 5

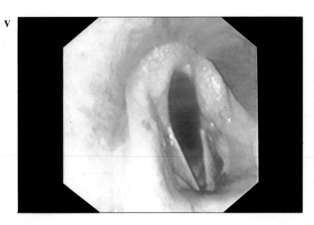

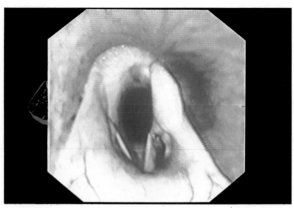

v Idiopathic laryngeal neuropathy (ILN) (Grade IV).
Note: No movement of left arytenoid in response to swallowing, nasal occlusion or exercise. Negative slap test on left arytenoid. Obvious axial displacement of arytenoid apex. Photograph taken mid-inspiration.

w Idiopathic laryngeal neuropathy (ILN) (Grade V).
Note: Severe axial displacement of arytenoids. Left arytenoid looks small. No movement. Negative slap test on left side. Arytenoid collapsed into airway during exercise and nasal occlusion.

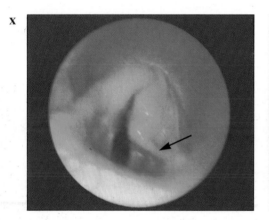

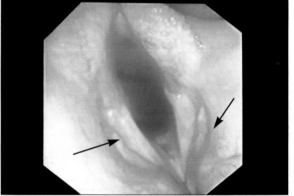

x Idiopathic laryngeal neuropathy (ILN) (Grade v) complicated by arytenoid chondritis.
Note: Flaccid nature of enlarged and edematous arytenoid. Cartilage flopped into airway at exercise and occluded *rima glottidis*. Severe exercise limitation and abnormal inspiratory noise ('roaring'). Flaccid and 'stretched' aryteno-epiglottic fold (arrow).

y Lateral laryngeal ventriculectomy (Hobday's Operation) (surgical 'treatment' of idiopathic laryngeal neuropathy).
Note: Lateral ventricles not present- replaced by white scarred areas (arrows).

Plate 5

z

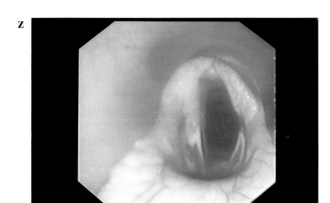

z Prosthetic laryngoplasty (McKay-Mark's Operation) (surgical treatment of laryngeal neuropathy) (at rest). **Note:** Neutral right (mobile) cartilage and fixed abduction of left cartilage. This extent of abduction is possibly slightly excessive and resulted in persist inhalation and coughing.

aa

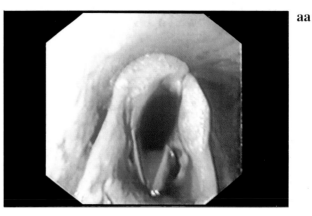

aa Prosthetic laryngoplasty (McKay-Mark's Operation) (surgical treatment of laryngeal neuropathy) (at exercise). **Note:** During exercise only the mobile right cartilage is abducted while the fixed left cartilage remains in its neutral or slightly abducted position. This degree of abduction in the left cartilage is approximately ideal - sufficient to allow an improved airway, no negative pressure collapse is possible and the airway is reasonably protected during swallowing.

bb

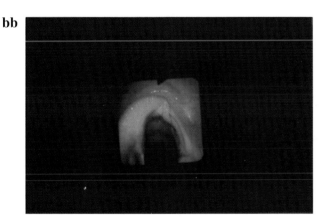

bb Partial arytenoidectomy (surgical treatment of laryngeal neuropathy and arytenoid chondritis). **Note:** Obvious arytenoid deficit.

cc

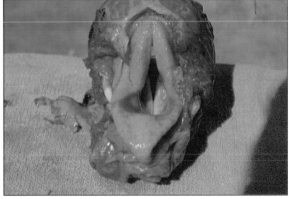

cc Right-side laryngeal neuropathy (Grade IV). **Note:** All such cases should be examined carefully for the presence of arytenoid chondritis.

There is usually little evidence of neurological or anatomical defects in these horses. Endoscopically the soft palate can be seen to lie above the epiglottis so that its free border is not visible and the free border of the soft palate is obvious, lying across the *aditus laryngis* (**Plate 5a**, page 111). Cases which have been subjected to surgical 'correction' of dorsal displacement of the soft palate by resection of the free border of the palate may easily be recognised endoscopically by the thickened rim of firm scar tissue along the free border (**Plate 5b**, page 111). Surgical excision is sometimes carried out in a wedge form (**Plate 5c**, page 111) in an attempt to prevent persistent dislocation following the surgery. In many of these cases, the epiglottis can no longer articulate effectively with the soft palate and more or less permanent dislocation is present). Individuals affected by **hypoplasia of the epiglottis (Plate 5k; Plate 5l**, page 113) show an increased tendency to recurrent or persistent dislocations consequent upon the inadequacy of the normally tight seal between the epiglottis and the soft palate. The diagnosis of pathologically significant dorsal displacement of the soft palate is frequently suggested by the behaviour of the horse at full gallop. However, confirmation may be difficult due to its intermittency and to the fact that it is often seen in sedated, normal horses, particularly after an endoscope has been withdrawn from the trachea. Dynamic airway studies during treadmill exercise have become a useful diagnostic aid in the recognition of clinically significant dorsal displacements of the soft palate.

Dorsal laryngopalatal dislocation (Plate 5d, page 111), which is caused by the displacement of the dorsal palatopharyngeal arch usually induces dysphagia, nasal regurgitation of food, coughing and respiratory compromise with abnormal noises at exercise. While it may be a developmental disorder of the fourth branchial arch, acquired displacements probably also occur. Endoscopic examination of the pharynx is the only effective means of diagnosis. The palatopharyngeal arch will be seen to be displaced rostrally to overlie the corniculate processes of the arytenoids (**Plate 5d**, page 111). The apices of the arytenoids will therefore, usually, not be visible. The extent of the displacement can be exaggerated by nasal occlusion, exercise or sedation. The condition is often mild in degree and may, then, have little clinical effect in young horses having little demand for airway efficiency. The firm muscular nature of the dorsal palatopharyngeal arch and the tension which is exerted within it, are sufficient to prevent effective abduction of the arytenoids when greater airflows are required. Indeed, the greater negative pressures during exercise merely serve to exaggerate the limitations of arytenoid abduction. The

greatest hindrance is, therefore, upon inspiration during exercise and inspiratory noises are prominent features of the condition. Expiratory noises are often present to a lesser extent. The diagnosis of this disorder is important in view of the poor prognosis which it carries. Simultaneous laryngeal neuropathy (**Plate 5u** *et seq.*, page 115) and other developmental defects including cleft palate and interventricular septal defects are sometimes found. In some cases it is possible to palpate an obvious deformity of the thyroid cartilage, having shortened lateral and posterior laminae (wings) which do not articulate with the cricoid cartilage. The *crico-pharyngeus* muscles are also commonly absent.

Epiglottic entrapment (Plate 5m, page 113) is another, relatively common, disorder of the larynx in which affected horses are reported to display abnormal respiratory (inspiratory and occasionally expiratory) noises at exercise. Cases show coughing and many have a distinct reduction in exercise tolerance. The entrapment is produced when the epiglottis becomes enfolded by the redundant, sublingual extensions of the aryteno-epiglottic folds which lie under the epiglottis (glosso-epiglottic membrane). Diagnosis of this condition is, again, dependent upon endoscopic examination of the pharynx but intermittent or occasional entrapment may not be reliably demonstrated on any particular occasion. The normal crenated edge and characteristic marginal, radiating blood vessels are lost to view although in many cases the outline shape of the epiglottis is still present (**Plate 5m**, page 113). The aryteno-epiglottic folds become abnormally prominent, extending between the base of the arytenoid cartilages and the entrapped epiglottis. The extent of the entrapment may vary from minute to minute and some apparently normal horses may be seen to entrap the epiglottis as they swallow (**Plate 5n**, page 114). In some mild cases, only the tip of the epiglottis may be entrapped. Extensive, long-standing entrapments often result in ulceration of the overlying mucosa (**Plate 5o**, page 114). On rare occasions the mucosa may even become disrupted and the free border of the epiglottis may be seen protruding through the fold. Entrapment may be asymmetrical, with only the tip and one lateral border of the epiglottis being lost to view. The caudal margin of the entrapping aryteno-epiglottic fold is however always visible. The presence of granulating ulcerations on the surface of the entrapped aryteno-epiglottic fold or on the apex of the epiglottis may support a diagnosis of intermittent entrapment. Lateral radiographs, particularly using xeroradiographic techniques, may also be used to identify the condition when the epiglottis will be seen to be prominent and,

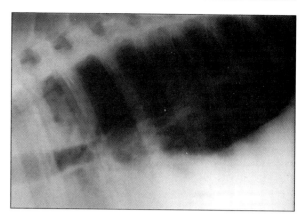

210 Inhalation pneumonia (radiograph).
Note: Marked radiodensity in anterior and ventral lobes of lung and reduced radiodensity in caudal and dorsal areas. Due to tracheal administration of liquid paraffin.

usually, somewhat shortened (**Plate 5p**, page 114). The intermittency of the disorder, however, makes this an unreliable diagnostic aid in many cases. There may be a greater tendency for epiglottic entrapment to occur in horses affected by hypoplasia of the epiglottis (**Plate 5k; Plate 5l**, page 113). The prognosis for horses with concurrent, persistent or frequent, intermittent dorsal displacement of the soft palate, or with obvious deformity of the epiglottis, is much worse as the underlying cause is usually not resolvable. In a few cases the disorder also occurs in association with sub-epiglottic cysts, and particularly with the more flaccid type in which there is an excess of redundant mucosa (**Plate 5i**, page 113). Traumatic or developmental deformities of the epiglottis (**Plate 5g**, page 112) may also result in either epiglottic entrapment or dorsal dislocation of the soft palate.

Combinations of the various pharyngeal and laryngeal disorders are relatively common in the horse. Thus, horses suffering from hypoplasia of the epiglottis might be affected by any or all of the disorders associated with the positional relationships of the epiglottis. **Concurrent epiglottic entrapment and dorsal dislocation of the soft palate** form a relatively common clinical entity. Similarly, **complete dislocation of the palato-pharyngeal articulation** results from a simultaneous dorsal displacement of the soft palate and rostral displacement of the palato-pharyngeal arch. The resulting endoscopic appearance is that neither the free margin of the epiglottis nor the apices of the arytenoid cartilages are usually visible. Although persistent or frequent complete dislocation would be regarded as of pathological significance, occasional milder dislocations observed during static endoscopy may be incidental (**Plate 5e**, page 112).

Clinically significant **inhalation of irritant or noxious chemicals** is unusual but horses involved in stable or vehicle fires frequently suffer from severe consequences of inhaled smoke or flames. Nasal irritation from chronic repeated inhalation of acrid smoke or chemicals induces an obvious rhinitis with nasal discharges which vary from serous (**Plate 6a**, page 120) to catarrhal (**Plate 6b**, page 120). In the later stages and where the problem persists for longer periods the discharge may be more purulent and the affected horse often develops a paroxysmal cough, due to pharyngitis and/or tracheitis. Smoke from burning plastic appears to be particularly dangerous to horses, creating a severe tracheitis and bronchitis and even, in some cases, necrotizing pneumonitis.

The **inhalation of dust particles, sand and other foreign bodies** is quite common in dry dusty conditions. While the nasal mucosa normally provides an efficient filter for larger, air-borne particles, at extremes of exercise it may be less effective. In most cases the mucociliary escalator will effectively prevent pulmonary contamination, and foreign matter within the trachea is often found incidentally (**Plate 4k**, page 104). Large amounts of food material in the trachea (**Plate 4l; Plate 4m**, page 104) are usually the result of dysphagia. It is remarkable how much tracheal contamination may occur in the rostral conducting airways without any apparent problem. However, when inhalation or misdirected nasogastric intubation result in large volumes of foreign matter in the lower airway, the affected horse is usually extremely ill, showing marked respiratory embarrassment with a bilateral, purulent, hemorrhagic nasal discharge having a necrotic, offensive odour (**Plate 6k**, page 122). Radiographic changes of **inhalation pneumonia** are characteristically restricted to the anterior and ventral lung lobes with the caudo-dorsal lobes showing evidence of hyperventilation (**210**). The extent of pulmonary involvement will depend upon the amount and nature of the contamination and the site of deposition. Thus, small volumes of liquid paraffin may contaminate large areas of the airway with catastrophic results, while saline or water usually has much less effect. Hypertonic solutions, such as 10% glucose or concentrated magnesium sulphate

Plate 6

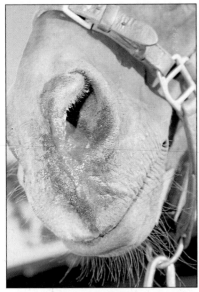

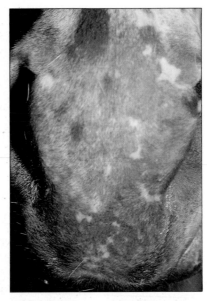

a Bilateral serous nasal discharge.
Differential Diagnosis:
i) Respiratory tract virus infection (early stage)
ii) Allergic/irritant rhinitis (eg smoke, noxious gas)
iii) Ethmoid hematoma (chronic, progressive)

b Bilateral catarrhal nasal discharge.
Differential Diagnosis:
i) Respiratory tract virus infection
ii) Chronic nasal irritation (smoke etc)
iii) Small airway disease (possibly postural)

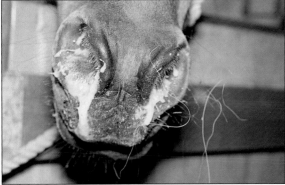

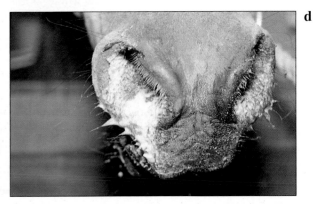

c Bilateral muco-purulent nasal discharge.
Differential Diagnosis:
i) Secondary bacterial infection following virus infection
ii) Strangles (*Streptococcus equi*)
iii) False strangles (*Streptococcus zooepidemicus*)

d Bilateral purulent nasal discharge (with blood).
Note: Differences left and right.
Differential Diagnosis:
i) Strangles (*Streptococcus equi*)
ii) Pharyngeal/guttural pouch abscess

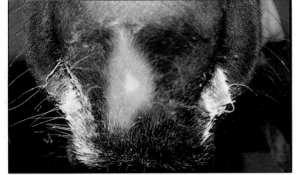

e Bilateral (chronic) purulent nasal discharge.
Differential Diagnosis:
i) Recovery phase of bacterial infection
ii) Bilateral primary sinusitis

f Bilateral epistaxis (fresh/transient).
Differential Diagnosis:
i) Nasal/facial trauma
ii) Skull trauma (eg fractured basisphenoid)
iii) Pharyngeal foreign body

g Bilateral (venous) epistaxis.
Differential Diagnosis:
i) Hemorrhagic diathesis (thrombocytopenia/ coumarin/warfarin poisoning)
ii) Purpura hemorrhagica (immune-mediated vasculitis)
iii) Guttural pouch mycosis (venous lesion) (usually unilateral)
iv) Exercise induced pulmonary hemorrhage (24–48 hours post exercise)
v) Disseminated intravascular coagulopathy (DIC)
(**Note:** Swelling of face and muzzle : case of purpura hemorrhagica.)

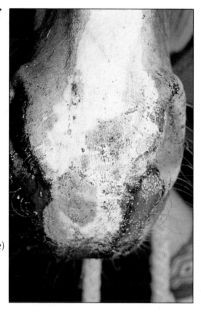

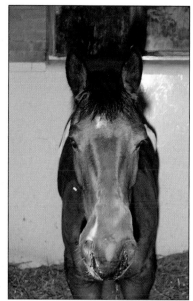

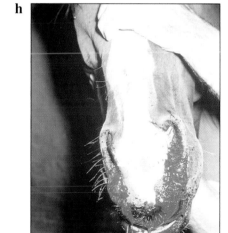

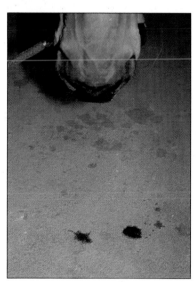

h Bilateral (arterial) epistaxis.
Differential Diagnosis:
i) Exercise induced pulmonary hemorrhage
ii) Guttural pouch mycosis (arterial lesion)

i Bilateral (postural) hemorrhagic nasal discharge (slight).
Differential Diagnosis:
i) Exercise induced pulmonary hemorrhage (48–72 hours post exercise)
ii) Pulmonary neoplasia

j Bilateral hemorrhagic nasal discharge (chronic, persistent).
Differential Diagnosis:
i) Pulmonary neoplasia (postural)
ii) Hemorrhagic diathesis
iii) Purpura hemorrhagica

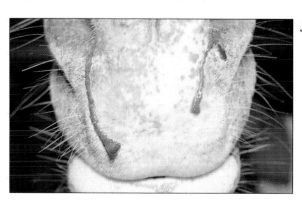

Plate 6

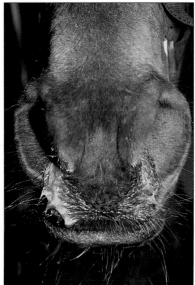

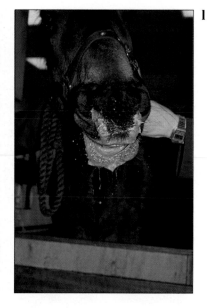

k Bilateral purulent-hemorrhagic nasal discharge (scanty) (with fetid odour).
Differential Diagnosis:
i)   Pleuritis
ii) Bronchopneumonia
iii) Gangrenous (inhalational) pneumonia
iv) Glanders
v) Tuberculosis

l Bilateral hemorrhagic serous nasal discharge (profuse).
Differential Diagnosis:
i)   Congestive heart failure (left side)
ii) African horse sickness
iii) Pulmonary edema
iv) Paraquat poisoning
v) Anaphylaxis

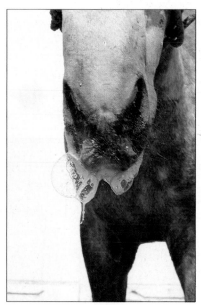

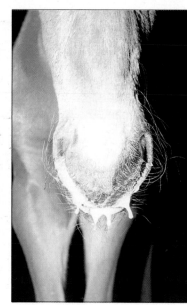

m Bilateral hemorrhagic serous nasal discharge (chronic, scanty, persistent).
Differential Diagnosis:
i)   Ethmoid hematoma (large lesion occluding both nostrils)
ii) Space occupying neoplasia in nasal cavities/paranasal sinuses (eq squamous cell carcinoma/polyp)
iii) Pharyngeal foreign body
iv) Acute allergic airway disease
v) Corniculate chondritis

n Bilateral milky nasal discharge (FOAL) (chronic, persistent).
Differential Diagnosis:
i)   Cleft hard palate
ii) Cleft soft palate
iii) Sub-epiglottic cyst
iv) Pharyngeal cyst (only rarely interfere with swallowing)
v) Botulism
vi) Guttural pouch tympany
vii) Strangles (*Streptococcus equi*)

Plate 6

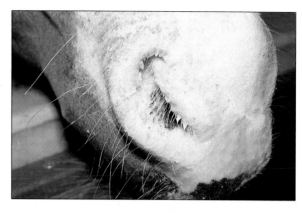

o Bilateral nasal discharge with food and saliva.
Differential Diagnosis:
i) Choke
ii) Esophageal stricture
iii) Neurological dysphagia (botulism, African Horse Sickness, heavy metal poisoning, guttural pouch mycosis, lathyrism, mouldy corn poisoning, encephalitis, rabies)
iv) Pharyngeal foreign body
v) Guttural pouch empyema
vi) Fracture stylohyoid bone

p Bilateral nasal discharge with food (scanty, chronic).
Differential Diagnosis:
i) Esophageal stricture
ii) Neurological dysphagia
iii) Cleft hard palate (small)
iv) Cleft soft palate
v) Pharyngeal neoplasia (lymphosarcoma, squamous-cell carcinoma)
vi) Esophageal dilatation (megaesophagus)
vii) Grass sickness
viii) Pharyngeal foreign body
ix) Pharyngeal paralysis

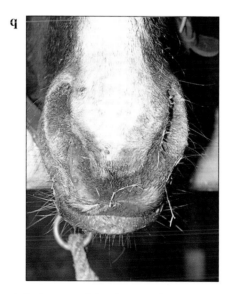

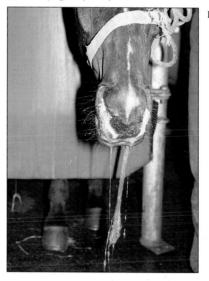

q Bilateral nasal discharge with food material (acute, persistent).
Differential Diagnosis:
i) Spontaneous gastric reflux (acid content) (intestinal obstruction)
ii) Grass sickness (acid or neutral)
iii) (Impending) gastric rupture
iv) Choke (neutral or alkaline)
v) Esophageal stricture
vi) Gastric (or esophageal) squamous cell carcinoma

r Dysphagia (Bilateral Nasal Discharge of water/food and saliva immediately following swallowing
Differential Diagnosis:
i) Choke (Intraluminal esophageal obstruction)
ii) Pharyngeal foreign body
iii) Pharyngeal paralysis (Rabies/ African Horse Sickness/ Guttural pouch mycosis/ Lead poisoning/ Grass Sickness/ Hypocalcemia/ Botulism/ Bracken poisoning/ Protozoal myeloencephalitis)
iv) Pharyngeal Lymphosarcoma

solutions, draw water from the circulation and result in a more serious effect than might otherwise be expected. Death, either directly from pulmonary obstruction or from the consequent necrosis or infection, is a common sequel to any such pulmonary contamination. At post mortem examination, a clear demarcation is usually present between the affected areas of lung and those relatively unaffected.

Horses suffering from either cardiac disorders complicated by **pulmonary hypertension**, such as congestive heart failure (**Plate 6l**, page 122), or infectious diseases including **African Horse Sickness** (*see* **215** *et seq.*) and **equine viral arteritis** (*see* **298**), or **pulmonary hypersensitivity and anaphylaxis**, or inhalation disorders (*see* **210**), are commonly complicated by pulmonary edema. Nasal reflux of large

amounts of fluid which is usually pale yellow and frothy, but which may be blood-stained (**Plate 6l**, page 122), is an obvious clinical feature. The lungs are usually moist or patently wet on auscultation and radiographic examination of the thorax will show a characteristic increase in the size of the pulmonary arteries, an increase in overall lung density and variable amounts of pulmonary consolidation and congestion. There may be concurrent pleural and/or pericardial effusion in any of these disorders. Non-cardiogenic pulmonary edema may also arise from electrocution, near-drowning and some poisons, notably with the weedkiller, paraquat. Post mortem examination of horses affected by pulmonary edema will reveal moist or wet lungs which fail to collapse fully (or at all).

Infectious Disorders

Viral Diseases: Upper and lower respiratory tract viral infections are some of the commonest infectious disorders encountered in the horse. Some of the important virus diseases are geographically restricted by epidemiological or other environmental factors while others are almost universal. Respiratory virus infections are a significant cause of acute illness in the horse and frequently predispose to secondary bacterial infections, and to possible subsequent small airway (allergic) diseases. In general, most of the common respiratory virus infections result in a similar clinical syndrome, with only minor variations associated with particular viruses. Almost all these infections induce some degree of coughing and nasal discharge. Most of them initially induce a serous nasal discharge (**Plate 6a**, page 120) which progress through catarrhal stages (**Plate 6b**, page 120) as recovery follows. If secondary bacterial infection is present the discharges become progressively more purulent (**Plate 6c; Plate 6d; Plate 6e**, page 120). The less virulent virus diseases are also commonly reported to cause reduction in performance or reduced exercise tolerance without any other overt clinical signs. Whilst single virus infections do certainly occur, complexes of virus and bacterial infections, in which several different pathogenic viruses and bacteria may be identified, are relatively common. In most such cases, a single pathogen may have been responsible for the initial infection but opportunist and commensal potential pathogens become increasingly significant. Diagnosis usually depends on the isolation of virus particles from pharyngeal swabs, and serological tests to confirm the increasing immunological response of the host to a particular virus.

The **equine influenza virus** complex and **equine herpes virus type-1 and type-4**, infections are possibly the commonest significant pathogenic virus infections encountered in temperate climates. Both diseases have a high morbidity amongst young horses, but have a low mortality in normal healthy horses. The clinical features of the diseases caused by the two virus complexes are largely similar with respect to the respiratory signs, although other systems may also be affected by some of the variants of these viruses. Affected horses are usually, however, acutely ill, with pyrexia, coughing and variable lymphadenopathy. In practical situations it is often not possible to positively identify the pathogen, especially when only a limited number of horses in a group is involved. In most cases the identification is then of academic interest to the owners of the horses, but may seriously influence epidemiological controls and vaccination programmes. Most individual cases affected by the common viruses will either have recovered or be suffering from complications by the time serological or other confirmation of the type of virus is available.

Equine herpes virus type-1 (**EHV-1**) and **type-4** (**EHV-4**) are common respiratory pathogens throughout the world. Although both types are universally important EHV-4 has been more frequently associated with respiratory disease alone. Severe epidemics of equine herpes virus infection are uncommon. A wide range of clinical syndromes is possible ranging from inapparent, through sub-clinical to severe, life threatening disease. The virus induces a marked rhinopneumonitis with serous ocular and nasal discharges (**Plate 6a**, page 120) and an obvious diffuse tracheitis (**Plate 4a**, page 102). A harsh,

211

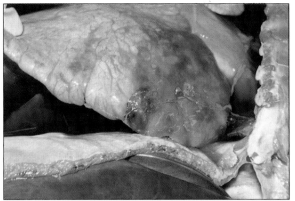

212

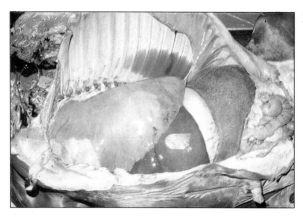

211 Equine herpes virus (Type-1/4) pneumonitis.
Note: Limited area of pulmonary consolidation of right apical areas of the lung. Pleural inflammation with fibrin adhesion and pleural exudate.

212 Equine herpes virus (type-1/4).
Note: Near-term aborted fetus.
Note: Enlarged spleen, perirenal edema, pleural effusion and congested solid lungs. Virus isolated from several organs.

non-productive cough during exercise, which is easily induced by tracheal or pharyngeal manipulation, is characteristic. Affected horses do not usually cough while at rest. Pulmonary involvement, which typically affects the most cranial parts of the lung **(211)**, is audible on auscultation. Once secondary bacterial infection develops the cough may become productive and the nasal discharge is more purulent **(Plate 6c**, page 120**)**. While EHV-4 probably only causes respiratory disease, EHV-1 may also cause abortion in the last trimester of pregnancy and this may occur between 3 weeks and 3 months after infection. It is also responsible for the well-recognised neurological disorder which affects adult horses, and is associated with an ischemic vasculitis within the spinal cord **(728)**. Mares with a prolonged interval between repeated exposures to EHV-1 virus seem to be at greater risk of both abortion and the neurological syndrome. Foals under 3–4 months of age, with normal levels of passive (maternal) immunity are usually only mildly affected, often with only serological evidence to support the diagnosis, but weanlings between 4 and 8 months of age may be more severely affected. Foals (and older horses) suffering from immune deficiency syndromes may be seriously affected. Death from a fulminating pneumonitis (*see* **211**) may occur. Foals infected *in utero* are usually stillborn but those born alive are usually weak and die shortly after birth, showing extensive pulmonary, pleural, hepatic and adrenal gland pathology **(212)**. Adult horses or foals suffering from any immunologic suppression, whether as a result of disorders of immune mechanisms or from concurrent temporary or milder disorders, may develop severe pulmonary disease which

may be life-threatening. More usually however, the diseases are detected serologically with limited clinical signs occurring simultaneously in a number of in-contact horses and confirmed by virus isolation techniques.

Influenza virus infection which is notably absent, at present, in Australasia, produces most of the typical signs mentioned above, but, in addition, often causes a marked conjunctivitis. While pulmonary involvement is usually minimal, certain strains of the virus (notably Influenza A-Equi type 1) have a more pneumotropic effect with more obvious pulmonary involvement. Cases of equine influenza usually have an acute onset of fever, depression and inappetence. An explosive, non-productive cough, which is present even when the animal is at rest, and lymphadenopathy, possibly accompanied by peripheral limb edema, are common signs. A marked tracheitis **(Plate 4a**, page 102**)** may be present, and, again, secondary bacterial infection is a frequent complication. This infection may have much more severe affects upon young foals, and particularly those with compromised immune status, than equine herpes virus infection. More rarely, severe effects on the lung and/or myocardium may be encountered. Horses affected by this virus group are probably much more susceptible to other respiratory pathogens, allergens and irritants, and may take some weeks, or even months, to recover fully from even mild infections. Confirmation of the pathogen is obtained from a rising antibody titre over the following two to three weeks and by virus isolation from pharyngeal swabs.

Young horses under 3–4 years of age, and occasionally older animals, which are examined endoscopically, are often found to have a prominent

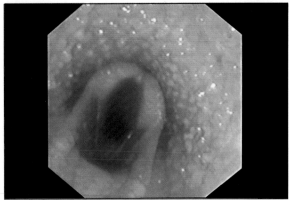

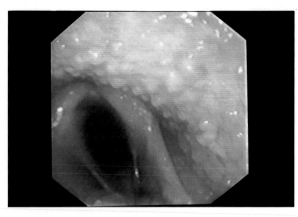

213 Chronic pharyngeal lymphoid hyperplasia (CPLH, pharyngitis, lymphoid follicular hyperplasia) (Grade IV). **Note**: Blister-like lesions over most of pharyngeal wall.

214 Pharyngeal lymphoid hyperplasia (CPLH, pharyngitis, lymphoid follicular hyperplasia) (Grade III). **Note:** Pustule-like lesions with catarrhal exudate over most of pharyngeal wall.

pharyngeal lymphoid hyperplasia (also known as **pharyngitis** or **lymphoid follicular hyperplasia**) covering more or less of the dorsal and/or lateral pharyngeal surfaces. Epidemiological evidence suggests that the condition is probably a result of complex viral and bacterial infections, particularly involving the equine herpes and equine influenza viruses. Interestingly, although the disorder is commonly encountered in Australasia there is no evidence of equine influenza virus in that region. The visible lesions vary in appearance and the condition is graded according to the distribution and numbers of lesions which are present. In Grade I hyperplasia the lesions are restricted to a limited area around the pharyngeal tonsil (dorsal pharyngeal recess), whereas Grade IV shows marked hypertrophy over a wide area of the pharyngeal wall, with particularly intense lesions in the area of the tonsil. The character of the individual lesions also varies. In acute cases small discrete red foci (often having a central depression) or blister/vesicle-like lesions (**213**) are present. Yellow-tipped conical lesions (**214**) are found in longer standing cases. The chronic (quiescent or recovered) form is represented by a few, small, flat, white follicles over the roof of the pharynx, often arranged in linear fashion (**Plate 5a**, page 111) and the absence of any surface exudate. It is not clear whether any particular clinical appearance represents more, or less, aggressive lesions, and furthermore, it is possible that the condition is a normal physiological/ immunological response to natural viral/bacterial challenges in the young horse. In most cases there are no detectable clinical signs. However, occasional animals are severely affected by active, edematous lesions covering the greater part of the dorsal and lateral

walls of the nasopharynx and possibly extending into the guttural pouches. Coughing, repeated swallowing and recurrent or persistent dorsal displacement of the soft palate (**Plate 5a**, page 111) are blamed on the condition. The more severe forms may also have a deleterious effect on exercise tolerance and milder forms might be responsible for lesser performance limitations. The disease is only diagnosed on endoscopic examination and the clinical signs attributed to it may not in fact be related to its presence.

There are numerous other virus infections which produce mild or moderate upper respiratory tract infections including **equine picornavirus** and **equine adenovirus**, but, typically, these are almost asymptomatic, except in immune-suppressed horses such as those affected by **combined immuno-deficiency syndrome (CID)**, and those affected by **pituitary-adrenal axis disorders** such as **Cushing's disease** (*see 362 et seq.*). In these, there may be catastrophic effects from relatively mild pathogens including viral (and bacterial) pneumonia, diarrhea and septicemia.

African Horse Sickness is, possibly, the most serious viral respiratory disorder of the horse. The disease is limited geographically to areas of Africa, the Middle East and Southern Europe and it causes widespread mortality (up to 95% or more) amongst susceptible populations of horses, mules and donkeys. The zebra may act as an asymptomatic carrier of the virus, and as such have possibly been responsible for the introduction of the disease into previously disease-free areas. Most countries where the disease is not present have strict regulations regarding its quarantine and control. African Horse Sickness is believed to be transmitted by nocturnal biting insects of the *Culicoides*

215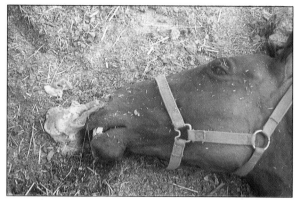

216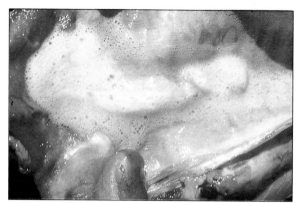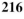

215 African Horse Sickness (pulmonary form).
Note: Profuse blood stained, frothy nasal discharge.
Differential Diagnosis:
i) Congestive heart failure
ii) Paraquat poisoning
iii) Anaphylactic shock
iv) Lightning / electrocution

216 African Horse Sickness (pulmonary form).
Note: Severe pulmonary edema with froth in airway resulting in death.

217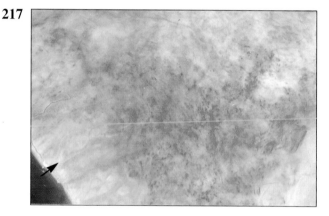

218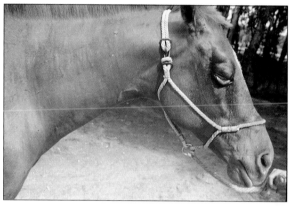

217 African Horse Sickness (pulmonary form).
Note: Pulmonary edema (mottling of lung) with prominent lymphatic vessels along margin of lung (arrow), petechial and ecchymotic hemorrhages over pleural surface.

218 African Horse Sickness (cardiac form) ('Dikkop').
Note: Swelling of head and neck and chemosis (edema of conjunctiva).

group, with *Culicoides imicola* being the most likely vector. There is a strong seasonal incidence which closely follows the prevalence of these insects. A variety of clinical syndromes may be encountered, which are dependent upon the susceptibility of the individual horse and the virulence of the strain of virus involved, particularly with respect to its pneumotropism. Four forms of African Horse Sickness are described, ranging from a peracute, rapidly progressive, highly fatal form, to a mild, almost inapparent respiratory infection. These various syndromes are, however, not well defined and it is not often possible to categorise a specific case into one or other of them. However, all but the mildest types show marked cardiac and respiratory involvement.

The clinical characteristics of the **peracute (pulmonary) syndrome** are largely the result of massive, catastrophic pulmonary edema, in which a profuse nasal discharge of yellowish, frothy liquid sometimes blood tinged **(215)** is present. Paroxysmal coughing, sweating and a high fever are prominent features. Death usually occurs between 4 and 24 hours after the onset of clinical signs. Post mortem examination confirms the presence of extensive accumulations of froth in the conducting airways **(216)** and marked pulmonary edema **(217)**. The lungs are water-logged, exude large volumes of protein-containing fluid, and fail to collapse.

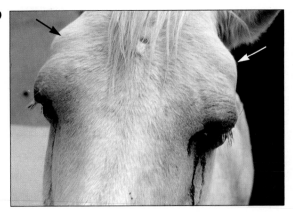

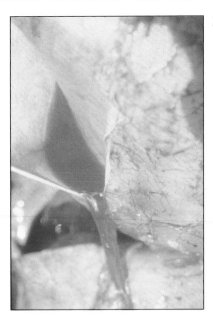

219 African Horse Sickness (cardiac form) ('Dikkop'). **Note:** Swelling of eyelids and supraorbital fossae (arrows), lacrimation.

220 African Horse Sickness (cardiac form). **Note:** Hemorrhagic pericardial effusion.

The sub-acute or **cardiac form of African Horse Sickness** has a somewhat longer course and is characterised by swelling (edema) of the head (**218**), neck, trunk and limbs. The temporal fossae and eyelids are usually grossly swollen (**219**). Prominent chemosis (conjunctival edema) is almost always present in cases which survive beyond 24 hours (*see* **218**). Cyanosis (**Plate 8b**, page 178), congestion (**Plate 8c**, page 178) and petechial hemorrhages (**Plate 8g**, page 179) are usually visible on mucous membranes. Clinically, cardiac tamponade secondary to pericardial effusion may be detectable. Cases which survive for a few days may develop a serious and profound pharyngeal paralysis (**Plate 6r**, page 123) in which nasal re-gurgitation of food and water is present. This latter sign may be made even more obvious by the fact that affected horses will often continue to eat and drink despite apparently severe distress and a high fever. While some cases of the cardiac form of African Horse Sickness survive, the mortality is nevertheless high, with many horses succumbing between 1 and 4 days after onset. Those surviving the first four days are usually destined to recover, provided that no secondary complications arise, and provided that they are not unduly stressed. Full recovery may, however, take months, or even years in some cases.

A **mixed form**, showing features of both the cardiac and pulmonary form is occasionally encountered. Usually, these are cases which have initially survived the cardiac form, but which subsequently develop a peracute, invariably fatal, pulmonary form. Sometimes it is seen in cases which survive the pulmonary form but

residual cardiac signs are prominent. Again, the course is usually fatal. Post mortem findings include severe hydrothorax, hydropericardium (**220**) and pulmonary edema (*see* **217**) with failure of the lungs to collapse. Extensive ecchymotic and petechial hemorrhages are present on the epicardium and endocardium. There may be significant amounts of peritoneal fluid which in some cases contains small numbers of red cells and while colic is not commonly encountered it may be difficult to eliminate the presence of serious intestinal complications.

The mildest forms of African Horse Sickness are probably the result of a non-virulent virus attacking a partially-immune host. In this form, which is often referred to as **horse sickness fever**, there may be few clinical signs apart from a mild and transient pyrexia, swelling of the eyelids and supraorbital fossae (*see* **219**), and occasional, transient dyspnea. Contrary to the more serious types, appetite in these horses is often depressed and the disease closely resembles the respiratory syndromes caused by equine herpes virus, equine influenza virus and equine viral arteritis (*see* **298**). A definitive diagnosis of African Horse Sickness can usually be established by virus isolation, serology and epidemiological features.

Bacterial Diseases: Foals under 6 months of age are particularly susceptible to infection with *Rhodococcus (Corynebacterium) equi*. Some diseased foals are found dead without a history of any respiratory or other premonitory signs, or die over the course of a few days from the onset of clinical disease. Most, however, show an insidious onset of a progressive respiratory disorder

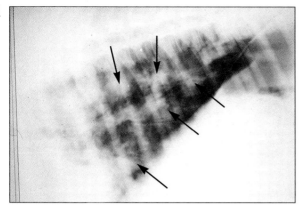

221 *Rhodococcus equi* (pulmonary form) (standing lateral radiograph).
Note: Multiple radiodense lesions throughout lung tissue (abscesses)(arrows).

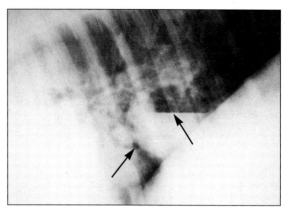

222 *Rhodococcus equi* (pulmonary form) (standing lateral radiograph).
Note: Few large abscesses in lung tissue. Some have ruptured into the airway and show air-fluid interfaces (Arrows).

attributable to suppurative bronchopneumonia. Initially, affected foals show a mild, intermittent pyrexia and progressive lethargy and weakness. There is often an elevated resting respiratory rate. The breathing pattern gradually becomes faster and more abdominal and foals may ultimately become patently cyanotic. A purulent nasal discharge and coughing are only rarely present. The growth rate is often poor, and although affected foals may be seen to suckle they are often weak and feed poorly. Even minor exertion may result in collapse. The development of obvious clinical signs is often delayed for some weeks (or even months) after initial infection, and this may make the prognosis difficult to assess. There are few pathognomic clinical signs, but auscultation of the thorax usually reveals prominent adventitious sounds consistent with bronchopneumonia. These include wheezing and crackling sounds and where there is a quantity of tracheal exudate an audible rattle, coordinated with breathing may be present. Thoracic percussion may detect areas of obvious consolidation and cases pleural effusion may be detected by an elevation of the ventral percussible border of the lung. Individual cases may develop a profuse, watery diarrhea and where this occurs with advanced respiratory signs the prognosis for recovery is much reduced, even when aggressive therapeutic measures are taken. In spite of the existence of extensive cecal and colonic lesions (*see* **225**), gross intestinal dysfunction is not common, however. Individual cases may be affected only with the intestinal form. Radiographic examination of the thorax reveals severe bronchopneumonia (**221**). Large, well defined, encapsulated or ruptured pulmonary abscesses

(**222**) represent the more advanced stages of the infection. The presence of pleural effusions represents a serious complication. Serial radiographic examination of the thorax is a useful aid in the assessment of disease progression, with progressive resolution of the pulmonary lesions indicating an improvement, and therefore a better prognosis. Individual cases may show a chronic, non-suppurative synovitis in one or more joints and/or uveitis, with an obvious aqueous flare and hypopyon (inflammatory debris in the anterior chamber of the eye) (*see* **642**). Bacteriological cultures from tracheal aspirates, feces or blood of affected foals almost always contain *Rhodococcus equi* bacteria and, although the organism can be isolated from the feces of some normal, apparently unaffected horses, pure cultures from feces or trachea and any bacterial content of the blood are significant. Hematological and biochemical changes, including elevations of plasma fibrinogen and absolute neutrophil and platelet counts, are helpful in establishing the clinical progression of individual cases and the earliest benefits from therapeutic measures, when falls in all of these parameters indicate an improving disease status. Once these values have persistently returned to normal, the foal is probably cured, particularly if there is simultaneous radiographic evidence of resolution.

Adult horses, and foals over 6 months of age, are solidly resistant to infection with *Rhodococcus equi*, unless the animal is severely immuno-compromised such as with the immune deficiency syndromes or with pituitary-adrenal axis disorders (*see* **362 et seq.**).

Post mortem examination of foals affected by the respiratory form of *Rhodococcus equi* infection will

223

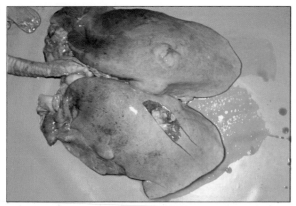

224

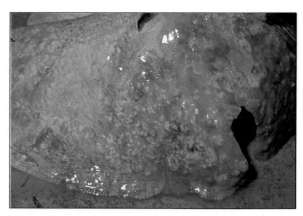

223 *Rhodococcus equi* (pulmonary form).
Note: Large numbers of abscess lesions in lung parenchyma. Abscesses were well encapsulated and contained creamy-yellow, purulent material.

224 *Rhodococcus equi* (pulmonary form).
Note: Miliary abscesses, probably developed as a result of septicemic dissemination into the lungs (compare with **223**).

Differential Diagnosis:
i) Septicaemia (salmonella spp., *E. coli*, actinobacillus spp.
ii) Tuberculosis

225

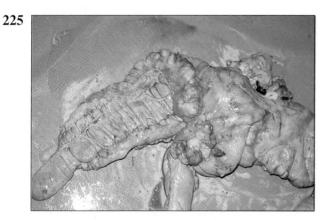

225 *Rhodococcus equi* (intestinal form).
Note: Foal presented with severe diarrhea. Large numbers of abscesses in mesentery and lymph nodes of colon and cecum. Lesions were also present in mesenteric lymph nodes at root of mesentery, and in the eyes. Miliary abscesses were present in the lungs (**224**).

confirm the presence of large and/or small well-defined abscesses within the lung substance (**223**) and/or miliary abscesses throughout the lung (**224**). The abscesses are characteristically well encapsulated and usually contain a caseous, purulent material. Cases having extensive intestinal involvement show large numbers of small (or larger) abscesses in the wall of the cecum and colon (**225**). Lesions may also be present in the mesenteric lymphatic vessels and associated lymph nodes.

Perhaps the most common bacterial infections of the respiratory tract of horses are those due to Streptococcal bacteria and *Streptococcus equi* and *Streptococcus zooepidemicus*, in particular. Infections with either (or both) of these bacteria are commonly encountered subsequent to respiratory (or other) virus infections,

when they are probably secondary opportunist pathogens. Both organisms can, furthermore, often be cultured from the respiratory tracts of apparently normal horses.

Streptococcus equi is the causative organism of the disease commonly referred to as '**Strangles**'. The condition may occur in horses of all ages, although those under 5 years of age are probably most susceptible and therefore most frequently affected by serious forms of the disease. The clinical signs depend largely upon the individual form which the infection takes in a particular animal, and are probably dependent upon the immune status of the host and the virulence of the bacterial strain involved. The organism can apparently survive well within macrophages in non-immune or partially immune horses and can furthermore be found in the respiratory

226

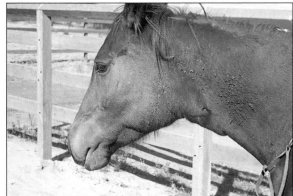

227

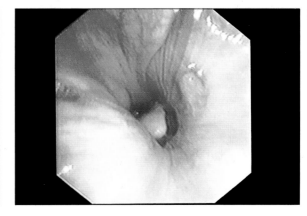

228

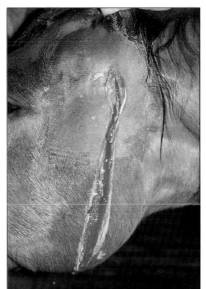

226 Strangles (*Streptococcus equi*).
Note: Massive pharyngeal and submandibular lymphadenopathy.
Differential Diagnosis:
i)   False strangles (*Streptococcus zooepidemicus*)
ii) Pharyngeal abscess/gangrene
iii) Pharyngeal emphysema/edema (tracheal rupture, disruption or dislocation)
iv) Anthrax
v)   Glanders

227 Strangles (*Streptococcus equi*).
Note: Lateral and dorsal pharyngeal compression due to pharyngeal lymphadenopathy.

228 Strangles (*Streptococcus equi*) (ruptured pharyngeal lymph node).
Note: Creamy yellow purulent exudate with some blood.

tract of apparently normal horses. The classical form of Strangles presents with gross lymphadenopathy of the pharyngeal, submaxillary and submandibular lymph nodes (226). This may be sufficient to result in serious, and often life-threatening pharyngeal respiratory obstruction. Endoscopic examination of the pharynx shows a markedly narrowed pharynx (227), with, more or less, dorsal pharyngeal compression (*see* 188), which is usually more severe on one side than the other. (This is the clinical feature which gives rise to the name Strangles.) Affected horses are febrile and frequently stiff about the neck, often being unable to feed from the floor, and holding their necks in extension in an attempt to provide some relief from the pharyngeal pain and respiratory obstruction which may be sufficient to warrant an emergency tracheostomy. The pharyngeal obstruction often causes dysphagia and food material, saliva and purulent exudates from the pharynx may appear at the nose. The enlarged lymph nodes ultimately

burst releasing a creamy-yellow pus, often with some blood (228). While some abscesses burst outwards, others may rupture into the pharynx or guttural pouches, producing a profuse purulent nasal discharge (possibly with some blood) (**Plate 6d**, page 120). A purulent discharge from the ostia of the auditive tube may reflect the stage of the infection in the pharyngeal lymph nodes, the discharges usually being hemorrhagic immediately after rupture of the abscesses, and purulent thereafter (229). Occasionally the discharge from guttural pouches or pharynx may be profuse. Milder forms of Strangles in which the extent of pharyngeal lymph node abscess formation is minimal and the systemic effects are much less dramatic, are increasingly recognised. Partially immune, or mature horses appear more likely to develop the milder forms. In these forms the infection with *Streptococcus equi* closely resembles infection with *Streptococcus zooepidemicus*.

'Bastard Strangles' represents the most severe

229

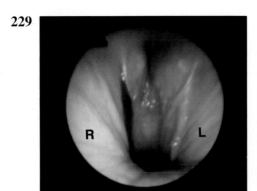

230

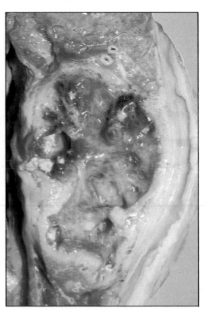

229 Strangles (*Streptococcus equi*) (endoscopic view of pharynx).
Note: Difference in discharges from guttural pouches indicating time differences to rupture of pharyngeal abscesses in guttural pouches. Discharge from left pouch is older than right.
Differential Diagnosis:
i) Guttural pouch mycosis (right)
ii) Guttural pouch empyema/diverticulitis (left)

230 Bastard strangles (*Streptococcus equi*).
Note: Extensive pulmonary abscess with multiple compartments and thick fibrous reaction.

231

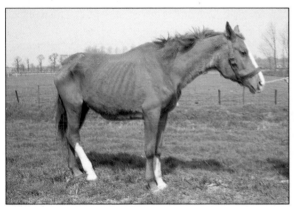

232

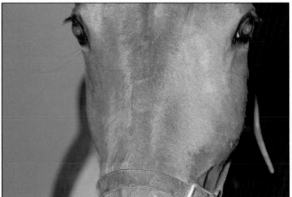

231 Bastard strangles (*Streptococcus equi*) (chronic form).
Note: Pharyngeal swelling, discharging abscesses, weight loss. Tracheostomy tube. Abducted elbow(s) associated with dyspnea. Ventral edema.

232 Maxillary sinusitis (rostral).
Note: Facial distortion.
Differential Diagnosis:
i) Maxillary sinus cyst
ii) Secondary sinusitis (due to periapical infection, or fracture of face)

complication of the classical form of Strangles described above, and may develop subsequent to it or independently. In this form there is 'metastatic' distribution of the organism to lymph nodes and organs other than those of the pharynx and head, presumably following inhalation or pyemic spread of the organism in an animal which is either immune-suppressed or fully susceptible. While large encapsulated, or miliary abscesses may occur in any site, the commonest locations are the lungs (**230**), liver, spleen, kidney and brain (*see* **730**). Abscesses may also develop in the skin (*see* **547**) and within synovial structures. Diffuse, multiple-organ abscesses result in a clinical condition which has serious systemic effects upon the horse. These include dramatic weight loss, ventral edema (**231**), debilitating and progressive dyspnea and inappetence. A severe anemia associated with chronic infection, and even death, from inanition and overwhelming infection, may occur. Endoscopic evidence for pulmonary involvement includes the detection of generalised tracheal purulent exudate (**Plate 4c**, page 102). Animals which show no improvement in their metabolic, physical and mental status following rupture of pharyngeal abscesses and aggressive therapeutic measures should be regarded as possible cases of 'Bastard Strangles'. A specific diagnosis may, however, be difficult to confirm in the live animal.

Infection with **Streptococcus zooepidemicus** and/or **Streptococcus pneumoniae** are relatively common and although both organisms can be isolated from the respiratory tract of a high proportion of apparently normal horses, they may become pathologically significant in particular circumstances. As neither organism can invade intact mucous membranes they are usually secondary pathogens requiring mucosal disruption within the respiratory tract before they can cause any pathological effect themselves. Severe exercise or respiratory stress from other causes, including other viral and bacterial infections, are common predisposing circumstances. Respiratory tract viruses which cause mucosal damage in the airways including equine herpes and equine influenza viruses are particularly common precursors to pathological infection with these bacteria (and indeed, with *Streptococcus equi*). The clinical signs for both organisms include those attributable to other types of respiratory disease including pyrexia, cough, purulent nasal discharges and lymphadenopathy ('**False Strangles**'). Enlargement of lymph nodes is usually restricted to those of the head and pharynx and may in some cases be sufficient to result in some respiratory obstruction. The complicating factors associated with *Streptococcus equi* infection such

as abscess and systemic dissemination do not usually occur with these organisms, although complicating superimposition of *Streptococcus equi* is relatively common. However, primary or secondary pleural infections (*see* **246**) and sinus infections (**232**) are probably more often associated with *Streptococcus zooepidemicus* and/or *Streptococcus pneumoniae* than with *Streptococcus equi*.

Secondary infections of the respiratory tract of the horse represent a very important group of disorders. **Infections of the paranasal sinuses and the guttural pouches** are particularly common. Infection of the maxillary (and/or frontal sinuses) may arise from direct extension from the nasal cavity or from infection associated with **tooth root disorders** (*see* **37,38**). In the latter cases there may be an associated foul-smelling breath, which is usually restricted to the ipsilateral nostril. The caudal root of the third cheek tooth (fourth premolar) and the roots of the fourth tooth (first molar) are usually located within the rostral compartment of the maxillary sinus. Infections associated either primarily as a result of bacterial infection extending from the nasal cavity, or secondarily related to disease of the roots of these teeth, usually result in swelling and facial distortion (*see* **232**). Only in exceptional circumstances does the rostral compartment of the maxillary sinus communicate with the caudal compartment; the two parts of the maxillary sinus draining independently into the nasal cavity through well defined drainage ostia high on their medial walls. The frontal and caudal maxillary sinus are connected through a wide intercommunicating ostium. The caudal compartment of the maxillary sinus contains the roots of the remaining upper cheek teeth. Infections within the caudal maxillary sinus result in a more caudal facial distortion and swelling. Frontal sinus infections seldom cause any facial distortion. A unilateral purulent nasal discharge is usually present (**Plate 7b; Plate 7c**, page 143). Radiographic examination of the sinus will usually reveal the presence of one or more air/fluid interfaces (fluid level) within the limits of the affected sinus (**233**), each associated with separate divisions within the frontal and/or maxillary sinuses. However, where the contents of the sinus have become inspissated, such distinct features may not be visible. Instead, diffuse and irregular opacities within the confines of the sinuses may be detected (*see* **195**). Endoscopic examination of the caudo-dorsal region of the ipsilateral nasal cavity may reveal fluid and/or purulent discharge descending from the drainage channel created by the converging ventral and dorsal conchae (**234**). This feature will, of course, only identify that the drainage is from either the caudal

233

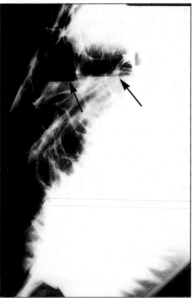

234

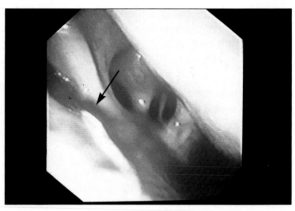

233 Maxillary sinusitis (caudal) (standing lateral radiograph).
Note: Horizontal air-fluid interfaces (fluid levels) (arrows) within limits of caudal maxillary sinus and the conchal component of the frontal sinus.

234 Caudal maxillary (and/or frontal) sinusitis.
Note: purulent material draining from channel created by converging dorsal and ventral conchae (arrow).

maxillary sinus or the frontal sinus (or both) as the two communicate freely and drain by a common ostium into the nasal cavity. In cases with occluded drainage ostia, particularly where there is an inspissated sinus content, trephination of the affected sinus will allow effective endoscopic examination of the contents and in many cases will establish the etiology. Direct visualisation of the tooth roots and the mucosa of the sinus is most useful in this respect.

Bacterial infections within the guttural pouch probably occur more frequently than is realised, both as a primary and secondary disorder. Mild infections associated with primary virus or mild bacterial infections frequently result in a diffuse catarrhal inflammation of the guttural pouch mucosa (**diverticulitis**) which can only be identified effectively through endoscopic examination. A diffuse 'velvet' appearance to the mucosal surface of the pouch with an apparent loss of detailed structure (**235**) is often recognisable in the more severe cases. The normal, clearly-visible, superficial blood vessels and nerves are lost to view under a velvety homogeneous blanket of catarrhal or purulent exudate and mucosal inflammation and edema (**235**). As soon as there is significant accumulation of inflammatory debris in the pouches, some swelling will become apparent in the parotid region (**236**). Usually, this is considerable and displaces the parotid salivary gland making it much

more prominent, but the location of the tendon of insertion of the *sternocephalicus* muscle may displace the swelling to a more ventral site than might be expected (*see* **236**). Endoscopic examination shows marked dorsal pharyngeal compression (**237**) which, particularly if the disorder is bilateral, may be sufficient to result in severe inspiratory dyspnea. The amount and character of the purulent material in each guttural pouch is often significantly different and consequently the pharyngeal distortion may be asymmetric, and, indeed, this will also be the case when only one pouch is affected. The contents are usually either fluid or solid and the amount of purulent material is largely dependent upon its consistency and the efficiency of drainage from the auditive (eustachian) tube. Most horses affected with diverticulitis or guttural pouch empyema will, however, show some accumulation of purulent material as the auditive tube does not drain from the most dependent part of the pouch. Furthermore, the auditive tube itself is commonly involved in the inflammatory process and is often, therefore, somewhat narrowed or even totally occluded. In most cases, even when the contents are very solid, purulent material will be seen to be draining from the ostium within the pharynx and the character of this may reflect the type of inflammation which is present (*see* **237**). Very liquid content (**238**) will, however, usually drain relatively freely, particularly

235

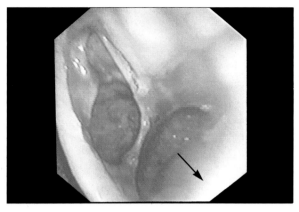

236

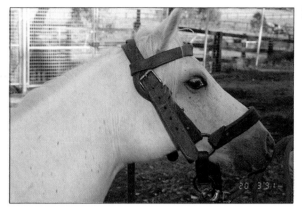

235 Diverticulitis.
Note: Loss of normally obvious anatomical structures within guttural pouch due to catarrhal exudate and fibrinous adhesions. Quantity of liquid purulent material in floor of medial compartment (arrow).

236 Guttural pouch empyema (Empyema of the diverticulum of the auditive tube).
Note: Swelling (non-tympanitic) below tendon of insertion of *sternocephalicus* m.
Differential Diagnosis:
i) Guttural pouch tympany
ii) Strangles
iii) Guttural pouch hemorrhage
iv) Parotid salivary mucocele
v) Parotid melanoma/melanosarcoma

237

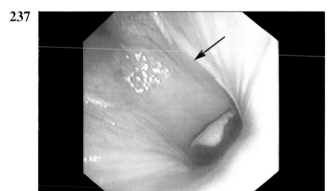

238

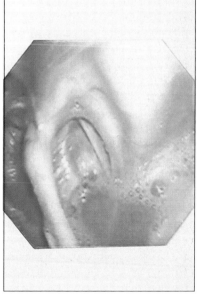

237 Guttural pouch empyema (empyema of the diverticulum of the auditive tube) (endoscopic view of pharynx).
Note: Purulent discharge from pharyngeal ostium of left pouch (arrow). Marked dorsal pharyngeal compression.
Differential Diagnosis:
i) Guttural pouch tympany
ii) Diverticulitis

238 Guttural pouch empyema (empyema of the diverticulum of the auditive tube) (endoscopic view of pouch).
Note: Very liquid contents, generalised diverticulitis with loss of normally obvious detailed anatomical features such as blood vessels and nerves.

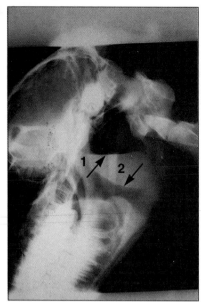

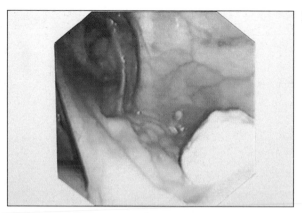

239 Guttural pouch empyema (empyema of the diverticulum of the auditive tube) (standing lateral radiograph).
Note: Very young foal (dental germ centres visible). Horizontal air-fluid interface (fluid level) visible (arrow 1). Dorsal pharyngeal compression (arrow 2).

240 Guttural pouch empyema (empyema of the diverticulum of the auditive tube) (endoscopic view).
Note: Caseated, purulent material on floor of medial compartment. Some loss of surface detail.

when the head of the horse is lowered, giving rise to a largely, posture-related nasal discharge which may be either bilateral or unilateral (in the event that only one pouch is affected). Profuse discharges from a single guttural pouch will often result in bilateral nasal discharge although there may be differences in amount in each nostril (**Plate 6c**, page 120). Where the content is fluid in consistency lateral radiographs of the pharyngeal region show both a fluid line, created by the air-fluid interface, and significant dorsal pharyngeal compression (**239**). Longer standing accumulations are often associated with progressive inspissation. More solid masses of purulent material with a caseous appearance may, therefore, be observed endoscopically (**240**), and radiographically. In these cases, of course, no fluid line will be shown on standing, lateral radiographs but dorsal pharyngeal compression and an ill-defined opacity in the floor of the pouch will be seen. In the event that the pouch is filled with purulent material, a diffuse opacity of the affected pouch(es) will be present with a particularly severe dorsal pharyngeal compression (**241**). Purulent exudates which have been present for very long periods sometimes form into discreet balls (known as **chondroids**) which are rendered more or less spherical by continued inspissation and the sustained tumbling against each other within the confines of the pouch (**242**). They may occur in considerable numbers or there may be relatively few larger masses. On occasion, their rattling movement may be audible as the horses head is

moved, and particularly during exercise. Radiographically the appearance will be dependant upon the number of chondroids present, the extent to which they fill the pouch and their relative density, but they are usually obvious as discrete circular structures or a diffuse opacity of the whole affected pouch with obvious dorsal pharyngeal compression. Occasionally, chronic inflammation of the pouches results in neuropathies related to dysfunction of the glossopharyngeal, vagus, facial and sympathetic nerves which lie within, or adjacent to, the diverticulum. The signs include dysphagia (**Plate 6r**, page 123), facial paralysis (*see* **689** *et seq.*) and Horner's Syndrome (*see* **697**). Erosion of major blood vessels within the guttural pouch is only rarely associated with bacterial diverticulitis but rupture of localised abscesses may result in catastrophic hemorrhage; presenting with signs more often attributable to guttural pouch mycosis (*see* **250** *et seq.*). A diagnosis of diverticulitis or guttural pouch empyema relies heavily upon endoscopic and radiographic examination although the clinical appearance may be strongly suggestive of the disorders. Where neither radiographic nor endoscopic facilities exist, it is still possible to introduce a rigid catheter into the guttural pouch and aspirate the contents.

The other site in which bacterial infection causes severe respiratory disease in the horse is the **pleural cavity**. Although the pleurae seem particularly susceptible to bacterial infection with *Streptococcus spp.*

241

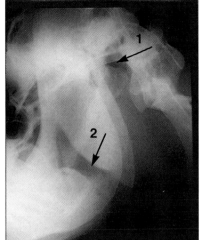

242

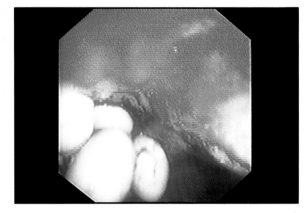

241 Guttural pouch empyema (empyema of the diverticulum of the auditive tube) (standing lateral radiograph).
Note: Diffuse opacity of both guttural pouches (no air present except at very top of one pouch- arrow 1). Dorsal pharyngeal compression (arrow 2).

242 Guttural pouch empyema (empyema of the diverticulum of the auditive tube) (endoscopic view). **Note**: Chondroids (inspissated and 'tumbled' purulent material). Generalised diverticulitis with loss of detailed structures such as blood vessels on mucosa.

bacteria, a wide variety of other organisms are also potentially very dangerous in this site. Usually, affected animals have suffered from a previous viral or bacterial respiratory tract infection coupled with stress, including transportation. The initial pleural inflammatory response (**pleuritis**) may be mild and pass unnoticed, but extensive purulent material develops rapidly thereafter and is often complicated by anaerobic infection. The condition is responsible for the development of intense parietal pain and affected horses are consequently reluctant to move and have a prominent abdominal component to breathing. They seldom cough but, when they do, this is soft and obviously painful and there may be an associated grunt, which may also be present at the end of expiration. There is frequently an obvious, foul-smelling, bilateral, purulent nasal discharge which is often flecked with blood or is overtly hemorrhagic (**Plate 6k**, page 122). Pressure applied between the ribs elicits marked pain and an obvious guarding response. The presence of anaerobic infection within the pleural cavity is accompanied by a severe depression and the nasal discharge becomes particularly foul. The elbows are often abducted and there may be considerable sternal (ventral) edema (**243**). Horses with extensive, fibrinous, pleural adhesions may show less pain than those in which the inflammatory response is still active and allows movement between the visceral and parietal pleural surfaces. Where the disorder has been present for some weeks a profound non-regenerative iron-deficiency-type anemia, will be noticed in most cases

(**Plate 8d**, page 178). The metabolic effects of the condition are usually serious, with poor, or very poor, oxygenation and progressive sequestration of protein and fluid into the pleural space. In such cases ultrasonographic examination, using a sector array head, is an extremely useful aid to the diagnosis, and the findings have a considerable bearing on the prognosis. Fibrin tags, locules of purulent fluid, fluid levels and adhesions between the visceral and parietal pleurae will usually be clearly demonstrated and provide evidence of a dangerous **pleuritis**. Radiographic examination of the chest is a useful adjunct to ultrasonography and will usually identify an obvious horizontal gas-fluid interface which can also be demonstrated by percussion, when the ventral percussible border of the lung will be significantly elevated (*see* **243**). However, the purulent material may not always be fluid in consistency and, furthermore, may be loculated into discreet areas making diagnosis more difficult. Under these circumstances thoracocentesis (**244**) and cytological and bacteriological examination of the pleural effusion are particularly useful. A discrepancy in the height of the fluid levels on the two sides, or differences in the character of the contents, or obvious differences in the ultrasonographic features are indicative of unilateral pleuritis (**245**). In many cases the two cavities will be affected to a different extent, and the infection will be of different duration. Where the disorder is relatively early in its development primary pleuritis usually involves only one lung (the right most usually), but progressive disruption of the

243

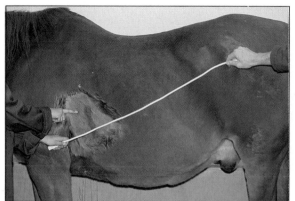

243 Pleuritis (pleural effusion).
Note: Normal ventral percussible border of lung shown by white tape. Elevation indicated by finger and site of aspiration. Ventral oedema and prepucial swelling.
Differential Diagnosis: (NB. volume and nature of contents very important)
i)   Mediastinal or pleural neoplasia
ii) Hydrothorax
iii) Hemothorax (ruptured thoracic vessels)
iv) Pyothorax (Bastard strangles, *Rhodococcus equi*, nocardiosis)
v) Chylothorax (ruptured thoracic duct)
vi) African Horse Sickness
vii)Congestive heart failure

244

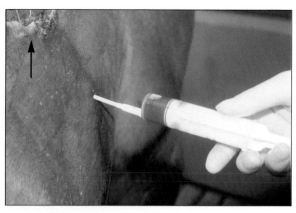

244 Pleuritis (pyothorax).
Note: Thorax opened due to chest injury (arrow) with fractured rib. Elevated percussible ventral border of lung. Ultrasonographic examination showed multiple loculated fibrinous lesions. Radiography showed distinct air/gas-fluid interface. Contents of pleural cavity hemorrhagic, purulent material with thick, creamy, cellular sediment.
Differential Diagnosis:
i)   Thoracic neoplasia (different radiologically, ultrasonographically and in character of exudate)
ii) Primary pleuritis

245

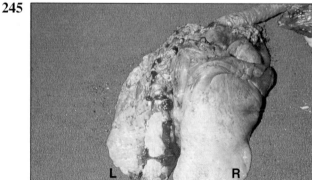

246

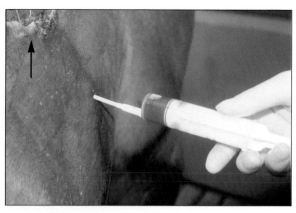

247

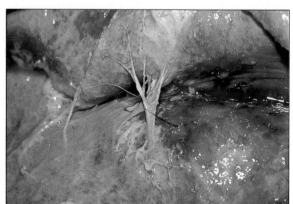

245 Unilateral pleuritis (left).
Note: Young horse. Condition followed upper respiratory tract infection and transportation. Pleural cavities obviously separate.

246 Fibrinous pleuritis.
Note: Both lungs affected but to different extent (pleural cavities separated).

247 Pleuritis (chronic).
Note: Dense fibrinous adhesions between visceral and parietal pleura.

mediastinum frequently results in fenestration of the mediastinum and extension to the contralateral cavity. In all cases involving pleural effusions, therefore, both thoracic cavities should be examined by all means at the disposal of the clinician and due note taken of any differences which are present. In cases of infective pleuritis, purulent material will be aspirated from the cavity, often, though not invariably, in large amounts (*see* **244**). Where anaerobic bacteria are present the material obtained by thoracocentesis frequently has a foul odour, which is reflected also in the breath. The fluid will be found to contain a high number of inflammatory cells, most of which will be degenerate, and which form a dense, beige-yellow deposit if the fluid is left to stand for a few minutes. Most other conditions with significant pleural effusions, such as hydrothorax and neoplasia, have sterile and odour-free pleural aspirates. Very large amounts of fluid which are rapidly replaced in an animal which shows no pleural pain are usually of neoplastic, metabolic or circulatory origin. While most cases of infectious pleuritis are the result of systemic or pyemic infection, others follow penetrating wounds of the chest wall (*see* **244**), rib fractures which may puncture the lung or may be open fractures, or from rupture into the pleural cavity of *Rhodococcus equi* or *Streptococcus equi* abscesses from within the lung substance. The presence of any pleural effusion is to be regarded as extremely serious and every effort should be made to establish the cause as early in the course as is possible. Dramatic deteriorations within hours or days are common in apparently mild cases of infective pleuritis which may initially affect only one cavity and may be clinically almost undetectable. A combined pleuritis and pneumonia is a most serious combination. A marked neutrophilia and elevations of platelet count and plasma fibrinogen concentration are indicative of an advancing inflammatory process and reductions may be used to assess the effect of therapeutic measures.

Post mortem findings in cases of infected pleuritis are variable according to the type of bacteria present and the duration of the condition. Usually, the pleural cavities of the horse are separated but in some normal horses and in most cases of pleuritis this division is incomplete. Infective pleuritis in young horses may initially affect one pleural cavity only (*see* **245**) (usually the right), or both cavities may be simultaneously affected (possibly to a different extent). Long-standing, infective pleuritis cases almost always affect both cavities to about the same extent. Inflammatory debris, fluid in consistency, are reflected in a distinct line of demarcation on the pleural surface whereas in other cases fibrin will be found over the entire pleural surface (**246**). Long-standing inflammation results in the development of extensive (often dense) fibrinous adhesions between the visceral and parietal pleurae (**247**). It is not always possible to establish the original cause of the problem, particularly as the course is rapid and secondary infections are particularly quick to establish themselves.

Young foals and, more rarely, older horses may develop **pulmonary abscesses** or more diffuse **pneumonia** following septicemic infections with organisms such as *Salmonella* spp., *Escherichia coli*, *Pasteurella* spp., and other Gram-negative organisms. Usually such abscesses are miliary in distribution (*see* **224**) and arise from diffuse embolic spread throughout the lung tissue.

Ingestion or inhalation of avian or bovine strains of tuberculosis has been responsible for the development of a chronic debilitating disease in which neck stiffness and localised or generalised lymphadenopathy are present. In the later stages of the disease, the horse is generally febrile (either persistently or intermittently) and the resting respiratory rate is high. The characteristic lesions in the intestine (**141**), spleen, mesenteric lymph nodes and lungs have a tumour-like appearance, being devoid of any caseating material and without well defined capsules.

Although the horse is apparently particularly resistant to infection with *Mycobacteria* spp., pulmonary tuberculosis is recognised in certain parts of the world where the disease associated with this bacterial species in other domestic and wild animals, is endemic. **Tuberculosis**, particularly attributable to *Mycobacterium avium*, in the horse may produce pulmonary or intestinal lesions, and occasionally affects other organs. A chronic, soft cough and weight loss with a bilateral, purulent nasal discharge with some hemorrhage (**Plate 6k**, page 122), typical of pulmonary abscess, are the most obvious signs of pulmonary involvement. Lesions in the vertebral bodies and involvement of the meninges and cord in the infective process may have severe consequences. The pulmonary lesions are characteristically miliary, granulomatous abscesses (*see* **224**). Lesions occurring in the intestinal wall are more often single, or few in number and are larger (**141**). Intestinal lesions are, in most cases, regarded as the primary lesion resulting from ingestion of the infective organism, from which miliary hematogenous spread occurs to the lungs and other organs.

One of the most feared primary contagious bacterial diseases of the horse, donkey and mule is **Glanders**; a disease which has been eradicated from large areas of the world, but which is still endemic in parts of Asia and the Middle East. Glanders has been described for many centuries and its severity and zoonotic nature have resulted in an almost universal fear of the disease. Most countries of the world have strict quarantine measures relating to the control of the infection and these have largely been successful in reducing the incidence and, in many places, completely eradicating it. The ease of world wide transportation of horses makes its recognition extremely important. The condition is caused by ***Pseudomonas (Malleomyces) mallei***. Pulmonary, nasal and cutaneous forms are recognised. All are more or less chronic in their course and characterised by the formation of nodules, ulcers and fibrous scars in the skin (*see* **550, 551),** and respiratory tract. **Acute Glanders** is rarely encountered in horses but donkeys and mules are often severely affected by this form. There are few pathognomonic features, but most cases have a tenacious, unilateral, hemorrhagic, mucopurulent nasal discharge, and obvious ulceration of the nasal mucosa. A marked, non-abscess forming lymphadenopathy of the glands of the head is a common feature (*see* **226**). The profuse discharge, and nasal and laryngeal edema induce severe respiratory obstruction. Death as a result of overwhelming bronchopneumonia, respiratory obstruction and septicemia follows in a few days. Horses are more commonly affected by the sub-acute or chronic pulmonary forms, which have an insidious onset, often lasting several months or even longer. In the early stages there may be few overt pathognomonic features with some cases showing only a mild, tenacious, catarrhal nasal discharge which can easily be mistaken for other respiratory tract infections. While, in some cases, the disease may remain in this form for long periods, any superimposed stress (or other disease) will usually result in an immediate development of the sub-acute form. Coughing, weight loss, intermittent or persistent fever, pneumonia and a high respiratory rate may be present. At post mortem examination, which is not without major hazard to the operator, characteristic abscesses and lesions in the respiratory tract, lung, spleen and liver will be present. In the chronic form the obvious nasal ulceration takes on a more benign appearance with a 'glassy' hue and is covered with thick, grey, semi-transparent, tenacious mucus.

Horses with the chronic form of glanders often appear to be remarkably well, and may show a normal enthusiasm for work for extended periods of time. There may be little indication of the potential danger of the nasal discharges, both for the horse itself, and in-contact equidae and humans. Ultimately however, the condition develops into either the naso-pulmonary form or into 'Farcy' (the cutaneous form). Here, ulcerative nodules, which discharge a brownish, honey-coloured pus containing small yellow or brown granules, occur on the nasal, pharyngeal and tracheal mucosae, and along cutaneous lymphatics, particularly over the face, neck (*See* **551**) and the medial thigh and hock regions (*see* **550**). Typically, the nasal lesions heal slowly, leaving a stellate scar. Horses affected with any of the forms of Glanders lose weight dramatically, and almost all will finally develop the true pneumonic form which terminates fatally. A few horses recover and return to normal health after a very prolonged convalescence, often lasting some years. In endemic areas the disease may be confused in its early stages with Strangles and other lesser respiratory viral infections, but while in a few cases the condition may remain mild for long periods, it seldom if ever resolves.

Melioidosis is a condition which closely resembles Glanders which occurs in the Far-East and northern parts of Australia, and is caused by ***Pseudomonas pseudomallei***. Definitive diagnosis of the disease is usually reliant upon post mortem examination and bacterial culture. Affected horses develop a fulminating bronchopneumonia, encephalitis and enteritis. While almost every case of melioidosis will be diagnosed in the acute stage, most cases will have been affected previously by an often, almost inapparent infection, which may have been present for months before the acute stage develops. The chronic form of the disease affecting the skin and the lungs is probably clinically indistinguishable from Glanders.

Fungal Diseases: The nasal cavity of horses may be affected by various fungal infections. **Phycomycosis** due to ***Conidiobolus coronata*** occurs predominately in the United States of America, occasionally in Australia, and rarely in other warm, wet climatic regions. Infection results in numerous small granulating ulcers or fissures in the rostral part of the nasal cavity (**248**). In some cases the size of the lesion and the associated inflammatory response may be sufficient to occlude the affected nostril. Cases are, consequently, presented for the investigation of respiratory stridor, exercise intolerance and/or chronic, unilateral, purulent, nasal discharge which may contain blood (**Plate 7e**, page 144). Air flow patterns through the affected nostril may be impaired and where the disease extends into the sinuses these may become dull-sounding on percussion. The lesions may be visualised directly or by endoscopy (*see* **248**).

The nasal lesions associated with ***Aspergillus*** spp. are commonly encountered in most parts of the world and **nasal aspergillosis** occurs in two main forms. **Non-**

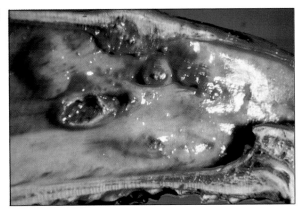

248 Conidiobolus coronata
Note: Ulcerated, nodular lesions in nasal mucosa
Differential Diagnosis:
i) Glanders
ii) Nasal aspergillosis
iii) Amyloidosis

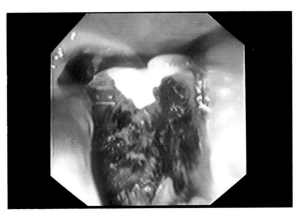

249 Nasal aspergillosis (invasive form).
Note: Wide destruction of nasal mucosa and underlying turbinate with minimal inflammatory margin of lesion. Catarrhal exudate with slight hemorrhage (and foul smell) (**Plate 7e**, page 144).

invasive aspergillosis results in a superficial proliferation of fungal mycelium over the surface of the nasal mucosa. Little clinical effect may be present and most such lesions are detected incidentally, although a mild yellowish mucoid nasal discharge may be encountered (**Plate 7c**, page 143). The more serious invasive or destructive form occurs on the mucosa of the nasal turbinates and occasionally within the maxillary or frontal sinuses. This form results in extensive destruction of the mucosa and the underlying bone (**249**). A surprisingly scanty, foul-smelling, unilateral, purulent nasal discharge, possibly containing some blood (**Plate 7e**, page 144) is usually present, reflecting the limited inflammatory response within the nasal mucosa around the active lesion. The erosive lesion is often black or very dark-red in colour and a fine white, or grey, mycelium can usually be seen over the surface (*see* **249**). Secondary bacterial infection is uncommon. While the larger lesions are pathognomonic for the condition, they may be very small and difficult to appreciate in some cases, and then culture from the nasal discharge or from the surface of the lesions is diagnostic.

Nasal cavity infection with ***Cryptococcus* spp.** also sometimes occurs, producing lesions within the nasal cavity. Fulminating often fatal pulmonary complications may arise. This fungus has a greater tendency to erode the underlying nasal conchal and septal bones, than do *Aspergillus* spp.. The nasal discharges are usually mucoid and sanguineous and have a foul odour which may also be confused with secondary sinusitis.

Guttural pouch mycosis represents one of the commonest mycotic infections of the horse occurring, primarily (but not exclusively), in areas of the world where preserved forages are fed. The disorder is recognised more commonly in Europe than elsewhere, but has been recorded sporadically in many parts of the world. Its effects range from highly fatal vascular (**250**) or serious neurological defects (*see* **693**) to remarkably little effect. The lesions are most commonly located on the mucosa of the roof of the medial compartment of the guttural pouch, medial and caudal to the petrous articulation of the hyoid bone (**251**). They may also be located on the lateral or medial walls (**252**) of the guttural pouches, and occasionally in other areas. The extent of clinical signs is variable according to the location of the invasive lesions, the depth to which the organism penetrates and the structures affected by the invasion of fungal organisms. *Aspergillus* species are most commonly involved, with *Aspergillus nidulans* being the single most common isolate. The character of the lesions reflects a similar invasive capacity as those it causes within the nasal cavity. The fungus appears to have an affinity for the walls of the major arteries and pre-existing aneurysm of the wall of an artery appears to provide a preferred site for the fungus. Alternatively, aneurysms may be a consequence of the fungal damage to the arterial walls. There are a number of other important structures which may also become affected, including nerves and veins which course through the guttural pouch or which lie directly under the mucosa of the roof of the pouch. Mild (**Plate 7g**, page 144) or more severe (**Plate 7h**, page 145), unilateral, epistaxis which is unrelated to

250

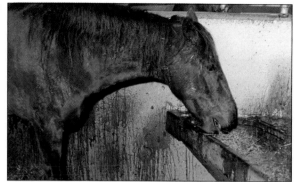

250 Guttural pouch mycosis (vascular form).
Note: Two previous minor epistaxis episodes preceded this catastrophic rupture of the internal carotid artery. Horse died within minutes.
Differential Diagnosis:
i)   Severe exercise induced pulmonary haemorrhage
ii) Ruptured pulmonary artery
iii) Rupture of major vessel in guttural pouch due to bacterial infection
iv) Rupture of carotid or maxillary verminous aneurysm

251

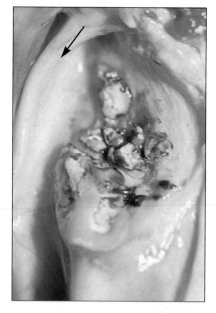

251 Guttural pouch mycosis.
Note: Lesion on free margin of hyoid bone in guttural pouch. Little inflammation around erosive and destructive lesion. Radiographs showed extensive bone destruction. Internal carotid artery unaffected (arrow).

252

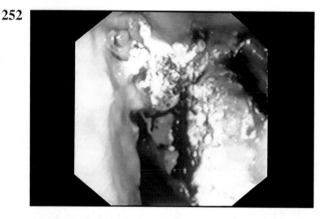

252 Guttural pouch mycosis (neurological form).
Note: Extensive invasion of roof of medial compartment, hyoid bone and medial wall. Severe neurological deficits present including unilateral pharyngeal (dysphagia), laryngeal (inspiratory dyspnea) and facial paralysis and Horner's Syndrome (corneal ulceration, sweating).

exercise, a unilateral, foul-smelling, mucoid, nasal discharge (**Plate 7c**, page 143) (**Plate 7e**, page 144) and pharyngeal paralysis (*see* **693**), with more or less dysphagia (**Plate 7j**, page 145) are the three most common clinical signs associated with the condition. Epistaxis is usually due to fungal erosion of smaller or larger blood vessels and in its most serious form, the wall of the internal carotid artery. Lesions on the lateral wall are often located over the external carotid artery and this may too become eroded and result in catastrophic hemorrhage. A single or repeated mild epistaxis usually involving scanty volumes of dark blood (**Plate 7g**, page 144) or a somewhat more obvious nasal bleeding (**Plate 7h**, page 145) is usually reported to precede a severe or extreme bilateral arterial epistaxis (**Plate 6h**, page 121) which may be precipitated by stress such as transport or restraint. The typical, scanty,

dark hemorrhages are probably due to the continued drainage of stale blood from the diseased pouch over the days/weeks following a mild episode of bleeding from an arterial or venous defect. More unusually a slight unilateral mucoid nasal discharge will be all that is detected clinically (**Plate 7e**, page 144) and in most of these cases the lesion has little effect upon blood vessels and correspondingly more upon the major nerves within, and adjacent to, the pouch. Endoscopic examination will usually identify at least some hemorrhagic discharge from the external ostium of the auditive tube within the pharynx. A single or several episodes of more severe hemorrhage, having an obvious arterial origin (**Plate 7i**, page 145), usually precedes a further, single, catastrophic and often fatal episode (*see* **250**). Although the lesion is usually unilateral the more severe epistaxis is invariably bilateral

Plate 7

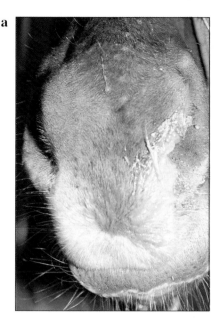

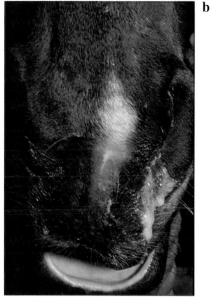

a Unilateral serous nasal discharge.
Differential Diagnosis:
i)   Nasal foreign body
ii) Ethmoid hematoma (early)
iii) Nasal trauma (mild) eg nasogastric intubation/endoscopy
iv) Nasal polyp
v) Sinusitis (primary, early)

b Unilateral purulent nasal discharge.
Differential Diagnosis:
i)   Maxillary sinusitis/empyema (primary/secondary)
ii) Guttural pouch empyema
iii) Maxillary sinus cyst

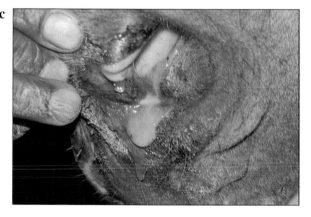

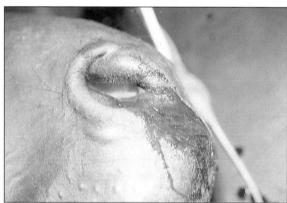

c Unilateral purulent nasal discharge.
Differential Diagnosis:
i)   Guttural pouch mycosis
ii) Nasal neoplasia (squamous cell carcinoma)
iii) Amyloidosis
iv) Nasal aspergillosis
v) Ethmoid hematoma

d Unilateral serosanguineous nasal discharge.
Differential Diagnosis:
i)   Ethmoid hematoma
ii) Nasal polyp
iii) Maxillary sinus cyst
iv) Nasal foreign body
v) Ulcerative rhinitis (viral respiratory infections)

Plate 7

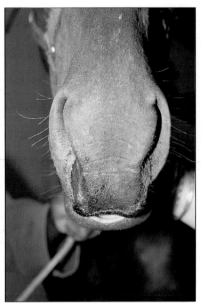

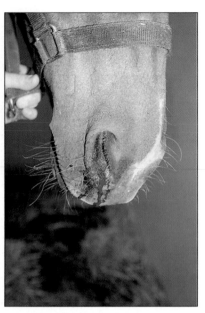

e Unilateral purulent-hemorrhagic nasal discharge.
Note: Some evidence of blood at left nostril).
Differential Diagnosis:
i)   Nasal amyloidosis
ii) Nasal aspergillosis (turbinate necrosis)
iii) Pharyngeal/guttural pouch abscess
iv) Conidiobolus coronatus (phycomycosis)
v)   Squamous cell carcinoma (nasal)
vi) Ethmoid hematoma

f Unilateral acute (mild) epistaxis.
Note: Splashing appearance.
Differential Diagnosis:
i)   Pharyngeal/nasal foreign body
ii) Nasal vein varicosity
iii) Trauma to nasal cavity (mild) (eg nasogastric tube or facial trauma)

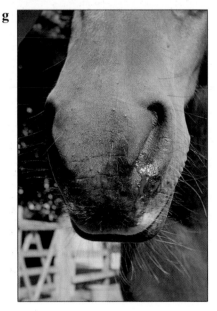

g Unilateral (venous) epistaxis (slow, scanty, dark, intermittent or persistent).
Differential Diagnosis:
i)   Guttural pouch mycosis
ii) Idiopathic/autoimmune thrombocytopenia (spontaneous bleeding)
iii) Exercise induced pulmonary hemorrhage (usually bilateral)
iv) Amyloidosis
v)   Nasal polyp
vi) Ethmoid hematoma

Plate 7

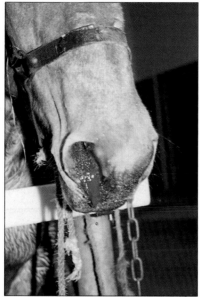

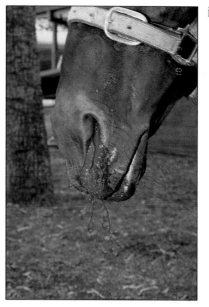

h Unilateral (venous) epistaxis (profuse, persistent).
Differential Diagnosis:
i)   Guttural pouch mycosis
ii) Exercise induced pulmonary hemorrhage (usually bilateral)
iii) Nasal polyp

i Unilateral (arterial) epistaxis (profuse).
Differential Diagnosis:
i)   Nasal trauma (internal) (e.g. misdirected nasogastric intubation)
ii) Guttural pouch mycosis (usually bilateral when arterial)
iii) Fracture of skull (basisphenoid/nasal/facial/maxillary)

j Unilateral nasal discharge containing food material.
Differential Diagnosis:
i)   Small cleft palate
ii)   Guttural pouch mycosis
iii) Ethmoid hematoma (on floor of nasal cavity/soft palate)
iv)   Protozoal myeloencephalitis
v)   Amyloidosis (extensive)
vi)   Fractured stylohyoid bone
vii) Pharyngeal neoplasia
viii) Pharyngeal foreign body

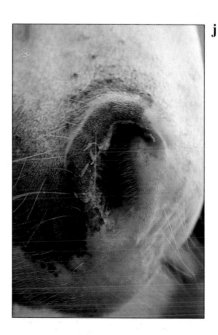

253

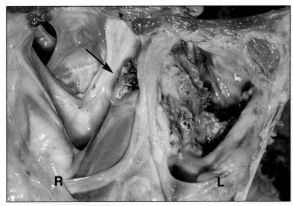

254

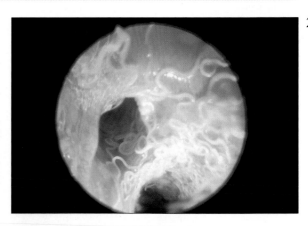

253 Guttural pouch mycosis (neurological form).
Note: Major lesion in roof of medial compartment of left pouch extended through mesial border to right pouch (arrow). All clinical signs were attributable to lesions in left pouch (*see* **693**).

254 Lungworm (*Dictyocaulus arnfieldi*).
Note: Most of the parasites shown here are larval forms. This is an exceptional burden for a horse.

and obviously arterial. It is usually impossible to specifically identify the site of the bleeding in even the less severe stages.

Where nerve tissue is invaded by the expanding fungal mycelia, horses may be more or less severely handicapped by **neurological deficits**, particularly where the pharyngeal components of the vagus and glossopharyngeal nerves are involved. **Pharyngeal paralysis** which is most often unilateral (*see* **693**), is the most common neuropathy. These effects are entirely understandable in view of the very vulnerable anatomical location of these nerves within the guttural pouch, and their proximity to the internal carotid artery, which appears to be the predilection site for the organism. Dysphagia, with, usually, a nasal discharge containing ingesta at one (**Plate 7j**, page 145) or both nostrils (**Plate 6o**, page 123), associated with **unilateral pharyngeal paralysis** and **Horner's Syndrome** (*see* **697**) are probably the commonest neurological signs associated with guttural pouch mycosis. Examination of the pharynx with an endoscope will often reveal evidence of neurological deficits which include persistent dorsal displacement of the soft palate (**Plate 5a**, page 111), saliva and ingesta in the nasopharynx, ipsilateral paralysis of the pharyngeal ostium of the guttural pouch (*see* **693**), and ipsilateral paralysis of the laryngeal intrinsic musculature (laryngeal hemiplegia) (**Plate 5u** *et seq*, page 115). The pharynx may have a narrow appearance, particularly on the affected side, due to the flaccidity of the pharyngeal muscles. The sympathetic trunk and cranial sympathetic ganglion may also be involved in the pathological process and damage to these is largely responsible for the development of Horner's Syndrome

in these cases (*see* **697**). **Facial nerve paralysis** (*see* **688**) may be present when the lesion affects the nerve situated under the mucosa of the dorsal aspect of the lateral compartment. A wide range of secondary effects may be present, including laryngeal hemiplegia, corneal ulceration, aspiration pneumonia, vestibular and sight deficits depending upon the extent of the neurological damage. Other signs include parotid pain, head shyness or head shaking and sweating. Interestingly, it is unusual to encounter both the neurologic (dysphagic) and hemorrhagic forms in the same animal at the same time.

Endoscopy of the early case shows the visible lesion of guttural pouch mycosis to be limited to the mucosal surface where it appears as a closely attached diphtheritic membrane. The colour and extent of the lesion may vary from small areas of yellowish-white nodules, to larger, white or grey lesions (*see* **251**) and ultimately to extensive dark, black, yellow or grey lesions located in the roof of the medial and lateral compartments and extending to the mucosa overlying the hyoid bone and the medial wall (*see* **252**). Whilst most lesions are limited to the roof of the pouch some may extend more widely. The floor is rarely involved even in extensive cases. In spite of the apparent erosive and invasive character of the fungus it is remarkable how little active inflammation occurs along the margin of the lesions (*see* **251**). Radiographic studies may be used to identify the extent of the condition and the amount of erosion of the hyoid bone and angiography may be useful in defining the location and extent of arterial wall involvement. Bilateral lesions are particularly unusual but may be encountered and while some of these are true bilateral lesions, most are due to extension through the medial septum (**253**).

Pulmonary fungal infection ('Farmers Lung') is probably most often due to the inhalation of spores which are, however, present in almost all circumstances in inspired air. The consequent development of pathological disorders of the lungs is very rare and usually only occurs when immuno-compromised or severely stressed animals, or those with significant intercurrent disease, are challenged with opportunist pathogens. The detection of pulmonary involvement including coughing, hemoptysis (coughing up blood) and radiographic evidence of extensive patchy pneumonia or solidification of lung tissue is suggestive of a diagnosis of fungal pneumonia. Pre-existing or concurrent fungal lesions in the nasal cavity or paranasal sinuses, from which *Aspergillus* spp. may be recovered (*see* **249**) are commonly present. Extensive fungal involvement with either *Aspergillus* spp. or *Nocardia* spp. organisms in the lungs and/or the pleural cavity may be a possible factor in the development of hypertrophic pulmonary osteopathy (Marie's Disease) (*see* **416, 417**).

Parasitic Diseases: The life cycle of *Parascaris equorum* in foals involves a period of lung migration and while the clinical effects of this migration have not been well defined, heavily infested young foals develop a marked productive cough, hyperpnea, loss of weight and very occasionally overt pneumonia. Endoscopic examination usually shows a profuse mucoid exudate within the trachea, in which the larvae may occasionally be identified. In many cases however the extent of the inflammatory response is marked while few parasites are present. A diagnosis of verminous (ascarid) pneumonia in foals may be confirmed when the adult parasites (*see* **142**) are identifiable (possibly through fecal eggs) and where specific treatment results in resolution. The condition is exclusively found in foals less than 4–6 months old, older horses being solidly immune unless immunocompromised.

Dictyocaulus arnfieldi, the **equine lungworm**, occurs in most parts of the world but is rarely responsible for disease in horses. It is relatively common in Europe and less so in North America, Africa and Australasia. The primary hosts for the parasite are probably the donkey and the tapir. In these species the parasite causes little or no harmful effect, apart from a mild but persistent, non-progressive, cough. Horses grazing the same pasture as donkeys may become infested and this results in a similar clinical syndrome but which is more severe, and is often capable of limiting the exercise ability of the host. In some cases the clinical syndrome is alarming and may be almost indistinguishable from allergic small airway disease (*see* **204**). Tracheal aspiration is commonly used to diagnose the disorder when a few parasites, or their eggs or larvae, can be identified in an exudate which contains large numbers of degenerate neutrophils and eosinophils. Endoscopic examination may identify the presence of adult or larval forms of the parasite (**254**). As the horse is not the definitive natural (preferred) host for the parasite, adult, egg-laying worms are less common than in the donkey and consequently examination of feces for larvae is often unrewarding. A specific diagnosis depends upon historical contact with donkeys, identification of the larvae (or eggs) in tracheal aspirations or in feces and a dramatic benefit from specific treatment.

Pulmonary hydatidosis, which represents the intermediate stage of the canine tapeworm, *Echinococcus granulosis* var *equinum*, is encountered relatively commonly as an incidental finding during thoracic radiography, when one, or more, radio-dense, cyst like structures may be seen. They may reach considerable size but their significance is equivocal. The presence of a thoracic lesion may be indicative of other (abdominal) lesions and where these are present in large numbers, particularly on or in the liver (*see* **173**) some metabolic effects are to be expected. The parasite is probably significantly different from the species which is responsible for infestation of sheep and humans, and the intermediate stage may be host-specific for the horse. It is certainly true that large numbers of parasitic cysts may be present without any detectable clinical effect.

Neoplastic Disorders

Primary neoplastic disorders of the respiratory tract are unusual but are of considerable importance. The classification of respiratory neoplastic disorders of the horse may be simplified into benign and malignant neoplasms. **Secondary, metastatic neoplastic infiltrations of the lung** of the horse are far more common than primary lesions, but even these are rare.

Nasal polyps are benign, usually unilateral, pedunculated growths on the mucosa of the nasal cavity. Non-specific signs occurring early in their development include various degrees of respiratory obstruction, and chronic, unilateral, serous, nasal discharges, possibly associated with hemorrhage **(Plate 7d; Plate 7g**, page 144). Some polyps are small, remaining clinically insignificant, and may be difficult to locate in the nasal cavity. Others rapidly expand rostrally and may even protrude from the nose **(255)**. Complete nasal occlusion may arise and some of the larger lesions, which protrude from the nose may occlude the nasal opening of the ipsilateral nasolacrimal duct causing epiphora (*see* **255**). They are usually pedunculated with surprisingly small origins within the nasal cavity. Lateral radiographs of the nasal region may be used to identify the full extent of the lesion with the largest showing a distinct air-fluid interface within the nasal cavity lying caudal to the caudal extremity of the mass. Retrograde endoscopy from a tracheostomy site or via the contralateral nostril may establish the site of origin and may on occasion be used to free the attachment and allow removal of the mass.

Previous interference or damage to cartilaginous structures in the respiratory tract may give rise to benign **chondromas**. They occur relatively frequently in the cartilages of the larynx, including the epiglottis **(256)**, trachea **(257)** and bronchi. Respiratory obstruction is usually the first evidence of their presence particularly those occurring within the larynx, which expand to occlude the airway (*see* **256**). Initially the main effect will be on inspiration but later expiratory difficulty will also develop. One of the commonest iatrogenic causes of **laryngeal chondroma** is the presence of a misplaced laryngeal prosthetic ligament. Where the mucosa of the larynx is perforated and the prosthesis lies in the lumen of the larynx there is a high incidence of localised infection (chondritis), granulation tissue and chondroma. Each of these may be responsible for more or less severe occlusion of the lumen. Small **chondroma masses in the trachea** (*see* **257**) have little clinical effect but when larger may cause obvious snoring sounds during both inspiration and expiration. It is unusual for tracheal chondromas to reach life-threatening size. While most such masses are probably the result of prior trauma (either through surgery or foreign bodies) others have developed without any history of such damage.

Ethmoid hematoma is a progressive, locally invasive and destructive mass occuring in the nasal cavity and/or the paranasal sinuses of mature horses, usually over the age of 8–10 years. They have a neoplastic-like appearance but are not recognised pathologically as true neoplastic lesions. The masses

255

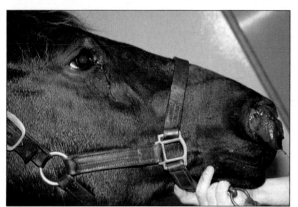

256

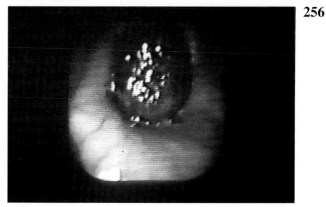

255 Benign nasal polyp (large).
Note: Lesion grew very fast, appearing within 7 days of the onset of a mild nasal obstruction with snoring. Occlusion of nasal punctum of nasolacrimal duct causing epiphora.

256 Laryngeal chondroma.
Note: Occlusive nature, dangerous respiratory obstruction necessitated emergency treatment.

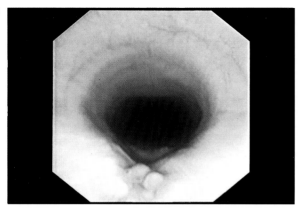

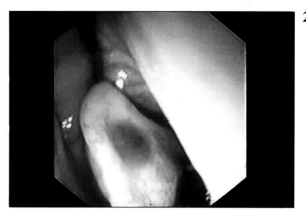

257 Tracheal chondroma.
Note: Lesions at site of old tracheostomy wound. Found incidentally.

258 Progressive ethmoid hematoma.
Note: Earliest lesion in mucosa of great ethmoturbinate bone.

vary widely in size and location, and may reach considerable size. They are rarely bilateral. The largest lesions are located in the ethmoidal labyrinth and these frequently have a wide base, whilst the smaller lesions, which are more often pedunculated, tend to originate from the floor of the nasal cavity or the mucosal surfaces of the paranasal sinuses. All forms of the condition are identical in their gross and histological appearance and their progressive tendency. The progressive nature of the lesions often results in physical distortions within the nasal cavity but they very rarely cause facial distortions. As the mass expands the surface mucous membrane ulcerates and a limited loss of blood occurs. This is often combined with an excess of mucus production from the area. Typically, therefore, the earliest clinical indication of ethmoidal hematoma is a mild, non-postural unilateral, intermittent, spontaneous, odour-free, serosanguineous (**Plate 7d**, page 143) or sero-mucoid nasal discharge. Where the nasal discharge is bilateral the history usually confirms that a unilateral hemorrhagic discharge has been present for some time. Careful examination of horses with bilateral serosanguineous nasal discharges or overt epistaxis due to ethmoidal hematoma will often reveal the discharge to be of different character and quantity in the two nostrils. Bilateral nasal discharge usually indicates that the lesion has progressed to occupy a large area of the nasopharynx with extension into the contralateral nostril. The nasal discharge may be present for months or years without causing any apparent harmful effect. Some horses have a mild, muco-purulent nasal discharge with less obvious hemorrhage, and only rarely are coughing, head shaking and a malodorous breath present. Where lesions are situated in the ethmoidal labyrinth they can usually be easily visualised endoscopically. The earliest

lesions appear as dark black patches on the mucosa (**258**). More advanced lesions which are accompanied by serous and hemorrhagic discharges appear as small (**259**), or larger, well-defined, grey-black, yellowish or yellow-green masses (**260**), often covered with a mucoid (*see* **259**) or serosanguineous (*see* **260**) exudate. Larger, dark-coloured lesions with a more invasive appearance, extending over a wider area (**261**), represent a more advanced stage. These often expand at a greater rate and may become serious with respect to blood loss and ipsilateral nasal obstruction (**262**). As the lesions progress in size they exert an ever-increasing effect upon the air flow through the nasal cavity and begin to distort the local anatomy. The serosanguineous nasal discharge typically becomes more persistent and ultimately may have a foul, necrotic smell which is usually indicative of necrosis of the mass itself or of underlying bone within the ethmoidal labyrinth or the paranasal sinuses. Stertorous respiration usually indicates that both nostrils have become invaded and these animals are usually severely compromised (**Plate 6m**, page 122). Lesions may even expand rostrally to the extent of protruding from the nostril (*see* **262**) or may progress caudally to interfere with swallowing. Less commonly masses may be located elsewhere, such as on the soft palate (**263**) or within the sinuses and those extending into the nasopharynx from the nasal cavity are associated with dysphagia, with food material, blood and mucoid discharges present at the nostril(s). Lateral (**264**) and ventro-dorsal radiographs of the head can accurately define the location and extent of the mass. Where the lesions are restricted to within the paranasal sinuses, clinical and radiographic definition may be more difficult and ventro-dorsal radiographs may be more useful in these cases. A diagnosis of progressive

259

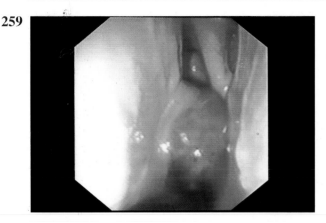

260

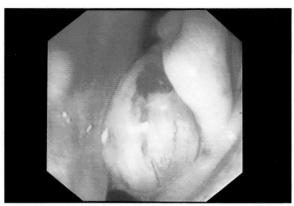

259 Progressive ethmoid hematoma.
Note: Mucoid exudate from small lesion in ethmoid region.

260 Progressive ethmoid hematoma.
Note: Serosanguineous discharge, yellowish lesion in ethmoid region, with hemorrhage.

261

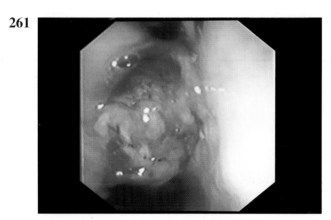

262

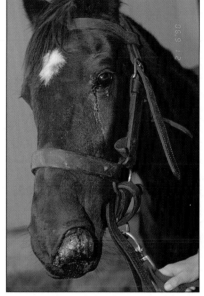

261 Progressive ethmoid hematoma.
Note: Larger, poorly defined, aggressive lesion with serosanguineous exudate and obvious bleeding.

263

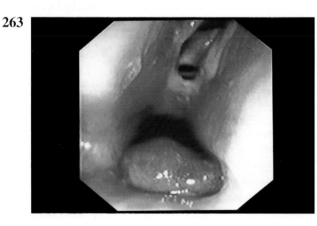

262 Progressive ethmoid hematoma.
Note: Very large lesion occluding left nostril. Occlusion of nasal punctum of nasolacrimal duct causing epiphora.
Differential Diagnosis:
i)   Benign nasal polyp

263 Progressive ethmoid hematoma.
Note: Unusual lesion on surface of soft palate.
Differential Diagnosis:
i)   Squamous cell carcinoma
ii) Lymphosarcoma (multicentric or cutaneous histiocytic form)

264

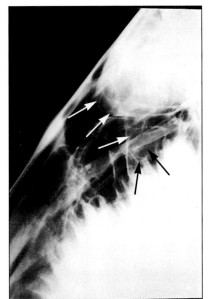

265

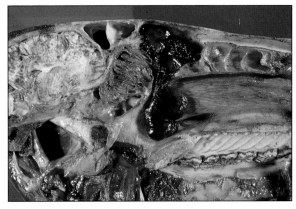

264 Progressive ethmoid hematoma (standing lateral radiograph).
Note: Diffuse radiodensity in nasal cavity rostral to ethmoturbinate. Outline of hematoma shown by arrows.

265 Progressive ethmoid hematoma.
Note: Invasive lesion extended into nasopharynx and maxillary and frontal sinuses from relatively small area of attachment in ethmoidal labyrinth. Dark, black colour due to high, stale-blood content.

266

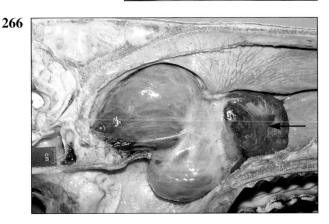

266 Progressive ethmoid hematoma.
Note: Large lesion incorporating entire ethmoid turbinate with broad attachment and extending into nasopharynx and both nasal cavities.

Note: greenish-yellow coloration due to blood pigments and smooth mucosal surface over most of the mass. One area of hemorrhage at rostral extent (arrow).

ethmoidal hematoma is relatively simple with the aid of endoscopy, but without either this or radiographic examination, a diagnosis should still be feasible, based upon a careful history and critical clinical examination to eliminate other sources of nasal hemorrhage. The treatment of the condition is at present entirely reliant upon surgery and the location of the origin is of paramount importance when considering an approach to the lesions.

Post mortem examination of the nasal cavity of horses affected by progressive ethmoidal hematoma shows their contents to be dark, partially organised blood clot (**265**). The origin of the lesion may be relatively small giving a pedunculated appearance (*see* **265**), in spite of an extensive mass of abnormal tissue. Many, however, have a much wider base covering a larger area of the ethmoidal labyrinth and pharynx (**266**).

Sinus cysts are single, or loculated, fluid-filled cavities with an epithelial lining which develop primarily in the maxillary, and occasionally in the frontal sinuses and which have some features in common with ethmoidal hematomas. They have, however, a more well-defined and predictable pathological appearance. As horses around 10 years of age are most often affected, a developmental etiology is unlikely, and they are therefore probably not similar to the maxillary sinus cysts encountered in young foals (*see* **181, 182**). Abnormal tooth root development may be a significant factor in their development, but many have no detectable dental attachments or structures. Affected horses show mild, progressive, facial distortions (**267**), unilateral, mucoid (**Plate 7a**, page 143) or mucopurulent (**Plate 7b**, page 143) nasal discharge. Varying degrees of respiratory obstruction related to progressive occlusion of the ipsilateral nasal cavity and distortion of the nasal septum, are present. The nasal discharges are rarely malodorous or hemorrhagic unless the masses become infected or cause necrosis of underlying bone.

267

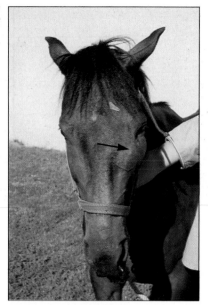

268

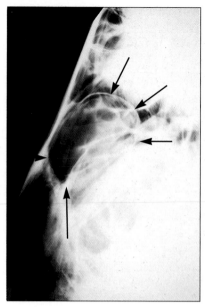

267 Maxillary sinus cyst (caudal) (left side).
Note: Facial distortion (arrow), endoscopy showed ipsilateral nasal occlusion. The lesion itself was not visible from the nasal cavity.
Differential Diagnosis:
i)   Primary/secondary sinusitis
ii) Developmental sinus cyst
iii) Mucocele
iv) Sinus/Ethmoid hematoma

268 Maxillary sinus cyst (caudal) (standing lateral radiograph).
Note: Obvious cyst-like structure with bony margin in the caudal maxillary sinus (arrows). Ventro-dorsal projections showed ipsilateral nasal occlusion and obvious deviation of the nasal septum. Many of these have multiple fluid levels due to the multiple compartments within the cyst.
Differential Diagnosis:
i)   Maxillary sinus empyema
ii) Mucocele
iii) Sinus/ethmoidal hematoma

Endoscopically, the ventral conches is usually edematous and thickened and may be obviously displaced to the extent that endoscopic examination of the more caudal regions is not feasible from the ipsilateral nostril. The lesion itself cannot be visualised without the help of trephination of the affected sinus, but percussion usually identifies an abnormal solidity. Standing lateral radiographs show a characteristic, multiloculated, cystic structure with a dense, bone-like margin, within the natural confines of the affected sinus (**268**). Numerous air-fluid interfaces are commonly visible within it. Ventro-dorsal radiographs confirm the considerable distortion of the nasal septum and show a well-defined density in the region of the affected sinus. Pathologically, sinus cysts of this type consist of an often dense, or even bony, capsule with a smooth spongy mucous membrane possibly containing incomplete plates of bone or tooth like material. The cyst contains an acellular, amber coloured, muco-viscid fluid and is quite unlike the purulent material associated with infected (primary or secondary) sinusitis. In some

cases, however, the drainage ostium of the affected sinus may become occluded and the cyst may then become infected and present clinical features normally associated with secondary sinusitis including a mucopurulent malodorous content.

Perhaps the commonest malignant neoplasm in the airways of the horse is **squamous cell carcinoma**. All forms are rare, but may affect the nasal cavity, sinuses, guttural pouches and pharynx. The clinical signs associated with any neoplastic disorder within the upper airway will probably be non-specific. Nasal discharges (often with blood) (**Plate 7e**, page 144) may be odour-free or, where bone is involved, may have a strong, necrotic odour. Airway obstructions are likely where the lesions are present in the nasal cavity, guttural pouches, paranasal sinuses or pharynx. Dysphagia may be encountered where they interfere with either the physical or neurological function of the pharynx. Masses located rostrally usually expand outwards producing facial distortions with little encroachment on the nasal cavity itself (**269**) whereas lesions occurring more caudally

269

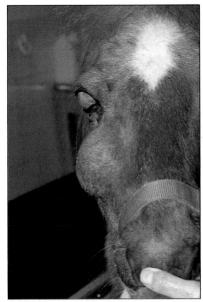

270

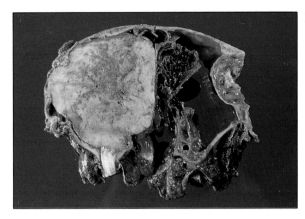

269 Squamous cell carcinoma (nasal).
Note: Lesion occurred rostrally in nasal cavity and caused obvious facial distortion but little nasal occlusion.
Differential Diagnosis:
i) (Rostral maxillary) sinusitis
ii) Periapical infection (upper first or second cheek tooth)

270 Squamous cell carcinoma (nasal).
Note: Lesion occurred caudally in the nasal cavity and extended into both ipsilateral maxillary sinuses. It caused severe nasal occlusion but limited facial distortion.
Differential Diagnosis:
i) Lymphosarcoma (multicentric or cutaneous histiocytic forms)
ii) Maxillary sinus cyst
iii) Maxillary sinusitis
iv) Ethmoidal hematoma (sinus)

271

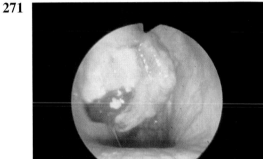

271 Squamous cell carcinoma (pharyngeal).
Note: Lesion occurred in dorsolateral wall of pharynx adjacent to pharyngeal ostium of the ipsilateral auditive tube. The lesion was itself of limited immediate importance but had resulted in a secondary diverticulitis and empyema of the guttural pouch with marked dorsal pharyngeal compression.
Differential Diagnosis:
i) Foreign body
ii) Pharyngeal abscess

272

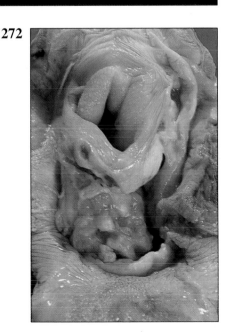

272 Lymphosarcoma (pharyngeal component of multicentric form).
Note: Lesion resulted in gross distortion and persistent dorsal displacement of the soft palate (**Plate 5f**, page 112). Severe dysphagia was present.
Differential Diagnosis:
i) Squamous cell carcinoma
ii) Foreign body

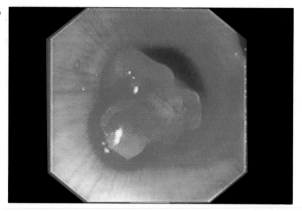

273 Undifferentiated bronchial carcinoma.
Note: Slow growing mass with extensive hemorrhage which pooled at thoracic inlet (**Plate 4j**, page 104). Resulted in chronic posture related nasal discharge containing dark, blood-stained serous fluid (**Plate 6j**, page 121). No coughing was present.

create correspondingly less facial distortion but more encroachment into the nasal cavity (**270**). The latter masses may result in significant and dangerous nasal occlusion when their expansion extends across the nasal septum (*see* **270**). Lateral and ventro-dorsal radiographs may be used to define both their extent and their effect on adjacent bony and soft tissue structures. Occasionally, local invasion occurs and, although they seldom metastasize from these sites, they may have severe local consequences.

Pharyngeal squamous cell carcinoma may arise in the roof of the pharynx (**271**) where it may exert deleterious effects on the guttural pouch or the underlying nerves or blood vessels. In other locations the lesions have variable effects related to their space occupying and disruptive effects on underlying or adjacent structures. Dysphagia and respiratory noises are commonly present where these lesions reach significant size.

Primary lesions of **lymphosarcoma** may also be found in the pharynx (**272**) where, as part of the multicentric form of the disorder, they may cause obvious and debilitating dysphagia with chronic, persistent, nasal regurgitation of food and saliva (**Plate 6p; Plate 6r**, page 123). Lesions associated with the cutaneous histiocytic form of the disorder also occur in the pharynx (*see* **592**), the skin of the muzzle and the mucosa of the nostrils (*see* **591**) which may be infiltrated with malignant tissue and obstruct the airway. Lesions of the multicentric form of lymphosarcoma originating in the lingual tonsillar tissue at the base of the tongue and involving the floor of the nasopharynx or the oropharynx, may displace the soft palate (**Plate 5f**, page 112) and consequently have marked effects upon deglutition and, once they become large, will also affect respiratory function.

Primary thoracic lymphosarcoma is probably the most common thoracic neoplasm, although thoracic neoplasia in the horse is generally very rare (*see* **320** *et seq.*).

Persistent, posture-related, bilateral, epistaxis (**Plate 6j**, page 121) accompanied by progressive dyspnea, increasing resting respiratory rate, and exercise intolerance may indicate the presence of **neoplasia within the conducting airways** (**273**) or the lungs. The nasal discharge is most often dark brown or red-black in colour (**Plate 6j**, page 121), indicative of the prolonged time the material has spent in the airway. Coughing and hemoptysis are rarely encountered even in severe cases. Lesions developing in the airway have considerable limiting effects upon the perfusion of lung distal to the lesion and the clinical effects of this are variable according to the extent of the obstruction and its locality. Percussion of the affected side may reveal areas of dullness associated with solidity. Endoscopically there is often a considerable pooling of blood and serous exudate in the thoracic inlet (**Plate 4j**, page 104) and the source of the bleeding can be traced to identify the site and character of masses growing into or within the airways (*see* **273**).

Primary pulmonary neoplasms are very rare in the horse and, with the possible exception of lympho-sarcoma, most thoracic neoplasms of the horses are **secondary metastatic tumours**. Clinical signs attributable to pulmonary lesions are not specific and many cases are largely asymptomatic until they reach an advanced stage.

Grey horses are liable to the development of **melanomas** (*see* **588**) which may affect many internal organs, including the lungs. There is some dispute over the true nature of many of these lesions. The lungs of some horses may contain many thousands of lesions, but it is still rare for them to exert any detectable clinical effect. Extension from the lung into the mediastinum or lesions developing directly in the mediastinum may reach sufficient size to obstruct lymphatic and blood vessels. **Melanotic lesions** are often present in the guttural pouches, and more particularly in the lateral

274

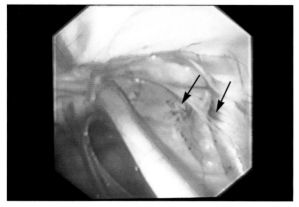

275

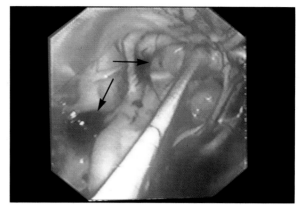

274 Melanotic hamartoma.
Note: Small, flat, irregular areas of black pigment grouped on walls of major arteries in guttural pouch (arrows).
Differential Diagnosis:
i)   Melanoma
ii) Petechial/ecchymotic hemorrhages (hemorrhagic diatheses)

275 Melanoma / melanosarcoma.
Note: Dark black, masses in lateral compartment of guttural pouch (arrows).
Differential Diagnosis:
i)   Melanotic hamartoma

276

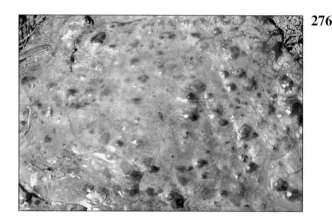

276 Secondary hemangiosarcoma (pulmonary metastases).
Note: Diffuse spread of lesions through lungs indicative of hematogenous metastasis.

compartment. At this site two distinct types of lesion can be identified. The first are benign-looking, flat, irregular patches of black pigment, often in large numbers and very small, located on the walls of the major vessels (**274**). These are probably not tumours but represent abnormal accumulations of normal cells (**hamartoma**). Larger, well-defined, tumour-like masses of black tissue represent the more serious, and more obviously neoplastic, disorder. These are often located high in the lateral wall of the lateral compartment (**275**) or, more rarely, in the medial compartment. The significance of these lesions is equivocal, but extension from the lateral wall of the guttural pouch to the parotid lymph nodes and lymphoid tissue in the salivary gland is possibly responsible for the externally obvious form of the disorder which is present in this structure (*see* **58**).

Malignant tumours (adenocarcinomata or squamous cell carcinomata) in any remote organ might be expected to result in secondary masses in the lung. Even secondary lesions will however, exert a significant effect on pulmonary function, although this may have limited clinical effects upon the horse in the early stages. Poor exercise tolerance, coughing, hemoptysis and a hemorrhagic nasal discharge (**Plate 6j**, page 121) may be attributable to primary or secondary pulmonary neoplasia but it is surprising how seldom these are presented, even in severe, invasive neoplasia. Primary sarcomas occurring in other organs such as kidney and muscle rapidly metastasise to the lung and clinically affected horses show hemothorax, anemia, dyspnea and chronic weight loss. Blood loss into the pleural cavity may be significant and detectable by percussion, radiography and thoracocentesis. However, the respiratory signs of this progressively deteriorating disorder may be less well defined, and thoracic radiographs may be required to confirm the presence of multiple, intrapulmonary, radio-dense ('cannon ball') lesions. The difficulties associated with thoracic radiography of the horse, however, mean that many of these cases (particularly where the lesions are very small) may not be detectable before death. At post mortem examination the lesions of any secondary tumour are usually evenly distributed through the lung **(276)**. Squamous cell carcinomas appear to result in little or no pulmonary interference, in spite of extensive infiltration, and no pleural effusions are usually encountered.

Further reading

Problems in Equine Medicine
Brown, C.M. (1989) Lea & Febiger, Philadelphia, USA
Current Therapy in Equine Medicine (1)
Ed Robinson, N.E. (1987), W B Saunders, Philadelphia, USA
Current Therapy in Equine Medicine (2)
Ed Robinson, N.E. (1992), W B Saunders, Philadelphia, USA

Manual of Equine Practice
Rose, R.J., and Hodgson, D.R. (1993)
WB Saunders, Philadelphia
Equine Clinical Neonatology
Koterba, A.M., Drummond, W.H., and Kosch, P.C. (1990) Lea & Febiger, Philadelphia, USA
Equine Respiratory Disorders
Beech, J. (1991) Lea and Febiger, Philadelphia, USA

4. Disorders of the cardiovascular system

Part 1: The Heart and Blood Vessels

Developmental Disorders

Serious and/or complicated congenital defects of the circulation such as **cardiac ectopia (277)** usually result in intra-uterine death but some cardiac and vascular anomalies may only become evident after birth, and sometimes much later when the animal starts to work. The incidence of congenital abnormalities of blood flow in the horse is low in comparison to other domestic species, but this may be a product of the high perinatal mortality which these conditions cause in affected foals. The significance of post mortem findings may be difficult to assess in the absence of prior clinical examination and such lesions encountered in dead foals should be interpreted with care. In-breeding may be responsible for the higher incidence of these defects in the Arabian breed, but embryological development may be significantly affected by infections or other insults during the early stages of gestation.

Defects of structure in the heart usually arise within the first 50 days of gestation, when the rate of development of the heart is maximal. Factors affecting the embryonic development during this time might be expected to have effects upon the heart and great vessels, in particular. The dramatic change to lung perfusion/circulation occurring at birth, also provides an opportunity for deficiencies of function to become apparent and so, factors affecting late gestation and the birth process, may also influence the incidence of defects, particularly with respect to the *ductus arteriosus* and *foramen ovale*. Unfortunately, it is not always easy to clinically separate the more sinister disorders from benign or physiological changes in foals or, indeed, in adult horses. Normal foals often maintain the patency of the *ductus arteriosus* for up to 72 hours after birth, and 'machinery-type' (continuous) murmurs audible after this stage, are probably best regarded as abnormal.

Ventricular septal defects are probably the most frequent congenital defect of the equine heart. Their size and position in the interventricular septum varies markedly with small defects situated high in the interventricular septum being most common. Ventricular septal defects link the left ventricle just below the right coronary cusp of the aortic valve, with the right ventricle, below the septal leaflet of the tricuspid valve and are best imaged by ultrasonography **(278)**. Defects

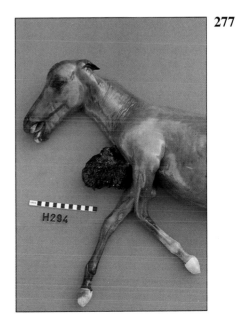

277 Ectopic heart (aborted fetus).

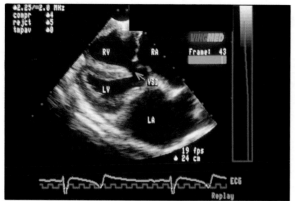

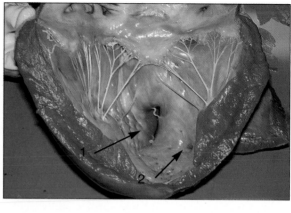

278 Ventricular septal defect (B-Mode Ultrasound). **Note:** Image taken from right side of horse, (right parasternal, long-axis view). Defect visible in septum just beneath tricuspid and mitral (bicuspid) valves (green arrow). This is the most common defect of this type. (LA = left atrium; LV = left ventricle; RV = right ventricle; RA = right atrium).

279 Ventricular septal defect. **Note:** Large (5cm x 5cm) defect in lower, muscular portion of septum (arrow 1) and second, small defect to the right of main one (next to cut surface of heart) (arrow 2).

are also found in the lower regions of the interventricular septum (**279**). Large septal defects are not usually compatible with extra-uterine life and most affected foals, therefore, die at, or immediately after, birth. Occasional cases however remain alive, and have obvious, persistent murmurs, associated with a marked thrill, which are usually easily audible during clinical examination. While the prognosis for small, isolated septal defects is fair, these lesions are also commonly present in conjunction with other complex disorders of the heart and great vessels which almost invariably carry a poor or hopeless prognosis. Horses with small septal defects (less than 2.5 cm diameter) may grow adequately and, apart from the presence of an obvious murmur, may be asymptomatic. However, they are more often stunted, and show a poor exercise tolerance. A history of lagging behind the dam or disinclination to play with other foals is often reported. Young foals with septal defects of clinical significance, often show a characteristic exhaustion when suckling and sometimes collapse (faint) during feeding or after only slight exercise. A persistent dyspnea and weakness with an inability or disinclination to stand for reasonable periods of time are often noted. Auscultation will reveal an obvious, loud, pansystolic murmur in the area of the aortic and tricuspid valves. The persistent, undulating, "machinery type" murmur has a marked precordial vibration (thrill) which radiates widely is audible on both sides of the chest, but is usually significantly louder on the right. The thrill can often be appreciated merely by palpation of the lower right thoracic wall. The murmurs usually become more prominent with exercise and rising blood pressure.

The positive identification of these lesions has been made relatively easy with the advent of ultrasonography which, with experience, can be used to clearly demonstrate the discontinuity of the septal wall (*see* **278**). The more sophisticated pulsed-wave, colour (Doppler) echocardiography, in which the flow patterns through the valves and septal defects can be readily appreciated, makes the extent of the defect and the consequent blood-shunting, obvious (**280**). Membranous, ventricular septal defects have an intermittent or incomplete effect, and may only become significant when the pressure gradient between the two chambers is altered. This type of lesion is often not audible except under the particular circumstances outlined (usually with increased or decreased blood pressure). Diagnosis is best confirmed by ultrasonographic examinations using Doppler methods. Major septal defects which shunt significant volumes of blood into the relatively lower-pressured, right side, result in gross right-sided enlargement and this may be detected on percussion or, more precisely, by radiographic and ultrasonographic examination of the chest.

Complex flow disorders of the heart, including the **Tetralogy of Fallot**, form the majority of the remaining developmental conditions of the equine heart. Many of the affected foals are born dead or die shortly after birth, having shown marked respiratory distress, polypnea and cyanosis. The foals may appear to faint spontaneously and collapse at the slightest exertion. Furthermore, affected foals which survive, grow poorly and their outlook for long term survival is very poor. A loud pansystolic murmur, with a prominent precordial thrill,

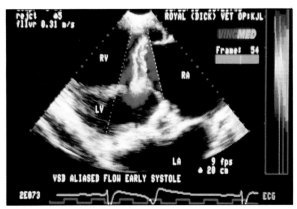

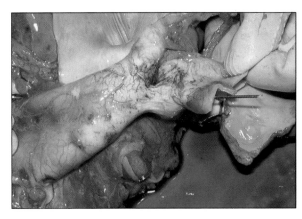

280 Ventricular septal defect (Doppler, colour flow-study).
Note: Blood flow coded red, flowing from left ventricle (LV) to right ventricle (RV) during systole. The signal has aliased, as shown by the central core change from red through to blue (i.e. travelling so fast that signal received as if traveling in the opposite direction).

281 Patent ductus arteriosus.
Note: A wire probe has been inserted from the aorta to the pulmonary artery, through the wide ductus arteriosus.

over the left base of the heart is audible and palpable. The defect may also be audible on the right side but is usually less intense on this side. Radiographic examination of the thorax will usually identify the grossly enlarged right ventricle and a very prominent ascending aorta. At post mortem examination a variety of complex distortions of anatomy will usually be identified. These anomalies are fortunately extremely rare.

Persistent cannulation of the ductus arteriosus, which in the fetus normally shunts blood from the pulmonary artery to the aorta, is an unusual neonatal disorder, occurring in foals less commonly than in other domestic animals. However, it is regarded as physiologically normal for a foal to maintain some shunting of blood in the opposite direction (i.e. from aorta to pulmonary artery) for up to 72 hours after birth. Persistence of the loud, continuous ('machinery') murmur, accompanied (usually) by a detectable thrill, beyond this age, is probably abnormal. Although the murmur may be easily audible on the right side, it is most obvious over the left side at the base of the heart, or slightly above this point. The foal may grow reasonably, but most cases show considerable exercise intolerance and are often noted to be reluctant to play with other foals and lag behind the dam. Older foals or adults affected with **patent *ductus arteriosus*** develop a progressive pulmonary artery hypertension and ultimately the pressures in the pulmonary artery and the aorta are equated and the murmur may become very faint. However, the increasing pulmonary pressure results in a reversion to the fetal blood flow pattern in

the advanced stages and the murmur, again, becomes clinically audible. The ultrasonographic appearance of this condition is diagnostic. Post mortem examination of affected horses shows the presence of a wide, patent *ductus arteriosus*, linking the pulmonary artery with the aorta (**281**).

Patency of the *foramen ovale* beyond the immediate post-natal period results in left-to-right atrial shunting of blood with consequent enlargement of the right atrium and overloading of the right ventricle. The *foramen ovale* is usually obvious in the heart of a new born foal and its detection at post mortem examination of young foals should be interpreted with care. Significant patency is usually accompanied by other cardiac abnormalities such as the well-recognised but rare **tricuspid valve atresia**. It is entirely understandable that an atresia of the tricuspid valve should be accompanied by a persistence of the *foramen ovale*, as the pressure in the right atrium would be expected to be higher than that in the left atrium and thus, the normal closure of the foramen would be prevented. Pulmonary perfusion is reduced and venous blood is shunted into the left side. A progressive cyanosis is the most prominent clinical feature of this condition with stunting, poor (or extremely poor) exercise tolerance and a secondary polycythemia (absolute increase, in numbers of red cells in the circulating blood).

Interatrial septal defects, arising in sites other than the *foramen ovale*, are much less common than their ventricular equivalents and, while in most cases the effects are obvious in the first few weeks of life, some cases show increasing lethargy and dyspnea at older ages. The defects present in a similar fashion to the patent *foramen ovale* syndrome. Tachycardia, mucous membrane pallor (with normal capillary refill time), jugular engorgement and a marked jugular pulsation are detected. A widely radiating murmur audible from both sides of the chest with an obvious (palpable and audible)

thrill focusing at the base of the heart is typical. Intercurrent atrial fibrillation develops in many cases and this may markedly alter the audible events. These defects may be identified positively before death by the use of ultrasonographic techniques particularly with the pulsed (Doppler) methods.

Non-Infectious Disorders

Acquired disorders of cardiac blood flow in the horse are relatively common but it is not always easy to identify the significant lesions from the purely incidental abnormalities of sound associated with normal turbulence in major vessels, or those functional sounds associated with other disease processes such as anemia, toxemia and shock. Audible murmurs which radiate across large areas of the heart field and those accompanied by a detectable thrill are, however, likely to be significant. Milder abnormalities of sound may or may not have any detectable effect on the function of the horse. It is the latter which provide the most diagnostic challenge to the veterinarian. Whilst sophisticated investigative methods are available for the investigation of the dynamics of cardiac function in the horse, most murmurs are detected simply by auscultation. The clinical significance of any heart 'defect' cannot, however, usually be based solely on this, and further studies should be performed to differentiate the functional (incidental) defects from the more sinister cardiac-related abnormalities which are likely to have a major bearing on the animals usefulness. The diameter of the major outflow arteries and the dynamics of cardiac contraction commonly result in physiological turbulence which may be audible as an ejection murmur. The relative pressures between the left and right sides and the resistance against which the respective sides have to pump, means that where there is increased resistance in the distal capillary beds the opportunity for murmurs increases. Thus, increased resistance to pulmonary artery pressure, arising from such diseases as chronic, small airway (allergic lung) disease, results in a progressively increased pulmonary pressure and a murmur may develop. Cardiac hypertrophy and alterations in the hemodynamics within the right side, then results in an increased severity of the murmur. Thus, murmurs may be a product of other disease processes which variously affect the viscosity of the blood and both the systolic and diastolic pressures. Furthermore, any defect in valvular integrity resulting from physical damage, distortion, or from increasing size of the cardiac annulus will also result in audible

murmurs and these may be further complicated by concurrent hemodynamic factors.

Mild valvular pathology, either **incompetence** or **stenosis**, is probably the most common cause of **significant** murmurs. These are sometimes accompanied by physiological disturbances of blood flow and exert consequent effects on the well-being and exercise capacity of the horse. In particular, defects of the **mitral valve** appear somewhat more likely to result in clinically significant murmurs. Mild, chronic, **progressive valvular disease** resulting in systolic murmurs, form the commonest group of acquired disorders of the equine heart. The murmurs are usually of low intensity, and the sounds remain localised over the affected valve. Serious valvular dysfunction results in poor exercise tolerance and prolonged recovery after exercise. There is usually a high resting heart rate which shows a poor recovery rate to normal resting levels following even limited exercise but some cases affected by apparently severe murmurs, show no detectable clinical effect on either performance or well being. Predictions of the expected effects of a particular murmur are therefore unwise. There may be moderate, or severe, exercised-induced pulmonary hemorrhage (*see* **200, 201**) (although by far the majority of horses affected by this condition have no detectable cardiac disease). The extent of the defect and the consequent effect upon blood flow patterns can be imaged clearly with the aid of pulsed (colour) Doppler echocardiography (**282**). Two-dimensional echo-cardiography may provide useful information in many cases of valvular insufficiency particularly when there are gross valvular defects and this technique can be enhanced with the addition of 'micro-bubble' contrast, injected intravenously during the procedure. Post mortem examinations most often reveals thickening and rounding of the free borders of the atrio-ventricular valves, with the left (mitral) valve being most often affected. Damage to the atrial wall adjacent to the site of the murmur may lead to roughening and inflammation in the wall. These sites are the so-called 'jet lesions'.

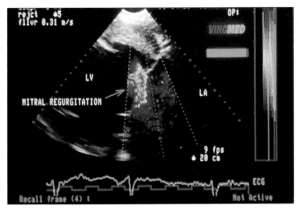

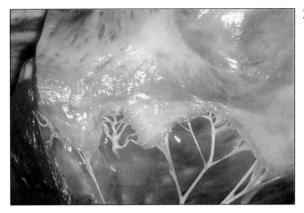

282 Mitral valve incompetence (colour flow dDoppler, ultrasound).
Note: Blood flow coded red, flowing from left ventricle (LV) to right atrium (LA) during systole. The signal has aliased, as shown by the central core change from blue through to red (i.e. travelling so fast that signal received as if traveling in the opposite direction).

283 Rupture of chordae tendinea (right commissural cusp of mitral valve).
Note: Also chronic thickening of free border of mitral valve leaflets.

Loud, widely radiating murmurs with an abrupt onset (usually during exercise) and a marked thrill, develop in cases where there is **rupture of one or more of the *chordae tendineae*** (tendinous strands running from the papillary muscles to the free borders of the atrio-ventricular valves). The mitral valve is most often affected (**283**). Fortunately, the condition is rare but is most often encountered in over-exercised horses and almost all affected animals die suddenly during or immediately after exercise, with obvious signs of congestive heart failure. Horses which are seen alive show an abrupt onset of severe respiratory distress, pulmonary edema, which is often audible and may be evident as a blood-stained, frothy, bilateral nasal discharge (**Plate 6l**, page 122), and cyanosis (**Plate 8b**, page 178). Although most affected horses die at the time of rupture or shortly after, or show severe, life-threatening congestive heart failure, a few are less affected. Ultrasonographic and pulsed wave (Doppler) examination of these cases will clearly establish the nature of the defect and the extent of valvular insufficiency (*see* **282**). The more sophisticated and detailed ultrasonographic techniques may also identify the specific ruptured cord and its associated papillary muscle. Long-standing cases develop pulmonary hypertension and right ventricular failure, which are clinically characterised by extremely poor exercise tolerance, persistent coughing, ventral edema, peripheral venous congestion and jugular engorgement. A relatively high proportion of horses affected by significant mitral valve lesions resulting from rupture of chordae or vegetative changes on the valves have concurrent atrial fibrillation. It is difficult to be certain whether, in some of these cases the electrical abnormalities are a cause or result of the valvular defects. Concurrent electrical disorders result in various bizarre audible sounds and it is often impossible to be certain of the underlying complex by auscultation alone. Careful post mortem examination of horses affected by rupture of the *chordae* will identify the ruptured chord(s). Most often the mitral valve is involved (*see* **283**). Multiple chord rupture is quite common and such a state inevitably results in catastrophic collapse of the circulation.

An equally dramatic cardiac failure is induced by **rupture of the cardiac annulus**. This highly fatal disorder results in gross distortion of the valvular integrity. While some cases may be seen alive, *in extremis*, with very high heart rates and severe congestive heart failure with extreme cyanosis and prominent, pulsating and engorged jugular veins, most cases are found dead.

Dilatation of the heart (dilated cardiomyopathy, cardiomegaly), resulting from gross, chronic distension of the chambers or muscular hypertrophy (or both) is a sequel to most forms of cardiac disease in the horse. The relative size of the heart can be assessed radiographically from upward displacement of the trachea (**284**) and/or obvious enlargement, which, for technical reasons in larger horses, is usually only radiographically evident from changes in the left side. Physiological cardiac hypertrophy is common in fit performance horses but this should not affect the relative position of the trachea in the chest.

Gross cardiac enlargement as a result of **idiopathic**

284

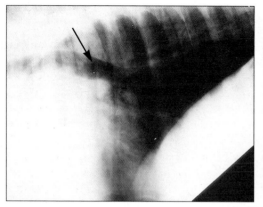

285

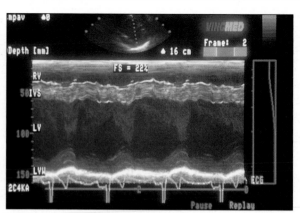

284 Dilated cardiomyopathy.
Note: Dorsal displacement of trachea (arrow) and enlarged caudal (left side) heart.
Differential Diagnosis:
i)   Heart-base tumours (very rare)
ii) Mediastinal/thymic lymphosarcoma

285 Dilated cardiomyopathy (M-mode ultrasound).
Note: Thin ventricular wall, poor compliance, valvular incompetence and enlarged left ventricle.

286

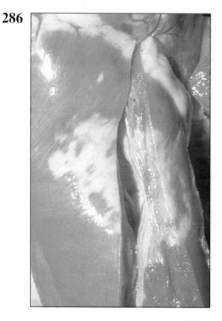

286 Myocardial fibrosis (infarct).

cardiomyopathy is accompanied by severe exercise intolerance, clinically detectable weakness, staggering and occasionally collapse, during or after exercise. Resting heart rates are elevated in most cases. Ultrasonographic assessment using M-mode may be used effectively to identify the thinner-than-normal atrial and ventricular walls, a loss of compliance (contractility) and a gross distension of the cardiac chambers (**285**). The disorder may arise without any explanation but horses deficient in dietary selenium and vitamin E may show marked evidence of enlargement and myocardial pallor associated with oxidant-induced myocardial necrosis at post mortem examination. Foals less than 1 month of age seem to be most liable to the disorder, whereas the myocardium of the adult horse appears to be more resistant, even in the face of prolonged, extreme deficiency. Horses suffering from the acute stages of myocardial degeneration often have intercurrent skeletal (and possibly smooth) muscle involvement and may be presented with all the clinical features of colic. Evidence for myocardial degeneration may be provided by estimation of the isoenzymes of creatine kinase. At post mortem examination the heart is pale, flabby and grossly distended.

Until recently myocardial disease was thought to be an infrequent condition in the horse, with the post mortem findings of **myocardial fibrosis** being of doubtful significance. With the advent of more sophisticated imaging and biochemical techniques, the diagnosis has been made with increasing frequency in the live animal and it is possible that it is of greater clinical importance than has been appreciated. **Myocardial dysfunction** arising from pathologically significant **intrinsic myocardial disorders** is responsible for poor cardiac performance and therefore for some cases of poor or reduced performance. The effects of myocardial disease on exercise are generally profound, with lethargy, weakness, staggering and, occasionally, even collapse and death. Clinically, tachydysrhythmias are encountered and there may be obvious signs of heart failure with audible irregularities and murmurs. Post mortem examination may show generalised myocardial pallor, which is sometimes ascribed to selenium and vitamin-E deficiency syndromes, or focal areas of fibrosis within the myocardium **(286)**. In many apparently normal horses, areas of myocardial fibrosis can be found **(286)**. These may represent focal areas of ischemia due to either intra-myocardial arteriosclerosis or other coronary arteriolar occlusive pathology, but are most often ascribed to parasitic migrations (**verminous embolism**), and in particular migrating strongyle larvae (and emboli) originating in the root of the aorta (*see* **307**). Viral, bacterial, toxic or traumatic disorders may also be incriminated in the etiology. Significant larger areas may be identified in association with **atrial fibrillation** and with some cases of sudden and unexpected death. It is unclear whether these areas are the result of occlusion of the coronary arteries. A particularly severe myocardial degeneration, necrosis and consequent fibrosis (in surviving horses) is associated with **monensin poisoning** (and other ionophore antibacterial agents, commonly added to sheep and cattle feeds).

Rupture of the aorta at its base (or the pulmonary artery) is a rare but important clinical syndrome in stallions in particular. Sudden death is usual although some survive long enough to allow the identification of extensive hemothorax or pulmonary bleeding (*see* **308**). Rupture of the aorta into the right atrium (aorto-atrial fistula) results in a catastrophic cardiac failure although death is often delayed for some hours and minor fistulation resulting in lesser degrees of arterial shunting may be present. The pressure gradient is such that the condition does not remain static and progression is to be expected. Cardio-aortic (dissecting) aneurysm results in aortic bleeding into the atrial and ventricular septal muscle and again a catastrophic loss of myocardial function with gross electrical abnormalities results in rapid death.

Rupture of the middle uterine or the ovarian artery occurs in the brood mare as a complication of foaling. Death occurring less than 24 hours after parturition is more usual than sudden collapse immediately after delivery. Rupture of the middle uterine artery within the broad ligament may result in the development of a large hematoma which may be sufficiently extensive to result in colic and clinically significant blood loss, without any overt signs of bleeding. Rectal examination will usually identify the lesion as a large discrete fluid filled mass lying cranial to the pelvic brim on one or other side (*see* **776**).

Rupture of mesenteric vessels, resulting in large hematomas within the mesenteric confines **(287)** are also encountered and may be the result of parasitic damage. This is a possible cause of colic. Obvious anemia is unusual but a blood stained peritoneal fluid (**Plate 2d**, page 46) usually encourages exploratory laparotomy, during which the hematoma is obvious.

Foals may be deprived of a significant proportion of their circulating blood volume if **cord separation is unduly hasty** and, while the direct clinical consequences of this occurrence may not be dramatic,

287

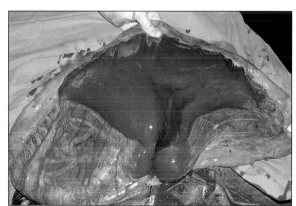

287 Mesenteric hematoma.
Note: Bleeding confined to mesentery.

288

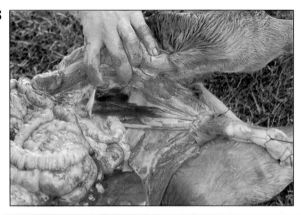

288 Rupture of umbilical artery.
Note: Foal died 5 minutes after assisted delivery following induced parturition.

289

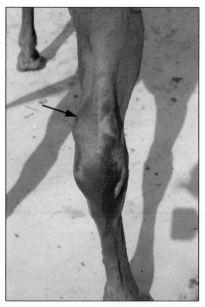

289 Arterio-venous fistula (developmental).
Note: Swelling on medial aspect of distal tibia (arrow). Pulsation and fremitus was obvious at the site.
Differential Diagnosis: [Should not really be confused with anything else]
i)   Distension of tarsal sheath (Thoroughpin)
ii) Bog spavin (distention of tibiotarsal joint)
iii) Hematoma

290 Arterio-venous fistula (acquired) (between carotid artery and jugular vein).
Note: Gross distension of right jugular vein. Prominent pulsations and fremitus palpable in mid-section of jugular groove. Jugular vein contained arterial blood. Right facial artery pressure low, with an almost imperceptible pulse. Left side normal but jugular vein also distended.
Differential Diagnosis:
i)   Congestive heart failure
ii) Anterior thoracic space occupying lesion

290

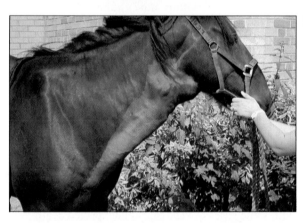

the secondary effects in relation to weakness in the early hours after birth may be serious. Rupture of the umbilical artery occurs in neonatal foals subjected to excessive cord tension at delivery **(288)**. Although the outward extent of hemorrhage may be relatively minor, it is often sufficient to result in death, particularly as a significant volume of the foals blood is usually left in the placenta. Overt hemoperitoneum may be present and detectable by abdominal paracentesis but in some cases there is none detectable and in these the hemorrhage is usually confined within the falciform and round ligaments (*see* **288**).

Peripheral arterial aneurysms or shunts (arterio-venous fistula) may be either congenital or acquired as a result of local trauma (often venipuncture). The **congenital shunts** occur almost anywhere including the distal limbs, and particularly at the hock **(289)**. They are usually incidental findings, having little or no pathological significance. Only lesions associated with the more superficial vessels are likely to be detectable. **Acquired shunts**, apart from those occurring between the heart and the aorta which have already been described, are almost exclusively the result of venipuncture or other trauma and usually, therefore, affect the superficial vessels. In all cases there is fremitus and swelling over the site, and the distal part of the affected vein may be grossly distended. Large lesions involving major vessels may result in disorders of cardiac flow and, ultimately, congestive heart failure. A **fistula between the carotid artery and the jugular vein** in the mid-cervical region is probably the commonest iatrogenic form of the disorder, and follows misdirected intravenous injections (of irritant drugs, in particular). The proximity of the carotid artery to the medial wall of the jugular vein makes inadvertent intracarotid injection relatively easy. The high pressure differential between the two vessels ensures that once a small fistula has been created it is likely to enlarge

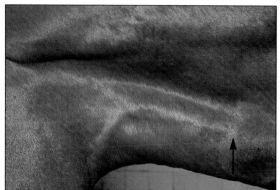

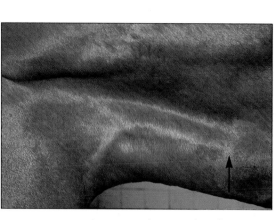

291 Disseminated intravascular coagulopathy (DIC) (jugular vein thrombosis).
Note: Jugular vein hard but neither painful nor hot on palpation. Site of venepuncture at arrow.
Differential Diagnosis:
i)   Jugular thrombophlebitis
ii) Abscess
ii) Congestive heart failure
iii) Anterior thoracic/mediastinal mass

292 Disseminated intravascular coagulopathy (DIC).
Note: Bilateral jugular occlusion caused obvious venous congestion of superficial facial veins which also became thrombosed.
Differential Diagnosis:
i)   Congestive heart failure
ii) Space-occupying lesion in anterior thorax or thoracic inlet
iii) Bilateral jugular thrombosis/thrombophlebitis from other causes

progressively and result in gross enlargement of the jugular vein(s) **(290)**. A diagnosis can be confirmed from the clinical appearance of a large pulsating jugular vein (often with fremitus at the site) and the presence of arterial (or nearly arterial) blood within the vein. The ipsilateral distal arteries (including the easily palpable posterior facial and facial arteries) have a very poor pulse pressure when compared to the normal side).

Thrombosis and thrombophlebitis are serious and common disorders in the horse. The etiology is of major significance in assessing the clinical importance of a particular case. **Spontaneous venous thrombosis** may occur as a result of **disseminated intravascular coagulopathy (DIC)**, **aorto-iliac thrombosis disease** and some systemic, viral and bacterial diseases. Thrombosis of a superficial vessel (usually the jugular vein) **(291)** is an unfortunate, common, sequel to venipuncture, particularly when the procedure is performed inadequately, or when strong concentrations of irritant drugs are administered, or when the patient is in a hypercoagulable state (such as occurs in the early stages of disseminated intravascular coagulopathy (DIC) or toxemia). It is also a common complication following the long term use of indwelling catheters and cannulae,

particularly when these are used for repeated administration of irritant or concentrated drugs. The etiology of such cases is probably a localised or diffuse endothelial inflammation affecting the vessel which predisposes to the adherence of fibrin, platelets and cells through the exposure of endothelial collagen. Extensive and compromising venous obstruction, particularly when both jugular veins (which are by far the most common sites for venous thrombosis) are involved, may have considerable circulatory consequences. Generalised venous engorgement and coagulation **(292)** and gross edema, venous distension and/or necrosis of the tissues in the distal capillary beds **(293)** are common sequelae. The recognition of the earliest (hypercoagulable) stages of disseminated intravascular coagulopathy in toxemic horses or those suffering from excessive blood loss, is of paramount importance for the clinician as it is succeeded by a dangerous and progressive hypocoagulative state.

Thrombosis (or other occlusion) of arteries has catastrophic effects upon the distal tissues, particularly where the collateral circulation is inadequate to maintain oxygenation. Thus occlusion of a digital artery in the limb by a neuroma may result in gangrene and sloughing of the foot. Occlusion of a major mesenteric artery (*see*

293

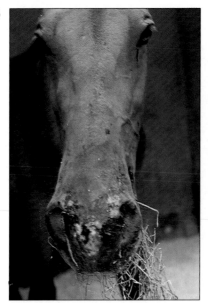

294

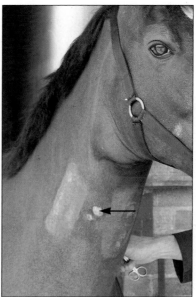

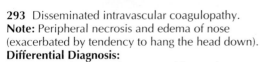

293 Disseminated intravascular coagulopathy.
Note: Peripheral necrosis and edema of nose
(exacerbated by tendency to hang the head down).
Differential Diagnosis:
i)   Systemic lupus erythematosus-like syndrome
ii) Bilateral jugular vein thrombosis/thrombophlebitis
iii) Local irritation/chemical or physical burns
iv) Photosensitisation (white areas only)
v)   Snake/spider envenomation

294 Phlebitis (with abscess).
Note: At site of infected perivascular injection (arrow).

146) may cause extensive and catastrophic ischemia whereas occlusion of a minor mesenteric vessel (*see* **147**) has less local effect. Occlusion of major veins whether through thrombosis or obstruction results in increased venous pressure on the capillary bed it serves. This causes edema and ischemia which result in further damage and progressive deterioration.

Inflammation of the veins or **thrombophlebitis** is most often the result of the perivascular injection of irritant substances, but may arise as a direct sequel to 'spontaneous' thrombosis. Where the extent of the inflammation is minimal, the reaction may be limited to a localised swelling and, where this is infected, it may develop into an abscess with proximal swelling (**294**) and heat. More extensive necrosis may follow perivascular injection of severely irritant drugs, in particular, and the extent of the necrosis and the consequent sloughing may be considerable (**295**). Damage to a jugular vein in these cases is usually of somewhat lesser importance than damage to the adjacent muscles of the ventral neck, the carotid artery, vago-sympathetic trunk and recurrent laryngeal nerves. Consequent ipsilateral laryngeal paralysis (**Plate 5u,** page 115), Horner's Syndrome (**695** *et seq*) and other circulatory effects may be present. In spite of apparently severe damage to the jugular vein and the carotid artery, the vascular effects are usually far-outweighed by the neurological consequences. The deposition of irritant substances and/or bacterial infection beneath (medial to) the jugular vein is more likely to result in neurological damage. Subcutaneous inflammation is often restricted to this site and often fortunately has little or no effect on the structures lying deep to the jugular vein. In cases in which there is little or no perivascular involvement there is correspondingly little or no swelling, and the vein is hard and painful. Thrombophlebitis is frequently complicated by sepsis and this may have serious systemic consequences, ranging from pyrexia, depression, endocarditis and embolic dissemination of infection or occluding thrombi. The risk of significant embolic disease increases dramatically where the site is infected due to an increased tendency for disruption of the thrombus. Thus distal swelling, extensive edema of the lower limbs, endocarditis (*see* **300,** *see* **301**) and pulmonary thromboembolism may develop.

The rate of development of **vascular occlusion and arterial damage** has a profound effect upon the extent of signs. Thus, slowly progressive occlusion of one (or

295

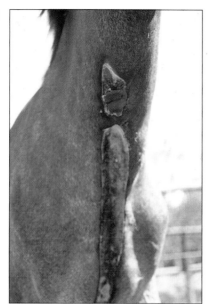

296

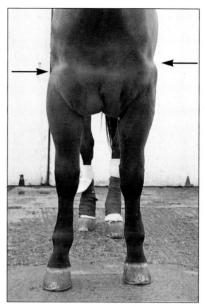

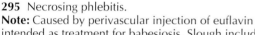

295 Necrosing phlebitis.
Note: Caused by perivascular injection of euflavin intended as treatment for babesiosis. Slough included jugular vein, carotid artery and vago-sympathetic trunk. Right side Horner's Syndrome and laryngeal paralysis were present.

296 Purpura hemorrhagica.
Note: Sharply demarcated edema of fore-limb at level of elbow (arrow). Severe serum exudate. Urticaria-like plaques present on limbs and trunk and neck. Petechiation of all visible mucous membranes **(Plate 8g)** and bilateral epistaxis with nasal swelling **(Plate 6g)**.

even both) jugular veins is usually adequately compensated by collateral circulation. In these cases swelling of extremities is less evident, although it is usually possible to identify distension of the superficial veins distal to the lesion (*see* **292**). Alternatively, rapidly developing, complete venous occlusion induces severe edema, which in the case of the jugular vein, is exacerbated by the tendency for the affected horse to hang its head down (*see* **293**). The type of disorder present may be accurately defined with the help of ultrasonographic examination and this should be employed in all cases of venous occlusion. Many cases of venous thrombosis resolve spontaneously over months or years with some effective cannulation of major and lesser vessels.

Diffuse vasculitis occurs fairly frequently in the horse as a result of immune-mediated, infectious and toxemic disorders. Most **equine vasculitis syndromes** have the characteristics of an **immune-mediated hypersensitivity** and arise secondarily to infectious, toxemic or neoplastic conditions or follow the administration of drugs or other chemicals. It is less commonly due to the direct action of viruses or bacteria on vessel walls. Perhaps the best recognised **immune-mediated vasculitis** is *purpura hemorrhagica* which, in the horse, in spite of its name, is a non-thrombocytopenic purpura (i.e. platelet numbers are

generally normal). It is most often encountered in young horses, some weeks after recovery from an upper respiratory tract virus or bacterial infection (in particular, equine influenza virus and/or *Streptococcus equi*). Some non-infectious causes have been identified, including the administration of drugs and vaccines. Affected horses have severe and often sharply demarcated, asymmetric, subcutaneous edema of the muzzle, face (*see* **Plate 6g**) and ventral abdomen, skin (*see* **517**) and limbs **(296)**. Warm, painful skin lesions, resembling urticarial plaques, are present on the trunk and neck. Extensive serum exudation from the inflamed and edematous skin lesions is a common sign and may ultimately result in extensive sloughing. Petechial hemorrhages may be visible in the skin (although this is usually difficult to identify) and in the mucous membranes of the mouth, eyes and vulva **(Plate 8g**, page 179). More extensive, ecchymotic hemorrhages may also occur in any mucous membranes **(Plate 8h**, page 179). Affected horses are often stiff and reluctant to move, giving the impression of laminitis, and may show marked respiratory distress due to obstructive edema of the upper respiratory tract. Anemia **(Plate 8d**, page 178) and spontaneous nasal bleeding (in spite of normal clotting profiles and normal platelet counts) **(Plate 6g**, page 121) are also encountered in some cases. A wide variety of apparently unrelated clinical signs including colic, weight loss, azotemia, lameness, dyspnea and ataxia may be encountered and are probably the result of organ involvement. The diagnosis is frequently difficult to confirm and is largely reliant upon historical and clinical features. The prognosis for cases of *purpura hemorrhagica* is very guarded, with some showing little or no response to treatment and others responding fairly well initially, only to relapse. Mortality may be high.

Photoactivated vasculitis is an interesting disease which is characteristically restricted to non-pigmented areas of the lower limbs. There are clear similarities but some notable differences between this condition and the forms of photosensitivity which accompany advanced hepatic disease (*see* **502**) or some plant poisonings (*see* **168**). The condition presents with a painful edema, erythema and serum exudation (**297**) in the non-pigmented skin of the lower limbs. Unlike the other forms of photosensitivity this condition does not affect white areas on other parts of the body. A diagnosis can be reached by biopsy when obvious vasculitis and thrombosis can be found in the superficial dermis. However, all horses showing evidence of photoactivated dermatoses should be carefully assessed for all the possibilities including hepatic failure.

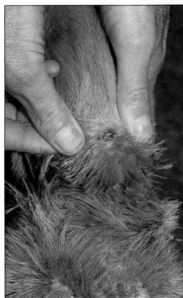

297 Photoactivated vasculitis.
Note: Exudative dermatitis with hemorrhagic foci, scaling and matting of hair on white leg extremities. No lesions on other white markings on face and body.

Infectious Disorders

Myocardial inflammation (myocarditis) may arise directly from intercurrent endocarditis or pericarditis. In many cases of myocarditis there is a detectable dysrhythmia with supraventricular or ventricular extrasystoles or atrial fibrillation. Many cases in which myocardial inflammation is suspected have no overt clinical evidence, and it is likely that many viral diseases (including equine herpes virus, equine influenza virus, African Horse Sickness etc) may be associated with some pathological inflammation. The significance of the myocarditis may be overshadowed by the more obvious clinical features but its importance should not be overlooked. Creatine kinase (CK) and lactate dehydrogenase (LDH) isoenzyme studies on horses suspected of having acute myocardial pathology may be helpful in supporting a diagnosis.

Viral Diseases: Equine viral arteritis virus is probably distributed worldwide, though little serological evidence of it has been found in Britain or Japan. While, in some parts of the world, this produces a severe and highly fatal disease, milder or completely inapparent infections, which are only detectable serologically, are more common. The clinical signs are the result of a panvasculitis and are similar, in most mild cases, to those caused by equine herpes and equine influenza viruses and to some extent those of the milder forms of African Horse Sickness (*see* **218**; *see* **219**). Affected horses show typical signs of upper respiratory tract virus infection with pyrexia, cough, palpebral edema (**298**), chemosis (conjunctival edema) and conjunctivitis with

298

299

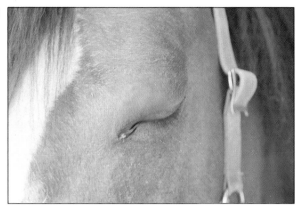

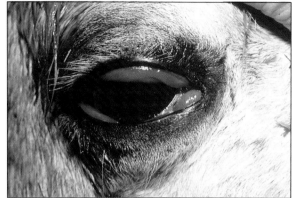

298 Viral arteritis.
Note: Edema of eyelids, no lacrimation.
Differential Diagnosis:
i)   Trauma
ii) Allergic responses (articaria)
iii) African Horse Sickness
iv) Purpura hemorrhagica

299 Viral arteritis.
Note: Chemosis, eyelid swelling, blood-stained lacrimation.
Differential Diagnosis:
i)   Trauma
ii) Circulatory impairment to head
iii) African Horse Sickness
iv) Babesiosis

lacrimation (**299**). The significant specific clinical signs are related to the panvasculitis and the consequent increased vascular permeability of small arteries and capillaries which results in blood stained tears (*see* **299**). There is commonly a prominent edema of the limbs, head and neck in a very similar way to African Horse Sickness. The ventral abdomen and the genitalia of stallions are often edematous. The severe forms of the disease present with many of the typical clinical signs of *purpura haemorrhagica* (*see* **296**), but are usually also febrile and show lacrimation, chemosis (edema of the conjunctiva), swelling of the eyelids, diarrhea and weakness. Petechial hemorrhages are commonly encountered in the mucous membranes (**Plate 8g**, page 179). Cutaneous edema and urticaria-like plaques are less common in viral arteritis than in *purpura haemorrhagica*. Abortion is a particularly common and serious effect of the virus. Secondary pleural and peritoneal effusions are present in the severe forms. Many infections are entirely subclinical without any overt clinical signs, only being detectable serologically. The similarity of this disease to several other conditions in which upper respiratory tract infections and/or vasculitis are present makes its diagnosis particularly important.

African Horse Sickness (*see* **215** *et seq.*) is also characterised by an extensive and diffuse vasculitis with petechiation and protein loss into tissues and organs. The clinical signs of the disease can be attributed almost completely to the development of an extensive and severe vasculitis in the lungs and other major organs.

Bacterial Diseases: Murmurs arising from **inflammatory and/or vegetative lesions** on the heart valves are unusual without a preceding **endocarditis**. Large, multiple lesions may cause valvular stenosis (which in practical terms only ever affects the aortic valve), but, more frequently, they result in **valvular insufficiencies** manifest by audible murmurs. **Valvular inflammation** arising, usually, from septicemia results in a very aggressive ulceration and inflammation of the valve leaflets (**300**) and although affected valves may not appear to be grossly thickened, there are serious consequences in relation to valve movement and the development of **valvular endocarditis** lesions which act as a focus for the accumulation of fibrin; extensive blood clots are commonly present attached to the damaged valves. While the majority of obvious valvular endocarditis lesions are found in the **mitral (bicuspid) valve**, the **aortic valve cusps** may develop a marked inflammation along their free borders (**301**). Again, this may act as a site of fibrin deposition and clot formation but in many cases this is an incidental finding of uncertain significance. Organisation of the fibrinous accumulations (with the enclosed bacteria) produces friable **vegetative lesions (302)**, from which infective emboli may be disseminated into the circulation. These have, therefore, considerable potential as sources of emboli, of both infective and non-infective types. Progressive organisation of the inflammatory foci in the valve leaflets has profound effects on valve closure and the site and type of the lesion may be of great importance. Smooth, long-standing and well organised

300

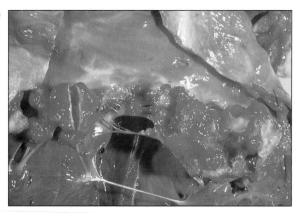

300 Bacterial endocarditis of left atrioventricular (mitral) valve (acute).

301

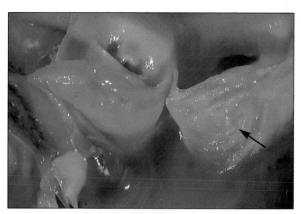

301 Bacterial endocarditis of aortic valve (acute). **Note:** Well-defined impact site on free borders of cusps (arrow).

302

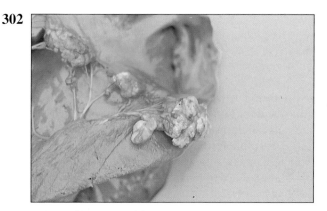

302 Bacterial endocarditis of left atrioventricular (mitral) valve (chronic, proliferative form).

303

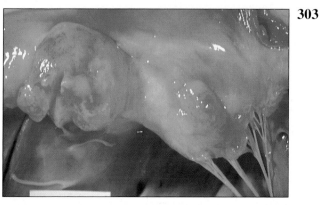

303 Endocarditis (chronic, fibrosing form). **Note:** Thickened valve leaflets.

thickening of the valve cusps typical of chronic valvular endocarditis (**303**) is somewhat less likely to result in serious embolism than the more irregular, friable lesions associated with acute bacterial endocarditis (*see* **302**). The latter is most often associated with septicemic infections with *Streptococcus equi* and other septicemic organisms. Lesions most often develop on the aortic or mitral valves. Although they do occur on the valves of the right side, the effects of emboli are likely to be less obvious, possibly even passing unnoticed. Lesions on the heart valves in foals affected with *Rhodococcus equi* septicemia are particularly unusual. Horses with bacterial endocarditis lose weight, are dull and have a characteristic recurrent, fluctuating pyrexia. Valvular insufficiencies may be obvious but sometimes are less audible. Shifting-leg lameness, resulting possibly from the embolic occlusion of endarteries in the sensitive laminae of the feet, and exercise intolerance, are often reported to occur.

Pericardial inflammation and/or infection is particularly uncommon in the horse. It may, however, lead to life-threatening cardiovascular compromise. Virus and bacterial infections are most commonly implicated and it is possible that subclinical pericardial inflammation may be a feature of some bacteraemic and viremic disorders of the horse. Primary pneumonia, pulmonary abscess, pleuritis or thoracic trauma (either blunt or penetrating) are associated with some cases of **pericarditis**. Although sepsis is by far the most common cause of pericardial inflammation, culture from the fluid (or even from the pericardium at post mortem examination) is frequently unrewarding. The clinical signs associated with the disorder vary according to the extent and nature of the exudate within the pericardial sac. Where the disease is secondary to respiratory tract disease, the respiratory signs may be prominent and the presence of concurrent pericarditis might easily be overlooked. In these cases there may be very limited volumes of pericardial exudate and its detection may be particularly difficult in the presence of overt and more extensive pulmonary or pleural pathology. **Extensive pericardial effusions (304)** result in diminished or

304

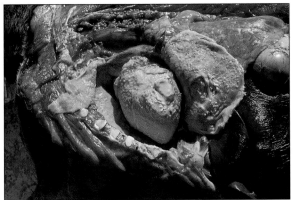

305

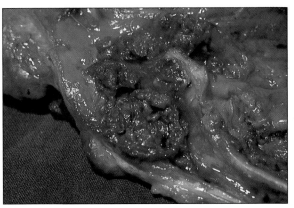

304 Suppurative pericarditis.
Note: Muffled heart sounds. Fluid detectable by ultrasonographic examination. Signs of congestive heart failure including jugular engorgement and pulsations, peripheral edema and very poor exercise tolerance. Persistent fever and endocarditis with shifting-leg lameness.

305 Verminous arteritis (cranial mesenteric arteritis).
Note: Proliferative reaction which contained parasitic (*Strongylus vulgaris*) larvae. Horse died of non-strangulating, infarctive colic **(See 146)**.

muffled heart sounds and evidence of cardiac tamponade (compression of venous return to the heart due to increased volume of fluid in the pericardium). The signs of tamponade are those of right-side cardiac failure, including prominent jugular distension and pulsation, tachycardia, poor pulse pressure (hypotension) and ventral edema. In some cases the apex beat of the heart may not easily be palpable, but a number of other conditions, including obesity and pleural effusions, may also have the same result. The definitive diagnostic method for the disease is the use of echocardiography where the thickened pericardium and the presence of variable amounts and consistency of effusion will usually be obvious. The electrocardiogram of horses affected with pericarditis shows a characteristically diminished QRS voltage and/or repeated variations in QRS amplitude which may be attributable to the movement of the heart within the distended pericardial sac. Thoracic radiography may also be used to demonstrate an enlarged, rounded cardiac silhouette but is limited by any concurrent pleural fluid and the technical problems of thoracic radiography in all but the smaller horses. Pericardiocentesis may be performed between the fourth, fifth or sixth left intercostal space mid way between the shoulder level and the sternum. This technique can provide useful information and is relatively easy and safe. Simultaneous ultrasound may provide accurate guidance for the aspiration needle. Normal pericardial fluid is limited in volume and contains few cells and a low protein, whereas in most cases of pericarditis, whether septic or not, both cell and protein content increase markedly. Post mortem

examination reveals a markedly thickened pericardial sac and the presence of exudate which may be purulent (*see* **304**) or partially organised and, in long-standing cases, fibrinous. There is commonly some intercurrent valvular endocarditis (*see* **300**; *see* **302**).

Parasitic Diseases: Lesions arising in the wall of the major arteries form an important group of disorders. Lesions occurring in the arteries are frequently attributable to the migratory habits of *Strongylus vulgaris*. Damage to the *tunica intima* of the cranial mesenteric artery and/or the aorta leads to damage which may either result in narrowing of the arterial lumen or to a localised (but often severe and extensive) **arteritis** surrounding variable numbers of larvae **(305)**. Destruction or disruption of the muscular layer of the arteries allows the development of a localised enlargement or ballooning (aneurysm) of the arterial wall. The commonest arteries involved in this process are the root of the **cranial mesenteric artery** (*see* **305**) and the renal arteries (*see* **349**). These probably being the definitive migration sites for the parasitic larvae. Rupture of either of these two arteries usually results in a catastrophic blood loss into the abdomen, and a profound anemia **(Plate 8e**, page 179) which has a typically acute onset. In some cases the extent of bleeding may be more limited and show almost no effect on mucous membrane colour. This is probably the most dramatic form of verminous arteritis but it is rare for these vessels to burst and rupture. Usually it is restricted to horses less than 6 years of age. Much more commonly, the localised inflammatory response results in embolic occlusion of larger or smaller mesenteric arteries and this results in

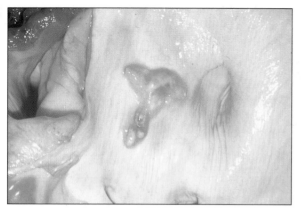

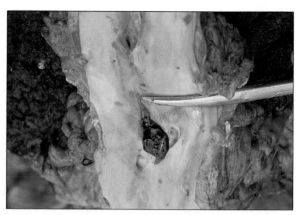

306 Verminous arteritis (lesion in aortic root).

307 Verminous arteritis (active lesion in thoracic aorta). **Note:** Blood clot adherent to wall of artery and larva visible (at end of pointer).

focal areas of ischemia of the jejunum (*see* **144**; *see* **146**), colon (*see* **147**) or cecum. The clinical consequences of this occlusion are heavily dependent upon the extent and efficiency of collateral circulation and upon the amount of devitalised intestine. Thus, remote arteries having poor or negligible collateral circulation, such as those supplying the pelvic flexure or the cecum, and large emboli which occlude major mesenteric arteries have the most severe clinical effects (*see* **146**). The result of this occlusive disorder is invariably thrombo-embolic colic but weight loss, diarrhea and milder, intermittent (or recurrent) colic may result where the extent of the occlusion is less marked in a particular locality and is more diffuse.

More remote migration of *Strongylus vulgaris* larvae may cause **infarction or inflammatory responses in the walls of the aorta** within the thorax (**306**) or in the wall of the **distal abdominal aorta** and its major branches to the hind limbs. In the former cases localised damage is found at post mortem examination as an area of inflammation on the surface of the vessel, often with an adherent blood clot and sometimes even a live larva (**307**). Rupture of the aorta between the right coronary sinus and the brachiocephalic trunk, which is the commonest site for aortic wall lesions due to parasitic migration, may occur when an aneurysm has developed in the wall at this site. A similar lesion sometimes arises in the wall of the pulmonary artery. Both of these are most frequently encountered in stallions. Cases of aortic rupture in stallions, however, often show no consistent evidence for a parasitic etiology. The condition usually follows breeding activity or fast work, and may be associated with dramatic rises in arterial pressure. It

results in a catastrophic hemothorax (**308**) or hemopericardium (or both). Occasionally, rupture of the aorta occurs into the right atrium (aorto-atrial fistula), or into the right ventricle and interventricular septum (cardio-aortic fistula). These conditions are associated with sudden and unexplained death, although an occasional case may survive long enough to be examined. Catastrophic ventricular tachydysrhythmias and peracute congestive heart failure are usually present. The horses are usually in severe distress, with massively elevated heart rates, extreme jugular engorgement and obvious jugular pulsation. A very obvious continuous murmur which is particularly intense during diastole and loudest on the right side of the chest may be detected but very high heart rates may preclude its accurate definition. The signs are those consistent with a massive left-right shunting of blood and/or extensive septal disruption.

Aorto-iliac thrombosis involving the distal aorta, its quadrification and the major hind limb arteries, is an important clinical disorder of unknown etiology. Affected horses show **intermittent claudication** (limping) which is characteristically brought-on, or aggravated by exercise. The extent of the clinical signs is largely dependent upon the speed of onset and the ultimate extent of the occlusion. True, **saddle-thrombus** occurring at the bifurcation of the aorta as a result of a massive, peracute occluding embolus, and resulting in complete occlusion of the iliac arteries is very rare in the horse. Affected animals have cold hind limbs and rapidly developing, complete hind-quarter paralysis. The slowly developing diffuse thickening of the distal aorta (**aortic 'thrombosis'**) , the aortic quadrification and the

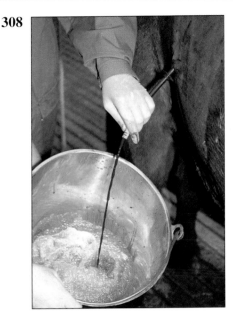

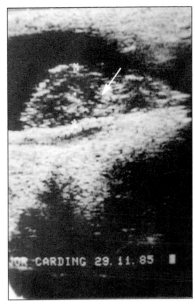

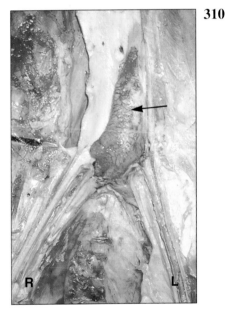

308 Hemothorax.
Note: Stallion suffering from acute onset of severe dyspnea and anemia. Drain inserted into pleural cavity. Both sides similar.

309 Aorto-iliac thrombosis (arteriosclerosis) (Ultrasonographic appearance).
Note: Narrowing of aortic diameter with dense fibrous thickening on ventral wall (arrow).

310 Aorto-iliac thrombosis (arteriosclerosis).
Note: Dense nature of tissue narrowing the aortic diameter (arrow). Marked asymmetry of occlusive lesion resulting in a more severe left iliac occlusion than right.

iliac vessels, characterised by narrowing of the arterial lumen is much more common. The clinically significant forms of the disorder are readily detectable by rectal and particularly by ultrasonographic examination (**309**). Affected horses are usually promising, young, entire or castrated males. They often have a performance expectation not matched by their work. This is often ascribed to a vague hind-leg lameness which is exacerbated by exercise. At rest, or light exercise, the affected horse is often apparently normal but more demanding work causes a well-recognised clinical entity. The extent of the thrombosis and narrowing is variable, often with one hind leg being more severely affected than the other (**310**). Bilateral cases in which there is little apparent difference between the hind legs are however encountered. The clinical signs are more obvious in unfit horses and those which have been rested for some weeks. With the onset of exercise, the horse may be seen to show a progressive deterioration of hind limb function. Severe cases may collapse or be reluctant to move or they may walk with an arched back and extended distal hind limbs. Most are obviously distressed by the condition. The affected musculature is painful. Sweating over the body and the less-affected leg may be severe in relation to the work performed. The affected limb is relatively cool and sweating is very limited. Very poor subcutaneous venous definition will invariably be present in the affected limb(s). A weak, or even absent, arterial pulse in the arteries of the distal limb may help to define the position and severity of the obstruction. Differences in peripheral pulse quality between the two hind limbs is usually strongly indicative of an occlusive lesion in the more proximal arteries although this may, of course, in some very rare cases, be due to other obstructive conditions. All of the typical signs are consistent with the reduced blood supply, which may be adequate when there is little or no demand upon circulatory efficiency. Immediately following exercise, affected horses commonly exhibit clinical signs of colic, often lying down, flank watching and stamping their feet. There may be muscle wasting over the hind-quarters although this is uncommon. A

definitive diagnosis may be achieved with careful rectal and ultrasonographic assessment of the pelvic arteries and by a painstaking comparison of the pulse quality in the distal limb arteries. Not all the branches of all the arteries will be affected equally, and some may be partially occluded, others may have no occlusion while others may be totally obstructed. Occlusive lesions which extend down to the major muscle branches of the hind limbs are relatively frequent. A detailed anatomical knowledge and careful clinical examination may define the extent of the problem. At post mortem examination the extent (*see* **310**) and the chronic, atherosclerotic nature of the lesion, can be appreciated. In most cases there is no evidence of a parasitic etiology. It is easy to understand why treatment regimes using anticoagulants are not usually effective but the etiology remains obscure.

Part 2: The Blood, Lymphatic Vessels and Lymph Nodes

Disorders of the blood and blood forming organs produce a limited number of clinically detectable signs, prominent amongst which are **anemia** (and its associated clinical effects), **bleeding** and **icterus** (and their associated implications). A wide variety of clinical disorders may ultimately present with apparently similar clinical features identified primarily by changes in the mucous membrane characteristics (**Plate 8a** *et seq.*, page 178). Accurate and careful clinical assessment will usually enable the clinician to establish a tentative diagnosis which may then be confirmed with the aid of

appropriate laboratory investigations. The responses of the equine erythron to decreasing numbers is notoriously slow and unspectacular and even long-standing cases of anemia may show only mild changes in circulating cell morphology and numbers. Nucleated red cells are very rarely encountered in peripheral blood and reticulocytes probably do not appear at all. The responses of the red and white cell series to disease processes are useful aids to the diagnosis of many diseases, but the changes are fickle and they should not be given undue significance without supporting clinical evidence.

Developmental Disorders

Congenital abnormalities of the blood and lymphatic system of the horse are, in general, very rare conditions. **Hereditary disorders of coagulation (hemophilia)** are, however, encountered in Thoroughbred, Standardbred and Arabian foals, and may be sex-linked to the male and genetically carried by apparently normal females. Clinical signs are attributable to a bleeding diathesis characterised by large vessel hemorrhage, usually including spontaneous hemorrhages into the subcutis, multiple hematoma formation (**311**) and a progressive (regenerative) anemia (**Plate 8d**, page 178) which ultimately becomes non-regenerative. Hemarthrosis (bleeding into joints) is also a common finding and

consequently both joint swelling and lameness are presented. Aspiration of blood-stained synovial fluid from more than one joint of a young foal is highly suggestive of the disorder, particularly when other evidence also exists. Colic, as a result of intra-abdominal bleeding, epistaxis, hemoptysis, depression and dyspnea are less common signs. Most of these conditions are certainly hereditary and laboratory evaluation will enable a definitive diagnosis to be made of the specific factor deficit. There is no cure for the disorder and the genetic implications should be considered before embarking on any factor-replacement therapy. Carrier females should be removed from the breeding population.

Combined immunodeficiency syndrome (CID) is a genetic, heritable disorder, primarily of the Arabian and Appaloosa breeds, which is the result of a complete failure to produce functional B and T lymphocytes. Most cases have normal cellular immunity and normal passive transfer of colostrally derived immunoglobulins at birth. Accordingly, affected foals are most often normal at birth, and grow and behave normally until the colostrum-derived passive immunity fades. At this time, usually at around 5–12 weeks of age the demand for intrinsic, active immunity is high, with natural challenges of virus and bacterial pathogens from the environment. Recurrent pulmonary infections (particularly with equine adenovirus, equine herpes viruses, equine influenza viruses, *Pneumocystis carnii* and *Streptococcus* spp) may, however, develop at any age, and while individual episodes may be overcome either by natural means or, more frequently, following therapeutic measures, respiratory, joint and enteric infections eventually overwhelm the foal. Affected foals

may be detected at an early stage by an almost complete absence of circulating lymphocytes and a failure of response to intradermal injection of phytohemagglutinin which is a strong attractant for lymphocytes. In normal foals, an obvious dermal lump develops following the injection. Foals in which the condition is diagnosed, have an extremely poor outlook, and although some do survive for up to 6–12 months, euthanasia is recommended. The condition is best regarded as invariably fatal and the genetic implications are of vital importance to the breeders of these unfortunate foals. Gross post mortem findings show marked hypoplasia of the lymph nodes, thymus and spleen.

A number of **specific immunodeficiency syndromes** are recognised in foals including specific deficiencies of individual gamma globulins and while one of these (transient hypogammaglobulinemia) is a transient disorder, all the others have the same potential outcome as the combined immunodeficiency syndrome, with minor variations in the extent of immunocompromise.

311

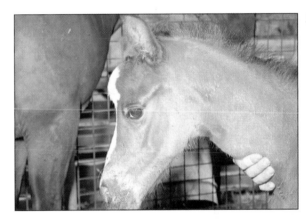

311 Hemophilia.
Note: Large (spontaneous) hematoma on forehead. Other hematomas on limbs and body. Foal very anemic, dull and lethargic. Specific factors (VII and VIII) deficient.

Non-Infectious Disorders

Neonatal isoerythrolysis (jaundiced foal) occurs in foals born to multiparous mares with specific anti-erythrocyte antibody which suckle the mare normally in the first 6 hours of life, thereby acquiring significant antibody to their own erythrocytes. The severity of the clinical signs, which usually develop between 12 and 48 hours of birth, is dependent upon the amount of specific anti-erythrocyte antibody absorbed. There may be a massive intravascular lysis of red cells, in which rapidly progressive lethargy, weakness, hemoglobinuria and death occur in a foal which was apparently normal at birth, and which had fed well within the first 2 hours from a dam producing high quality colostrum.

Clinically obvious anemia and hemoglobinuria resulting from the catastrophic destruction of red cells in the circulation may be the first and only presenting signs before death. Other causes of rapidly developing, progressive anemia such as blood loss from ruptured arteries, should also be considered. In cases which survive for some hours, or in lesser affected foals, profound icterus is usually observed (**312**). The icterus is often made more striking by the intercurrent anemia (**Plate 8f**, page 179). The foals will often show lethargy and yawn repeatedly. Any exertion or excitement is accompanied by an inordinate increase in both heart and respiratory rate and some even collapse during minimal

312

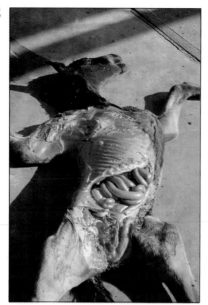

313

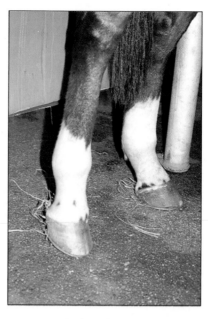

312 Neonatal isoerythrolysis.
Note: Intense (whole body) icterus in a foal which died 3 days after birth. No hemoglobinuria seen.

313 Sporadic lymphangitis ('Monday-Morning Leg').
Note: Edematous swelling (pits on pressure) resolved easily following short walking exercise. Recurred regularly while horse was stabled.

exercise. A jugular pulse may be present and the severe reduction in blood viscosity may result in an obvious hemic heart murmur. Erythrocytes from affected foals, diluted in plasma or saline (1:4), will often be seen to clump on a slide. Such a dilution of the red cells reduces the possibility of rouleaux formation which may give the impression of clumping/ agglutination. Repeated blood samples should be examined from suspect foals both prior to, and subsequent to, the institution of therapeutic measures which may include blood transfusion and immunosuppressive drugs. Mildly affected foals seldom require intensive and aggressive therapy and, indeed, such an approach may be contra-indicated. Foals surviving for 5 – 10 days are usually destined to survive. The prepartum detection of significant anti-erythrocyte-antibody in the mare is suggestive of the development of a possible compatibility problem, and such a foaling should be monitored particularly carefully, ensuring that the foals red cells are tested for compatibility with the mares serum at birth, prior to any nursing. The condition is much more likely to develop in mares which have had previous foals affected by the condition and is very rare in primipara. At post mortem examination the carcass is usually patently icteric (*see* **312**) with a large rounded liver.

A number of other clinical syndromes associated with auto-immune processes occur in the horse including **autoimmune hemolytic anemia** and **immune-mediated thrombocytopenia**. In contrast to the hemolytic disease of newborn foals, immune-mediated, **(autoimmune) hemolytic anemia** in adult horses is rare. The condition may be primary, in which antibody is produced directly against the animals own erythrocytes, or secondary when antibody is produced against other antigens which become adherent to erythrocytes. The former state is particularly rare, while the latter is somewhat commoner and is usually associated with more severe underlying disease such as septicemic infection and lymphosarcoma, or follows drug administration. Some infectious agents have been thought to be responsible for the development of red-cell-antibody but it is most likely that this is a product of antigen adherent to erythrocytes. Most often the progression of this disease is slow and insidious, with a long-standing, chronic anemia. Pallor (**Plate 8d**, page 178), weakness and poor exercise tolerance, are the major presenting clinical features. Icterus and hemoglobinuria are rarely present, presumably as the destruction of red cells takes place within the reticuloendothelial organs and is therefore extravascular. The most specific test for the disorder is the direct Coombs test using patient red cells and a specific anti-equine globulin. A positive test supports the diagnosis that the red cells are coated with immunoglobulin, complement or both. However a negative test is not conclusive, due possibly to technical difficulties with the procedure or to prior, intrinsic destruction of all the coated red cells in the circulation at that time.

Immune-mediated thrombocytopenia is, again, most often associated with other pre-existing infections (such as upper respiratory tract infections), or other serious intercurrent disease such as lymphosarcoma or chronic infectious processes. In many cases, however, no other condition can be identified at the time of presentation. The onset of the clinical syndrome is characteristically insidious and the signs of hemorrhagic diatheses are often the most obvious presenting features. Thus, mild or occasionally more severe, spontaneous intermittent or persistent, unilateral (*see* **Plate 7g**, page 144) or bilateral (*see* **plate 6g**, page 121) epistaxis is a common finding and occurs when the platelet count falls sufficiently. As one of the primary functions of the platelets is the maintenance of the vascular endothelial integrity, dramatic reductions in their numbers result in the development of petechial (**Plate 8g**, page 179) or larger, ecchymotic (**Plate 8h**, page 179) hemorrhages, which are most prominent on the more stressed mucous membranes of the nasal cavity, pharynx and vulva. Hyphema (bleeding into the anterior chamber of the eye) (*see* **616**) and micro-hematuria are commonly encountered but may easily be overlooked. There are usually few other signs of overt illness, but spontaneous and/or trauma-induced hematomas and prolonged bleeding from injection sites or minor cuts may be encountered. Chronic (persistent) bleeding commonly occurs into the lumen of the intestine and results in significant, detectable blood and blood products in the feces. The response to corticosteroid therapy is highly supportive of the diagnosis but the specific detection of antiplatelet antibodies is definitive. However, the latter tests are insensitive and are, at present, poorly defined for the horse. The absence of hot, painful, skin swellings helps to differentiate the disorder from *purpura hemorrhagica* and the absence of febrile response and other systemic signs of illness preclude infectious causes of anemia.

Idiopathic thrombocytopenia, in which no underlying explanation (either immunological or infectious or iatrogenic) can be found, also occurs in horses. The disorder presents in the same way and the clinical course follows the same pattern as the auto-immune disorder but fails to show any response to therapy. Bone marrow examination is a useful, under-utilised, means of assessing the response to all of these conditions.

Horses which are stabled for long periods of time, and in particular those which are immobile during such confinement, either due to voluntary or enforced immobility, are often found to have swollen ('filled') distal limbs (**313**). The hind legs are often particularly affected and the swelling may be considerable in some cases. The condition, known as **sporadic lymphangitis** or **'Monday-morning Leg'**, can readily be differentiated from the more sinister causes of distal limb edema by the fact that rapid resolution usually follows even short exercise, and no underlying disease process is present. As its colloquial name implies, it is commonly seen on a Monday morning after a rested weekend in a stable.

Disseminated Intravascular coagulopathy (DIC) is a serious and life-threatening disorder of coagulation characterised by extensive fibrin deposition in the microcirculation of capillary beds with consequent ischemia in the major organs and body tissues. Many disease conditions including toxemia, peritonitis, pleuritis, shock, septicemia, and extensive hemorrhage, are implicated in the development of the disorder. It is a particularly common complication of strangulating intestinal obstructions and of the septicemic diseases of foals. The normal horse has a relatively inhibited coagulation mechanism and usually does not follow the typical course for the disorder in other species. In the early stages there is a hypercoagulable state which arises, primarily, from the effects of collagen exposure in small blood vessels and capillaries. Extensive activation of clotting mechanisms result in widespread intravascular coagulation which is usually first manifest at sites where venepuncture has been carried out. **Jugular thrombosis** (*see* **291**; *see* **292**) in response to venepuncture is usually the commonest manifestation of the early stages of the condition. The progressive and overwhelming consumption of clotting factors and the metabolites arising from the destruction of fibrin (fibrin degradation products, FDP) in the bloodstream (which are themselves intensely anticoagulant) combine to result in the development of a markedly hypocoagulable state. Bleeding from even minor surgical wounds and venepuncture sites and spontaneous hematoma-formation indicate the onset of the advanced hemorrhagic stages. Petechiation and ecchymotic hemorrhages on mucosae (**Plate 8h**, page 179), inner pinna, retina (in foals), melena and epistaxis (**Plate 6g**, page 121) form the overt clinical signs of the condition. Damage to the kidney or other internal organs, may ensue from the development of thrombi, ischemia and bleeding within the capillary beds, resulting in further damage and further collagen exposure. Laboratory

Plate 8

a

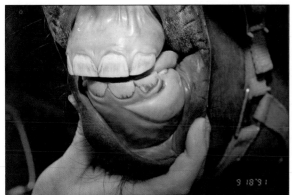

b

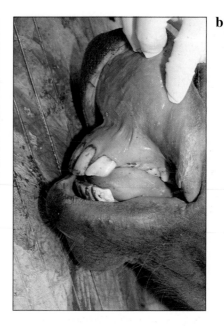

a Normal pink oral mucous membranes.
Note: Yearling foal with ossifying fibroma of the jaw.

b Cyanotic mucous membranes.
Note: Horse dying of gastric rupture as a result of severe strangulating jejunal obstruction.
Differential Diagnosis:
i)   Circulatory compromises/congestive heart failue
ii) Respiratory obstructions/failure
iii) Severe endotoxemia
iv) African horse sickness

c

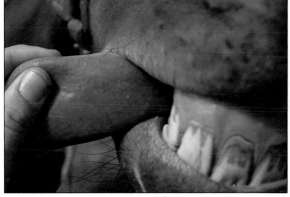

d

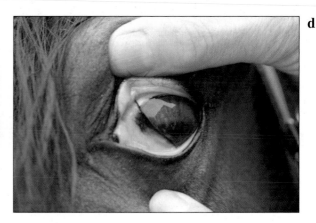

c Congested mucous membranes.
Differential Diagnosis:
i)   Endotoxemia
ii) Circulatory obstructions
iii) Congestive heart failure
iv) African horse sickness
v)   Acute renal failure

d Mild anemia.
Differential Diagnosis:
i)   Blood loss
ii)   Hemolytic diseases (Usually rapidly progressive)
iii) Bone marrow suppression e.g. Chronic infection, iron deficiency (usually slowly progressive)
iv)   Deficiency disorders
v)   Clotting disorders
vi)   Malabsorbtion syndromes
vii) Lymphosarcoma
viii) Equine infectious anemia

Plate 8

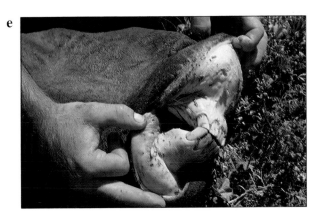

e Severe anemia.
Differential Diagnosis:
i)   Blood loss (obvious or not obvious)
ii) Severe bone marrow depression

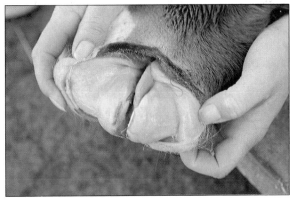

f Mild anemia with icterus.
Differential Diagnosis:
i)   Neonatal isoerythrolysis
ii) Babesiosis
iii) Equine infectious anemia (adult horses)

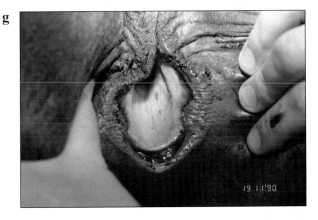

g Petechiation.
Differential Diagnosis:
i)   Hemorrhagic diatheses
ii)   Thrombocytopenic purpura
iii) Purpura haemorrhagica
iv)   Septicemia
v)   Toxemia
vi)   Vasculitis (systemic lupus erythematosus-like syndrome of horses)
vii) African Horse Sickness
viii) Viral Arteritis
ix)   Equine infectious anemia

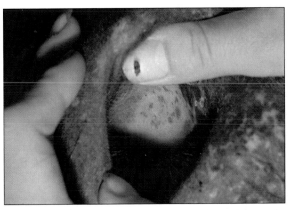

h Ecchymotic hemorrhages.
Differential Diagnosis:
i)   Vasculitis (immune mediated and infectious)
ii) Toxemia
iii) Hemorrhagic diatheses
iv) Immune-mediated thrombocytopenia
v)   Systemic lupus erythematosus-like syndrome

methods may be useful in supporting the diagnosis, but ultimately the clinical features are obvious. The diagnosis represents one of the most serious complications of many equine disease processes and action should be directed towards both this and the underlying disease process.

Incompatible blood transfusions and the **administration of biologically derived products** have been implicated in the development of **Theiler's Disease** (*see* **162**; *see* **163**). Blood transfusions are most often used in the treatment of blood-loss conditions and hemolytic disease in the foal but are also occasionally used in adult horses. Gross incompatibility of blood administered to a recipient results in anaphylaxis and/or the catastrophic lysis of red cells. The latter state closely resembles the isoerythrolytic syndrome of young foals (*see* **312**). Restlessness, respiratory distress (hyperpnea), urticarial plaques (*see* **509**) and occasionally collapse are early indications of incompatibility of transfusion solutions.

Infectious Disorders

Chronic infection (and other persistent immune stimulant conditions including neoplasia) is one of the commonest causes of **non-regenerative anemia** in both foals and adult horses. Pleuritis, pneumonia, chronic internal abscesses and neoplasia are potentially responsible for the development of a typical **iron-deficiency anemia** which arises from a lack of available iron, although total body-iron is usually normal. Affected horses show a profound progressive microcytic, hypochromic anemia with little or no bone marrow response. Deficiencies of other nutrients are supposedly responsible for the development of clinically important anemia but it is unlikely that, in the absence of underlying disease, horses ingesting a normal diet will be found to be deficient in any of the more significant nutrients.

Nutritional deficiency of protein, iron, folate, vitamin B$_{12}$, copper and cobalt have all been implicated in chronic progressive anemia in foals and adult horses. In both adults and foals normal dietary components are usually sufficient in all these respects but dietary deficiency or failure of absorbtion and chronic infections may affect the availability of one or more of them. Anemia associated with acute, massive blood-loss in the absence of overt bleeding from wounds etc, is usually the result of internal bleeding which in the foal may be from gastric ulceration (*see* **94**), or from the rupture of one or more of the major blood vessels (*see* **288**; *see* **Plate 8e**, page 179). Significant blood loss may arise in young foals from premature rupture of the umbilical cord. Bleeding into the internal cavities renders most of the iron temporarily unavailable to the animal, although a significant proportion of the red cells may be re-introduced into the circulation via the lymphatic vessels.

Viral Disease: Equine infectious anemia (EIA) is a virus disease transmitted by blood-feeding arthropods, which occurs worldwide, but which has been effectively controlled in some areas. Infection produces a number of different clinical syndromes, ranging from an almost in-apparent, sub-clinical form through a chronic form, to a peracute, life-threatening disease. Animals, once infected, appear to remain viremic for the rest of their lives. The acute syndrome is usually associated with the first episode of infection and is clinically similar to that caused by equine viral arteritis (*see* **298**) with transient petechial hemorrhages (**Plate 8g**, page 179) and fever. Recurring cycles of fever and progressive anemia (**Plate 8d**, page 178), ventral and dependent edema, icterus (*see* **158**; **Plate 8f**, page 179) and weight loss are typical of the disease. The severity of the anemia increases with each succeeding

314

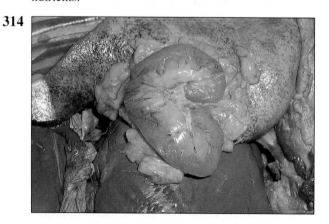

314 Equine infectious anemia.
Note: Pale and enlarged kidney and grossly enlarged spleen (possibly related to barbiturate euthanasia).

315

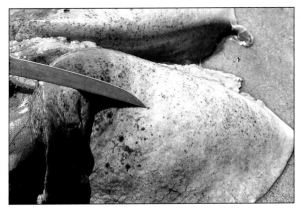

315 Neonatal septicemia (*Actinobacillus equuli*). **Note:** Generalised petechiation of all body surfaces including this pleural surface. Further petechiation in retina and obvious uveitis (*see* **640**).

viremic, febrile episode and while successive episodes are usually milder, the disease progresses inexorably. Consequent severe, prolonged anemia results in organ failure which, along with the anemia, may be detected at post mortem examination (**314**). The clinical signs usually become less severe with time but any stress may result in the development of an acute or peracute episode. The agar gel immunodiffusion test (Coggin's Test) is extremely sensitive and very easily performed, and has been largely responsible for the control and eradication of the disease over large areas of the world.

Bacterial Diseases: Bacterial septicemia is most often encountered in newborn foals, and particularly in premature or dysmature foals, and those in which there are complicating factors associated with gestation, parturition or their immediate post-natal adaptation and management. Infection with organisms including *Actinobacillus equuli*, *Salmonella* spp, *Streptococcus* spp, and other (particularly Gram-negative) bacteria, result in the development of the **neonatal septicemia syndrome**. In the early stages of the infective process the signs are often subtle with lethargy, weakness and poor suckling. Localising signs are unusual at this stage and severe disease may be present before there is any overt clinical evidence of abnormality. Congested mucous membranes, petechial hemorrhages in the pinnae and sclera, uveitis (*see* **640**), diarrhea and seizures are encountered. Infections and swellings of the urachus and/or umbilicus (*see* **334**) and joint swellings (*see* **433**), with radiographically detectable infective arthritis or physeal abscesses (*see* **431**) affecting one or more joints, are typically present. The foal is febrile and become progressively more lethargic and depressed. Diarrhea is a common feature (*see* **133**). A diagnosis may be particularly difficult to reach in the early stages, when therapeutic measures might be expected to be of assistance, and the use of blood culture techniques may be most useful. All foals affected by septicemic disorders, whether severe or not, should be assessed for their immune status with respect to passive immunity. A high proportion of foals with poor colostral absorption develop infections and many of these become septicemic. At post mortem examination extensive petechiation (**315**), possibly as result of a disseminated intravascular coagulopathy, and multiple organ involvement are detectable.

An important septicemia of foals under the age of six months is that due to *Rhodococcus equi*. The clinical features of the disease are usually restricted to respiratory (see **221** *et seq*) and alimentary (*see* **225**) signs, but joints and other organs including the eye may be involved.

Septicemic infection with *Streptococcus equi* causes the so-called 'Bastard Strangles' (*see* **230**; *see* **231**).

The horse is as sensitive as other species to infection with *Bacillus anthracis* which occurs throughout the world and **anthrax** is, in most places, a notifiable disease, carrying statutory implications. Feed, contaminated by the infective spores, or biting insects, may infect the individual animal. It is usually a sporadic peracute or acute disease in the horse. The route of infection appears to have an effect upon the form which the infection takes. Infection by insect transmission causes hot, painful, edematous, subcutaneous swellings at the site of infected bites. In some cases a single, non-healing, discrete, skin carbuncle with a characteristic necrotic centre is encountered without any systemic effects, and in these the course may be prolonged. Ingestion of spores is followed by colic and enteritis and these cases usually die after a fulminating, febrile septicemic course lasting only a few hours. Acute fever, petechial or ecchymotic hemorrhages (**Plate 8h**, page 179), severe depression, dyspnea and diarrhea may be encountered. Extensive inflammation and edema of the head and neck in particular (**316**) are signs of the subacute form of the disease. Animals dying of anthrax often have hemorrhagic nasal and anal discharges and the carcass undergoes particularly rapid autolysis. A

316

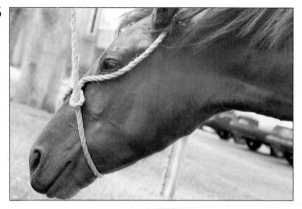

316 Anthrax (*Bacillus anthracis*) (septicemic form).
Note: Edematous swelling of neck and throat. Dyspnea and very high body temperature.
Differential Diagnosis:
i)   Strangles
ii) African Horse Sickness
iii) Disseminated intravascular coagulopathy (DIC)
iv) Guttural pouch empyema
v)   Guttural pouch tympany
vi) Bilateral jugular vein occlusion/thrombosis
vii) (Bilateral) thrombophlebitis

317

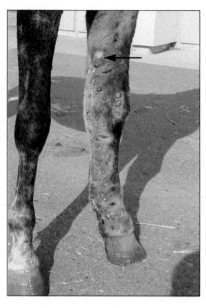

317 Ulcerative Lymphangitis.
Note: Corded lymphatic vessels and purulent discharge from ulcerated site (arrow). Chronic thickening and exudate over distal parts of limb.

diagnosis may be confirmed by the finding of the characteristic spore forming short chains of bacilli in peripheral capillary blood smears. Smears should be obtained from the edema fluid or directly (by impression) from lesions in the skin where these are present. The disease is transmissible to man and appropriate care must be taken to ensure the safety of the handlers and the adherence to local regulations relating to the disease.

Ulcerative lymphangitis is a bacterial infection of the cutaneous lymphatic vessels, most commonly involving the hind limbs, and usually associated with *Corynebacterium pseudotuberculosis*. Other organisms including *Streptococcus equi*, *Rhodococcus equi* and *Pasteurella hemolytica* have been isolated from some cases. Bacterial contamination of superficial wounds usually precedes the development of skin nodules along the course of the lymphatic vessels which ulcerate and drain onto the skin surface (**317**). Where the condition is long-standing and, more particularly where it is due to *Corynebacterium pseudotuberculosis*, there is usually a massive and extensive fibrosis and local and distal edema (**318**). A very similar appearance is presented in cases of sporotrichosis, due to infection with the fungus *Sporothrix schenkii* (*see* **560**), Farcy (Glanders) due to *Pseudomonas mallei* (*see* **550**) and pythiosis (*see* **562**), which also appear to track along lymphatic vessels in skin and sub-cutis and which present with chronic, discharging, ulcerated, dermal nodules.

Protozoal Diseases: Protozoal infections in the

horse form an important group of diseases in various parts of the world. In general, they require the presence of suitable vectors for transmission between animals and most are therefore species specific and seasonally and geographically restricted.

Potomac horse fever is a seasonal disease due to *Ehrlichia risticii* and which is geographically restricted to limited areas of North America. The disease has some enigmatic features relating to its transmission and epidemiology and appears to occur in a number of different circumstances affecting horses in different ways. A short disease course lasting from one to three days with soft ("cow-pat") or diarrheic feces due to an acute typhlocolitis, accompanied by fever, general malaise and anorexia are seen in the milder forms of the infection. Colic and profuse watery diarrhea may be seen in more severe cases and endotoxemia and laminitis are common sequelae from which horses seldom recover. While the diagnosis cannot be confirmed from the clinical features alone even the laboratory tests are difficult and sometimes misleading.

Equine babesiosis (piroplasmosis) is an acute or chronic disease caused by either *Babesia caballi* or *Babesia equi* (or both), and is transmitted by ticks, primarily of the *Dermacentor* spp (including *Dermacentor nitens*) or *Rhipicephalus* spp (including *Rhipicephalus sanguineus*). While *Babesia caballi* causes a milder (and often inapparent) disease and has an almost world-wide distribution where vectors exist,

318

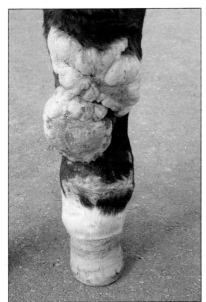

319

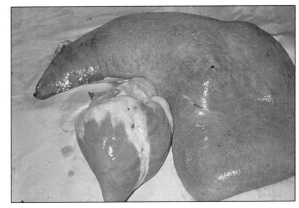

318 Chronic (ulcerative) lymphangitis
Note: Extensive fibrosis and distal edema of (hind) leg.
Differential Diagnosis:
i)   Exuberant granulation tissue
ii) Botryomycosis
iii) Glanders (Farcy)

319 Babesiosis (*Babesia equi*).
Note: Enlarged, pale and flabby appearance of heart and splenomegaly (easily detected per rectum).

the smaller *Babesia equi* causes a more recognisable and serious disease and is more restricted geographically. The clinical effects of either infection are largely similar, varying only in degree, and are dependent upon the degree of immunity of the host. In endemic areas most horses are symptomless carriers in a premune state, and overt infection may only emerge when the balance between the host and the parasite is altered, especially if the host-immunity is allowed to wane or is reduced by stress, such as that associated with racing, transportation or pregnancy. The clinical signs of **acute babesiosis** include fever, depression and icterus (*see* **158**), which is rendered more prominent by the intercurrent anemia (**Plate 8f**, page 179). Moderate supraorbital edema is a common sign (*see* **299;** *see* **218**) and terminally, this extends to peripheral and dependent edema of the limbs and ventral abdomen. Hemoglobinuria is uncommon in spite of the colloquial name 'redwater'. Infected red cells are removed by the spleen which is often grossly enlarged (**319**) and this can be recognised during rectal examination. Fetal foals may be infected with *Babesia equi* and are sometimes born with a severe, often overwhelming, parasitemia. They are febrile and icteric from birth and mortality is particularly high. In endemic areas **neonatal babesiosis** may be confused with neonatal isoerythrolysis syndrome (*see* **312**) and Tyzzer's disease (*see* **171**). Post mortem examination of horses with overt piroplasmosis reveals a grossly enlarged spleen and a pale flabby heart (*see* **319**). Most major organs are pale, degenerate and/or icteric.

Obvious edema of the renal capsule is usually present.

Trypanosomal infections of the horse present different clinical signs depending on the infective organism. With the exception of ***Trypanosoma equiperdum*** which is transmitted venereally and causes **Dourine** (*see* **861**), the other organisms require specific vectors for transmission and are therefore geographically restricted to areas where these occur. Infection with ***Trypanosoma brucei***, which is transmitted by tsetse flies (*Glossina* spp.), is restricted to areas of north and central Africa and causes the disease known as **Nagana**. Recurrent pyrexic episodes of variable severity are accompanied by anorexia, dramatic weight-loss and progressive hind-quarter weakness with ataxia. The superficial lymph nodes are enlarged and may be visible from a distance. Ventral edema, particularly of the prepuce, scrotum and lower limbs, anemia with tachycardia, and dyspnea are typical signs of the disease but these closely resemble the signs of babesiosis. Conjunctivitis, epiphora and photophobia are sometimes present. The diagnosis may be confirmed from peripheral (capillary) blood smears when the parasites can be readily identified. In many cases however, the extent of parasitemia is low in circulating blood and thick smears or serological methods or cerebrospinal fluid examination are then helpful.

Surra is a trypanosomal infection due to ***Trypanosoma evansi*** and is particularly important in India, but has been found in other parts of the world. It is transmitted by biting flies (and possibly other insects) and occasionally by injudicious re-use of needles and syringes. The signs are indistinguishable from Nagana.

Metazoan Diseases: Equine cutaneous oncho-cerciasis (*see* **586**) represents the clinical syndrome which arises from infection with the microfilaria of *Onchocerca cervicalis*. A large number of apparently normal horses are known to harbour the blood-borne microfilaria. Pruritic skin lesions develop in affected horses over 2–3 years of age, due to nests of the parasites (and/or their death) in the capillary beds of the skin (and particularly that of the ventral midline, forehead, pectoral area and withers). The parasite is transmitted by biting flies of the *Culicoides* spp. A diagnosis of onchocerciasis is hard to establish and the effect of therapeutic measures may be a useful aid to the diagnosis.

Neoplastic Disorders

The major primary neoplastic disorder of the blood and blood forming organs is **lymphosarcoma**. The name is given to a variety of myeloproliferative tumours that occur in the lymphoid tissues and are associated with the malignant expansion of lymphocytes and their precursor cells. Lymphosarcoma in its various forms is probably the commonest internal neoplasm in the horse and is certainly the most frequent tumour of the hemopoietic system. It is probably the most common neoplastic cause of death in the horse. While most lymphocytic cells occur in the lymph nodes, spleen, intestinal walls, bone marrow and pharynx, they are also present in lesser numbers in almost all tissues. Therefore, tumours involving lymphocytes are possible in almost all sites including the skin and the central nervous system. Four more-or-less distinct equine lymphosarcoma syndromes are recognised. These are:

a) the generalised form (*see* **272**),
b) the alimentary form (*see* **155**; *see* **156**),
c) the mediastinal form (*see* **320** *et seq.*) and
d) the cutaneous form (*see* **591** *et seq.*).

With the exception of the cutaneous form, metastasis of the primary tumours is particularly common and consequently, multiple organ involvement is frequent. Where secondary (metastatic) tumours are present clinical signs may be attributable to (multi-)organ failure and are very variable. Horses of all sexes, ages and breeds are liable to the condition and, while most cases are to be found in middle aged horses (4–15 years of age), younger and older horses are by no means precluded. The general signs of lymphosarcoma of all the forms are similar, with depression, progressive weight-loss, peripheral and dependent edema (*see* **321**), diarrhea (particularly in the diffuse intestinal form) (*see* **134**) and intermittent, recurrent, pyrexic episodes at variable intervals. Secondary effects, including immune-mediated hemolytic anemia and thrombocytopenia, are sometimes the first and most obvious clinical manifestations.

Interference with vascular or lymphatic circulation, by enlarged lymph nodes in the abdomen or thorax results in localised edema and accumulations of fluid within the body cavities. This fluid often contains cells of diagnostic value. Hypoalbuminemia, hyperfib-rinogenemia and gammopathies are good supportive laboratory findings in all forms of the disease. Plasma calcium concentrations are often, but not always, significantly elevated. In some cases of lymphosarcoma, the hematological and biochemical findings may be disappointing in relation to the severity of the underlying pathology. With the exception of the cutaneous form the rate of progression is usually rapid, with significant deterioration apparent within 2–4 months, at most.

i) **Generalised (Multicentric) Lymphosarcoma**:
The most frequently affected tissues are lymph nodes, liver, spleen, intestine, kidney and lung. The clinical signs are very variable and depend heavily upon the organ(s) most affected. Obvious peripheral lymphadenopathy is usually presented in these cases. Physical enlargement of lymph nodes induces secondary respiratory signs, dysphagia (*see* **272**), exophthalmos (*see* **662**). Signs attributable to organ dysfunction such as icterus, colic, weight loss, and particularly anemia (**Plate 8d**, page 178) are common.

ii) **Alimentary (Intestinal) Lymphosarcoma**:
This form occurs in two well recognised ways:

a) **Diffuse intestinal lymphosarcoma:** (*see* **155**)
This is the most common of the alimentary types and is more prevalent in younger horses than the focal form. Horses affected have a grossly impaired intestinal absorptive capacity which is caused by diffuse intestinal infiltration by abnormal blast cells. Weight loss, peripheral and dependent edema, lethargy and ascites are common signs. Recurrent pyrexia is a frequent finding and, in the later stages when the cells invade and affect the water absorptive capacity of the cecum and

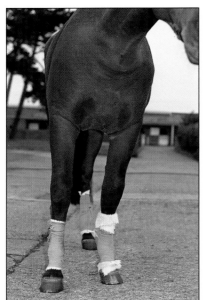

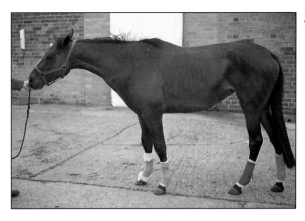

320 Thoracic (mediastinal) lymphosarcoma.
Note: Edema primarily affecting front right limb, shoulder and neck. Jugular engorgement was also present.

321 Thoracic (mediastinal) lymphosarcoma.
Note: Forelimb, neck and ventral edema giving the impression of a relatively well developed fore-quarter. Hind-quarter weight loss.

colon, diarrhea is often present. Metastases are slow to develop but grossly enlarged mesenteric lymph nodes at the root of the mesentery are often palpable per rectum. Diagnosis may be supported by a particularly slow/poor absorption of glucose (or xylose) from the intestine during a glucose (xylose) absorption test. Abdominal fluid frequently contains cells of diagnostic value and rectal biopsy may occasionally be diagnostic and is easy to obtain. A definitive diagnosis is often, however, only possible from biopsy specimens obtained from the intestine at laparotomy.

b) **Focal intestinal lymphosarcoma:** (*see* **156**)
The general signs of lymphosarcoma are also present in this form. Post-prandial abdominal pain, as a result of non-strangulating (sometimes partial or intermittent) small intestinal obstruction, is a presenting sign and, with weight loss, is often the first overt clinical evidence of the disease. Rectal palpation frequently identifies significant mesenteric lymph node enlargement at the root of the mesentery and sometimes the intestinal mass(es) may be appreciated. Rectal biopsy is not often of diagnostic value but significant blast cells may be found in peritoneal fluid. Laparotomy is often the best method of making the diagnosis.

iii) **Mediastinal Lymphosarcoma**:
The progression of this form is usually particularly rapid. Clinical signs of thoracic involvement are attributable to circulatory effects of masses within the mediastinum and include coughing, dyspnea or tachypnea, and exercise intolerance. There is usually some obstruction of one or both jugular veins, and the thoracic lymphatic ducts are frequently obstructed. Consequent edema of, at first, one forelimb (**320**) and then both, with jugular engorgement and edema of the head and neck (**321**) are typical. Owners might report the forequarters to be "good" and the hindquarters to be "poorly developed or wasted" (**321**) under the misguided impression that the forelimb and head/neck signs are less significant than the hindquarter sign of weight loss (and possibly) ascites. Massive pleural effusion of clear or hemorrhagic fluid (**322**) which is replaced almost as fast as it is withdrawn, is characteristic. It is not unusual to remove up to 35 litres of the fluid from the chest only to have to repeat the procedure within 12–24 hours. The fluid contains cells of diagnostic value in almost all cases. Although the site of the most obvious lesions is in the cranial parts of the thorax (**323**), the disorder seldom involves the thymus except in very young horses. Extensive tumour masses in the mediastinum and its associated lymph nodes may be found at post mortem examination (**324**). In some cases the malignancy extends to the dorsal thoracic (*see* **323**) and abdominal lymph nodes and hind limb edema, ascites and diarrhea may then be present.

iv) **Cutaneous (Histiocytic) Lymphosarcoma**: (*see* **591** *et seq.*)
Multiple cutaneous nodules, which may be firm or fluctuant, or may resemble edematous plaques, which may ulcerate, are found all over the body (*see* **591**).

322

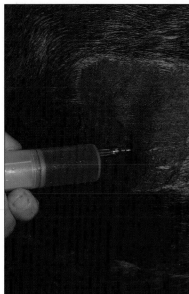

323

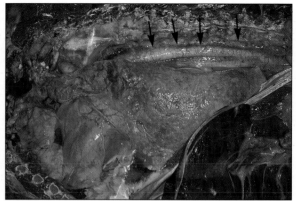

322 Thoracic (mediastinal) lymphosarcoma (thoracocentesis).
Note: Blood-stained, clear fluid aspirated from both sides of chest. A total of over thirty litres was removed. The same volume was removed 24 hours later. The fluid contained large numbers of neoplastic cells. Immediate relief of dyspnea followed pleural drainage. Horse was anemic and showed intermittent pyrexia and an elevated serum calcium concentration.

323 Thoracic (mediastinal) lymphosarcoma.
Note: Multiple large tumour masses at thoracic inlet and in mediastinum. Extensive lymph node enlargement with secondary tumour masses in dorsal thoracic chain (arrows).

324

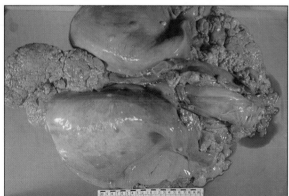

325

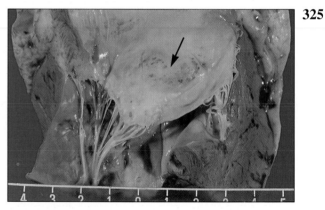

324 Thoracic (mediastinal) lymphosarcoma.
Note: Extensive mediastinal tumour masses.

325 Secondary (metastatic) lymphosarcoma.
Note: Well-defined lesion in leaflet of left atrioventricular (mitral) valve (arrow), responsible for valvular insufficiency and audible murmurs. Primary lesion in mediastinum.

326

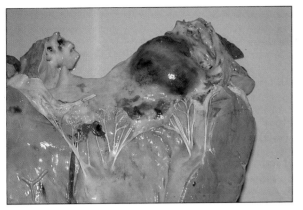

327

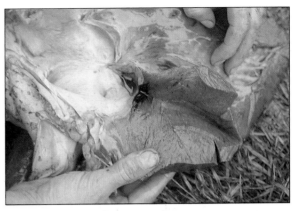

326 Secondary (metastatic) Hemangiosarcoma.
Note: Several lesions are visible, the largest of which is situated at the base of the left atrioventricular (mitral) valve and was responsible for valvular insufficiency. Major lesions detected by ultrasound examination.

327 Secondary (metastatic) Melanoma.
Note: Lesion situated in interventricular septum was probably responsible for bizarre electrical conduction deviations.

Similar lesions are found in the pharynx (*see* **592**) and nasal cavity where they may induce dysphagia and respiratory obstructions respectively. This is the only form of lymphosarcoma which may take a protracted course and metastases seem particularly slow to develop.

Horses are rarely leukemic in any form of lymphosarcoma, but both acute and chronic forms of leukemia do sometimes occur. The clinical signs of myelogenous leukemia are very similar to those of lymphosarcoma and this disorder can often be more readily diagnosed as marked hematological alterations, including the presence of circulating blast cells in massive numbers, can be found. Plasma cell (multiple) myeloma in horses between 3 months and 25 years of age, resulting in a detectable monoclonal gammopathy, again induces similar general signs but shifting-leg lameness, renal failure, hemorrhagic diatheses and chronic, intractable infections are usually present to a variable extent.

Secondary lymphosarcomatous tumours may develop in almost any organ including the liver, spleen, kidney and heart (**325**).

The diagnosis of lymphosarcoma, and related lymphoproliferative and myeloproliferative disorders, often presents the clinician with considerable difficulties in that many of the signs are non-specific and, as the disorder carries a hopeless prognosis, antemortem confirmation is very desirable. Suitable biopsy specimens from affected tissues (including tissue aspirates from lymph nodes, pleural, pericardial or abdominal fluids) is the only satisfactory and definitive way of confirming the diagnosis at present.

Primary hemangiosarcoma occurring in the walls of blood vessels within muscles and elsewhere are very inclined to metastasise to remote sites and lesions may therefore occur in any or all of the major organ systems, including the lung (*see* **276**), myocardium and heart valves (**326**) and liver (*see* **175**). Chronic and persistent blood loss and impaired circulation within body cavities results in massive accumulations of blood stained fluid (**Plate 2h**, page 47) and/or hematuria and melena. Ultimately, such blood loss commonly results in the development of disseminated intravascular coagulopathy and chronic, blood-loss anemia (**Plate 8d**, page 178).

Primary neoplastic disorders of the heart are very uncommon, but secondary lesions may develop in the myocardium, epicardium, endocardium or within the pericardial sac. The commonest lesions are those of lymphosarcoma (*see* **325**), hemangiosarcoma (*see* **326**) and melanoma (exclusively in grey horses) (**327**). Lesions occurring in and around the heart valves (*see* **325**, *see* **326**) produce valvular distortions and murmurs are audible. Ultrasonographic examination will detect the thickened and distorted valve and incompetent valve closure but will not usually identify the type of lesion present. Masses within the myocardium, such as melanoma (*see* **327**) and lymphosarcoma, may be asymptomatic but, particularly where these are located in the interventricular septum or at either the sinuatrial or interventricular node, may induce serious irregularities of electrical activity and consequent arrhythmia, including atrial fibrillation and ventricular ectopic contractions, and may be responsible for sudden and unexpected deaths.

Further reading

Current Therapy in Equine Medicine (2)
Ed. Robinson,N.E. (1987) W B Saunders, Philadelphia USA

Current Therapy in Equine Medicine (3)
Ed. Robinson,N.E. (1992) W B Saunders, Philadelphia USA

Problems in Equine Medicine
Brown,C.M. (1989) Lea & Febiger, Philadelphia USA

Veterinary Clinics of North America (Equine Practice) (Cardiology)
(1985) Volume 1 W B Saunders

Veterinary Clinics of North America (Equine Practice) (Clinical Pathology)
(1987) Volume 3 W B Saunders

Manual of Equine Practice
Rose & Hodgson (1993) W B Saunders

5. Urinary tract disorders

While the incidence of clinically significant disorders of the urinary tract of the horse is less than in many other species, pathological changes are quite frequently recognised at post mortem examination and it is possible that subclinical urinary tract disease passes largely unnoticed. Foals are markedly more prone to renal disease than adult horses, and this may be associated with the neonatal maladjustment syndrome and septicemic disorders. Normal horse urine has a markedly cloudy appearance, particularly towards the end of the flow, due to the very high calcium carbonate content, and is frequently mucoid or viscid in consistency. The general signs of urinary tract disease are associated with variations in the volume of urine produced and abnormalities of micturition including abnormal frequency of urination, or dysuria (difficulty or pain during or after micturition). Abnormalities of the lower urinary tract such as cystitis and urethritis in the horse are often not accompanied by easily recognisable alterations in frequency of urination or volume of urine or altered appearance of the urine. In common with some other organ systems, damage to the urinary tract organs may be reflected clinically in a limited number of ways. Thus the clinical appearance of different disorders may be similar and the specific identification of organic disease may prove to be an exacting task. Furthermore, the kidney itself has a very large functional reserve and damage may only become clinically obvious when over 70% of the available tissue is non-functional. The implications of this fact for diagnosis and therapy of renal disease are particularly important as the opportunity for therapeutic measures has often been lost before clinical disease is recognised. The clinical signs seen in urinary tract diseases in the horse are also dependant upon the specific structure affected and the extent of the effect upon its function.

The physical assessment of the urinary tract has largely been restricted to rectal examination, but this has severe limitations. Only the caudal extremity of the left kidney is usually palpable, the right is almost always not palpable unless grossly enlarged or displaced. The use of transrectal or percutaneous ultrasonography has considerably widened the scope for the physical examination of the kidneys and ureters. Abnormalities of the kidney, however, may be accompanied by marked non-specific signs including weight loss and inappetence. Although there may, sometimes, be distinctive clinical features, the diagnosis of many of the urinary tract diseases frequently relies upon supportive clinical pathology.

Developmental Disorders

Congenital or hereditary disorders of the kidneys and ureters are particularly unusual in the horse. Agenesis, hypoplasia and ectopic ureters have been encountered. Unilateral disorders of this type are likely to be incidental findings at post mortem examination whereas bilateral disorders are likely to result in recognisable, if non-specific, clinical signs or the early demise of the foal, possibly even intra-uterine death.

Perhaps the commonest, and most important, congenital disorder of the urinary system of the horse is the **patent/ruptured bladder syndrome**. This is particularly common in Thoroughbred male foals, but it is also recognised in most other breeds from time to time, and may also affect occasional female foals. Clinical signs of a patent bladder characteristically develop between 1–3 days after birth, the foal having been normal up to this point. Astute handlers might, however, have recognised the reduced or absent urinary output from an early age. The earliest sign is usually frequent straining attempts with a crouching or squatting posture (**328**). Affected foals show progressive abdominal distension (*see* **328**) and a palpable fluid thrill may be detected across the abdominal cavity. In some cases rupture of the bladder possibly occurs at a somewhat later age, and this is particularly so in foals with septicemic infections. It is possible that these represent an aggravation of relatively minor defects which have had little effect upon the well-being of the foal up to the time the septicemia developed. Radiographic examination invariably shows obvious fluid characteristics with a uniform ground-glass appearance of the abdomen. However, the addition of positive and negative (air) contrast can be most useful in identifying the condition definitively with a clear air-fluid interface and increased contrast density of the fluid (**329**). Cardiac dysrhythmias and convulsions are associated with the progressive hyperkalemia, hyponatremia and azotemia. Abdominal paracentesis

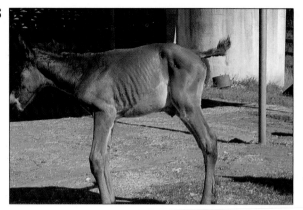

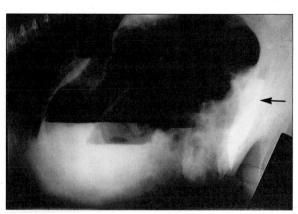

328 Patent (ruptured) bladder syndrome.
Note: Ventro-flexed back, crouching during attempts to urinate. Abdominal distension.
Differential Diagnosis:
i)   Retained (impacted) meconium
ii) Atresia coli
iii) Atresia ani

329 Patent (ruptured) bladder syndrome (double-contrast, standing, lateral radiograph).
Note: Air fluid interface in abdominal cavity. Air injected into bladder via bladder catheter escapes into abdominal cavity creating a gas cap, while contrast medium escapes from bladder (some is retained in bladder – arrow) and increases the radiodensity of the dependent urine in the abdominal cavity.

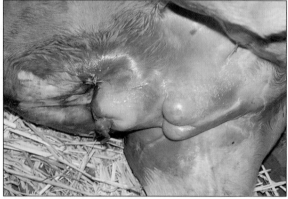

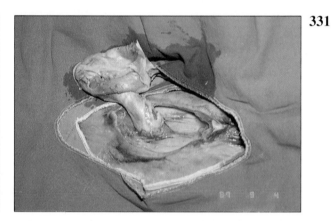

330 Patent (ruptured) bladder syndrome.
Note: Urine forced into urachus and inguinal canals by persistent straining. Urine dribbling from urachus and extensive sheath edema.

331 Patent (ruptured) bladder syndrome.
Note: Extensive necrosis of umbilical stump as a result of subcutaneous leakage of urine. (Photograph taken during surgical exploration of persistent urine dribbling).

produces a clear, yellow fluid with all the visible and biochemical characteristics of urine. Creatinine concentrations in the fluid which are much more than twice as great as those of blood are supportive of the diagnosis of uro-peritoneum. Some urination may still occur in spite of the discontinuity of the bladder wall, particularly where the defect is limited in size and, in some cases, there may be a reasonable flow of urine. However, in spite of the passage of some urine, the persistent straining often results in gross swelling of the sheath and in some advanced cases, straining will force significant amounts of urine down the inguinal canals and result in swelling of the scrotum and prepuce (*see* **330**). Necrosis of the umbilical stump and adjacent skin

is a common sequel in neglected cases (**331**) and particularly those which strain inordinately. Straining also results in urine being forced out through the urachus and swelling of the umbilicus with urine contamination of the ventral abdomen and thighs often occurs in severely affected foals (*see* **331**). Signs of colic (rolling and frequent lying-down) and progressive dullness, lethargy and inappetence, over several days are usually encountered. The speed with which this condition becomes clinically significant, and the severity of the clinical signs, depend largely upon the extent of the bladder defect, which may vary in both size and pathological appearance. In some cases the bladder defect is large (**332**) but in others it may be very small,

332

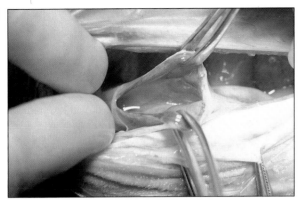

333

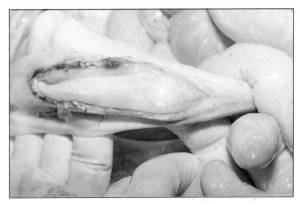

332 Patent (ruptured) bladder syndrome.
Note: Extensive Bladder defect in dorsal wall with no hemorrhage or inflammation along the margins of the defect.

333 Patent (ruptured) bladder syndrome.
Note: Extensive bladder defect in dorsal wall of bladder with marked hemorrhage along margins, indicating traumatic etiology.

334

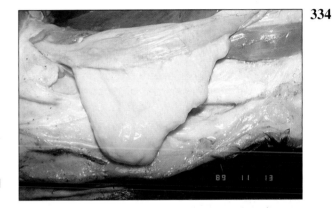

334 Umbilical vein sepsis.
Note: Diagnosis is easily confirmed by ultrasound examination.

becoming obvious only when the bladder is distended. Although its etiology is obscure it has been suggested that it is a result of parturient rupture of the bladder, particularly when the urachus has closed early resulting in an overdistended bladder at birth. However, a developmental failure of the closure of the dorsal bladder wall has also been suggested. While most defects are located in the dorsal wall, their pathological appearance may vary. In some cases the margins of the defect are smooth, rounded and show no evidence of recent traumatic rupture (*see* **332**), supporting the hypothesis of a developmental defect. In other cases a hemorrhagic margin can be seen along part or all of the defect (**333**) suggesting a traumatic tearing of the bladder wall. In view of the wide and short urethra of the female it seems unlikely that the pathogenesis involves obstruction of the urethra and traumatic/over-distension disruption in female foals.

The **subcutaneous leakage of urine** into the skin around the umbilicus may arise from the ruptured bladder syndrome or from urachal leakage as a result of a **damaged urachal stalk**. Foals which strain for whatever

reason appear more likely to develop this disorder. Urine infiltrates extensively into the subcutaneous tissue of the ventral abdomen (*see* **330**) and even extends into the flank folds in the more severe, long-standing cases. In contrast to the relatively minor inflammatory effects of urine within the peritoneal cavity, urine in these sites results in severe, local necrosis of both the skin and the urachus (*see* **330**). Extensive sloughing of the skin of the ventral abdomen is a common, serious sequel.

The persistent dribbling of urine from the umbilicus in a neonatal foal should alert the clinician to the possibility of a **patent urachus** (*see* **331**). The disorder is more common in debilitated foals or those with an underlying septicemia. Furthermore, where the urachus fails to close adequately at birth, the patent structure provides a portal for the entry of bacteria, and local abscess, particularly of the umbilical vessels (**334**) or even septicemia may result. Ascending infections from the urachus into the bladder (and thence to the ureters and kidneys) and from the umbilical vessels into the general circulation have particularly serious systemic consequences.

Non-Infectious Disorders

The urinary tract of the horse is not liable to be traumatised from external damage, with the possible exception of the patent bladder syndrome in foals described above. However, horses which are repeatedly catheterised may suffer from **bladder perforation**, particularly where there is an intercurrent cystitis (**335**). More unusually, the bladder may rupture as a result of severe and total urethral obstruction such as might occur with **urethral calculi (336)**, which is effectively restricted to the male. Bladder rupture has also been encountered as an accident of parturition. In all these cases the presence of free urine in the abdominal cavity (sometimes with blood-staining and inflammatory cells) may be detected by paracentesis and, again, the speed with which the fluid accumulates depends upon the extent of and reasons for the rupture. Progressive azotemia and hyperkalemia are common sequels to any disruption of the urinary tract within the abdomen. However, it appears that peritonitis is not a common feature, the peritoneum appearing to tolerate the presence of urine fairly well, unless there are complicating bacteria present.

Displacements of the urinary bladder are effectively limited to the female. The most common of these disorders is **bladder eversion**, where the bladder is everted through the urethra and the mucosal surface is then visible at the vulva (**337**). The vesico-ureteral openings, from which urine will be seen to issue in pulses every few minutes, may be readily visible on the dorsal surface. **Urinary bladder prolapse** usually occurs through a tear in the vaginal wall at parturition and in these cases the smooth reddish serosal surface is visible (**338**). This is distinctly different from the mucosal surface visible in bladder eversion. By contrast to the free issue of urine in the everted bladder, in these cases, the bladder is unable to empty due to the kinking of the urethra and, consequently, the organ may become grossly distended and may ultimately rupture. Both of these conditions are most often associated with, and accompanied by, tenesmus (excessive involuntary straining) such as might occur during or after normal or assisted parturition, dystocia, colic due to small colon obstructions, rectal prolapse and vaginitis, or perineal lacerations occurring during foaling. It is unusual for neurological disorders of the bladder, or cystic calculi to result in displacements of this type. Mares affected with either condition will also strain incessantly as a result of the displacements, thereby making matters considerably worse, and possibly inducing secondary rectal prolapse and gross perineal edema. Persistent tenesmus of this type is exhausting and affected mares become very tired after a relatively short period.

Loss of neurological control of bladder function may be encountered in several neurological disorders including **cauda equina neuritis** (*see* **709** *et seq.*), **equine herpes virus-1 neurological syndrome (728)**, sorghum or sudan grass poisoning and other traumatic, inflammatory or neoplastic conditions affecting the spinal cord or peripheral nerves in the sacral and caudal lumbar regions. It may also follow a difficult parturition or caudal epidural anesthesia. In most of these circumstances bladder dysfunction is not the only sign

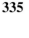

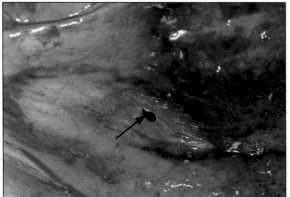

335 Bladder rupture (arrow).
Note: Repeated catheterisation for paralytic bladder syndrome resulted in traumatic rupture and uroperitoneum. Severe peritonitis followed.

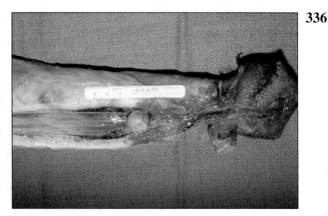

336 Impacted urethral calculus.
Note: Caused fatal rupture of bladder. Inflammatory focus and necrosis around calculus.

337

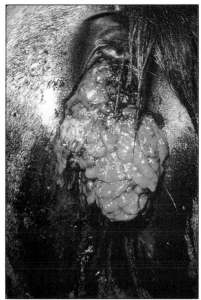

338

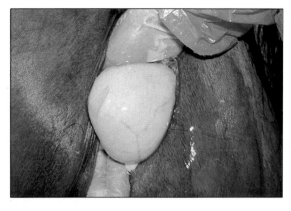

338 Bladder prolapse.
Note: Exposed serosal surface of bladder. Bladder prolapsed through vaginal tear following dystocia and assisted delivery. Bladder continued to fill, no urination possible. Mare became exhausted rapidly due to continued straining.
Differential Diagnosis:
i) Bladder eversion
ii) Impending parturition (amnion/chorioallantois)
iii) Prolapse of intestinal loop

337 Bladder eversion.
Note: Exposed mucosal surface of bladder and vesico-ureteral openings which continued to produce urine.
Differential Diagnosis:
i) Bladder prolapse
ii) Impending parturition (amnion/chorioallantois)
iii) Prolapse of intestinal loop.

which is present, and neurological and other deficits are frequently detectable. The most prominent sign of the **paralytic bladder syndrome** in the male is urinary incontinence with intermittent or continuous dribbling of small volumes of normal urine resulting in urine-scalding of the hind limbs **(339)** and extensive preputial inflammation and excoriation. In mares, exercise, coughing or vocalisation may result in spurting of urine from the urethra and persistent dribbling of urine results in perineal excoriation and crystallization of urine in the hair of the caudo-medial thigh **(340)**. Rectal examination reveals a very large, flaccidly distended bladder. Catheterisation of affected horses results in a relatively clear initial flow of urine but there is usually a very dense sediment in the dependent part of the bladder. The development of sabulous urolithiasis, made up of a homogeneous sludge of calcium carbonate and cellular and mucoid debris in the bladder, carries a poor prognosis as this is usually secondary to serious and long-standing bladder paralysis. Endoscopic examination of the bladder is usually required to identify the presence of extensive sabulous urolithiasis but supportive evidence can be gained from ultrasonographic examination per rectum.

While the prevalence of **obstructive disorders of the urinary tract** of the horse is low, they form an important group of conditions with potentially serious consequences. Most urinary tract obstructions can be attributed to one or other form of **urolithiasis** and this can occur at any site in the urinary tract. The pathogenesis of urinary calculi is uncertain, but it is likely that some underlying metabolic or inflammatory process precedes their development. The reason for the differences in the appearance of the two commonly encountered types of calculus are, similarly, not clearly understood. They are usually, however, composed largely of calcium carbonate, often with various additional inorganic components including magnesium, phosphate, ammonium and/or oxalate ions.

Urethral calculi are the preserve of the male horse, as the long narrow urethra is far more likely to become obstructed by relatively small calculi than the short widely dilatable urethra of the mare. Relatively small calculi passing down the male urethra may lodge either in the pelvic segment of the urethra, near the ischial arch, or in a more distal portion of the urethra (often in the penile urethra) (*see* **336**). Some cases result in a

339

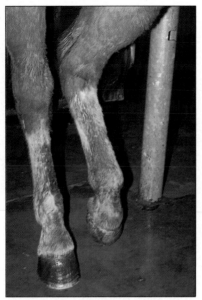

340

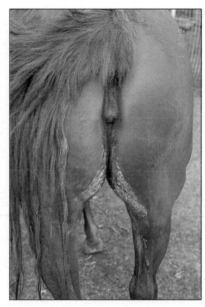

339 Paralytic bladder syndrome (gelding).
Note: Urinary scalding of hind legs due to urinary incontinence.
Differential Diagnosis:
i)   Cystic calculus
ii) Cystitis
iii) Urethral calculus
iv) Penile or preputial neoplasia
v)   Sorghum poisoning
vi) Cauda equina neuritis
vii) Spinal or sacral trauma
viii) Equine herpes virus-1 neurological syndrome
ix) Urethritis

340 Paralytic bladder syndrome (mare).
Note: Urinary scalding of perineum and extensive crystalline deposits on caudo-medial thigh due to evaporation of urine being dribbled out continuously (for 5 months).
Differential Diagnosis:
i)   Cystic calculus
ii) Cystitis
iii) Vaginal/cervical or uterine inflammation/infection or neoplasia
iv) Sorghum poisoning
v)   Cauda equina neuritis
vi) Spinal or sacral trauma
vii) Equine herpes virus-1 neurological syndrome
viii) Parturition injury

complete **urethral obstruction** and this may have extremely serious consequences. In others dysuria (difficult, painful urination) is present with blood in the urine which is passed in small amounts and which may dribble from the prepuce. Bladder rupture, severe colic and gross metabolic disturbances are encountered in males which have a **total urethral obstruction**. Persistent and strong straining efforts are made, often accompanied by small amounts of blood at the end of the penis. The penis is often protruded for prolonged periods while the horse maintains a posture of urination. Rectal examination reveals a very large, extremely tense bladder which is obviously different from the flaccid distension encountered in the paralytic bladder syndromes. Eventually bladder rupture and uro-peritoneum will inevitably arise. Attempts to pass a urethral catheter are frustrated by a complete obstruction at the site. Rectal, ultrasonographic and particularly, endoscopic, examination may identify the site and

character of the obstruction. Where the obstruction is partial some urine is passed and under these circumstances the bladder may be not become seriously distended and the clinical signs are correspondingly milder. However, tenesmus and urethral bleeding are frequently present, leading to blood staining of the hind legs (**341**). Catheterisation may under some circumstances be possible but the obstruction is usually sufficient to prevent this. The successful passage of a urethral calculus is almost always accompanied by urethral ulceration which may be obvious endoscopically. Urethral calculi lodging at the urethral process should not be confused with concretions of smegma in the urethral fossa, which can sometimes become large and very firm. Careful examination will easily define the difference between these two conditions.

Cystic calculi are the commonest clinically significant form of urolithiasis in the horse. Males are far more frequently affected clinically, than females, but

341

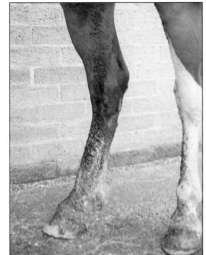

342

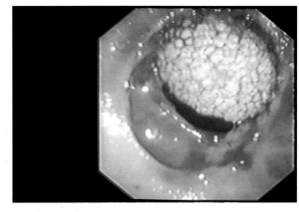

343

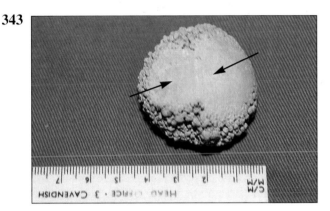

341 Cystic calculus (male).
Note: Urine and blood staining of hind legs due to persistent bleeding from urethra and frequent attempts at urination. Urine obviously hemorrhagic following exercise.
Differential Diagnosis:
i)   Urethral calculus
ii) Squamous cell carcinoma of prepuce/penis
iii) Hemorrhagic disorders of urinary tract
iv) Renal neoplasia
v)   Cystitis
vi) Accessory gland inflammation (bulbo-urethral glands)

342 Cystic calculus (endoscopic view).
Note: Spiky calculus partially enclosed in diverticulum at anterior pole of bladder. Obvious cystitis with mucosal edema and hemorrhage.

343 Cystic calculus.
Note: Facets (arrows) indicating the presence of at least two more calculi.

large and/or numerous calculi may also be present in mares. Affected horses have a history of dysuria and hematuria with prolonged posturing and grunting during urination. Flows of urine may be abruptly terminated and short squirts accompanied by pain (strangury), are frequently voided. Persistent dribbling of bloody urine results in the contamination of the hind legs of geldings (*see* **339**) and in perineal excoriation and crystalline deposition in mares (*see* **341**). Cystic calculi are almost always very readily appreciated during rectal examination and may also be visualised endoscopically, when the extent of bladder inflammation and the number and type of the calculi can be determined (*see* **340**). In some cases multiple calculi can, during rectal examination, be felt to be rubbing against each other, rather like a bag of stones. The use of ultrasonography has also proved useful in the detection of cystic calculi when a sharp hyper-echoic structure may be detected within the bladder but it may be difficult to identify anything further about the number and character of the calculi present. Most cystic calculi are rough surfaced, moderately friable, yellowish and spiky (*see* **342**; **343**) and these result in significant bladder inflammation (*see* **342**). Even in the most mildly affected horses, sensitive biochemical detection methods will, almost always, identify blood in the urine. Urine passed by horses affected with this type of stone immediately following exercise is characteristically intensely hemorrhagic and this is almost pathognomonic of cystic calculus. The smoother (often multiple) type of calculi are very hard, white or yellow in colour and cause less local bladder inflammation. Where more than one calculus is present, even in those cases affected by the rougher forms of stone, smooth surfaces (facets) may be present on the calculi (**343**). Surgeons should examine any calculi removed from the bladder carefully to establish whether there are others. Within the bladder, a calculus may, furthermore, be located in a diverticulum which is usually in the most cranial portion of the bladder (*see* **342**).

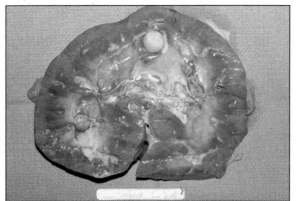

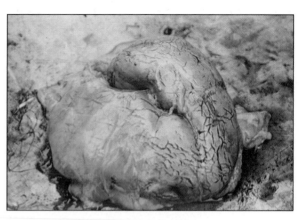

344 Renal calculi.
Note: Numerous small calculi in renal parenchyma and single larger calculus in renal pelvis associated with local renal medullary compression and distortion of cortex and renal outline.

345 Acute renal failure.
Note: Grossly enlarged right kidney with extensive capsular ruptures. Horse suffering from severe endotoxemia of 3 days duration. Anuria and progressive biochemical evidence of renal failure.

Renal calculi, which are often multiple and which may be present in both kidneys develop within the renal pelvis or the kidney substance (**344**) where they may be smooth or they may conform to the shape of the renal pelvis at that site. They are often asymptomatic being incidental findings at post mortem examination. However, a significant proportion of cases affected by unilateral or bilateral renal calculi have other, concurrent, urinary tract disease such as pyelonephritis, renal hypoplasia or neoplasia. Sometimes vague back pain, hematuria, which can be traced endoscopically to one ureter, or even failure to perform up to expectation, may be associated with the stones but, unless they are extensive and bilateral, signs of renal failure will not usually be present. The diagnosis of calculi in the renal substance, renal pelvis or ureter is generally confirmed by percutaneous or transrectal ultrasonographic examination. The detection of a calculus in one kidney may be a strong indication that the contralateral kidney is also affected.

Ureteral calculi are particularly rare and the loss of patency of one or both ureters may be detected by endoscopic examination of the vesiculo-ureteral openings when the normal pulsatile urine release, which usually occurs at about one to two pulses per minute, may be lacking. Complete ureteral obstruction results in a unilateral hydronephrosis which may be detectable during a thorough rectal examination but seldom causes any detectable signs of renal failure. Ascending infection into an inflamed and compromised ureter, however, has serious consequences with pyelonephritis and renal failure ultimately affecting both kidneys.

The causes of **renal failure** in the horse are poorly defined, although hemodynamic, toxic, infective and obstructive causes have been identified. **Acute renal failure** may be caused by a wide variety of non-infectious and infectious agents. Many poisonings, such as those caused by heavy metals and certain drugs may cause nephrosis while certain infectious diseases, including equine infectious anemia, equine herpes virus-1 and bacterial septicemia may cause nephritis and glomerulonephritis to varying degrees. While it is likely that hemodynamic disorders, including disseminated intravascular coagulopathy (*see* **291** *et seq.*), acute (particularly infectious) diarrhea, endotoxic shock and extensive hemorrhage or fluid loss resulting in hypovolemic shock, are the most common cause of acute renal failure, it is often not possible to establish the original cause of the renal insult. In most of these cases the onset of renal failure may be less dramatic than the primary instigating disorder, but is often more serious in the longer term. Clinical and biochemical evidence of renal failure is often only present when over 75% of the available renal tissue is non-functional and so the onset of clinical renal failure may be delayed for months or years after the original insult, particularly where this was mild. Acute or chronic renal failure as a result of **immune-mediated glomerulonephritis** is more often identified at post mortem examination but may, rarely, cause overt clinical signs, which are not specific for this type of renal failure. Many chemicals, particularly the inorganic salts of heavy metals such as lead, arsenic and mercury, are known to result in damage to the kidneys or to the related structures of the urinary tract. Some aminoglycoside antibiotics, including neomycin and gentamycin, and some non-

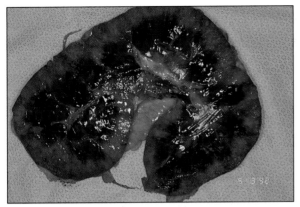

346 Acute renal failure.
Note: Amorphous appearance of kidney with extensive hemorrhage and loss of architecture due to severe endotoxaemia and hypovolemia over 3 day period. Oliguria and hematuria were present.

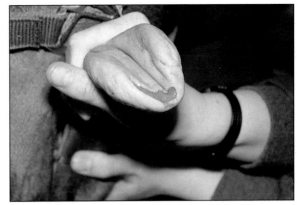

347 Acute renal failure - tongue ulceration.
Differential Diagnosis:
i)   Physical trauma
ii) Loss of oral sensation (self inflicted trauma)
iii) Plant fibres, awns
iv) Chemical burn

steroidal anti-inflammatory drugs, such as phenylbutazone, also have well recognised nephrotoxic effects. Many plants, including the oak (*Quercus ruber*) and its acorns, are liable to induce tubular degenerations within the kidney when ingested in quantity. Almost all these poisonings result in clinical signs which are associated with acute renal failure and reflect a dramatic and extensive renal damage involving more than 75% of the renal tissue. Pathologically the condition is recognised by acute tubular necrosis which results in oliguria (or anuria) and terminally a severe intravascular hemolytic crisis is encountered. In terminal cases, limited, or sometimes excessive, amounts of urine are passed containing obvious red-brown pigment which is identifiable as hemoglobin but which closely resembles myoglobin (*see* **471**). The specific clinical signs of acute renal failure are vague and limited to depression, anorexia and a marked brick red discoloration of the mucous membranes (**Plate 8c**, page 178). Dysuria, laminitis (*see* **409** *et seq.*), peripheral/dependent edema, colic, and diarrhea may be present. Rectal examination may, in about half the cases, detect the presence of an enlarged, edematous and often painful kidney, which at post mortem examination may have a ruptured renal capsule (**345**). A soft, amorphous kidney may also be identified and this finding reflects a dramatic loss of renal architecture (**346**). The latter state is most often encountered after severe hemodynamic or hypovolemic/shock syndromes, complicated by profound, acute, renal failure. Ultrasonographic examination, renal biopsy and renal function tests may be required to confirm the diagnosis. Serum creatinine and calcium

concentrations are useful biochemical indicators of renal failure, both being markedly elevated within a relatively short period. Serum urea concentration is a somewhat less reliable index of renal failure in the horse.

Chronic, progressive renal failure is recognised as a clinical entity in horses over 5 years of age and can be the result of glomerular or tubular disease (or both). Clinical signs of chronic renal failure in horses under 4–5 years of age are more likely to be the result of **renal hypoplasia** than acquired renal disease. Enlargement of the kidneys may be the result of cystic kidney disease, neoplasia or chronic pyelonephritis. In most cases the etiology of chronic renal failure cannot be established definitively as the original insult may have occurred some months or even years previously. Infectious and obstructive disorders resulting in pyelonephritis, hydronephrosis and other inflammatory renal disease ultimately progress to chronic renal failure, which represents the end stage of all these disorders. Horses affected by chronic renal failure have pronounced weight-loss and inappetence, which has no other obvious cause. Polyuria, polydipsia, laminitis and intermittent pyrexia are typically vague but important signs of the condition. Oral ulceration which initially affects the tip of the tongue (**347**), 'furring' of the tongue (*see* **164**), excessive dental tartar (*see* **32**), hypertension and the development of ventral edema (*see* **161**) consequent upon loss of protein in the urine and severe hypoproteinemia, are some of the signs which may be present. Rectal and ultrasonographic examination will usually identify dense, small kidneys which are seldom

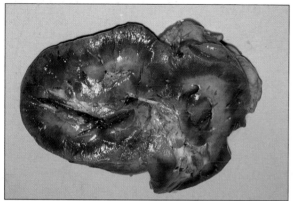

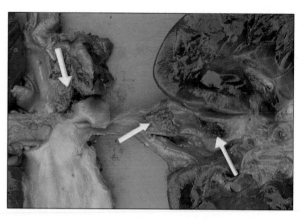

348 Chronic renal failure.
Note: Dense, contracted, irregular renal cortex. Polyuria with clear urine of low specific gravity.

349 Verminous arteritis of renal artery.
Note: Due to migration of *Strongylus vulgaris* larvae which were visible (arrows). Rupture of the renal artery at the renal hilus occurred causing abdominal bleeding and colic.

painful. The results of biochemical examination of blood from horses suffering from chronic renal failure may be somewhat disappointing with normal or slight elevations in the creatinine and calcium (and urea) concentrations. Significant elevation of plasma creatinine concentration supports a poor prognosis. The most dramatic hematological changes are likely to be related to loss of albumin from the blood (protein-losing nephropathy). Urine produced by horses with chronic renal failure is usually dilute (with a specific gravity between 1.008 and 1.014), and the urine is usually clear and watery, containing little or none of the cloudy, mucilaginous character encountered in the normal horse. At post mortem examination the kidneys are small, dense and fibrotic with a narrow cortex (**348**).

The only vascular disorder of consequence in the urinary tract of horses is **rupture of a renal artery** which is usually due to verminous arteritis, possibly as a result of migrating *strongyle* larvae (**349**). Clinically affected horses show moderate, persistent colic over a course of several days, and most often have free blood in the peritoneal cavity which can be detected by abdominocentesis. Hemorrhage may however be more restricted in some cases with retroperitoneal bleeding which may remain localised or extend into the diaphragm and sublumbar muscles. Where this is present some horses show a synchronous diaphragmatic flutter. In some cases the extent of blood loss may therefore be limited and the signs of the disorder are restricted to mild or recurrent colic and progressive anemia. Jaundice may be present where the capacity of the liver to excrete hemoglobin by-products is exceeded. In this event there will be an elevation of the total and the unconjugated bilirubin.

Infectious Disorders

Viral Diseases: The renal manifestations of **viral disorders** occurring in the horse are varied but are usually not the most obvious immediate presenting sign of the disease. The large functional reserve makes immediate renal failure unusual, but long term renal consequences of virus-induced damage may be more common than is appreciated and chronic renal failure may eventually arise from relatively minor viral diseases.

Bacterial Diseases: Bacterial septicemia, in foals affected by septicemic *Actinobacillus equuli*, *Salmonella* spp, *Escherichia coli* and *Klebsiella* spp. in particular, frequently results in multiple pyemic abscesses within the kidney parenchyma (**350**). The significance of these foci is probably limited but, in the event that the foal survives the initial episode, the possibility of chronic renal failure and secondary pyelonephritis remains.

350

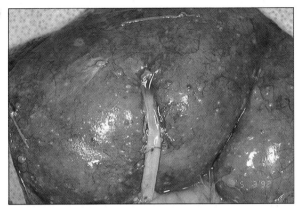

351

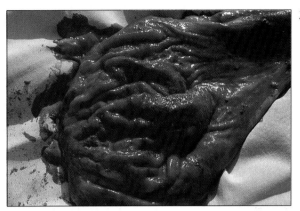

350 Renal abcess.
Note: Multiple pyaemic abscesses encountered in a 10 day old foal with Actinobacillus equili septicaemia.

351 Chronic Cystitis.
Note: Due to paralytic bladder syndrome and repeated catheterisation. Bladder wall very thin and distended.

The urinary bladder is strongly resistant to infection in normal horses as a result of both the repeated flow of urine through the organ which tends to dilute and flush out any residual bacteria, and the natural mucosal/epithelial resistance to the ingress of bacteria. Other factors tending to inhibit bacterial proliferation in the bladder include local secretory immunoglobulins and the varying pH of the urine. **Cystitis** is, therefore, uncommon as a primary disease, most cases being secondarily associated with bladder calculi in the male and to vestibular and vaginal infections in the mare. Conditions which result in urinary stasis, including urethral or cystic calculi or the paralytic bladder syndrome, are possibly the commonest causes of cystitis. The shorter female urethra possibly accounts for the relatively higher incidence of cystitis, when compared to the male horse. The clinical signs are the result of an intercurrent urethritis and frequent painful attempts at urination with prolonged straining, and small, dribbling amounts of urine passed frequently. While in some cases the urine may look normal, an abnormal appearance is usually a significant finding, with blood, protein and significant bacteria present. Those cases arising secondarily to neurogenic bladder disorders often have a flaccid, thin and hemorrhagic bladder wall **(351)** and the urine is often, then, intensely hemorrhagic. Rupture of the inflamed, distended bladder occurs more frequently than when the bladder is largely normal. During rectal examination the bladder may be painful but a small bladder may be difficult to palpate. Ultrasonographic examination may be used effectively to identify both the location and the extent of bladder wall thickening. Cystitis is frequently a chronic disorder and prolonged treatment regimes are essential. Relapses are common as bacteria remain dormant in the bladder wall.

Ascending or hematogenous bacterial infection may result in a severe obstructive inflammation of the ureters with consequent **hydronephrosis** and **pyelonephritis (352)**. Ascending infections usually develop from bladder infection and/or stasis while hematogenous infection usually extends directly down the ureters from the kidney and renal pelvis. In foals, infection may also arise from urachal infection (*see* **334**) and ascend via the bladder into the ureters and the renal pelvis. While the majority of cases arise from ascending infection, in adult horses descending infection from pyelonephritis (usually a consequence of *Corynebacterium* spp) is occasionally responsible for the development of cystitis. Pyelonephritis on its own may be unilateral or bilateral although the latter is more common. Chronic pyrexia, weight loss and malaise are the usual vague clinical signs. Alterations in urine character and appearance are commonly present but in unilateral cases the urine may be apparently normal and biochemical parameters of renal function may also be totally normal. The bladder is invariably affected and cystitis is a common complication. Percutaneous or transrectal ultrasonography is a most useful aid to the diagnosis of pyelonephritis. Examination *per rectum* reveals a grossly thickened and tortuous ureter on the affected side(s). At post mortem examination the extent of the infective process may be appreciated **(353)**. It is usual for the renal pelvis to be markedly affected (*see* **352**).

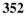

352

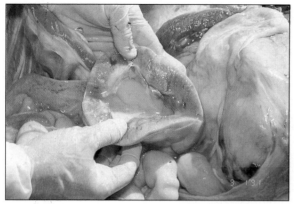

353

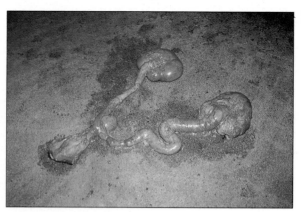

352 Pyelonephritis / Hydronephrosis.
Note: Two-week-old foal, arose as a result of chronic ureteral obstruction due to bacterial necrosis.

353 Pyelonephritis (bilateral).
Note: Uniform enlargement of ureters which were palpable *per rectum*.

Neoplastic Disorders

Primary neoplastic disorders in the urinary tract are extremely rare. Secondary neoplastic lesions arising from metastatic spread are encountered, with lymphosarcoma and hemangiosarcoma **(354)** being the most frequent.

354

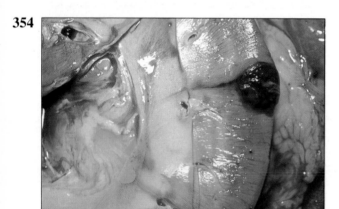

354 Hemangiosarcoma (secondary metastasis) in kidney.
Note: Primary lesion in renal artery, many other secondary tumours in other organs.

Further reading

Current Therapy in Equine Medicine (2)
Ed Robinson, N.E. (1987), W B Saunders, Philadelphia, USA
Current Therapy in Equine Medicine (3)
Ed Robinson, N.E. (1992), W B Saunders, Philadelphia, USA

A Review of 38 equine cases and discussion of diagnostic parameters. Proc. 31st Annual Convention of the American Association of Equine Practioners page 635. Adams, R. and McClure J.J. (1985)
Manual of Equine Practice Rose and Hodgson (1993) W B Saunders

6. Disorders of metabolism, nutrition and endocrine diseases

Developmental Disorders

Immaturity of the adrenal glands and concurrent abnormalities of the placental nutrition have been identified as a possible cause of prolonged gestation or dysmaturity (foal born at full term but with all the attributes of prematurity) (*see* **676** *et seq.*).

Non-Infectious Disorders

Starvation is a common disorder of neglected horses in all parts of the world. The metabolic consequences of significant nutritional deprivation are extensive and varied. A single animal affected in a group may suffer from effective deprivation in the presence of food for social reasons, there being no physical or medical reason for the failure to ingest the food. This is relatively common in confined herds of horses which receive all their food as preserved fodder, fed particularly at irregular intervals. One animal in a group (or on its own) having access to normal quantities of food may be metabolically deprived through inability to eat, chew, swallow or make effective use of ingested food material. Horses which are in poor condition may therefore not necessarily be starved. However, it is likely that where several horses in a herd are found in similarly poor bodily condition, the availability of nutritious food or any food may be limited. Individual horses in a group may however, suffer from starvation when they are subjected to dominance behaviour from more aggressive or dominant animals in the group. Horses suffering from starvation are able to tolerate considerable and prolonged deprivation without marked effects, and it is often only the extremes of nutritional deprivation which exert significant metabolic effect in terms of specific deficiencies of minerals, vitamins or other nutrients.

Deficiencies of specific components of the nutritional requirement of horses include protein, carbohydrate, vitamins and minerals. Persistent low protein diets result in low plasma albumin concentrations and, although this is theoretically possible as a result of pure dietary inadequacy, most horses showing the secondary effects of low circulating protein such as peripheral and dependent edema (*see* **161**), are suffering from other underlying organic disease such as liver failure (*see* **159** *et seq.*) or absorptive (*see* **134**) or other digestive disorders. Diffuse inflammatory changes such as lymphosarcoma (*see* **155**) in the small intestine lead to malabsorption of one or more of the nutritional components. The function of the equine large colon is such that food material needs to be retained therein to allow effective bacterial digestion of otherwise undigestible plant material and disorders which affect the motility or the absorptive function of the large and small colon inevitably have a dramatic effect upon the nutritional status of the horse.

Recognised deficiency disorders in the horse involving the supply or availability of mineral components of the diet include **calcium, phosphate, selenium, iodine** and some vitamins. These are most obvious in young growing animals, where the demand for minerals is high and some of the deficiency conditions may be present at birth. The metabolic effects of calcium and/or phosphate and/or vitamin D deficiency are interrelated and also involve the function of the thyroid, parathyroid and kidney. The control of calcium and phosphate concentrations in the circulation and in bones and other structures is therefore complex.

Hypocalcemia is most often seen in those animals having an abrupt, exceptionally high demand for calcium, such as the pregnant or lactating mare, but may also be significant in the exhausted horse. In the former, lactation tetany is occasionally encountered. Affected mares are depressed, sweating, ataxic or weak, and often develop marked muscle fasciculations. Pharyngeal paralysis resulting in dysphagia (**Plate 6r**, page 122) and/or marked inspiratory dyspnea is a frequent complication. In common with the hypocalcemia of exhaustion, mares may develop a synchronous diaphragmatic flutter, in which one or both sides of the diaphragm

355

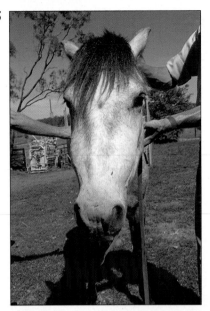

355 Osteodystrophia fibrosa (Big head, Bran disease, Millers disease).
Note: Bilateral thickening of the flat bones of the skull.
Differential Diagnosis:
i) Maxillary sinusitis
ii) Maxillary cysts
iii) Edema of the head (circulation deficits)

356

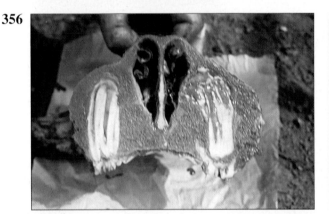

357

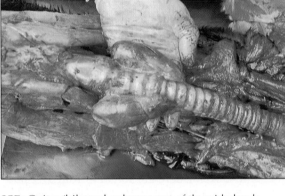

356 Osteodystrophia fibrosa (Big head, Bran disease, Millers disease).
Note: Dramatic hypertrophy of maxillary bones and distortion of dental arcade.

357 Goitre (bilateral enlargement of thyroid glands which is not due to neoplasm).
Differential Diagnosis:
i) Benign hyperplasia
ii) Neoplasia (C-cell tumour, adenoma)
Note: both of these are usually unilateral.

may be seen to contract suddenly and in synchrony with the heart beat, giving an appearance of hiccups. Flaring nostrils, tachycardia and, often, a very high body temperature are further signs that the disorder is more serious than merely spasms of the diaphragm. Poisoning with the Blister (Cantharides or Spanish-Fly) Beetle and chronic pancreatic degenerative disease also show marked hypocalcemia which may be manifest initially by synchronous diaphragmatic flutter.

The high reserve of calcium and phosphate in the bones of mature horses means that **calcium deficiency** may be present for weeks or years before bone defects are induced. **Phosphorus deficiency** affects the skeleton

in a very similar fashion but the growth of young foals suffering from specific phosphate deficiency is more markedly affected. A depraved or capricious appetite, with the affected animal eating tree bark or wooden posts, is also associated with fibre and phosphate deficits. The consequent ingestion of foreign objects may have secondary effects upon gut function or may lead to other, more serious, disorders such as botulism (*see* **735**) or choke (*see* **64** *et seq.*).

Nutritional secondary hypoparathyroidism (ostedystrophia fibrosa) is one of the oldest known diseases of the horse, and is colloquially known as 'Bran Disease', 'Big-Head', or 'Millers Disease' (**355**). This skeletal disorder results from sustained ingestion of large amounts of wheat bran (or other foods containing very high phosphate concentrations relative to calcium). Ingestion of substances which bind out the available calcium, such as phytic acid in wheat-bran, or oxalate in tropical pasture grasses in Australia and North America, renders the calcium less available and results in a further relative oversupply of phosphate. The most obvious manifestation of the disease is the development of a marked thickening of the flat bones of the head (**355**) due to the more or less symetrical laying down of cartilage in place of bone (**356**). Although young growing horses are most severely affected older horses are also subject to the condition. Shifting-leg lameness due to tendon and ligament avulsions, micro-fractures or even more serious pathological fractures, are commonly the first sign of the disease. The extent of cartilage deposition and the consequent weakness of the alveolar attachments of the molar teeth is a serious effect of the disease (*see* **356**). Ultimately, cachexia develops, which is primarily a consequence of pain and physical obstructions to mastication.

Iron deficiency results in the development of anemia and, although primary deficiency is rare, chronic infections or internal neoplasia often result in the secondary development of a dramatic, progressive and typical (microcytic, hypochromic) iron-deficiency anemia. In these horses the total body iron is invariably normal but the availability is severely impaired by the complex of inflammatory processes. Horses which suffer from a prolonged microcytic, hypochromic anemia without evidence of bone marrow activity should be investigated thoroughly for a possible underlying infectious or neoplastic disorder.

Adult horses are largely unaffected by **copper deficiency** and seem more tolerant of molybdenum excess than are ruminants. Some evidence for mild copper-deficiency related anemia in adult horses has been described and some cases of poor performance in racing horses have responded to the oral or parenteral administration of copper compounds. In foals, ill-thrift, stiffness, enlarged joints and flexural and angular limb deformities have been identified.

Iodine concentrations in soil and plants in specific areas of the United States of America and in other parts of the world are known to be low. **Dietary deficiency of iodine** results in the development of goitre (chronic symetrical bilateral enlargement of the thyroid glands which is not due to a neoplasm). Some plants, including most *Brassica* spp., are also goitrogenic through a tendency to reduce the availability of dietary iodine. The foals of iodine deficient mares are sometimes born dead, often with an obvious goitre (**357**). Thyroid hormones exert significant effects on many tissues and therefore, deficiencies may be responsible for a variety of clinical effects. **Hypothyroidism** has largely been overlooked as a possibly important clinical syndrome. However, it has been linked to developmental abnormalities of foals including prematurity and defects of ossification of the skeleton. Hypothyroidism developing in foals early in gestation is possibly also associated with failure to establish normal respiratory function at birth, whereas if the disorder develops in later gestation, lethargy, loss of suckle, muscular weakness, long coat hair, and goitre are present. Contracted tendons at birth (*see* **373**), collapse of tarsal bones with consequent sickle-hock posture (*see* **377**) are also possibly related to the condition. In young horses hypothyroidism is characterised by the development of hair growth abnormalities which develop after the foal-coat is shed. In adult horses, hypothyroidism may not be accompanied by an obvious goitre or any detectable skin or hair defects, but vague and recurrent myopathies and poor performance may represent one of the clinical effects of the condition. Very obvious lethargy and weight-gain in formerly thin (normal), energetic horses, with (or without) obvious bilateral goitre and with both low circulating thyroid hormones and a poor response to thyroid stimulation tests, and which subsequently respond to the administration of thyroid hormones, may be assumed to be cases of hypothyroidism. Generalised, irregular, progressive alopecia, particularly over the head, forelimbs and hindquarters may be present in some adult horses affected by hypothyroidism. The use of skin biopsies may be helpful but is not a definitive diagnostic procedure.

While most cases of **goitre** in young foals are a result of iodine deficiency, some may be associated with **excessive iodine** supplementation to pregnant mares. In these, long hair, muscle weakness, flexural deformities and gross limb abnormalities (*see* **373**) may be encountered. Affected foals may be born at full term, but show characteristic signs of prematurity i.e. are dysmature. The similarities between foals born to iodine deficient mares and those born to mares receiving excessive amounts are remarkable but are physiologically logical. Excessive dietary iodine depresses the stimulation of the gland and the conversion of inactive thyroid hormones to the active ones.

Increased thyroid size is often encountered in older horses, in particular, but these are seldom functional enlargements. Usually the enlargements are unilateral and they may reach considerable size (**358**). While most such enlargements are the result of **hyperplasia**, some

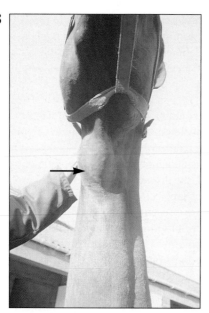

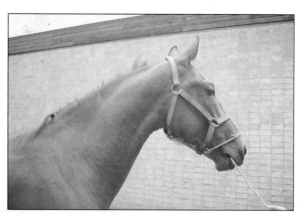

358 Thyroid hyperplasia (benign).
Note: Unilateral enlargement of thyroid (arrow). No detectable clinical effect. Normal thyroid function tests.
Differential Diagnosis:
i)   Thyroid adenoma
ii) Cystic hyperplasia
iii) C-Cell tumor

359 Selenium poisoning (chronic).
Note: Loss of mane hair and thinning and alopecia of facial hair.

360 Selenium poisoning (chronic).
Note: Loss of tail hair. Minimal effect on body hair.

are **adenomas** of the thyroid glandular tissue. Usually, very large, unilateral thyroid swellings are hyperplastic tissue and do not under most circumstances result from any goitrogenous tendency. Most adenomas are small and many are detected incidentally at post mortem examination. Dramatic enlargements of the thyroid gland are more likely to be caused by **C-cell tumours** which may reach alarming size, but which are often very small, and have a characteristic discrete, yellow appearance. C-cell tumours and small adenomas are frequently identified incidentally at post mortem examination of older horses. The metabolic effect of any of the thyroid enlargements is usually minimal in spite of obvious increases in size of one of the thyroid glands. It is therefore usual to identify the changes incidentally. The cosmetic aspect of thyroid enlargements in older horses is usually of greatest concern. Functional tumours, particularly of the C-cell type, are however,

potentially of pathological and physiological significance affecting the relevant metabolic processes, including calcium metabolism. **Hyperthyroidism** is an extremely rare disorder in the horse.

Selenium deficiency, with or without reduced availability of vitamin E, is known to result in the development of a well defined clinical syndrome in horses. While the extremes of deficiency possibly cause **White Muscle Disease**, subclinical deficiencies may be responsible for a wide variety of vague, but sometimes serious muscle dysfunctions, some of which are possibly responsible for poor or inadequate performance in racing. A group of myopathies involved in the exertional rhabdomyolysis – azoturia (paralytic myoglobinuria) complex (*see* **470**; *see* **471**) have been equivocally ascribed to selenium deficiency. Foals with serious selenium deficits may develop dilated cardiomyopathy (*see* **284**; *see* **285**). Young animals affected by selenium

361

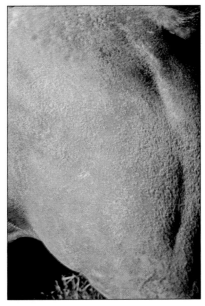

361 Anhidrosis.
Note: Typical lacklustre, moth eaten appearance of hair coat. Horse imported to tropics showed poor performance and inability to sweat after single profuse episode of sweating.

deficiency may show signs of colic and tachycardia and have all the signs of an acute, intestinal, non-strangulating lesion and this may be attributable to dysfunction of both intestinal (smooth) muscle and to concurrent cardiac muscle dysfunction. The response of some of these animals to selenium supplementation is often disappointing and a diagnosis based upon the clinical signs and supportive laboratory tests, carries a very guarded prognosis.

Selenium poisoning is a serious and increasingly common occurrence and although most instances are the result of ingestion of plants which concentrate selenium (*see* **500**), others are the result of over-enthusiastic dietary supplementation. Loss of mane (**359**) and tail (**360**) hairs, laminitis with sloughing of the hoof (*see* **498**; *see* **499**) and nervous signs including blindness, staggering gait and collapse may be encountered. Confirmation of the disorder is often very difficult to establish without selenium assay of major organs (and in particular the liver).

Biotin and/or methionine deficiencies have become a recognised entity associated with defective horn genesis. The relationship between these two essential vitamins is unclear, but some horses having poor hoof-wall quality (*see* **415**) show dramatic improvements when these substances are supplied as long-term dietary supplements.

Anhidrosis is a condition of inability to sweat in response to heat or catecholamine release. It characteristically affects horses which are moved to hot climates from milder, temperate regions but it may develop spontaneously in native horses in hot humid climates such as the Gulf States of the United States of America and the coastal areas of northern Australia and the Middle and Far East. Up to 20% of horses, whether native or not, may be affected in some areas. The onset of the condition is not always associated with poor acclimatization or the type of work, being precipitated, in some cases, merely by the onset of hot humid weather. Prior exposure to such conditions may have occurred and there are few clear circumstances in which it may not occur in hot climates. A single episode of profuse sweating before the onset of anhidrosis is often reported in acclimatising horses, and this is then accompanied by a dramatic reduction in water intake and loss of body condition. While in most cases the onset is abrupt and complete there are cases in which it develops gradually and affects some areas of the body more or less than others. Nostril flaring, a high respiratory rate and a very high body temperature, in the absence of any sweating, is usually all that is seen. The skin of chronically affected horses is dry with a 'moth-eaten' appearance (**361**), excessive scaling and some pruritus. Polydipsia, polyuria, and loss of condition are sometimes found. Biochemical analysis of electrolyte and other parameters are often disappointing and seldom assist the diagnosis.

362

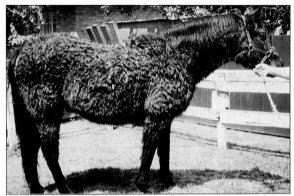

363

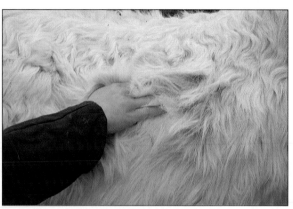

362 Pituitary adenoma (Cushing's disease).
Note: Excessive, curly coat in mid summer. Sweating and weight loss accompanied by polydipsia and polyuria. Hyperglycaemia and glycosuria were present.
Differential Diagnosis:
i) Hyperlipidemia (no coat-related signs)
ii) Diabetes mellitus (very rare)
iii) Acute/chronic renal failure (rare)

363 Pituitary adenoma (Cushing's disease).
Note: Abnormal length and density of coat. Sweating obvious when examined.

364

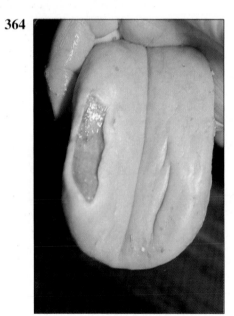

365

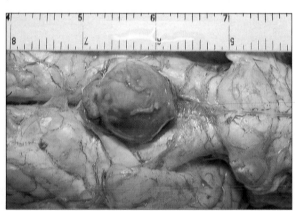

364 Pituitary adenoma (Cushing's disease).
Note: Buccal ulceration, with very limited inflammatory response.
Differential Diagnosis:
i)   Dental abnormalities
ii) Neurological (sensory) disorders of cranial nerve V
iii) Fracture of mandible/hyoid bone
iv) Dysphagia (central or peripheral origin)
v)   Renal failure

365 Pituitary adenoma (Cushing's disease).
Note: Large, easily identified mass in *pars intermedia* of pituitary gland. Tumours may also be very small with profound effects or larger and non-functional.

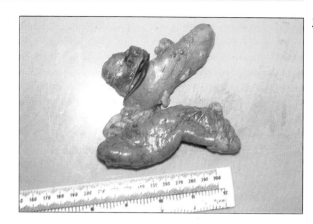

366 Pituitary adenoma (Cushing's disease).
Note: Secondary adrenal hyperplasia.

Neoplastic Diseases

Whilst primary (pancreatic) diabetes mellitus is extremely rare in the horse, a secondary diabetic status is characteristic of pituitary and adrenal neoplasia with **tumours of the *pars intermedia* of the pituitary gland** being relatively common in horses over 15 years of age. Rare cases may occur in younger horses but the greatest incidence is in horses over 20–25 years of age. Mares are more often affected, but this may reflect the greater population of mares in the older age groups and some studies have shown males to be at least as often affected. Typically, the first evidence of pituitary - adrenal axis disease is polyuria and polydipsia, although these might easily pass unnoticed in many cases, particularly in older horses which are not exercised regularly or examined closely. Elevated blood glucose and glycosuria are common findings and a diagnosis of diabetes mellitus may therefore be suggested. Hirsutism (abnormally dense, hairy coat) **(362)** commonly develops in the early stages. The hair coat is abnormally long, curly, brittle, and its density is exceptionally high **(363)**. Normal seasonal shedding of the coat does not occur and the horse remains hirsute in the summer months. Sweating and weight loss may be detectable on close examination, but may be missed under the heavy, shaggy coat. Abnormally high plasma cortisol concentration is found in about 50% of affected horses, and this has important secondary consequences, including hyperglycemia, a marked tendency to superimposed viral and bacterial infections and worm and ectoparasite infestations. Respiratory infections, infections of tendon sheaths and joints, buccal ulcers **(364)** and cutaneous abscesses are common. Even relatively minor wounds either heal very slowly or fail to heal at all. Dramatic weight loss, muscular weakness and lethargy are present. The reproductive cycles of mares are interrupted or abnormal in duration, and some affected mares even produce milk

without pregnancy. Many develop recurrent episodes of laminitis **(409 *et seq.*)** and/or colic in the later stages of the disease. Some show significant hyperlipidemia (*see* **165**) with a marked insulin resistance, while others may develop hypertrophic osteopathy (*see* **416**; *see* **417**). Bulging supraorbital fat pads may also be suggestive of the disorder but in common with many of the signs described may, equally, not be connected. Confirmation of the diagnosis is largely based upon the clinical features which are typical and upon the characteristic biochemical changes. Failure of dexamethasone suppression and abnormal response to adreno-corticotrophic hormone are typical but may not be shown in all cases. The presence of glycosuria and the response of the plasma cortisol to thyroid stimulating hormone are strongly supportive of the diagnosis. Computed tomography may be used to positively identify the mass but realistically, a definitive diagnosis may only be possible in many cases post mortem.

At post mortem examination, horses with **pituitary adenomas** are usually in poor condition and extensive parasitism may be present (including infestation with ascarids, which are particularly rare in normal, adult horses). A variably-sized, discrete tumour of the *pars intermedia* of the pituitary is often very obvious **(365)**. However it may be very small, even in some severely affected horses. Larger masses usually expand dorsally and exert pressure on the posterior lobe of the pituitary and the hypothalamus. This may explain the loss of thermoregulation and, in some cases, defects of vision and deranged carbohydrate metabolism. The adrenal gland is markedly hypertrophied **(366)**.

Tumours of the adrenal medulla (pheochromocytoma) are rare. Most cases occur in horses over 10–15 years of age. Weight loss, sweating, muscle tremors, laminitis and a high resting respiratory rate with flaring of the nostrils are encountered, as would be expected when abnormally high concentrations of endogenous catecholamines are present. One of the most significant clinical features of this condition is paroxysmal hypertension. A dramatic and unexplained increase in heart rate and force produces a hard bounding pulse and the heart beat may even be audible from a distance. Obvious mydriasis (pupillary dilatation) is usually present during these episodes and the animal may sweat profusely. The lesions responsible for this clinical syndrome are often surprisingly small, usually being well-encapsulated and nodular in appearance and located at one or other pole of one adrenal gland. Similar masses may be found incidentally at post mortem examination apparently having no functional effect. The contralateral gland is usually normal in appearance.

The clinical effects of **ovarian disorders** are possibly the most obvious of the endocrine abnormalities. **Granulosa cell tumours** in the mare are a relatively common disorder with characteristic hormonal changes and consequences upon cyclicity and upon the development of abnormal secondary sex characteristics (*see* **765 et seq.**).

In the stallion testicular tumours (*see* **845**) are unusual but where present often have effects upon the fertility of the horse but seldom influence behaviour.

Further reading

Current Therapy in Equine Medicine (2)
Ed Robinson, N.E. (1987), W B Saunders, Philadelphia, USA
Current Therapy in Equine Medicine (3)
Ed Robinson, N.E. (1992), W B Saunders, Philadelphia, USA
Problems in Equine Medicine
Brown, C.M. (1989) pub. Lea & Febiger, Philadelphia, USA

Manual of Equine Practice
Rose, R.J., and Hodgson, D.R. (1993)
WB Saunders, Philadelphia
Equine Medicine and Surgery 4th ed. Eds Beech, J. and Garcia, M.C. (1991) Diseases of the Endocrine System, page 1737. Colahan, P.T., Mayhew, I.G., Merritt, A.M., and Moore, J.N. American Veterinary Publications, Goleta, California

7. Musculo-skeletal disorders

Developmental Disorders

A wide variety of skeletal deformities occurs in horses, although individually most are rare. The importance of such abnormalities rests both in their heritability, and their immediate and long-term effects upon posture and locomotion. Even if severe the consequences of these deformities may not be life-threatening, but they may lead to significant disorders of gait as the animal grows or comes into work.

Deviations and distortions of both the skull (*see* **3**) and the axial skeleton are encountered. The latter include various degrees of **lordosis (367)** and **kyphosis**, where the vertebral column deviates abnormally in a ventral or dorsal direction respectively. While such defects are visually dramatic, there is commonly little or no material effect upon the growth or natural behaviour of the horse but they will become important when parturition or ridden work is required. The subsequent use to which the horse is to be put affects the prognosis of these cases, with most being unsuitable for riding or driving work. Other defects which are included in the clinical category of spinal deformities are vertebral column **torticollis (wry neck)**, **scoliosis (368)**, and some less dramatic deformities of the axial skeleton such as deformities of the coccygeal vertebrae. Most deviations of the axial skeleton are sporadic occurrences and there is little evidence of heritability. The defects are usually obvious at birth and may show remarkable improvement over the early weeks of life. Such defects are thought to be the result of fetal malpositioning when, during the later rapid phases of growth, fetal movement is naturally suppressed. However, many other factors may be involved and the more severe deviations may be the result of growth deformities, arising from a number of factors such as maternal viral or bacterial infections, or toxemia during gestation.

Occipito-atlanto-axial malformation is a well recognised but rare, inherited abnormality primarily affecting Arabian foals. Many affected foals are stillborn, but some appear normal at birth and develop progressive and severe neurological deficits, ranging from ataxia to tetraplegia, in the first days or weeks of life. An occasional affected foal will show obvious neck deviations, without any apparent neurological deficits. However, most of these cases carry the neck extended and in some cases, an audible click may accompany spontaneous movement or manipulation of the atlanto-axial region. The clinical condition is associated with a deformity of the odontoid process of the axis. Radiography will reveal various anomalies of structure and position but usually the atlas and occiput are fused and the *dens* is characteristically hypoplastic **(369)**. The true extent of the deformity can be identified at post

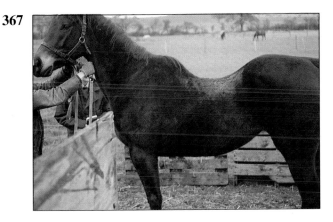

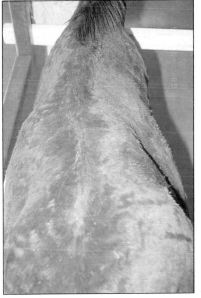

367 Lordosis (developmental ventral deviation of the vertebral column).

368 Scoliosis (developmental lateral deviation of the vertebral column).

369

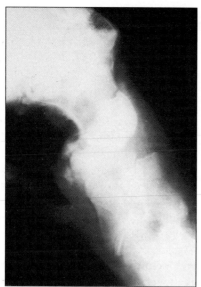

370

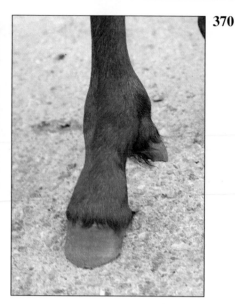

369 Occipito-atlanto-axial malformation.
Note: Abnormal shape of occiput, atlas and axis and hypoplastic dens.

370 Polydactyly.

mortem examination when the fusion of the atlas and occiput is obvious, the wings of the atlas are severely hypoplastic and the axis takes on the shape of the atlas.

Polydactyly is a relatively common developmental abnormality with little clinical significance, although cosmetically it is generally regarded as unacceptable. The extent of the defect may be variable from the presence of a small hoof like structure on the fetlock to a full extra digit articulating with the metacarpus (**370**). The full extent of the abnormality may be assessed from radiographs. It is rare for more than one extra digit to occur on one leg, and bilateral polydactyly does occur.

Cervical vertebral malformation(-malarticulation/ -instability) syndrome is a common and important developmental disorder of young horses between 4 months and 4 years of age. Although fast-growing, well-fed, Thoroughbred, colt foals are most often affected, the condition may be encountered in any horse of any breed, at almost any age. The disorder is typically seen in animals which have grown well, and which are subjected to neck trauma or unusual exercise regimes. Thus, it is frequently recognised when yearling or two year old colts, which are in excellent (often overweight) bodily condition, and growing particularly fast, are first given exercise under the saddle. The clinical signs of the disorder are attributable to dynamic or static compression of the spinal cord. While some cases have a true stenosis of the spinal canal, others develop a static stenosis as the result of new bone production around the intervertebral joints, and a further group develop a dynamic stenosis as a result of vertebral instability, allowing the vertebral body to compress the cord as the neck is flexed. In this last group the underlying pathology has often been present from the first few months of life, but the clinical signs are not apparent until the deviation of the vertebrae, and consequent compression of the cord, results in detectable neurological deficits. Any of the intervertebral joints in the cervical region may be involved, but lesions are most commonly located between the second and third, third and fourth (**371**), and fifth and sixth cervical vertebrae. Multiple lesions, involving more than one site in a particular case are also possible. The clinical manifestations are frequently subtle in the earliest and mildest types, and cases may require a very thorough neurological examination before a diagnosis can be supported or refuted. Progressive ataxia / incoordination of the hind limbs or, less commonly, all four limbs, is usually the first evidence of the disorder which is aptly called the '**Wobbler Syndrome**'. Acute onset tetraplegia is also possible when affected horses are subjected to trauma, sufficient to result in gross disruption of the unstable articulations between the third and fourth, or between the fourth and fifth cervical vertebrae. However, a progressive course of increasing apparent clumsiness, with a base-wide stance, having an insidious onset, is the more usual clinical syndrome. Horses in which gross bony deviations are present often show marked neck deviations which are more typical of cervical vertebral fractures or dislocations. More usually, the clinical signs are limited to neurological deficits relating to posture and locomotion. Postural deficits may be evident, with the animal showing little or no ability to correct abnormal positions of the limbs. Characteristic hind quarter swaying and hind-limb circumduction are usually detectable at an early stage. These are exacerbated by turning or backing, and may be made particularly obvious by flexing or extending the neck during movement. In some cases, an indication of the presence of a neurological deficit can be confirmed by an excessive wearing of the toe, resulting from dragging of the feet (the combined effect of a flexor weakness and a proprioceptive deficit). The affected horse may easily be dragged off-course with minimal effort applied to the tail or mane during forward movement. Although many cases show both fore- and hind-limb deficits, usually, the more dramatic signs are in the hind-limbs. In some long-standing cases, the signs may be, apparently, limited to the hind limbs. Where the fore-limbs are affected significantly, ataxia and spasticity, which can be exaggerated by uphill or downhill slopes, and a marked 'tin-soldier' gait (dysmetria) may be seen. In these cases, the weakness of the postural reflexes in the distal parts of the limbs are compensated by exaggerated movements of the more proximal joints. It is not usual for neck pain to be present. Although an area of hypoalgesia may be detected in the dermatome supplied through the affected vertebral outflow, the skin-twitch reflex is generally regarded as being poor in the cervical region in the normal horse, and interpretation of hypoalgesia is therefore difficult. Radiographic studies are often disappointing unless myelography is performed. However, in severe cases, even standing lateral projections may show evidence of vertebral canal stenosis due to wedging of the two adjacent vertebrae. Abnormalities of the intervertebral articular processes, subluxation of an individual or a number of vertebrae, pathological enlargement of vertebral growth plates, or gross distortions and luxations in cases complicated by trauma, may also be radiologically detectable without contrast studies. The use of myelography may facilitate the diagnosis of significant lesions (*see* **371, 372**), but recovery from general anesthesia in some horses suffering from cervical vertebral instability may be complicated by severe, life-threatening vertebral displacement and cord compression. Static stenosis of the cervical vertebral canal usually affects somewhat older horses and is most often located between pairs of lower cervical vertebrae. The compression of the cord in these cases is unaffected by flexion or extension of the neck with neither exacerbation nor relief of the symptoms being induced. In these cases the proliferation of the bone of the dorsal articular facets, the synovial tissues of their joint capsules and the ligaments at the vertebral junction, may contribute to the compression. Like cases of dynamic stenosis, the underlying cause is probably a developmental instability of the vertebrae relative to each other. Cases in which the static compression is due to physeal inflammation of the articular processes of the cervical vertebrae often have concurrent, obvious physitis (*see* **392, 393**) of the long limb bones (particularly of the distal radius). At post mortem examination the extent of the damage to the cord may be minimal but narrowing of the cord at the site of the lesion and some evidence of local bruising are usually detectable.

371

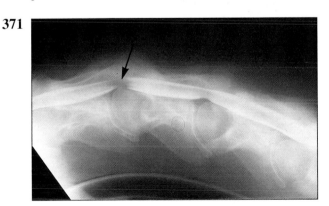

372

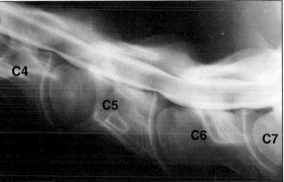

371 Cervical vertebral malformation(-malarticulation/-instability) syndrome (Wobbler syndrome) (myelogram). **Note:** Compression (narrowing) of spinal canal between third and fourth cervical vertebrae (arrow). Compare with normal compression of ventral column of vertebral canal between fourth and fifth cervical vertebrae.

372 Cervical vertebral malformation(-malarticulation/-instability) syndrome (Wobbler syndrome) (myelogram). **Note:** Compression (narrowing) of spinal canal between fifth and sixth cervical vertebrae. This is a somewhat unusual site. Compare with normal compression of ventral column of vertebral canal between fourth and fifth cervical vertebrae.

Congenital deformities of the limbs and joints (arthrogryposis) are relatively common. These developmental defects are usually obvious from birth and may cause significant dystocia. The extent of deformity ranges from mild deviations of limb position, resulting from relatively minor deformities in the long bones, to gross distortion of the bones, joints, ligaments and tendons of the limbs, with consequent severely restrictive, **postural deformities (373)**. It is more usual for the front legs to be involved, although hind leg deviations are sometimes encountered, either on their own, or in conjunction with fore-limb distortions. It is unlikely that the disorders are the result of genetic factors, although they are more often encountered in Thoroughbred horses and in the small European draught breeds. They are generally regarded as accidents of gestation, possibly associated with developmental infections, toxins and nutritional deficiencies or excesses. In spite of their relatively high incidence, a definitive etiology and pathogenesis has not been established. In most cases no apparent cause can be identified, and fetal malpositioning is then commonly blamed for the misshapen axial or appendicular skeleton.

Complex deformities involving one or more of the joints are common, while all the unaffected joints are apparently normal. Although most such cases are mild and affect single joints, more severe, clinically significant, deformities are encountered (*see* 373). Radiographic changes are often marked but the interpretation of the radiographic appearance may be particularly difficult as a result of both the technical difficulty of obtaining suitable projections and the immaturity of the centres of ossification. These abnormalities are often complicated by the co-existence of flexural and soft tissue deformities and the complex of distortions and deviations is referred to as the '**contracted foal syndrome**', a name which embraces all the possibilities. In some cases, joints are completely fused, having no mobility at all **(374)**, while others have a limited range of movement or grossly abnormal movements. Most such cases carry a poor prognosis, although some affected foals grow well and are apparently normal in most other respects. Complex developmental deformities involving skeletal, cardiac and other defects are frequently found concurrently. The presenting deformities are generally regarded as cosmetically unacceptable and, furthermore, increasing bodyweight frequently results in collapse and increasingly exhausting muscular effort during movement.

Newborn foals of all breeds are frequently born with either contraction of the soft tissues resulting in flexural contraction and distortion of the affected joint(s) or, more commonly, laxity of one or more of the major limb tendons. **Flexor laxity (375)** is particularly common in heavy breeds such as the Shire, Percheron, Suffolk Punch and Clydesdale, but is by no means restricted to this class of horse. It is, however, probably less prevalent in miniature breeds. The hind limbs are usually more severely affected than the fore limbs. The extent to which individual foals are affected varies markedly, but it is usual for both left and right limbs to be affected

373

 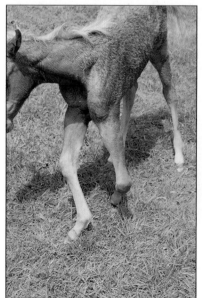

373 Contracted foal syndrome.
Note: Multiple developmental flexural and angular deviations of both fore limbs. Assisted parturition (dystocia). Possible iodine deficiency. Goitre present

374 Severe developmental carpal flexion with fusion.
Note: Wasting of shoulder and forearm muscles and both front legs markedly shorter than normal. Foal delivered normally by mare without assistance.

374

375

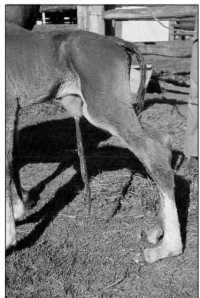

376

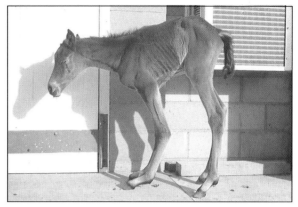

375 Flexural laxity (newborn foal).

376 Carpal collapse (newborn, dysmature foal).
Note: Concurrent flexor laxity in forelimbs, hind limbs normal.

377

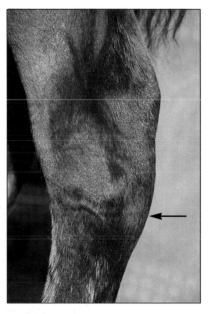

378

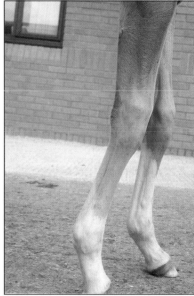

377 Tarsal collapse (central tarsal).
Note: Excessive strain and thickening of plantar ligament (arrow).

378 Carpal contracture (flexural deformity – mild).

more or less equally. Some show only a very slight dropping of the fetlock while others may walk on the palmar aspect of the pastern with the palmar fetlock on the ground. Flexor laxity is particularly common in premature foals (gestational age of less than 320 days), or dysmature foals (foals of normal or prolonged gestational age having the characteristics of prematurity). There may be accompanying signs of muscular weakness or intercurrent systemic illness in the more severely affected foals. Skeletal ossification, assessed radiographically, is often found to be poor. While most flexor laxity improves rapidly, resolving spontaneously within days of birth, it may persist, particularly when it is associated with concurrent systemic disease or prematurity, and may then exert more serious and possibly permanent secondary effects upon joint development and limb posture (**376**).

Collapse of carpal (*see* **376**) and/or **tarsal bones** (**377**) is relatively common in premature or dysmature foals, and is further evidence of the associated incomplete or defective ossification and abnormal weight distribution on the developing bones. The inadequacy of ossification may be appreciated by radiographic examination, when one or more carpal

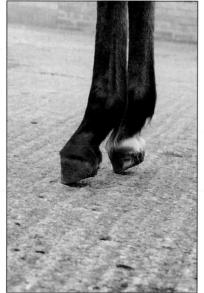

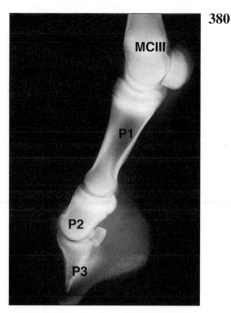

379 Developmental contracture of deep digital flexor tendon.
Note: 'Ballet-dancer' posture.

380 Developmental contracture of deep digital flexor tendon.
Note: Same foal as 379, two weeks later. Normal fetlock and pastern joint positions with marked flexion of distal interphalangeal (coffin) joint. Abnormally long heel, due to loss of wear.

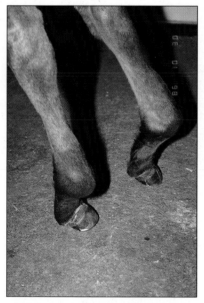

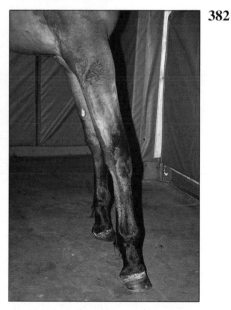

381 Flexural deformity (associated with bilateral extensor tendon rupture).

382 Developmental contracture of superficial digital flexor tendon.
Note: (Some contracture of deep also). 'Bowstring' appearance with upright fetlock and pastern but (nearly) normal foot position relative to the floor.

(usually the radial, third or fourth carpal) or tarsal (usually the central or third tarsal) bones have an obvious lack of ossification and a deformed shape. Ossification of these bones is, normally, well advanced at birth, and in the event that this is retarded or abnormal the pressure of standing upon the soft cartilage is often sufficient to cause distortion. Foals which are born prematurely would be expected to have a higher propensity for this collapse, in view of the poorer ossification and poorer cartilaginous strength present in these animals. Clinically the condition can be easily recognised by the abnormal angles adopted by the forelimb (in the case of carpal collapse) (*see* **376**) or the hind limb (in the case of tarsal collapse) (*see* **377**). Concurrent flexural deformities and other developmental defects, such as arthrogryposis and torticollis, may be found in the worst affected foals. More complex skeletal deformities may be accompanied by other defects of neurologic or cardiac function and/or palatoschisis (cleft palate).

Relatively mild **flexural deformities**, resulting from an apparent contracture of the flexor tendons, may also result in abnormal postures. These commonly affect the carpus (**378**), tarsus and distal limb joints (**379**). The pathogenesis of contractures of the flexor tendons is uncertain but it has been found to be particularly associated with hyperplastic goitre (*see* **357**), giving the impression that it might be related in some cases to iodine status and particularly to excessive dietary intake. The relationship between the disorder and these factors is not clear and many foals are born with flexural deformities in the absence of any discernible etiology. Contracture of flexor tendons may be a consequence of fetal malpositioning or of a discrepancy of growth between the flexor tendons and ligaments and the long bones of the limb. **Carpal flexural deformity** (*see* **378**) is, however, sometimes more complicated than this as efforts to lengthen the tendons by surgery are frequently unrewarding. In the worst of these cases (*see* **374**) the carpus cannot be extended even when all the soft tissues are sectioned. It is clear that they may therefore sometimes be related to joint defects and these are then included in the contracted foal complex described above.

An obviously upright ('ballet-dancer') posture (*see* **379**), to the extent that the foal is forced to walk on the toe or even on the dorsal hoof wall, is encountered where the length of the **deep flexor tendons** in the cannon region is reduced relative to the length of the cannon itself. Radiographically the digit is usually normal, with normal metacarpo-phalangeal (fetlock) and proximal interphalangeal (pastern) joints, but the distal interphalangeal joint is seen to be markedly flexed (**380**).

The severity of the disorder in the new born foal is variable and the natural, rapid growth of the metacarpals (or more rarely, the metatarsals) and radius serves only to aggravate the extent of the flexion of the digit (*see* **379**).

Rupture of the extensor tendons (**381**), occurring simultaneously or incidentally, will also result in a dramatic over flexion of the fetlock. In these cases, further flexion results in excoriation of the dorsal aspect of the pastern. In common with the acquired flexural deformities, which are characteristic of the growing foal, these may reflect a growth discrepancy between the lengthening of the bones and the tendinous structures. Where the bone grows faster than the tendons can stretch, the consequent 'bowstring' effect will inevitably result in the development of a flexural deformity. The disorder is therefore recognised at birth and during other rapid growth phases, such as around normal weaning age (**flexural deformity of the distal interphalangeal joint**) or at 12 – 18 months of age (**flexural deformity of the metacarpo-phalangeal joint**). Even the so-called acquired flexural deformities of foals are possibly related to the development of the bones, tendons and ligaments and may be regarded as developmental disorders. In most acquired cases, the foals are growing particularly well, and either the deep or superficial flexor tendons (or in rare cases) both are affected by an inability to lengthen at the same rate as the limb bones. In the former case, there is relative **shortening of the deep flexor tendon** between its attachment on the palmar aspect of the third phalanx and the attachment of the carpal check ligament at the level of the proximal third of the cannon. This typically results in a 'ballet-dancer' stance (*see* **379**). In cases involving the **superficial flexor tendon** there is relative shortening of this structure between the palmar aspect of the radius at the level of the proximal (radial) check ligament, and the attachment of the superficial flexor tendon on the palmar aspect of the first and second phalanges. This results in flexion of the fetlock joint leading to an upright pastern with an abnormal fetlock angle but a normal or near-normal, distal interphalangeal (foot) posture (**382**). Combined deep and superficial contracture which, with varying ratios of involvement, are relatively common, results in a very upright fetlock posture with a strong tendency to walk on the dorsal hoof wall and thereby cause gross foot deformities culminating in the development of a 'club-foot' (*see* **451**). Acquired flexural deformities are sometimes found in association with other developmental and growth disorders such as osteochondrosis (*see* **397**) and physitis (*see* **392**). It is believed that pain causes reduced weight bearing and an

383

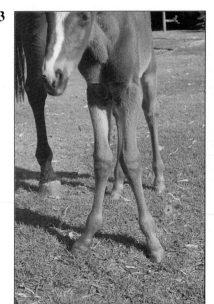

384

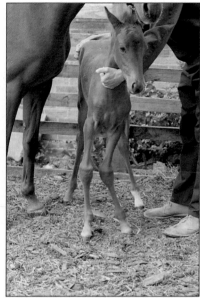

385

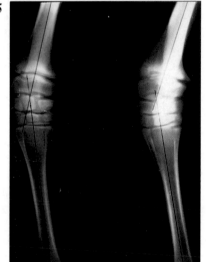

383 Bilateral carpal valgus ('Knock-knees').
Note: Slight fetlock valgus also present.

384 Combined carpal valgus-varus deformity ('windswept').
Note: Valgus in left leg worse than varus in right leg.

385 Combined carpal valgus-varus deformity ('windswept').
Note: Same foal as 384. Valgus in left leg (deviation 25°), varus in right leg (deviation 17°).

reduction in the stretching of soft tissues which culminates in tendon contractures on the painful limb and over stretching on the normal limb from excessive weight bearing. Foals showing any form of flexural deformity should be carefully examined to establish whether there are any underlying reasons for the condition before embarking on therapy.

Angular deformities of limb joints, particularly of the knee (carpus), hock (tarsus) and fetlock (metacarpophalangeal joint), are frequently encountered in rapidly growing foals and are regarded as a developmental disorder although there are significant etiological possibilities relating to management and nutritional factors. All breeds are liable to the disorders but the Thoroughbred and the Quarter Horse seem particularly prone to them. The deformities are most associated with loss of coordinated growth across the physis of the radius, tibia or third metacarpal and this results in lateral or medial deviations of the limb at these sites. **Carpal valgus** occurs when the metacarpus deviates laterally as a result of accelerated growth of the radius medially. This gives the foal a 'knock-kneed' appearance (**383**). The opposite situation (**carpal varus**) results in a 'bow-legged' appearance, with medial deviation of the

386

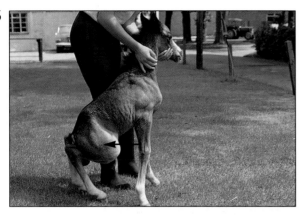

386 Bilateral congenital lateral luxation of patella.
Note: 'Kangaroo' posture. Thickened appearance of limb behind stifle and patella visible caudal to stifle (arrow) with quadriceps muscle acting as flexor of stifle.

metacarpus as a result of rapid growth of the lateral aspect of the radius. Deviations at the fetlock similarly result from abnormal growth of the cannon at the distal metacarpal physis, and are usually valgus deformities. Commonly only one limb is involved, but in some cases both may be similarly affected (*see* **383**). Occasionally a foal may have a valgus deformity of one limb and varus on the other, giving a 'windswept' appearance **(384)**. Although deviations occurring at the fetlock are usually less dramatic in appearance, they are regarded as being more urgent, as growth in the distal metacarpal physis ceases at an earlier age (3–4 months) than growth in the distal radial physis (9–12 months). Once the growth plate has closed, the potential for therapeutic intervention involving growth acceleration/retardation is lost. Even before physeal closure, the extent of the deviation may be such that there is exceptional weight bearing on the concave side and much less on the convex. This results in a slower growth rate (and often premature closure) of the physis on the 'short' side of the joint. Thus, the condition becomes progressively worse, and effective therapeutic measures are correspondingly less feasible. Significant deviations of these types may be encountered in new born foals, when it is presumed they are the result of mal-positioning *in utero*, but those deviations developing spontaneously in foals between 2 and 6 weeks of age may be a result of complex interactions between nutritional, traumatic, physical, conformational or exercise factors. Radiographically, the origin and extent of the deviation can be defined by the location and angle of intersecting vertical lines drawn through the middle of the radius and the third metacarpal **(385)**. The extent of physeal pathology may also be assessed (*see* **385**).

Congenital lateral luxation of one, or both, patellas is a rare but important clinical syndrome, resulting in a loss of stifle extension ability **(386)**. The extensors of the stifle become, effectively, flexors as the tendon of the quadriceps is displaced with the patella to behind the femoro-tibial joint. In some cases, the condition is due to significant hypoplasia of the lateral trochlear ridge of the femur, but this is not always present. Affected foals are unable to extend the stifle effectively, and cannot, therefore, stand without assistance. Muscular effort, which is often very energetic, during attempts to stand results in further flexion of the stifle and produces a characteristic kangaroo gait and appearance **(386)**. The stifle region in these foals may appear thickened by the laterally displaced patella on the affected side(s), which may also be visible (*see* **386**) and palpable. In unilateral cases, the signs may be less obvious.

Shetland ponies, in particular, suffer from a congenital, heritable, **lateral luxation of the patella** which appears, in most cases, to have little or no limiting effect upon their movement. Palpation of the stifle during walking, allows detection of an obvious displacement of the patella. Usually the luxation is not sufficient to result in any disabling loss of extensor ability, and affected ponies are often quite capable of normal work. Some individuals may, however, become disabled in the event that a more demanding work regime is expected, and furthermore, as they become older, some degree of osteoarthritis is almost inevitable. Radiographs (and particularly, dorso-proximal, (skyline) views) may demonstrate the dislocation or sub-luxation and a poorly developed trochlear groove on the femur.

Bones and joints

Non-Infectious Disorders

387

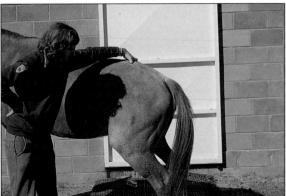

387 Sacroiliac joint/ligament strain/displacement.
Note: Unnatural response to applied pressure in sacral region. Normal horse arches back in response to focal pressure over croup.

388

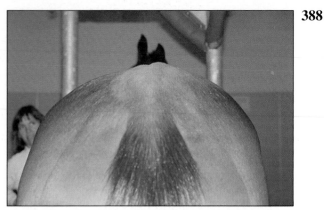

388 Sacroiliac joint/ligament strain/displacement.
Note: Discrepancy in height of sacral and iliac tuberosities (left lower than right) were noted. Left gluteus muscle mass wasted i.e. left side affected.
Differential Diagnosis:
i)   Chronic pain from (degenerative) joint disease of hip, stifle or soft tissue damage or pelvic fracture
ii) Previous exertional myopathy
iii) Traumatic or ischemic myopathy
iv) Lumbar nerve disorders
v) Equine protozoal myeloencephalopathy
vi) Cauda equina syndrome
vii)Damage to sacral plexus or to peripheral pathways of gluteal and femoral nerves

Traumatic injuries are amongst the most common disorders affecting the musculo-skeletal system. The use to which horses are put often results in severe and abnormal strains on bones, joints, ligaments, tendons and muscles. Furthermore, damage to peripheral and central nervous tissues will inevitably affect the function of muscles and the maintenance of normal posture and structural symmetry. There is clearly a vast range of traumatic possibilities and it is not within the scope of this book to provide a definitive description of all of these.

   Subluxation (dislocation or sprain) of the sacro-iliac articulation is an unusual but often diagnosed disorder. The clinical manifestations of the condition usually include chronic and subtle changes in hind limb action and/or pain associated with the movement of the pelvis. Many affected horses are presented with a history of poor exercise tolerance and vaguely restricted hind limb function. A history of back pain, resentment to weight applied to the back, and a tendency to collapse

behind when the sacroiliac region is palpated (**387**), is often reported. In the normal horse pressure applied to the lumbar spine results in ventroflexion and pressure applied to the sacral and sacrococcygeal region (croup) causes a strong reflex dorsiflexion of the spine. Cases of sacroiliac strain produce obvious variations in this behaviour (*see* **387**). This may not, however, be related solely to this disorder and any condition which is associated with 'back pain' may have the same result. Resentment to saddling has also been attributed to the back pain complex, which includes lumbar myopathy, overriding or 'kissing' (dorsal) spines and sacroiliac inflammation. Unilateral sacro-iliac lesions are far more often encountered than bilateral lesions. Sometimes the extent of the displacement at the sacro-iliac articulation is sufficient to result in an obvious dropping of the iliac crest relative to the sacrum, and of the position of the *tuber coxæ* (external angle of the ilium) (**388**). Disuse atrophy of muscle groups associated with the pelvis (*see* **388**) may exaggerate the discrepancy. A diagnosis may

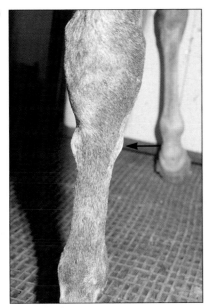

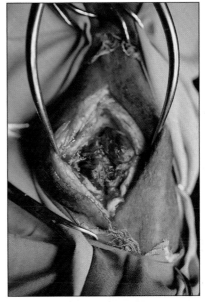

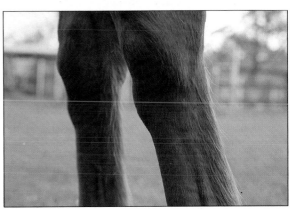

389 Bilateral 'splints' (high) (arrow).

390 Subperiosteal hematoma.
Note: Painful, hot swelling developed spontaneously on the distal cannon in a 2 year old Thoroughbred. Radiographically showed as lucent area under the periosteum. The lesion was curetted and the horse made an uneventful recovery.

391 'Bucked shin'.
Note: 'Bumpy' dorsal outline of cannon. Lesions very painful on palpation but little effect on gait.

be supported by the use of articular analgesia of the affected joint but the changes associated with the condition in relation to muscle atrophy may make this an unrewarding approach in many cases. Where there is an obvious deformity the diagnosis may be made more easily and with greater conviction. Thermal imaging equipment and gamma scintigraphy may be used to identify regions of excessive heat and deep inflammation but in many cases the disorder is only identified after an exhaustive post mortem examination and subsequent histopathological examination of the structures associated with the sacro-iliac articulation.

Traumatic injuries to the limbs are particularly common and in most cases are acute in onset and have obvious clinical or radiographic features which render their diagnosis relatively simple. The more subtle, relatively innocuous changes which occur in the periosteum or the interosseous ligaments are sometimes difficult to identify in the early stages.

The splint bones of both fore and, to a lesser extent, the hind limbs are liable to the development of **exostoses** in response to direct trauma or to spontaneous inflammation arising in the periosteum and the interosseous ligaments. In most cases the result is of little clinical significance in spite of considerable bony enlargement (**389**) but occasionally the local reaction may become sufficiently large to interfere with the tendinous and ligamentous structures of the palmar/plantar metacarpus/metatarsus. This is more likely when the reaction occurs in the more proximal reaches of the cannon (*see* **389**). The reaction is generally limited to the periosteum of the splint bones and their ligamentous attachments to the cannon bone, and it seems likely that it is a result of tearing, or of trauma applied to the periosteum. Hard training, poor conformation and malnutrition, with poor hoof care, may also predispose to the development of '**splints**'. The lesions are particularly common in young, growing

219

392

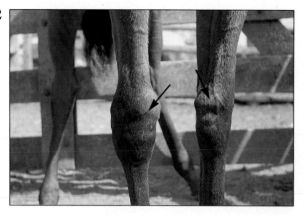

393

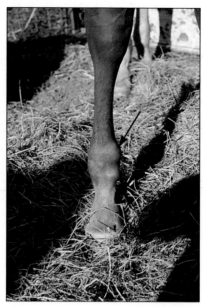

392 Radial physitis (physeal dysplasia).
Note: Obvious enlargement of radial physis most severe medially (arrows) and causing a mild carpal-varus deformity.

393 Metacarpal physitis (physeal dysplasia).
Note: Obvious enlargement of metacarpal growth plate, particularly medially (arrow). No apparent deviation of fetlock.

horses. More rarely, horses suffer from fractures of the splint bones as a result of direct trauma and the lateral splint of the hind limb is particularly prone to this injury. Horses with acute splint bone fractures will often rest the leg in slight flexion, and in fresh fractures there is invariably prominent local swelling centred over the affected bone. This may extend into the adjacent suspensory ligament and flexor tendons. The small size of the bones and the fact that they are most liable to kicks and over-reaching means that many of these fractures are comminuted, and some are compound (open). Subsequent infection, osteomyelitis and sequestration of fragments are common developments of compound splint bone fractures. The extent of these complications is usually identifiable radiographically.

Periostitis and micro-fracture of the dorsal metacarpus is a relatively common disorder of young, fast-gaited horses, particularly where the going is hard. The so-called '**Bucked-Shin**' complex of disorders also includes those cases with sub-periosteal hemorrhages in the metacarpal bones (**390**) in the absence of any identifiable fractures in the underlying cortical bone of the diaphysis. Micro and saucer fractures, and sub-periosteal hemorrhages are common sequels to treadmill work, particularly where the treadmill has a steel back plate on the running surface. Careful radiological examination may identify saucer-shaped fractures of the dorsal cortex of the cannon, and longer-standing lesions have a characteristic "bumpy" or uneven appearance along the dorsal aspect of the cannon bone (**391**). Palpation in the acute stages is painful and resented

although, usually, minimal gait alteration is present. Affected racing horses often show reduced performance without any detectable lameness.

Inflammatory changes within the physis of any bone, including the cervical vertebrae and the long bones of the limbs, may be nutritional in origin or the result of trauma. The latter group of conditions includes non-displaced, physeal fractures and physeal damage without fracture. Inflammation of the physis is known as physitis or physeal dysplasia. Clinically the disorder is recognised by pain, heat and swelling over the major physeal plates of the distal radius (**392**) and fetlock (**393**). Radiographically the disorder is easily recognised with a widening and asymmetry of the metaphysis and usually obvious metaphyseal sclerosis. The cortices of the long bones often show asymmetric thickness, due to the altered stresses placed upon the limb by alteration in angle and consequent modified weight bearing between the medial and lateral sides of the bone. This may result in the development of aquired angular deformities (carpal varus or valgus). While the condition is most obvious in the long bones, it is often present as a generalised bone disease in young growing horses. However, the major clinical effects are associated with the long bones and the cervical spine. The generalised forms are probably the consequence of complex nutritional and management factors complicated, in some animals, by hereditary aspects, possibly related to growth rate; heavy, fast-growing horses seem particularly prone to the disorder. Diets containing high phosphate and low available calcium concentrations

394

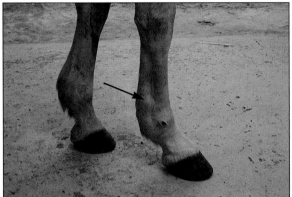

395

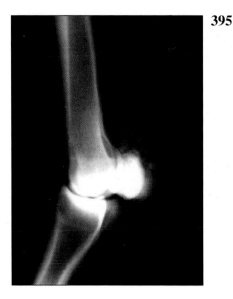

394 Bilateral (proximal) sesamoiditis (chronic). **Note:** Gross swelling around sesamoids, filling of digital sheath creating an apparent bowed tendon (arrow).

395 Proximal sesamoiditis (latero-medial radiograph). **Note:** Extensive new bone and lysis of sesamoid with calcification of suspensory ligament.

have been implicated in some outbreaks of the condition, but it is likely that the pathogenesis is more complicated than this.

Inflammation of the proximal sesamoid bones (**sesamoiditis**) is an osteitis, probably caused by abnormal strains placed upon the fetlock as a result of excessive loads on the suspensory and distal sesamoidean ligaments. The clinical features of the disorder are similar to those associated with fracture of these bones. Usually the inflammation is most severe over the abaxial surface of the affected bone(s). Mild, local swelling usually gives way to a firm, often marked, local swelling (**394**). Pain is often relatively mild, but may be more obvious with manipulation, and a markedly reduced flexion ability is commonly encountered. Radiographs taken 3 weeks or more after the onset of the condition show a distinctive diffuse loss of radiodensity in the bones themselves and new-bone formation extending into the associated ligamentous attachments (**395**). It is common for calcification/ossification to occur within the suspensory ligament and/or the distal sesamoidean ligaments.

Bone cysts are radiographically obvious cystic structures, in the subchondral region of limb bones in particular. Their significance is equivocal, with many being identified incidentally. It is likely that they represent a failure of normal ossification, and, as such, are the clinical manifestation of a disorder of cartilage maturation to bone. They are most often encountered in the medial condyle of the distal femur (**396**) and the distal end of the first phalanx (**397**). They are also found in the small bones of the carpus and tarsus and sporadically in a variety of other sites. Current knowledge suggests that bone cysts are of functional significance only if they are in communication with the adjacent joint. However, those close to a joint surface (*see* **396**), but not in communication, may become significant if trauma or increased work causes fracture of the subchondral bone plate.

Failure of normal endochondral ossification under the articular cartilage of a joint, resulting in failure of continuity of the cartilage over the lesion, is termed **osteochondritis dissecans** (OCD). In this disorder, there is a dissecting split in the cartilage which results in the formation of separate osteochondral fragments in the joint. Characteristically affected joints develop joint effusion (**398**), and the horse shows variable lameness, ranging from severe to almost undetectable. Common sites for the development of OCD include the femoropatellar (stifle) (*see* **398**), the tibiotarsal (hock) (**399**), the metacarpo-phalangeal (fetlock) and scapulo-humeral (shoulder) joints. However, any joint may be found to be affected (including the articulations of the cervical vertebrae). Radiographically the lesions of OCD result in defects in, or irregular outlines of, the joint margins, with or without subchondral fragments or bone fragments floating freely within the joint ('joint mouse'). Arthroscopic examination may reveal a fragment attached to the margin of an obviously abnormal area of the joint surface (**400**), or a focal articular surface defect with a floating osteochondral fragment. Even relatively minor lesions of OCD result in considerable joint distension (*see* **398, 399**). Examination of the synovial fluid from these joints reveals minimal inflammation;

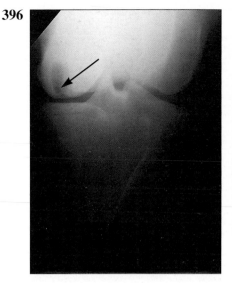

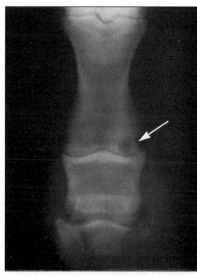

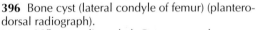

396 Bone cyst (lateral condyle of femur) (plantero-dorsal radiograph).
Note: Stifle very distended. Cyst apparently communicating with lateral femoro-patellar joint (arrow). Synovial fluid very watery but free of cells.

397 Bone cyst (distal extremity of first phalanx (long pastern bone) (arrow).
Note: No apparent connection with fetlock joint. Defect in overlying bone laterally. Joint not enlarged but slight lameness which was resolved by intra-articular anesthesia.

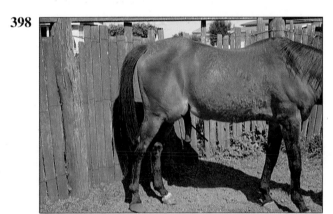

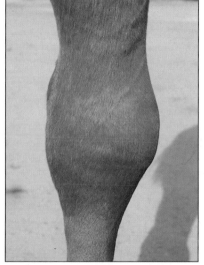

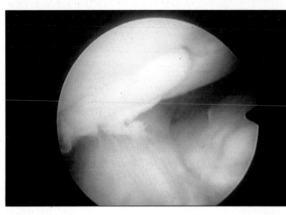

398 Osteochondrosis (osteochondritis dissecans) (lateral femoropatellar joint) stifle effusion (arrow).

399 Distension of tibiotarsal joint (Bog spavin).
Note: Pouching out anteromedially.
Differential Diagnosis:
i)   Osteochondrosis
ii) Infective arthritis
iii) Distention of tibial sheath (Thoroughpin)

400 Osteochondrosis (osteochondritis dissecans) (lateral femoropatellar joint) (arthroscopic view).
Note: Well defined abnormal cartilaginous lesion on lateral trochlear ridge of femur. Bone to right of picture is the patella.

401

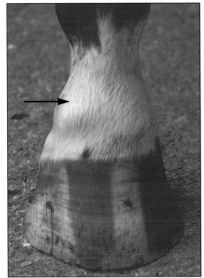

402

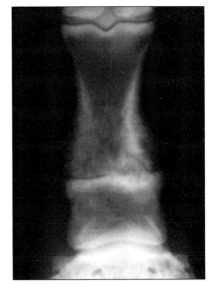

401 Degenerative joint disease (proximal interphalangeal joint) (high ringbone) (arrow).

402 Degenerative joint disease (proximal interphalangeal joint) (high, articular ringbone) (same horse as **401**).
Note: Extensive lytic and new bone formation in proximal interphalangeal (pastern) joint with narrowing of joint space and sclerosis of proximal end of second phalanx (short pastern bone).

there is a loss of viscosity and a moderate increase in protein, but it is unusual to encounter significant elevations in the cell count.

One of the possible consequences of OCD and, indeed, of some bone cysts is a progressive degeneration of the joint surface and a persistent lameness. This is termed **degenerative joint disease (DJD)** or **osteoarthritis** and, while OCD is one cause of this progressive disorder, it is by no means the only one. Traumatic fractures, dislocations and the consequences of joint infection, even after the bacteria are eliminated, may all lead to DJD. Horses affected by DJD show lameness, pain on manipulation of the joint and swelling of the affected periarticular area (**401**). If the lameness is severe, there may be secondary effects on other structures including weight bearing laminitis in the contralateral limb. The disorder represents the end-stage of a number of pathological processes, and it is characterised by changes in both the joint architecture, the synovial membrane and the synovial fluid. The changes typical of this condition develop most rapidly in the high motion joints such as the tibiotarsal and the femorotibial joints, whilst in low motion joints such as the distal intertarsal and tarso-metatarsal joints, the onset and progression may be insidious. Generally the response to DJD in the low motion joints such as the interphalangeal joints is towards the production of new

bone whereas in high motion joints the joint surfaces are more severely affected. In protracted cases, involving low motion joints, the characteristic changes are usually obvious radiographically (**402**). However the condition can be difficult to identify in the acute case, such as that which occurs in racehorses when there may only be superficial and subtle changes in the joint integrity. A diagnosis may rely upon exhaustive radiography, scintigraphy, arthroscopy and analysis of joint fluid as well as the response to selective (intra-articular) analgesia.

The hock is particularly sensitive to pain, and even minor injury to bones or synovial structures results in gross joint distension and marked pain. The pain may be sufficiently severe, even as a result of relatively minor intra-articular inflammation, to lead to severe lameness and dramatic weight loss. **Effusion of the tibiotarsal (hock) joint** (commonly referred to as '**Bog Spavin**') (*see* **399**) is a response to a wide range of intra-articular lesions. These include fractures, bone cysts, osteochondrosis, inflammatory arthritides or degenerative joint disease. The distal intertarsal and tarso-metatarsal joints are classified as low-motion joints, and these bear the brunt of the concussive forces transmitted up the limb. They are subjected to compression, torsional and tensile forces during normal movement. This not only makes them more liable to

403

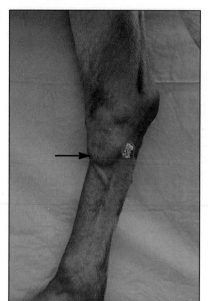

404

405

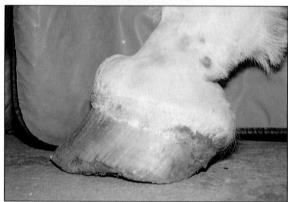

403 Degenerative joint disease (distal tarsal joints) (Bone spavin).
Note: Distinctive bony swelling over distal intertarsal and tarso-metatarsal joints on medial aspect of hock (arrow). Horse previously lame but resolved over 6 months.

404 Degenerative joint disease (distal tarsal joints) (Bone spavin) (dorsolateral-planteromedial oblique (45°) radiograph).
Note: Extensive bridging new bone formation on medial aspect of hock over distal intertarsal and tarso-metatarsal joints (arrow).

405 Degenerative joint disease (distal interphalangeal joint) (Pyramidal disease, Buttress foot).

fracture, but also to osteoarthritic degeneration. **Osteoarthritis** and **periostitis** of the low motion, distal inter-tarsal and tarso-metatarsal joints of the hock is referred to commonly as 'spavin'. Initially, the lameness is mild. The affected horse has a tendency to drag the foot, producing prominent wear at the toe. Progressive joint deterioration results in radiographically apparent narrowing of the joint spaces and periarticular new-bone production. Ultimately this may lead to an obvious bony swelling known as '**Bone Spavin**' on the medial aspect of the hock (**403**), which is readily identified radiographically (**404**) by use of appropriate (dorso lateral-planteromedial oblique 45°) projections. While most cases of tarsal osteoarthritis result in this characteristic bony change, some show little or no overt evidence of any physical abnormality in spite of moderate or severe lameness. The latter condition is commonly referred to as '**Occult Spavin**'. Such cases show irrefutable clinical evidence of hock lameness following the use of intra-articular analgesia, and the cause of the problem may (or may not) be identifiable radiographically. Radiographically some lesions are found to be of a predominately lytic character, in which the joint space is wide and irregular and there is an irregular loss of radiodensity in the subchondral bone of the affected tarsal bones. Once osteoarthritic changes have resulted in ankylosis of the affected joints, lameness is usually no longer detectable. The presence of a large bony swelling on the medial aspect of the distal tarsal region (*see* **403**) is usually indicative of spontaneous ankylosis, and, while it may appear unsightly and somewhat alarming, paradoxically the prognosis for such animals is good.

New bone formation which occurs on the distal end of the second phalanx (short pastern bone) and on the proximal end of the third phalanx (coffin bone) is called 'low ringbone'. This commonly involves the extensor process of the third phalanx and is encountered in

406

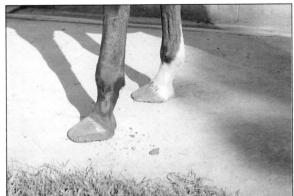

407

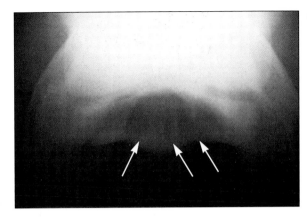

408

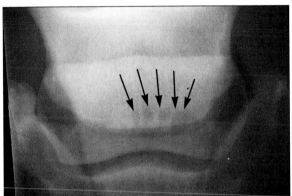

406 Navicular disease (podotrochleosis) (broken hoof pastern angle).
Note: Low heel - long toed posture with upright pasterns.

407 Navicular disease (podotrochleosis) (Flexor/tangential projection radiograph).
Note: Enlarged vascular channels (arrows).

408 Navicular disease (podotrochleosis) (60° dorsoproximal projection radiograph).
Note: Enlarged lollipop, and flask like vascular channels (arrows).

fractures and degenerative conditions of the bone and the distal interphalangeal (coffin) joint. From the clinical appearance alone it is not usually possible to establish an etiology, but horses with high heels and short toes, and particularly where these are present with a stilted or 'choppy' stride are particularly prone to its development. Affected horses are often lame with a shortened stride length and a prominent heel based action (presumably in an attempt to reduce tension and concussion in the dorsal structures. An extensive swelling at the dorsal portion of the coronary band creates the so-called '**Buttress Foot**' (**405**). Radiographically there is variable new bone formation in and around the pyramidal (extensor) process and this often extends onto the dorsal aspect of the second phalanx (pastern bone). The condition is regarded as a form of degenerative joint disease and carries a poor prognosis.

Navicular disease (podotrochleosis) is one of the commonest causes of lameness in adult horses, and while Thoroughbred and Quarterhorse geldings are most often affected, the disease may affect all types and ages of horse, including ponies. It is however particularly rare in heavy horses. Although the hind legs may be affected, the disease principally is a condition of the fore-feet. Whilst hereditary factors may be involved in the

etiology, management factors are probably at least as important in most cases. Faulty conformation, arising either from genetic reasons or mismanagement with respect to foot care, and concurrent exercise on hard surfaces, are implicated. The latter factors may be of greater importance in ponies than in larger breeds. The long-toed, low, flat-heeled horse (**406**) appears to be particularly liable to the condition. Affected horses often have a history of an insidious onset of progressive lameness, which is characteristically intermittent in the early stages. Lame horses which are rested after exercise display an increased lameness on further exercise, but, at least in the early cases, lameness will often be noted to work-off with exercise. There is a tendency to rest the affected foot in a slightly flexed position with the toe pointed. Pressure applied to the heel region is resented. During movement, the toe tends to land first and the anterior phase of the stride is reduced, possibly in an attempt to avoid heel pressure. Bruising of the sole at the toe and increased vascularity of the sole are common findings, resulting from the abnormal foot placement. Heel contraction, as a result of reduced heel pressure, is a common sign, and long standing cases may show marked foot contraction with increased concavity of the sole in both dorso-palmar and latero-medial planes.

409

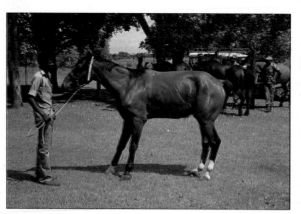

410

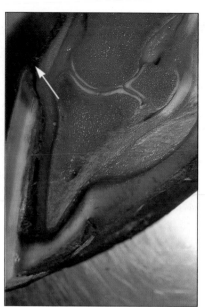

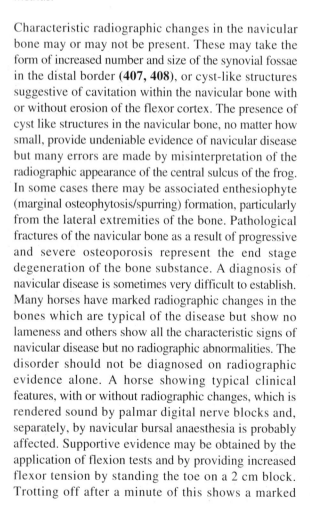

409 Laminitis (acute) (characteristic posture).
Note: Forefeet probably worse affected than hind. Very reluctant to move.

410 Laminitis (peracute, toxic form).
Note: Extensive disruption of laminar attachments and blood discharge from coronet (arrow). Little pedal bone rotation. Mare suffering from severe toxemia as a result of a retained fetal membranes (placenta) and consequent metritis.

Characteristic radiographic changes in the navicular bone may or may not be present. These may take the form of increased number and size of the synovial fossae in the distal border (**407, 408**), or cyst-like structures suggestive of cavitation within the navicular bone with or without erosion of the flexor cortex. The presence of cyst like structures in the navicular bone, no matter how small, provide undeniable evidence of navicular disease but many errors are made by misinterpretation of the radiographic appearance of the central sulcus of the frog. In some cases there may be associated enthesiophyte (marginal osteophytosis/spurring) formation, particularly from the lateral extremities of the bone. Pathological fractures of the navicular bone as a result of progressive and severe osteoporosis represent the end stage degeneration of the bone substance. A diagnosis of navicular disease is sometimes very difficult to establish. Many horses have marked radiographic changes in the bones which are typical of the disease but show no lameness and others show all the characteristic signs of navicular disease but no radiographic abnormalities. The disorder should not be diagnosed on radiographic evidence alone. A horse showing typical clinical features, with or without radiographic changes, which is rendered sound by palmar digital nerve blocks and, separately, by navicular bursal anaesthesia is probably affected. Supportive evidence may be obtained by the application of flexion tests and by providing increased flexor tension by standing the toe on a 2 cm block. Trotting off after a minute of this shows a marked increase in the lameness. The use of gamma scintigraphy has been used effectively to establish the site of active lesions in horses without any apparent radiographic lesions. The prognosis for horses affected with navicular disease is guarded, but careful farriery will probably prevent its progression and, indeed, may improve many cases.

One of the most serious and most frequently encountered conditions affecting the equine foot is **laminitis**. Inflammatory changes, occurring in the sensitive laminae of the foot, result in a characteristic clinical syndrome. Laminitis may develop in response to a number of etiological factors including over-ingestion/engorgement of grain, ingestion of plant-derived chemicals having vasoactive effects, endotoxemia, the administration of corticosteroids and, in some cases, excessive weight bearing (such as arises when one foot or leg is unable to carry weight) or severe and repeated foot concussion. Lack of regular exercise in fat ponies has been identified as a common etiological factor. **Secondary laminitis** occurs in a wide variety of disorders affecting the horse including septicemia and toxemia, and it is also a common complication in aged horses with pituitary adenoma. However, in some instances, no convincing explanation can be found, while, in others, apparently unrelated concurrent medical or surgical disorders may be implicated. Single feet may be affected, particularly when the etiology is related to excessive weight-bearing. Laminitis is a complex disorder affecting a wide range of organs and tissue

411

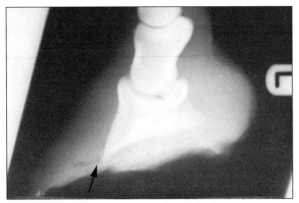

411 Laminitis (acute) (lateral radiograph).
Note: Obvious pedal bone rotation (approximately 20°).
Gas tract visible in sole from penetration of pedal bone
(arrow).

412

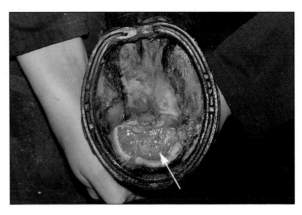

412 Laminitis (chronic with acute superimposition).
Note: Pedal bone rotation, solar penetration (arrow).

systems, in which the most obvious clinical signs are
related to the feet. The pathology is usually associated
with vascular disease, where the blood supply to the foot
is impaired. The development of arterio-venous shunting
and decreased capillary perfusion in the laminae of the
foot result in the development of ischemic necrosis of
the laminae. Regardless of the different etiological
possibilities, the clinical signs are very similar and are
easily recognised. Peracute, acute and chronic forms are
encountered, although most chronic cases are recovering
or recovered acute cases. However, occasionally the
chronic form develops insidiously, and in other cases
acute episodes may be superimposed upon the chronic
stage. In its acute phases severe pain is usually present.
Usually both front feet, or all four feet, are affected with
equal severity, although the extra weight carried by the
fore limbs makes the disease more obvious in these.
Where the fore feet are more severely affected the horse
will usually lean back onto its hind legs with its forelegs
stretched out in front (**409**). Where all the feet are
severely/equally affected the horse may adopt a
'rocking-horse' stance with all four feet brought together
under the abdomen. In severe cases, the horse may lie
down for long periods and show a marked reluctance to
rise. Dorsal recumbency with the feet held upwards may
also be seen. All cases are extremely reluctant to move.
Shifting weight from one foot to the other and resting
the feet in turn, are commonly seen. Mild cases may be
made to walk with relative ease, but their action has a
characteristic heel-toe movement where the heel is
placed down first and the foot is lifted quickly, giving a
shuffling, stilted gait. Mild cases will often walk without
much encouragement, but are very reluctant to trot.
Clinical examination in the acute stage reveals the
affected feet to be hot and painful, and a characteristic

bounding pulse can usually be palpated in the palmar
digital arteries. The clinical signs may be affected by the
presence or absence of intercurrent disease, but most
horses with acute laminitis show rapid respiration and
high heart rates, as well as signs of toxic shock.
Progressive necrosis and disruption of the venous plexus
and laminae of the foot result in separation of the hoof
from the underlying pedal bone (**410**). It is quite
common to encounter coronary bleeding as a result of
the severe disruption of the laminae and pooling of
stagnant blood between the sensitive and insensitive
laminae (*see* **410**). Downward rotation of the pedal bone
within the hoof (**411**) results from a combination of
dorsal laminar separation and continued tension on the
deep flexor tendon. The action of the horse while
moving exerts even greater tension on the flexor tendon
as the animal attempts to take more and more weight on
the heels. Once the pedal bone starts to rotate the process
is continued by the persistent flexor tension and the
force of weight applied to the dorsal aspect of the distal
interphalangeal joint. Continued pressure applied to the
foot may drive the dorsal, solar margin of the pedal bone
through the sole of the foot (*see* **412**) but, even without
this, some distortion of the sole, showing either a focal
bulging of the sole dorsal to the point of the frog (**413**),
or a general solar convexity, is apparent. Paring of the
sole will invariably reveal extensive subsolar bruising
and hemorrhage (*see* **412**). Gross disruption of the
laminar attachments in the most acute cases (usually
those suffering from severe toxemia) allows the pedal
bone to sink without much rotation, within the hoof.
Cases in which this occurs have a distinctive depression
at the coronary band (*see* **410, 413**). In severe cases the
hoof, may separate completely, or there may be
separation of the coronet over limited areas (*see* **498**).

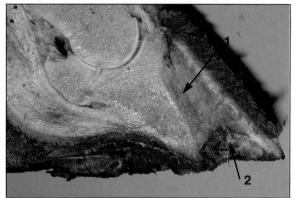
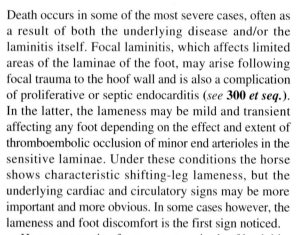

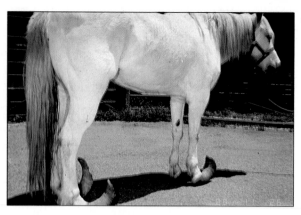

413 Laminitis (Sinker) (acute on chronic).
Note: Distinct depression at dorsal coronet. Finger could be pushed in behind coronary margin. Prominent laminar wedge (arrow 1) and solar penetration. White line at toe very wide with foreign matter wedged into it (arrow 2)

414 Laminitis (chronic) (turkish slippers).
Note: Excessive growth of horn at heels with slower than normal growth at toe. The white line was very wide with grit etc wedged into it. Pedal bone rotation of 15˚.

Death occurs in some of the most severe cases, often as a result of both the underlying disease and/or the laminitis itself. Focal laminitis, which affects limited areas of the laminae of the foot, may arise following focal trauma to the hoof wall and is also a complication of proliferative or septic endocarditis (*see* **300** *et seq.*). In the latter, the lameness may be mild and transient affecting any foot depending on the effect and extent of thromboembolic occlusion of minor end arterioles in the sensitive laminae. Under these conditions the horse shows characteristic shifting-leg lameness, but the underlying cardiac and circulatory signs may be more important and more obvious. In some cases however, the lameness and foot discomfort is the first sign noticed.

Horses recovering from an acute episode of laminitis, and those in which repeated mild episodes have occurred, may be found to be suffering from chronic forms of the disorder. In these cases the changes are usually milder and somewhat less painful. Superimposed acute episodes may occur at any stage. The chronic form is characterised by pedal bone rotation, a compensatory thickening of the dorsal hoof wall caused by excessive growth of laminae to form a laminar wedge, a convex sole (*see* **413**) and dramatic widening of the white line at toe. Diverging rings on the hoof wall, in which the spaces between the rings at the heel are wider than those at the toe (*see* **499**), will often be found. A typical heel-toe gait is present, although the extent of this depends largely upon the severity of the disease at the time of examination. Persistent heel walking, together with a faster hoof growth at the heels than at the toes, often results in the development of long overgrown 'Turkish-slippers', in which the walls of the hoof adopt a tubular form (**414**). The extent of chronic (and acute) changes

in laminitis may be quantified radiographically by using a protractor to measure the pedal bone rotation. The prognosis may be assessed from this and the extent of the lameness. The thickness of the dorsal wall may also be indicative of the chronicity of the particular case. Horses which suffer from repeated episodes of laminitis related to diet or to other environmental or management factors remain liable to it and their prognosis depends heavily upon the care and attention provided both to the feet and to the underlying causes.

Selenium toxicosis in horses results from the over-administration of dietary supplements or, more often, from ingestion of plants (such as *Astragalus bisulcatus*, *Morinda reticulata* and *Stanleya pinnata*) which concentrate selenium from the soil. Affected horses show hair loss (*see* **359, 360**) and marked effects upon the quality of the hoof wall. Horizontal 'growth lines' (*see* **499**) and coronary separation typical of severe chronic laminitis are usually present (*see* **498**).

'Seedy toe' is a common secondary effect of the widening of the white line and the heel-toe action of laminitic horses, which tends to force the dorsal hoof wall away from the sole still further, and may represent a serious secondary consequence of laminitis (*see* **413**). In some cases the disorder develops without any laminitic complications and small pieces of grit or other foreign matter is progressively wedged into the white line. Pressure and subsequent infection may cause moderate or severe lameness. The normally thin white line becomes separated, and foreign material is forced into the space by the pressure of the weight of the horse. Any conditions which result in widening of this zone, or which tends to force the two structures apart, such as overgrown toes (*see* **415**) and laminitis (*see* **413**), will

415

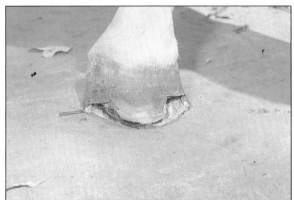

417

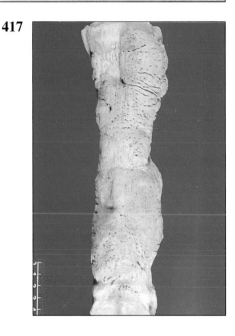

416

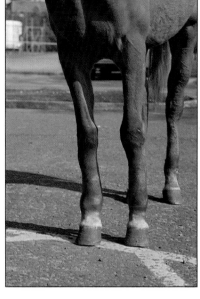

415 Seedy Toe.
Note: Breaking away of dorsal hoof wall and foreign matter wedged in between the sensitive and horny laminae. Horn quality was poor and responded to careful farriery and biotin and methionine supplementation

416 Hypertrophic osteopathy (Marie's Disease).
Note: Symmetrical enlargement of long bones. Lesions were painful on palpation. No thoracic lesions were found at post mortem examination.
Differential Diagnosis:
i) Fluorosis

417 Hypertrophic osteopathy (Marie's Disease) (same case as **416**).
Note: Irregular new bone growth particularly at the distal and proximal ends of the cannon bone. No joint involvement.

predispose to the development of the so-called 'seedy toe' (**415**). The condition is readily recognised when an affected foot is prepared. Although the lesion may appear to be of minor consequence, the extent to which the foreign material penetrates between the hoof wall and the sensitive laminae is often considerable. The full damage may often only be appreciated by lateral radiographs of the foot.

While most seedy toe cases are a result of laminitis or of poor hoof care, poor hoof quality is a contributing factor in some cases as well as in other hoof wall defects such as sandcracks. The quality of the hoof wall varies widely. Some hooves are inordinately soft and more elastic than normal, while others are very hard, brittle and flaky (*see* **415**). In either case, it may be difficult to establish the cause of the problem, but nutritional

deficiencies of vitamins (such as methionine and/or biotin) and essential oils may be responsible. Shoe retention in these horses is often poor, with a tendency for the hoof wall to crack away from the retaining nails.

Hypertrophic osteopathy (Marie's Disease, pulmonary osteopathy) is an unusual disorder of the horse characterised by progressive symmetrical, proliferative, periosteal new bone formation. The long bones of the limbs are most often and most obviously affected (**416**), but the axial skeleton and skull may also show similar changes, although these are often more difficult to demonstrate. While the disease is well recognised in other domestic animals, as a result of pulmonary or other intrathoracic pathology, often the condition in the horse is not accompanied by any obvious underlying disease. However, some cases are

418
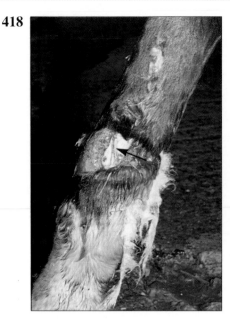

419
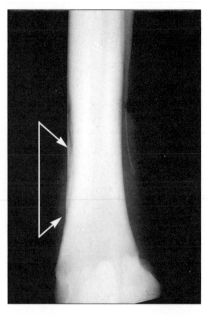

418 Periosteal injury (medial distal cannon).
Note: Due to leg being trapped between a gate and the gate post. Arrow indicates likely site of sequestrum development.

419 Bone sequestrum (same horse as **412**, six weeks later).
Note: Sequestrum (arrows). Also fractured lateral splint bone.

found to have long-standing abdominal or thoracic, neoplastic or inflammatory foci; pulmonary tuberculosis or other intrathoracic infections, such as pleuritis, and abdominal or thoracic neoplasia, such as lymphosarcoma, are the most common instigating factors. The clinical signs are related to the underlying cause (if this can be established) and to the periosteal hyperostoses (**417**). The condition is often painful, and particularly so to palpation of the bones. Local edema of soft tissues is commonly present. The radiographic appearance is characteristic, although the extent of the changes is not always marked and some areas may be more affected than others. Some cases apparently resolve spontaneously, while others resolve following satisfactory treatment of any underlying disease processes. However, as many cases have no detectable concurrent disorder which might be responsible, or have serious, untreatable underlying disease, many affected horses gradually, or sometimes rapidly, deteriorate and are then killed.

Disruption of the periosteal blood supply to an area of bone, through direct trauma, may result in the development of a **sequestrum** which, in due course, becomes separated from the underlying healthy bone. This process is much more likely if the wound is open and infected (**418**). Initially the extent of bony damage may appear to be minimal, with apparently insignificant damage to the periosteum, but the consequent sequestrum is often surprisingly large (**419**). The

separation of the piece of necrotic bone may be slow and this is a common possible explanation for failure of apparently minor wounds to heal satisfactorily. Wounds complicated by the presence of necrotic pieces of bone fail to heal, leaving a chronic discharging sinus and/or extensive overlying exuberant granulation tissue in which deep clefts can often be seen. Unless the offending sequestrum is sloughed out naturally or removed, the wound will continue to discharge, in spite of the best efforts of the attending physician and the use of potent antibiotics.

The foot of the horse is subject to a wide range of traumatic disorders. The horn of the hoof is frequently **avulsed**, as a result of **wire injuries** in particular, and while the appearance of such an injury is often alarming (**420**), provided that the coronary band and underlying structures of the foot are unaffected, the outlook is generally fair. Over-reach injuries in the region of the bulb of the heel may tear the heel away from the underlying tissue (**421**), but in many cases the area is only bruised. Repeated damage of this type results in marked thickening of the skin, and often some degree of **ossification** of the underlying **collateral cartilages** (*see* **422**). Damage to the horn and skin over the heels often results in separation, and the ingress of infection.

Ossification of the collateral cartilages of the forefeet ('**Sidebone**') (**422**) is most often encountered in horses with poor digit conformation, but is a common finding in apparently normal, heavy-draught horses.

420

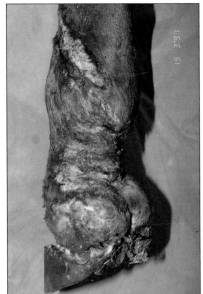

421

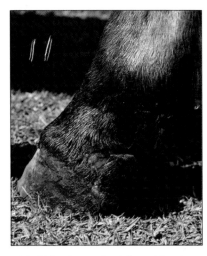

420 'Wire laceration' (lateral heel, pastern and cannon). **Note:** 12 year old Quarterhorse stallion. Hoof sloughed but after 18 months treatment the stallion returned to stud duties.

421 Over-reach Injury.

422

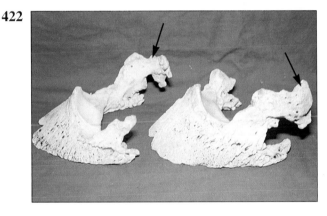

422 Sidebone (bilateral). **Note:** Lateral cartilages (arrows) affected worse in a heavy draught horse with a base narrow posture. Condition very easily palpated and obvious radiographically.

Base-narrow horses (ie those whose feet are close together while having a normal chest width), and base-wide horses, are prone to developing unilateral sidebones on the lateral and medial collateral cartilages respectively. Horses with very upright digit postures also show a relatively high incidence of lateral cartilage ossification. Direct damage to the cartilages by wire cuts (*see* **420**) or over-reaching injuries (*see* **421**) may also result, ultimately, in the development of sidebone. Sidebones are rarely encountered in the hind feet except following traumatic injuries. Ossification of the lateral cartilages, itself, is unlikely to be a primary cause of lameness, but the changes may arise as a consequence of underlying pathology of which lameness is an integral feature. Clinically, affected horses have prominent collateral cartilage(s) on the affected side(s) of the foot, often being palpable above the coronet and obvious radiographically in both dorso-palmar and latero-medial projections.

Traumatic injuries to the heels, and particularly when these include injuries to the lateral cartilages, result in gross deformities of the foot in the most protracted cases (**423**). These arise as a result of failure to use the heel of the foot during walking and consequent heel contraction, as well as horn growth defects arising from coronary band damage (*see* **490**). The consequent foot distortions are often severe (*see* **423, 491**), although in many cases the disability is surprisingly limited.

Hoof defects, arising from damage to the germinative tissue at the coronet, are common consequences of trauma at this site. Although the coronary band injury may seem relatively innocuous the resultant hoof defect ('**Sand Crack**') may extend from the coronet to the solar margin and persist for life (*see* **492**). In many cases, abnormal movement between the two sides of the crack results in persistent inflammation in the underlying sensitive laminae and infection is a common sequel. Affected horses often suffer from chronic intermittent lameness and repeated localised infective foci.

423
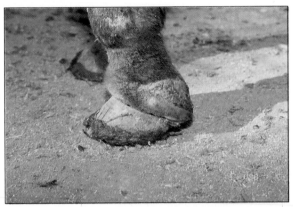

424
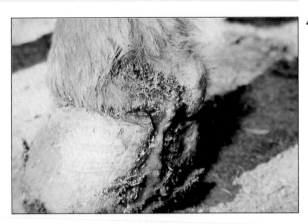

423 Foot injury (wire wound).
Note: Repair complicated by deep and superficial flexor tendon contracture.

424 Quittor (infection/necrosis of lateral cartilage).
Note: Lesion was present without alteration for 12 months. No apparent lameness.

Infectious Disorders

Bacterial Diseases: Bacterial infection and/or necrosis of the collateral cartilages ('Quittor') results in a chronic discharging sinus above the coronet on the affected side **(424)**. Gross foot deformities with coronary band defects result from a very long-standing, non-healing damage to the cartilages, with severe consequences upon the other structures of the foot. In spite of a relatively small drainage sinus, the extent of damage to the cartilage may be considerable and in some cases the entire cartilage is affected. Palpation of the affected area is usually painful, but in long-standing cases this may not be so. Likewise lameness may be mild or marked, and some cases may show little or no evidence of the condition for months or even years. The prognosis for horses affected by necrotic infected lateral cartilages depends largely upon the extent of the infection. They seldom resolve without aggressive surgical treatment and indeed may extend quickly into the underlying distal interphalangeal (coffin) joint and/or digital sheath. In these circumstances the outlook becomes dramatically worse. A diagnosis may be assisted by radiographic examination of the area with a metal probe inserted into the draining tract and by sampling fluid from the adjacent synovial structures.

Ill-fitting shoes, or an over-long interval between shoeing, may result in excessive pressure being applied over the 'seat-of-corn' (that portion of the sole between the bars and the wall of the hoof) and the development of a foot 'corn'. As the hoof grows, the heel of the shoe is drawn forward and medially, to lie directly over the sensitive tissue rather than over the wall of the hoof **(425)**. Pressure at this site frequently causes bruising **(bruised heel/corn)**, which may be obvious when the foot is cleaned and prepared **(426)**. Sustained damage, associated with the accumulation of foreign matter such as sand particles and bedding between the sole and the shoe, may allow the site to become infected **(infected/septic corn) (427)**. Typically, these 'corns' are very painful. If they are neglected, infection may result in extensive tracking into the soft tissues of the foot and ultimately present with a discharging sinus at the coronet or, as is more often the case with 'corns', over the bulb of the heel.

Poor hoof care and persistently wet conditions underfoot, particularly associated with wet, deep-litter bedding systems, often permit the development of a necrotic, foul-smelling bacterial infection of the clefts and central sulcus of the frog known as '**thrush**'. The region is poorly ventilated and bacteria, such as *Spherophorus (Fusobacterium) necrophorum*, multiply readily in the deepest crevices of the clefts of the frog. Characteristically, affected horses are not lame in the early stages, but foul-smelling black or grey necrotic hoof material can be found deep in the clefts. The infection may ultimately penetrate into the soft tissues of the foot, and result in a dramatic lameness and extensive under-running and separation of the sole. More serious deep infection, involving the deep structures of the foot, may also develop, resulting in severe foot sepsis. Infection of the deeper structures of the foot, such as the distal interphalangeal (coffin) joint,

425

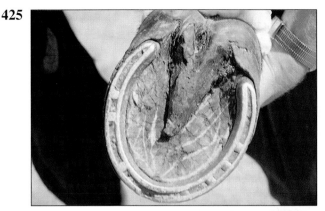

426

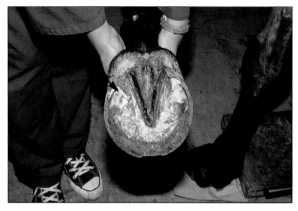

427

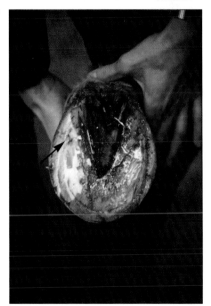

425 Poor Shoe Fit.
Note: Heel not supported and foot growth has dragged the heel of the shoe over the 'seat of corn'. Horse was lame until shoe removed.

426 Corn (same horse as **419**).
Note: Bruising in lateral heel (arrow).

427 Septic corn
Note: Purulent discharge from 'seat of corn' after exploring painful focus (arrow). Discharging tract was present at bulb of heel.

and extensive bone degeneration, may develop as a result of extension of the infection leading to even more serious consequences.

Foreign body penetration of the sole is a very common problem in the horse. The consequences range from insignificant to life threatening and such penetrations are almost always infected. The specific location of the foreign body, its length and its nature have an important bearing upon the prognosis and subsequent treatment. **Puncture wounds of the sole** may cause osteitis, fracture or necrosis of the digital cushion or third phalanx (with possible sequestration). Penetrations at the white line are frequently associated with infections which track up the wall and produce a discharging sinus at the coronet. The middle third of the sole and particularly the area around the frog at this site **(428)** is perhaps the most dangerous area for penetrations by sharp foreign bodies such as nails, thorns and glass shards. The underlying deep digital flexor tendon and its sheath and the navicular bone and its bursa are most liable to infection as a result. Deeper penetration results in infective contamination of the distal interphalangeal (fetlock) joint. The only protective mechanism for these structures is the dense fibroelastic digital cushion and the frog itself. Penetrations may appear to be innocuous initially but the consequences are possibly extremely serious. These include infectious tenosynovitis of the digital sheath and infection of the navicular bursa and/or the coffin joint. Infection within any of these synovial structures carries a poor or very poor prognosis. This is often associated with infective osteitis of the navicular bone **(429)** or fractures of the navicular bone **(430)**. Horses with serious penetrating wounds of the sole usually show immediate lameness but, particularly where the foreign body is no longer present this may be slight or even inapparent until infection is well established and is by then, commonly life-threatening. Severe lameness with or without

428

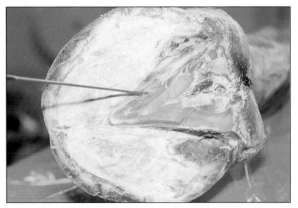

428 Solar penetration (middle third of frog).
Note: Nail removed immediately three days previously. Probe could be passed approximately 3cm into tract. No apparent discharge but severe lameness.

429

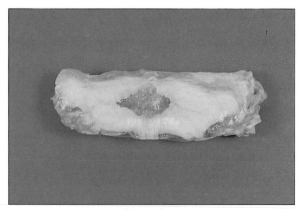

429 Septic osteitis of navicular bone (same horse as **428**).

430

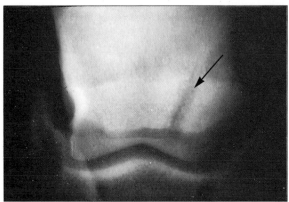

430 Fractured navicular bone (arrow) (60°dorsoproximal oblique radiograph).
Note: Due to penetrating nail 5 days previously

431

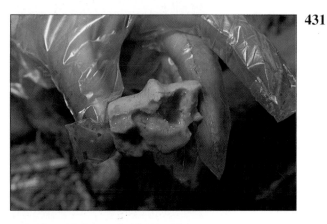

431 Physeal abscess (with joint ill).
Note: Septicemic salmonellosis in 40 day old foal. Severe osteolysis and erosion into fetlock joint.

draining sinuses at the coronet following sole penetration(s) should be regarded extremely seriously and every effort should be made immediately to explore the full extent of the problem.

Bacterial infections of the bones, as a result of hematogenous spread or direct introduction of bacteria, result in **osteomyelitis** when the infection involves the cortex and the medullary cavity or **infective osteitis** when it arises from the outer surface of the bone. The former is most often encountered in septicemic conditions of foals (*see* **433**), when **metaphyseal abscesses** develop with extensive local bone destruction. Active and severe infection at this site often extends to the growth plate, and the adjacent joint resulting in **septic arthritis (431)**. In other circumstances the development of osteomyelitis is usually a result of open fractures, and it represents an unfortunate sequel to

internal fixation of fractures. **Infective osteitis** commonly occurs in the extremities, possibly as a result of the paucity of overlying, protective soft tissues. Damage and infection of the periosteum (*see* **418**) may result in loss of vitality of the bone and sequestrum formation (*see* **419**). It is sometimes difficult to establish whether infection is a major aspect of the formation of sequestra and most such lesions are probably caused by vascular compromise resulting from periosteal damage/ separation.

Infection of joints and other synovial structures, such as tendon sheaths and bursae, represents a very serious and common clinical problem. Gross, open articular wounds are an obvious site for entry of bacteria as a result of damage to joint capsule pouches and tendon sheaths **(432)**. However, relatively small innocuous-looking wounds at sites which might not,

432

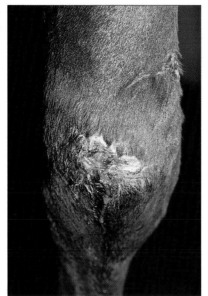

433

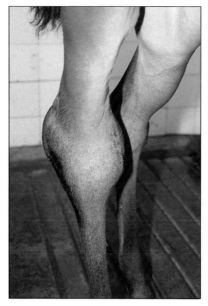

432 Open carpus joint.
Note: Small amounts of synovial fluid.
Generalised swelling of joint.

433 Joint ill (infective arthritis of hock) (septicemic sequestration).
Differential Diagnosis:
i) Osteochondrosis (osteochondritis dissecans)
ii) Bog spavin
iii) Periarticular infection

ordinarily, suggest involvement of the joint or tendon sheath, may result in an extremely serious synovial infection. Egress of synovial fluid (*see* **432**), even in very small amount, indicates that a synovial structure is open, and is therefore almost certainly infected. Sequestration of blood-borne bacteria into the synovial structures is relatively common, particularly in the foal. (*see* **433**). Iatrogenic septic arthritis or tenosynovitis are common sequels to contaminated intra-synovial injections (particularly when these include cortico-steroids or local anesthetic drugs) and/or aspiration of synovial fluid. Initially, lameness associated with joint infection may be mild, but it rapidly progresses to a total, non-weight-bearing lameness. Infected joints become grossly swollen by synovial effusion (**433**), hot and painful, and, in foals, systemic illness with fever, inappetence and depression are common. Swelling of the periarticular soft tissues is frequently present (**434**) which may be somewhat misleading unless the underlying synovial structure can be assessed accurately. Some joints such as the hock, shoulder and carpus are

particularly painful when infected, and dramatic weight loss, sweating and recumbency may be associated with this. Synovial fluid obtained from infected joints or tendon sheaths is turbid and contains large numbers of inflammatory cells, a high protein concentration and, often, obvious floccules of proteinaceous matter. Long-standing cases show extensive periarticular fibrosis and new bone formation with destruction of articular surfaces and underlying bone which is obvious radiographically.

Infection of synovial structures is always extremely serious, and without prompt, aggressive treatment the prognosis for return to normal function is, at best, poor. The identification of synovial fluid in the discharge from a wound is not always easy and it may be confused with partially clotted plasma and serum. Progressive changes in the synovial fluid may provide an accurate index of the progression or resolution of joint infection and inflammation. Radiographic evidence of cartilage or bone destruction is particularly serious and indicates the likely rapid development of degenerative joint disease (*see* **402**).

434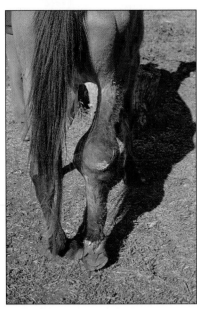

435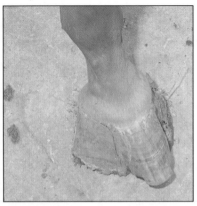

434 Septic arthritis (chronic).
Note: Extensive peri-articular fibrosis.

435 Keratoma.
Note: Deformity of dorsal hoof wall.

Neoplastic Disorders

Neoplastic diseases of the bones and joints of the horse are particularly rare when compared to other domestic animals.

A **keratoma** is a horn tumour which develops in the inner aspect of the hoof wall. The growth may vary in diameter from a few millimetres up to 2–3 centimetres. Some extend only a short way up the hoof wall while others reach from coronet to sole. While some are regular and cylindrical in shape, others are triangular, and still others are irregular. They may be the result of chronic irritation at the coronary band or within the laminae, but some develop without any apparent reason. While many are present for prolonged periods without causing any discomfort, others cause lameness from pressure on the underlying sensitive laminae of the foot. The hoof wall often has an abnormal shape (**435**) and, while most occur at the toe (*see* **435**), they commonly develop in the quarters (**436**). They are frequently difficult to identify clinically, and relatively innocuous distortions of the white line at the site (*see* **436**) may be the only indication of a problem. In some cases fistulous tracts extend between the coronet and the toe along the lesion and these are the animals which show the most dramatic consequent lameness. Radiographically, a characteristic appearance is seen, with a well defined area of resorption of the underlying pedal bone.

436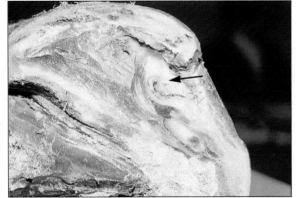

436 Keratoma.
Note: Defect at white line (arrow).

Tendons, Ligaments, and Bursae

Non-Infectious Disorders

The tendons, ligaments and bursae of the horses are subjected to considerable forces in the course of natural movement, and the uses to which the horse is put and its management make diseases and disorders of these structures relatively common. Many of the conditions relate directly to trauma or to excessive tension, and there is, therefore, an almost infinite variety of possibilities. The clinical consequences of the traumatic rupture or straining of a tendon or ligament are directly dependent upon the function of that structure and the extent of the damage.

Rupture of the common digital extensor tendon occurs most frequently as a bilateral condition in neonatal foals (*see* **381**), when the condition is obvious at or immediately after birth. Acquired rupture occurs at any time after birth and is commonly sited within the tendon sheath, and it shows immediately as a fluctuant swelling over the dorso-lateral aspect of the carpus (**437**). While in some cases the swelling may be the most obvious sign, there is often an extreme compensatory over-flexion of the carpus and fetlock as a result of secondary over-contraction of the flexor tendons (*see* **381**). In other cases, the rupture appears to be secondary to existing flexural deformities resulting in excessive tension on the extensor tendons. Careful examination

should permit identification of the disrupted and distracted ends of the extensor tendon in the sheath and ultrasonographic examination may be particularly useful in identifying the site of the disruption. Other developmental defects including carpal and tarsal collapse may be encountered at the same time.

Rupture of the *extensor carpi radialis* tendon in adult horses also occurs. Many cases are the direct consequence of trauma, with over flexion of the carpus being the most likely factor. Others may be a residual effect of rupture at a younger age but often no etiology can be established. In these cases the clinical signs are less obvious, with subtle gait changes and local swelling of the tendon sheath. However, it is often possible to see the ends of the tendon, as fluid accumulations are frequently minimal, particularly where the condition has been present for some time (**438**). Long standing cases show a marked and distinctive atrophy of the *extensor carpi radialis* muscle on the dorsum of the forearm (**438**). Ultrasonographic examination may be used to good effect in the diagnosis of the condition and the location of the distracted ends of the tendon. The prognosis for these animals is reasonable with many performing reasonably well and adapting well to the loss of carpal extension ability.

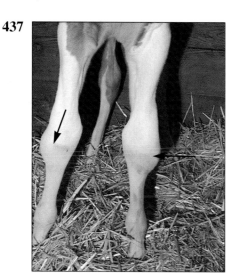

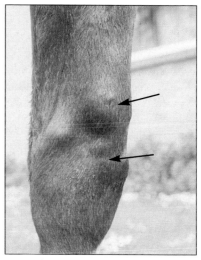

437 Common extensor tendon rupture (bilateral).
Note: Characteristic swelling on dorso-lateral aspect of carpus (arrows).

438 Extensor carpi radialis tendon rupture (old)
Note: Disrupted ends of tendon visible (arrows)(and palpable) and atrophy of the *extensor carpi radialis* muscle giving a hollow appearance to the forearm.

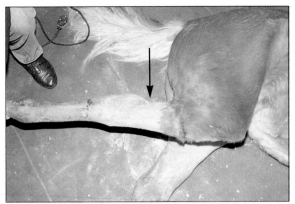

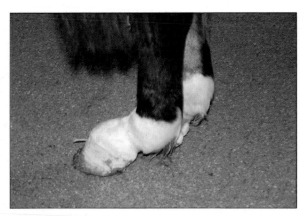

439 Peroneus tertius rupture.
Note: Characteristic ability to extend hock while flexing the stifle. Characteristic dimpling of Achilles tendon (arrow).

440 Superficial digital flexor tendon rupture.
Note: Dropped fetlock with normal foot position relative to the floor. Fetlock does not fall to the floor under weight bearing.

Other tendons in which traumatic rupture occurs relatively commonly include the *gastrocnemius* (Achilles) tendon, the tendon of the *peroneus tertius*, and the superficial flexor tendon of the hind limb. Tendons in which degenerative changes are present, either as a result of infection, disuse, trauma (resulting in edema and hemorrhage within the substance of the tendon), ischemia (secondary to digital neurectomy or from over-tight bandaging), are more liable to rupture than normal healthy tendons. However, it is not always possible to explain tendon ruptures in any of these ways and spontaneous disruption does apparently occur. Direct over extension of the flexor tendons as a result of over extension of the fetlock under racing conditions has been established as a possible cause.

In the hind limb, the origins and insertions of the gastrocnemius and the superficial flexor tendons are closely related. Proximal to the point of the hock the combined structures are known as the common calcanean tendon. Usually the **gastrocnemius tendon ruptures** before the superficial flexor tendon and results in 'dropping' of the hock with excessive angulation at the hock joint. Injuries resulting in **complete severance of the common calcanean tendon ('Hamstring' severance)** have a dramatic effect upon the function of the limb, with severe dropping of the hock and complete inability to bear weight. Bilateral rupture of the common calcanean tendon may occur during extremes of effort and particularly during recovery from falls.

Rupture of the *peroneus tertius* tendon produces a classical clinical syndrome in which the integrity of the reciprocal apparatus, which ensures the normal coordinated flexion of the hock and stifle, is lost. The hock may be extended while the stifle is flexed (**439**).

Whilst this manipulation is performed, a characteristic dimpling of the common calcanean tendon is visible. The condition is encountered after falls at speed, following violent struggles to free a trapped leg or following traumatic injuries to the cranial region of the limb below the stifle. It also occurs relatively frequently following the use of casts extending up to the mid tibia. Horses with a ruptured *peroneus tertius* tendon have a characteristic shuffling gait, in which the foot consistently fails to clear the ground as a result of reduced hock flexion. There is often marked wearing of the toe of the affected leg. In chronic cases little or no pain is usually encountered.

The extensor tendons of both fore and hind limbs are liable to **traumatic division**, often due to wire-laceration injuries, which occur most often on the dorsal aspect of the cannon. While the clinical appearance may be dramatic, the injury has less long-term effect on the gait of the horse than flexor tendon injuries. The inability of the horse to extend the digit may result in stumbling and toe-dragging and the animal may even 'knuckle-over' at the fetlock. Weight bearing is normal once the foot is placed in its natural position, and animals soon learn to compensate for the loss of extensor function by developing a 'flicking' action of the foot during motion.

Spontaneous or traumatic disruption of the superficial flexor tendon of either the fore or the hind limbs results in a dropping of the fetlock under weight bearing, without it touching the ground. The animal maintains a normal hoof position relative to the floor (**440**). Traumatic injuries to the superficial flexor tendon of the fore limb usually occur in the mid cannon region as a result of over-reaching by the hind limb, particularly

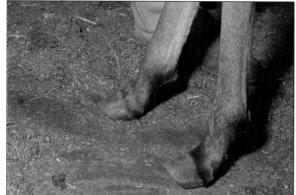

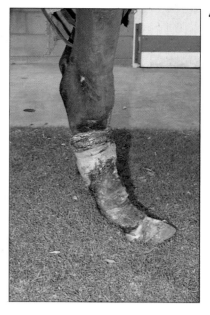

441 Deep digital flexor tendon rupture (spontaneous).
Note: Fetlock in normal position. Toe lifts under weight bearing.

442 Traumatic division of superficial and deep flexor tendons.
Note: Fetlock dropped but does not collapse under weight bearing and toe lifted. Suspensory apparatus intact.

when the latter is shod. This is a relatively common racing injury, and although there may be an apparently minor skin wound, the consequences upon the tendon are usually serious. A similar injury may occur to the hind limb during racing when the fore-foot of a following horse strikes the cannon region of the lead horse. The superficial flexor tendon of the hind limb is often subject to laceration when the horse backs into a sharp object. Under these conditions, the wound is usually obvious and it is complicated by simultaneous damage to the deep flexor tendon and possibly the suspensory ligament.

Traumatic rupture of the deep flexor tendon in the cannon region may occur spontaneously or as a result of lacerations occurring in the mid-cannon or pastern regions. In the latter cases the superficial flexor is necessarily involved. Traumatic laceration of the deep flexor tendon alone, in the palmar/plantar pastern area is a relatively common injury, as a result of stepping onto sharp objects. Although the size of the wound may be small the damage to the underlying tendon (and digital sheath) is often very serious and presents the same signs as rupture of the tendon in the cannon region. Excessive strain may also lead to spontaneous rupture of the deep tendon near its insertion on the third phalanx. However, the cord-like nature of the tendon makes spontaneous rupture less likely than in the superficial tendon and most cases of deep flexor rupture, in the absence of any other injury, are probably secondary to degenerative changes within the tendon substance, either from pre-existing strains, or infection in the tendon itself or in adjacent tissues and synovial structures. Where the

deep flexor tendon, only, is ruptured, the fetlock is maintained in its normal position relative to the leg, but, when the limb bears weight, the toe will be seen to lift off the ground (**441**).

Traumatic severance of both deep and superficial flexor tendons occurs quite frequently in both fore and hind limbs, and is usually the result of lacerations in the mid-cannon region (**442**). In the hind limb, severance above the point of the hock has the same result, and additionally it will result in a loss of hock extension ability. Injuries below the carpus or hock result in a combination of the expected signs, with dropping of the fetlock (which in the absence of simultaneous division of the suspensory ligament does not fall to the ground under load), and lifting of the toe under weight-bearing conditions (*see* **442**).

Complete severance or disruption of all the supporting structures of the palmar/plantar cannon, results in complete collapse of the distal limb. The fetlock falls to the ground when the animal takes weight on the limb and the toe is lifted.

Spontaneous disruption/collapse of the suspensory apparatus alone in the absence of concurrent flexor tendon rupture, with or without concurrent proximal sesamoid fractures, is a common cause of acute breakdown in racing Thoroughbreds and in foals, particularly of heavy breeds. It is usually the result of extreme over-extension of the fetlock, especially where this occurs in conjunction with weakness or disease of the proximal sesamoids or their ligaments. Clinically, the fetlock is grossly swollen, and the horse is severely lame. Weight bearing results in immediate sinking of the

443

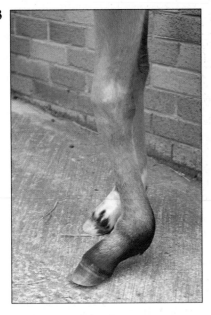

444

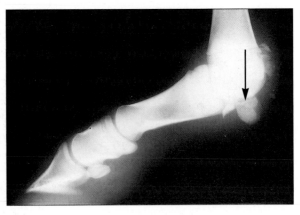

443 Disruption of suspensory apparatus.
Note: Foot and pastern position normal, but fetlock sunken (over-extended), swelling of fetlock region.

444 Disruption of suspensory apparatus.
Note: Abaxial fracture of proximal sesamoids (arrow), over extension of fetlock and subluxation of proximal interphalangeal (pastern) joint.

fetlock to the ground with obvious over-extension but the foot remains in its natural position (**443**). In some cases, the breakdown can result from rupture of the distal sesamoidean ligaments. The loss of the supporting ligaments may result in concurrent subluxation of the pastern joint (**444**). Radiographically the condition has a distinctive appearance and is often associated with (bilateral) abaxial fractures of the sesamoid bones. Concurrent rupture of the digital arteries carries a poor or hopeless prognosis.

Less severe **strains or sprains of the superficial flexor tendon(s)** of the fore-limbs, are extremely common in high-performance horses which work at speed. The resulting strain-induced inflammatory response may affect the body of the tendon (tendinitis), or the tendon and tendon sheath (tendosynovitis) where the sheath is present in the vicinity of the damage. Fatigue and inadequate training may form part of the pathogenesis, and some cases may be due to ischemia in horses exercised with non-elastic or over-tight bandaging. Sudden changes in underfoot conditions may also be responsible in some cases. The mid-cannon region of the superficial flexor tendon is most commonly affected. At this point, the tendon has its least diameter and has no enveloping tendon sheath, and it seems likely that the load per unit area (which is maximal at this point) is of importance in the pathogenesis of the condition. The more proximal damage results in concurrent tendosynovitis of the carpal sheath, while more distal injury affects the digital sheath and the palmar annular ligament. While most superficial flexor tendinitis results from over-stretching, some cases

follow direct blows such as occur in over-reaching injuries. The clinical features will depend upon the extent of the damage, with the mildest forms producing only slight local changes in temperature, mild, localised swelling and correspondingly mild lameness. Some cases may even show no obvious lameness. More severe tendinitis and tendosynovitis is characterised by marked pain, heat, swelling and obvious lameness. During the acute phase the digit is usually rested in partial flexion. Ultrasonographic examination of the acutely inflamed, sprained superficial (or deep) flexor tendon shows a characteristic loss of echogenicity, with non-echoic areas of fluid (either blood or edema) within the substance of the tendon in the affected area (**445**). In the later stages of repair ultrasonographic examination may also be used to detect and assess the extent of adhesions between the flexor tendons and the carpal or digital tendon sheath, which represent one of the more serious consequences of tendosynovitis. The affected tendon can be seen to be grossly swollen (bowed) (*see* **447**). One of the common causes of severe tendinitis of the flexor tendons, and in particular of the superficial flexor tendon, is the use of over-tight bandages, especially where the bandage is placed on a "cold" limb prior to exercise and where the bandage has no innate elasticity. The paucity of soft tissues in the metacarpal area means that swelling of the limb under a non-elastic bandage during exercise results in a marked reduction of blood supply to the skin. The blood supply to the tendon itself may be somewhat less important over short periods but severe ischemic necrosis and extensive sloughing may follow from such a practice (**446**). While the skin might be expected to

445

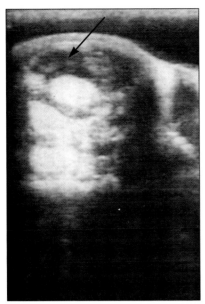

446

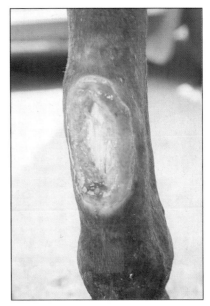

445 Superficial flexor tendonitis (ultrasonographic appearance).
Note: Superficial flexor tendon grossly thickened with fluid and dense fibrous tissue (arrow), lying above normal deep flexor and suspensory (interosseus) ligament. Lesion 3 weeks old.

446 Necrotic tendinitis.
Note: Due to over-tight bandaging during exercise. Healthy granulation tissue and remnants of superficial digital flexor tendon in mid cannon. 8 weeks post injury.

heal rapidly in most circumstances, any damage to the tendons is likely to be slow to appear and extremely slow to heal. Healing can only be expected when no necrotic tendon tissue is present, and any delayed healing in this site may, furthermore, result in exuberant granulation tissue.

Following the acute stages of tendon disorders, extensive scarring develops within the damaged portions, producing the typical **bowed tendon (447)** often encountered in racing horses, and particularly in steeplechasers.

Annular ligament constriction (*see* **457**) may be seen in conjunction with chronic tendinitis in the distal cannon area.

Infected or septic tenosynovitis is extremely serious, and is a frequent consequence of open wounds but is most unusual without such injuries.

Stress injuries may also affect the suspensory ligament, and the check ligament of the deep flexor tendon. **Inflammation of the inferior (accessory, sub-carpal) check ligament** of the deep flexor tendon, results from over-extension of the digit. The characteristic pain, heat and swelling is centred upon the proximal third of the cannon between the suspensory (interosseus) ligament and the deep flexor tendon **(448)**.

Lesser (subclinical) trauma to the flexor tendons,

particularly when this is repeated over extended periods, may induce no detectable changes in the tendons themselves. However, it commonly results in a mild degree of concurrent tenosynovitis, particularly of the digital sheath, which shows as a tense, fluid accumulation within the sheath. Digital tenosynovitis is frequently seen in the hind limbs of jumping horses or hunters, and a characteristic tendinous 'windgall' ('windpuff') may be easily recognised **(449)**. The extent of the filling is defined clearly by the natural extent of the digital sheath, with swelling being obvious between the branches of the suspensory (interosseus) ligament and the superficial flexor tendon, and extending up to the distal third of the cannon bone **(449)**. This swelling should not be confused with that of the palmar pouch of the fetlock joint which lies dorsal (anterior) to the suspensory (interosseus) ligament **(450)**. Horses with a sloping pastern conformation seem particularly prone to tendinous windgalls, and may in addition have a fetlock joint effusion ('articular windgall'). The latter creates a similar fluid filled structure dorsal to the suspensory ligament which does not extend as far proximally as the tendinous windgall. Some horses which have an upright conformation on the hind limbs and/or which have worked particularly hard may have both articular and tendinous windgalls (*see* **450**). The presence of these

447

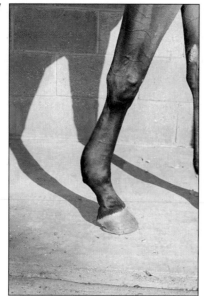

448

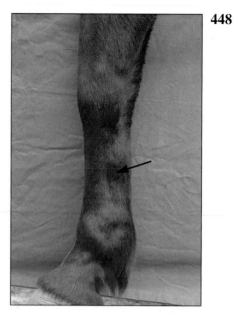

447 Superficial flexor tendonitis (chronic) ('low bow').

448 Proximal (sub-carpal) check ligament desmitis (arrow).

449

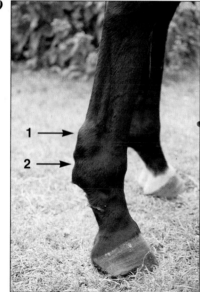

450

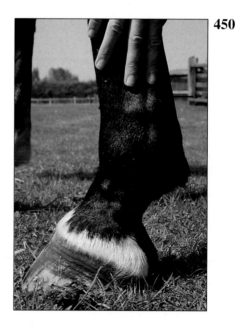

449 Tenosynovitis of digital sheath (mild) ('tendinous windgall', 'windpuff').
Note: Swelling caudal to suspensory ligament and extending up to level of splint button (arrow 1). Well defined cut-off at proximal end and at level of fetlock annular ligament (retinaculum) (arrow 2).

450 Effusion of fetlock joint ('articular windgall') and digital sheath ('tendinous windgall') (mild).
Note: Soft, fluid swellings separated by suspensory ligament. Tendinous windgall filling (below index finger) higher than palmar pouch of fetlock joint (anterior swelling below middle finger).

451

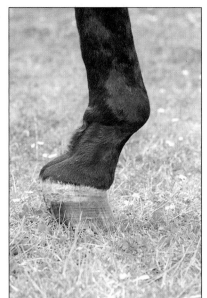

452

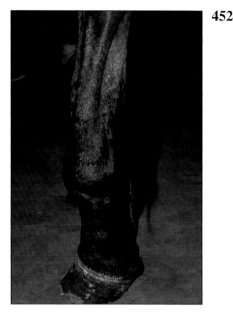

451 Acquired deep flexor tendon contracture with club foot.
Note: Normal fetlock and pastern joint posture.

452 Acquired superficial flexor tendon contracture.
Note: (Near) Normal foot position relative to floor. Fetlock and pastern joints flexed. Increased tension visible in long and lateral extensor tendons.

blemishes does not necessarily relate to lameness and, indeed, many working horses are so affected without any history of any lameness or weakness associated with the limbs.

Injuries involving the flexor tendons and their related check ligaments and tendon sheaths, chronic heel pain with consequent reluctance or inability to place weight on the heels, or disruption of the extensor tendons, may result in an **acquired flexor tendon contracture**. Most such cases involve the deep flexor tendon and the consequences may be a severe, function-limiting, flexion of the distal inter-phalangeal joint and the development of a club foot (**451**). In such cases the pastern conformation is usually normal (unless the superficial flexor tendon is simultaneously affected). Where the superficial flexor is affected on its own, the fetlock joint is held in an abnormally flexed position, and the pastern may be seen to be upright while the foot remains relatively normal in its relationship with the ground (**452**). The extensor tendons are often then under considerable tension and may rupture spontaneously allowing a severe fetlock flexion to develop (**453**). Where both tendons are affected simultaneously, both conformational defects will be present and result in a severe and often irresolvable malformation. Acquired ruptures or lacerations of the extensor tendons commonly result in secondary contraction of the flexor structures and often, the consequent flexion of the

fetlock joint is extremely serious (*see* **453**). Many of the acquired flexural deformities are slow to develop and, while they are often treatable in the early stages, severe and long-standing contractures may be irresolvable. The consequences of a grossly abnormal foot posture in particular are far-reaching with permanent deformity of the internal structures of the foot.

Dislocation of the superficial flexor tendon from the summit of the *tuber calcis* (luxation of the superficial flexor tendon) is a common injury, particularly of jumping horses. The dislocation occurs when the medial attachments of the tendon over the point of the hock (which appear to be weaker than the lateral attachments) rupture and allow the tendon to move laterally. Severe swelling, particularly over the point of the hock, occurs immediately, and it may be difficult to establish the diagnosis in the early stages without recourse to ultrasonography. The condition may be confused with a severe 'capped hock' (*see* **460**) but, when the swelling subsides, the tendon can always be identified visually or by palpation, lying over the lateral aspect of the calcaneus (**454**). The tendon can usually be restored to its normal position with the hock in extension, but it immediately displaces again on flexion. Initially, affected horses may be severely lame, but with prolonged rest they may regain some semblance of normality. The condition is sometimes accompanied by fractures of the calcaneus (fibular tarsal bone), and both

453

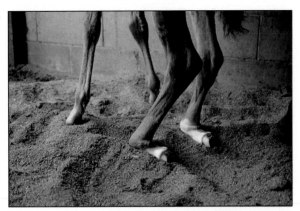

453 (Bilateral) severe contraction of flexor tendons (associated with rupture of extensor tendons).

454 Lateral luxation of superficial flexor tendon.
Note: Superficial flexor displaced laterally (arrow). Prominent proximal extremity of fibular tarsal bone (calcaneus). Minimal swelling indicating chronic lesion.

454

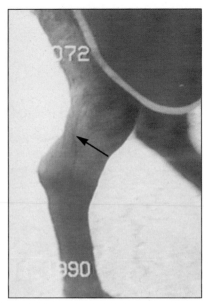

455

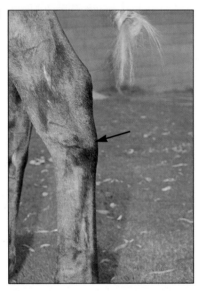

455 Desmitis of plantar ligament of the hock (curb).
Note: Swelling on plantaro-lateral aspect of hock at level of chestnut (arrow). 'Sickle-hocked' conformation.

radiographic and ultrasonographic examination should be employed to establish the extent of the damage in acute cases. Occasionally the lateral supporting band is affected, and the displacement is medial and these cases have a markedly worse prognosis.

Sprains of the plantar ligament of the hock ('**Curb**') are commonly encountered in horses with poor hind limb conformation. Typically affected horses have a 'sickle-hocked' and 'cow-hocked' appearance. An excessive angle of the hocks while at rest and outward rotation of the stifles results in a marked, persistent increase in the tension applied to the plantar structures of the hock, and in particular to the plantar ligament. In foals, this posture may be the result of a partial or complete collapse of the central and/or third tarsal bone(s) (*see* **377**). The clinical appearance of inflammation of the plantar ligament is termed a 'curb', and is manifest by an obvious swelling on the caudo-lateral aspect of the hock at the same level as the chestnut (**455**). Initially the condition is painful and obvious signs of inflammation are present. However, this stage is often missed, and a dense fibrous swelling at the site is more usually encountered. The clinical appearance is characteristic and while most are regarded as blemishes, underlying conformational problems may be serious with respect to the work capacity of the horse.

456

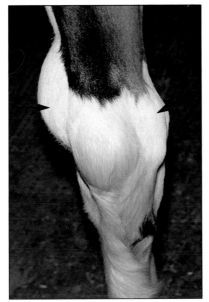

457

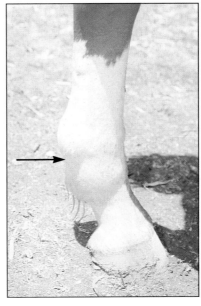

456 Distension of tarsal sheath ('Thoroughpin').
Note: (Communicating) Swellings lateral and medial aspects just anterior to point of hock (arrows).
Differential Diagnosis:
i)   Tenosynovitis of deep flexor tendon and sheath
ii) New bone formation on *sustentaculum tali*
iii) Bog spavin (distension of the tibio-tarsal joint)
iv) Septic arthritis of tibio-tarsal joint

457 Contracture of palmar annular ligament of the fetlock (annular ligament syndrome).
Note: Notched appearance on palmar aspect of fetlock (arrow) above the ergot created by combination of ligament contraction and by effusion in digital sheath.
Differential Diagnosis:
i) Bowed tendon (low) (tendinitis)
ii) Severe tenosynovitis of digital sheath.

 Gross distension of a synovial sheath, as a result of idiopathic tenosynovitis, in the absence of any apparent pain or lameness, or obvious outward sign of inflammation, occurs in the sheath of both the common digital extensor tendon over the carpus (particularly of foals) and in the tarsal sheath. The tarsal sheath surrounds the deep digital flexor tendon of the hind limb, and idiopathic synovitis of this results in gross distension which is known as 'Thoroughpin'. Whatever the cause of the tenosynovitis, there is a similar large, tense, fluid distension, both medially and laterally, dorsal to the calcaneus (**456**). Pressure applied to the swelling on one side will result in corresponding enlargement of the other, confirming that the two are interconnected. 'Thoroughpin', is significantly different from the swelling found in chronic distension of the tibio-tarsal joint (Bog spavin) (*see* **399**), in which the swelling is lower and pouches antero-medially. A similar appearance is, however, present when the *sustentaculum tali* develops a rough new-bone surface. The consequent physical damage results in secondary chronic tenosynovitis and the tarsal canal itself also becomes narrowed, thus emphasising the extent of the tendon sheath distension. While, in most idiopathic cases, the onset of the distension may be insidious and

lameness is then unusual, the chronic tenosynovitis as a result of **degenerative changes on the *sustentaculum tali*** is almost always very painful. The condition is refractory to treatment and the horse is consequently permanently lame. It is of importance therefore to establish the presence or absence of these changes by use of radiographic projections which 'skyline' the *sustentaculum tali* including the planterolateral-dorsomedial oblique and the planteroproximal-planterodistal (flexed) views. Ultrasonographic examination is also particularly useful where there is generalised swelling which makes palpation difficult.

 The **annular ligament of the fetlock** is a tough, fibrous and thickened portion of the fascial sheath and forms a tight retaining structure around the palmar (plantar) aspect of the fetlock, known as the palmar (plantar) retinaculum. The ligament is sufficiently dense and inelastic to prevent any enclosed structure from swelling significantly and, therefore, damage to, and swelling of, the enclosed tendons may result in ischemia of those structures. Any trauma resulting in contraction of the annular ligament of the fetlock might therefore be expected to have marked effects upon the enclosed tendons - even when these are, themselves, normal. Tendinitis of the superficial flexor tendon in the area of

458

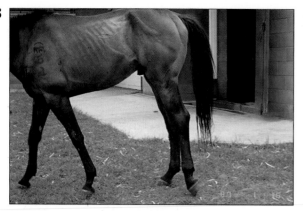

459

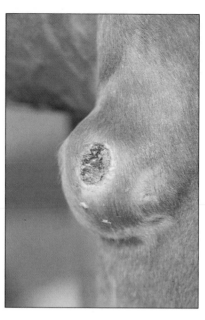

458 Upward fixation of patella.
Note: Limb locked in extension as the horse attempts to draw the limb forward. Flexed fetlock and pastern while stifle and hock joints are fixed in extension.

459 Olecranon bursitis (Capped elbow, Shoe boil).
Note: Prominent swelling over point of elbow. Note wound from persistent shoe pressure during recumbency.

the distal cannon or any direct trauma to the palmar (plantar) aspect of the fetlock may result in scarring and constriction of the annular ligament and an effective narrowing of the fetlock canal. The result is a continuing cycle of damage and healing, and continued contraction. Horses affected by **annular ligament constriction** are often lame. The lameness will usually become worse with exercise as the tendons become warm and swell (even slightly). Local anesthetic agents injected aseptically into the digital sheath often result in a temporary abolition of most of the lameness. Long-standing, idiopathic annular ligament constriction, and that which arises secondarily to tendinitis, often results in adhesions between the tendons, the digital sheath and the annular ligament. In nearly all cases there will be an obvious distension of the digital sheath proximal to the annular ligament, and in some cases the superficial flexor tendon will be thickened (either as a result of the condition or as part of its etiology). These changes can often be identified by ultrasonographic examination. When viewed laterally, the fetlock often has an obvious notch, which is further emphasised by the fluid distension of the tendon sheath above it (**457**).

Swelling of the flexor tendons in the carpal sheath or contraction of the carpal retinaculum (often secondary to an accessory carpal bone fracture) may result in a similar problem on the palmar aspect of the carpus. This is frequently referred to as the **carpal tunnel syndrome**.

Upward fixation of the patella occurs when the stifle joint is fully extended and is encountered particularly in stabled horses which on rising, extend one or other leg backward in a stretching effort. Also, horses having a 'straight' hind-leg conformation (straighter than normal at the stifle and hock) show a high predisposition to partial, or complete, upward fixation of the patella. However, in some cases, trauma, lack of muscular fitness, and poor body condition may also be significant. The disorder is characterised by an abrupt, momentary or complete, recurrent locking of the limb in an extended position (**458**). The stifle and hock cannot flex but the fetlock is normal, although usually the fetlock is flexed with the toe resting on the ground (*see* **458**). Momentary, milder forms of the condition are manifest by an apparent 'catching' or clicking of the stifle during movement without the limb becoming fixed in extension. These cases will often be noted to drag the toe and will invariably be reluctant to walk up and down slopes. At the trot, the foot may be seen to hesitate momentarily, as it leaves the ground. In some cases the signs are very intermittent and/or subtle. The 'locking' may only be shown for limited numbers of strides, the gait then becoming quite normal. In cases of complete fixation release of the entrapped medial patella ligament from the medial trochlear groove is often accompanied by an audible snapping sound. The condition is commonly bilateral, although one side may be more severely affected than the other. The clinical features of the disorder are almost pathognomonic and section of the medial patellar ligament results in a dramatic and complete resolution, although in so doing any underlying conformational abnormality is not corrected.

460 Capped hock (traumatic bursitis). **460**

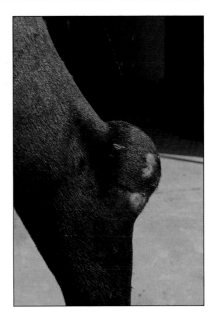

In those young horses in which the condition develops as a result of loss of muscular condition a conservative approach involving muscle toning and fitness, is sometimes effective.

Synovial bursae occurring naturally, or those acquired in response to persistent insult, act as cushions between two moving parts, or at points of unusual pressure, such as between bony prominences and tendons. Naturally formed bursae are present in constant positions and are present before birth, while the acquired bursae are usually formed subcutaneously over bony prominences such as the olecranon and the calcaneus (*tuber calcis*). The formation of an **acquired bursa** is usually in response to persistent pressure over bony prominences and, although they may be large, they are seldom inflamed under normal circumstances.

Acquired subcutaneous bursae commonly develop over the olecranon (**459**) of draught breeds in particular, a condition known as 'capped elbow'. In some cases, the skin over the area is traumatised and the acquired bursa may become infected ('**shoe boil**') (**459**). The small natural bursa which lies under the tendon of the *triceps brachii* muscle is seldom affected. In most cases these are formed in response to direct trauma - often from the shoe or hoof when the animal is lying down. Horses which remain recumbent for any reason are also liable to the development of this bursa. Gaited or Standardbred horses may cause damage to this area during exercise.

A large acquired **carpal bursa** often develops as a result of direct and repeated trauma, associated with lying down on hard surfaces such as concrete or from habitual banging of the knee onto stable doors. At this site the skin overlying the bursal swelling is usually thickened, and the lining of the bursa may become thickened giving a firm, rather than a fluid-filled, texture.

Another common site for acquired bursa formation is over the point of the hock ('**capped hock**') (**460**). Again, this is usually the result of trauma from kicking out against a wall or trailer tailgate, and may develop very rapidly. Although in some cases there is a transient mild lameness, most are not lame. Occasionally they arise without any obvious predisposing cause at sites in which traumatic injuries are not common and no surface evidence for trauma can be found. These may be a result of leakage of synovial fluid from adjacent joints or tendon sheaths, and may reach considerable size. Acquired superficial bursae are seldom painful and, unless they attain great size, or become infected, they remain cold and painless. Bursae of this type are very difficult to treat effectively. In the event, that they become infected and/or burst, they often fail to heal, discharging copious amounts of infected fluid and may then become significant causes of lameness. Exuberant granulation tissue is a common sequel.

Inflammation of deep bursae (bursitis), such as that under the tendon of origin of the *Biceps brachii* tendon are much more painful than the acquired superficial bursae, possibly because of their (usually) deep location and their cushioning function. **Bicipital bursitis** is most often encountered in draught horses with ill-fitting collars and are probably the result of direct trauma and persistent pressure. Like most other deep bursae there are few outward signs of the problem although lameness is often marked.

Infectious Disorders

Bacterial Diseases: Infection involving tendons and tendon sheaths is a relatively common clinical problem associated with wounds, particularly of the distal limb (*see* **446**).

Inflammation of bursae, in response to infection or trauma, results in bursitis. Infection of natural bursae is more unusual because they usually have deeper locations. However the **atlantal bursa**, which lies between the *ligamentum nuchae* and the *rectus capitis dorsalis major* muscle, is liable to both aseptic inflammation and to infection, either spontaneously or more commonly from wounds in the poll area, a condition known as '**poll evil**'. Initially the bursa is swollen, the head is held extended, and movement of the head and neck is strongly resisted. Persistent inflammation of the bursa results in progressive thickening of the bursal membrane. Ultimately this extends to the funicular portion of the *ligamentum nuchae*, and the bursa ruptures onto the surface. Necrosis and infection of the ligament and the bursa result in a non-healing, chronic, discharging, fistulous condition. This has a characteristic appearance, and discharges a clear serosanguineous exudate or (in older lesions) a creamy, yellow purulent material (**461**). Historically, this condition (and fistulous withers) were often associated with primary systemic infection with *Brucella* spp. or *Actinobacillus* spp. bacteria, but once the affected bursa ruptures, secondary, complicating bacteria are often involved.

The **supraspinous bursa**, which lies between the dorsal spines of the third and fourth thoracic vertebrae and the *ligamentum nuchae*, in the withers, may, similarly, become infected by hematogenous spread or by direct inoculation via a wound in the area. *Brucella abortus* has been identified as being the major cause for this infection, but this is probably less significant nowadays and a wide variety of bacterial species may be involved. The inflamed bursa increases in size and, with the considerable forces applied to the surface by the *ligamentum nuchae*, enlarges into the tissues of the withers. The horse is usually reluctant to move, and marked pain and swelling is evident on palpation of the withers. Eventually the bursa bursts onto the skin. **Fistulous withers** is characterised by the presence of chronic discharging sinus tracts between the bursa and the skin, most often producing profuse quantities of cloudy, serosanguineous and flocculant, infected exudate (**462**). Contrast radiographic studies may be used to identify the full extent of the problem and the possibility of concurrent osteomyelitis or sequestra arising from traumatic damage to the spines of the thoracic vertebrae. However, care must be taken in interpretation, as separate centres of ossification of the dorsal spinous processes of the cranial thoracic vertebrae are usually irregular in appearance, and this should not be misinterpreted as a sign of bone infection. Most cases which show multiple, discharging sinuses over the withers do not, in fact, involve the supraspinous bursa

461

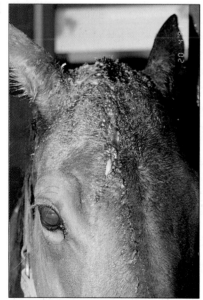

462

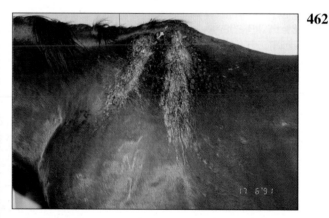

461 Poll evil.

462 Fistulous withers.
Differential Diagnosis:
i) Infected sinus tracts (not involving supraspinous bursa)
ii) Sequestration of dorsal thoracic spines (osteomyelitis / osteitis / fracture)

and therefore are not truly fistulous conditions. In these circumstances there is frequently an extensive network of sinus tracts extending between the muscles of the withers. Necrosis of the *ligamentum nuchae,* and dorsal spines of the cervical vertebrae is responsible for the chronicity of the exudate. In the treatment of these conditions meticulous surgical debridement and drainage are paramount.

Infection or inflammation of sub-tendinous bursae, such as those occurring between the navicular bone and the deep flexor tendon or under the origin of the *biceps brachii* muscle, are typically extremely serious. The pain which results from pressure of the tendon on the bursa will result in severe lameness and may produce a typical stance as the animal attempts to relieve the pressure on the bursa by appropriate limb placement.

Neoplastic Disorders

There are no significant neoplastic disorders of the tendons and ligaments of the horse and secondary tumours within these are also not reported.

Muscles and Associated Structures

Non-Infectious Disorders

Traumatic injuries to the muscles of the horse are many and varied. Disruption of muscle masses without concurrent breaks in the skin present two major clinical syndromes. Where the muscles of the abdominal wall are ruptured, an **acquired hernia (rupture)** may develop **(463)**. While in many cases these appear to cause little difficulty, complications may arise when abdominal viscera become entrapped within the hernia and more particularly when these become incarcerated therein.

Rupture of muscles, occurring as a result of excessive or violent contraction, may cause obvious distortion of the muscle belly itself when there is simultaneous rupture of the muscle sheath (epimysium). More often such disruption causes little overt swelling, with the

hemorrhage and disruption remaining within the sheath. Under these circumstances, healing is accompanied by scarring, fibrosis and possibly by calcification. Individual muscles undergoing fibrous metaplasia following this type of injury may ultimately become severely wasted (*see* **699, 711**). **Traumatic damage to the** *semitendinosus, semimembranosus* **and /or** *biceps femoris* **muscles** may be unnoticed at the time, or may be considered to be of minor importance, but subsequent scarring and fibrosis, and the extension of fibrous scarring between these muscles, may result in the development of the disorder known as **fibrotic/ ossifying myopathy**. Ossifying myopathy is a development and complication of the fibrotic stages of the disorder. Clinically the *semitendinosus* muscle is the

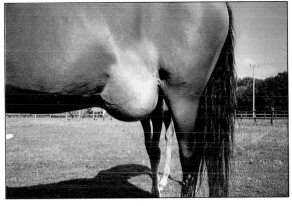

463

463 Ventral abdominal rupture.
Differential Diagnosis:
i)   Abscess
ii) Neoplasia
iii) Acquired bursa
iv) Hematoma

464

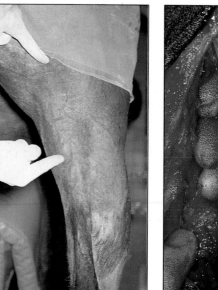

465

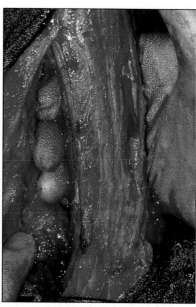

464 Fibrotic myopathy (*semitendinosus* muscle).
Note: Dense fibrous band palpable in this area.

465 Fibrotic myopathy (same horse as **464**).
Note: Belly of *semitendinosus* muscle replaced by dense fibrous tissue band. Extensive adhesions to *biceps femoris* m.

most important muscle involved. Adhesions developing between it and the *biceps femoris* m. limit its action by partially restricting the anterior phase of the stride. The foot of the affected limb is suddenly pulled caudally, moments before ground impact would normally occur and the foot is slapped to the ground, giving a characteristically shortened stride and sound to the gait. Clinical examination will identify an area of obvious firmness on the caudal aspect of the limb at the level of, and/or just above, the stifle (**464**). Surgical exploration of the affected muscle shows it to be markedly fibrosed (**465**) with little or no obvious muscle tissue and limited or extensive adhesions between this and the underlying *biceps femoris*. Occasionally a very similar congenital condition is detected in neonatal foals. However, in these cases, although the clinical appearance is entirely typical, few (or no) adhesions can be found and no fibrous thickening of the muscles is present. The developmental disorder probably represents a restrictive myopathy rather than true fibrotic change.

More dramatic **wounds**, involving the laceration of skin and underlying muscles are common in the horse (**466**). While the damage may look dramatic, the consequences are often surprisingly limited, with healing and wound contracture occurring rapidly in the absence of complicating factors such as sequestration of bone or foreign matter, infection and/or excessive movement. Generally, wounds involving large amounts of muscle

are better prospects for spontaneous healing (**467**) than those occurring in areas where no, or limited, underlying muscle is present such as the distal limb (*see* **486**, **487**) and those wounds complicated by other damage such as to tendons and joints (*see* **420**).

Loss of muscle mass in the horse may be a consequence of starvation when the loss is general, but specific groups of muscles may undergo **atrophy** in response to trauma, myopathy, denervation (*see* **699**) (*see* **209**) and chronic disuse (*see* **388**). **Disuse atrophy** is generally slow to develop whereas **neurogenic atrophy**, following total neurectomy, is much more rapid and would be expected to affect all the muscles supplied by a particular nerve (*see* **700**). However, gradual neuronal degeneration such as that affecting the recurrent laryngeal nerve in cases of **idiopathic laryngeal neuropathy (Plate 5u**, page 115) may correspond with a gradual, progressive atrophy of the associated muscles (*see* **209**). Disuse atrophy of muscles usually relates to underlying pain or disability syndromes, often associated with musculo-skeletal disorders (*see* **388**, **438**). The identification of the cause of obvious and severe, long-standing muscle atrophy may be particularly difficult and may require sophisticated means of measuring both nerve and residual muscle function.

The development of palpable **calcification of muscle** may occur secondarily to severe muscle damage.

466

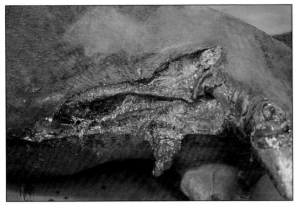

466 Traumatic muscle injury

467

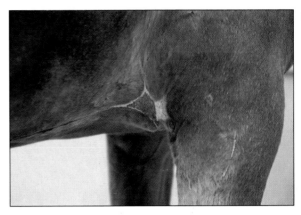

467 Traumatic muscle injury (same horse as **466** and **467** 7 weeks later).
Note: Wound healed uneventfully after 7 weeks with minimal treatment and minimal scarring was present.

468

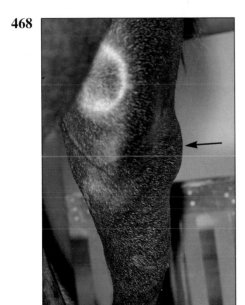

468 Tumoral calcinosis.
Note: Discreet swelling on lateral aspect of limb at level of stifle joint (arrow).

469

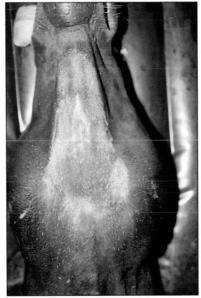

469 Masseter myopathy.
Note: Severe bilateral swelling of masseter muscles. Jaw held firmly closed, only possible to examine and open mouth under general anaesthesia. Blood selenium concentration very low.

Tumoral calcinosis (*calcinosis circumscripta*) occurs in young horses, over the lateral aspect of the gaskin, in particular, close to the femoro-tibial joint (**468**). The mass is usually non-painful, freely moveable over the underlying structures, and usually has no apparent harmful effect upon the horse. The lesion, which may be identifiable radiographically, may be attached to the joint capsule of the stifle joint but more commonly it lies beneath the aponeurosis of the *biceps femoris* muscle and lateral fascia of the limb. The lesions usually contain dense white, gritty calcified granules, within a creamy-white, paste-like material.

Inflammation and swelling of muscle masses without any predisposing cause such as trauma or ischemia, occurs rarely. It is accompanied by acute pain, and obvious difficulty with function. **Masseter myopathy** in which the masseter muscles become grossly swollen and intensely painful, is a rare disorder, affecting adult horses kept under poor management and nutritional conditions. Affected horses have an abrupt onset of

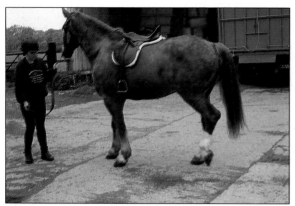

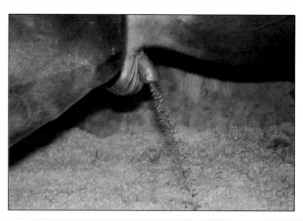

470 Exertional myopathy (exertional rhabdomyolysis, azoturia, myoglobinuria, tying up syndrome).
Note: Horse transfixed 20 yards from stable door. Sweating, particularly over left gluteal region.

471 Exertional myopathy (myoglobinuria).
Differential Diagnosis:
i)   Terminal renal/hepatic failure
ii) Haemoglobinuria (intravascular erythrolysis from babesiosis, autoimmune hemolytic disease, etc)
iii) Intra-abdominal or intra-thoracic bleeding
iv) Phenothiazine poisoning
v) Oak leaf/acorn poisoning

anorexia, the masseter muscles are obviously swollen (**469**) and are intensely painful. Manipulation of the mandible is resented strongly, and the lower jaw may be held slightly open or firmly closed. Simultaneous cardiac and diaphragmatic dysfunction (including synchronous diaphragmatic flutter, are found, and this disorder is (somewhat equivocally) associated with inadequate selenium and vitamin E metabolism and white muscle disease. Recovered horses may seem relatively normal for a limited time, but profound masseter atrophy (*see* **737**) is a common sequel.

Nutritional myopathy (dystrophic myodegener-ation, nutritional myodegeneration, white muscle misease) is a well-recognised clinical syndrome, which mainly affects foals up to 7 – 9 months of age, but occasionally affects older horses. In some cases it has been attributed to deficiency of vitamin E and/or selenium. In the foal syndrome, there is a non-inflammatory degeneration of muscle which characteristically affects the skeletal, diaphragmatic and cardiac muscle. Affected foals are weak and may be unable to rise. Cardiac rhythm irregularities, myocardial degeneration, and sudden death as a result of abrupt cardiac failure are encountered. The disorder is often difficult to diagnose without recourse to laboratory methods (including lactate dehydrogenase and creatine kinase isoenzyme studies). At post mortem examination, skeletal muscle and myocardium are found to be obviously pale and the diaphragm is commonly dark and diffusely fibrosed.

In the adult horse, the relationship between vitamin E and selenium and the myopathies of exercise is not well established. However, a group of **exertional myopathies (paralytic myoglobinuria, exertional rhabdomyolysis, tying-up, azoturia)** in the adult horse, presenting a variety of clinical syndromes, are a common and important group of disorders. The disorder most often affects fit, working and performance horses. Mares and heavily muscled horses appear to be more commonly affected. A similar condition may be encountered in unfit horses subjected to unaccustomed, severe exertion. Classically, the most severe myopathies were described as occurring within the first few steps, following a few days rest, on full rations (Monday morning disease) when a dramatic peracute muscle stiffness and spasm develops, particularly affecting the gluteal and/or loin muscles. The horse is transfixed, showing extreme pain, with sweating (**470**), shaking, tachycardia and polypnea within moments of leaving the stable. Where one limb is affected it is rested and palpation of the affected muscles, which may include both fore and hind limb masses, reveals a board-like hardness, with pain and heat. Urine sometimes becomes a dark red-brown in colour (**471**) due to the presence of large amounts of the muscle pigment, myoglobin. The tubular accumulation and precipitation of vast amounts of myoglobin in the kidney, particularly where the urine is acidic (as is often the case in these horses), may result in the rapid onset of oliguria, anuria and acute renal failure. Recovery from the most serious forms of the condition usually takes some days or weeks, and, during this time, the horse cannot usually be moved without

472

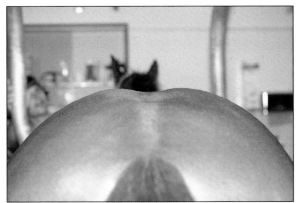

473

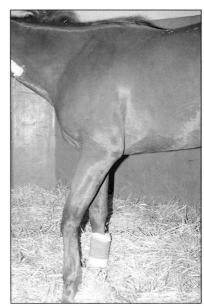

472 (Bilateral) gluteal myopathy.
Note: Gluteal muscles grossly swollen (and painful) following prolonged anesthesia in dorsal recumbency.

473 Triceps myositis (myopathy).
Note: Leg rested in partial flexion, triceps muscle flaccid, painful.
Differential Diagnosis:
i) Radial paralysis
ii) Brachial plexus inflammation
iii) Fractured olecranon
iv) Origin of triceps muscle torn from scapula.

risk of further muscle damage and repeated bouts of rhabdomyolysis in the same or different muscle masses. Horses will usually return to normal activity, but individual masses of muscle which have been severely affected may not heal normally. Marked loss of muscle bulk, as a result of atrophy or fibrous metaplasia, is common following the worst forms (*see* **711**).

Less severe forms of **myopathy** occur commonly in performance horses and have much reduced clinical signs. A very minor form of exertional myopathy occurs in racing horses when, during extremes of exercise, they may appear to cramp-up, slowing their pace and showing only minor, transient discomfort. Some horses 'tie-up' even after limited work, showing stiffness, cramps and walking on tip-toes with the hind legs. These cases often recover rapidly, and while some habitually develop the condition, many have no obvious reasons for its development under any particular circumstances. Muscle enzyme levels are sometimes elevated but in other cases no changes are apparent. These are anecdotally associated with electrolyte imbalances but on most such occasions no significant hematological evidence for this can be found. 'Sludging' of red cells in the capillary beds of muscles may also be involved.

Myopathy due to prolonged recumbency is relatively common, and represents a complication of general anesthesia, in heavy horses in particular. Characteristically the condition affects the dependent muscles. Thus, heavy animals maintained in dorsal recumbency develop an ischemic myopathy in the lumbar muscles, while the muscles of one fore or hind limb (or both) may be affected in those held in lateral recumbency for extended periods. The clinical features of such a myopathy are obviously related to the specific muscles affected and the extent of the damage. Affected muscle masses may be hard, hot and grossly swollen (**472**) but may, equally, be normal in appearance while being extremely painful and non-functional. In the forelimb, the triceps mass is the most commonly affected and although it is seldom grossly swollen as a result, muscle function is severely compromised (**473**). Affected horses present with a lameness and weakness which is very similar in appearance to radial paralysis (*see* **702**). Indeed there may also be components of neurological dysfunction at the same time and it is often difficult to be sure which is the more prominent. Typically, the onset of the clinical effects of these myopathies are present immediately or shortly after recovery from anesthesia. Muscle enzyme levels are almost always very elevated and careful clinical assessment is imperative to establish the cause of the condition and its extent.

Venomous snakes and spiders occur world-wide and the effect of their toxins is varied. Many have profound neurological and/or circulatory effects but many also have strong cytotoxic properties. Most such bites are also infected by pathogenic bacteria and lead to localised myonecrosis (**474**). As the effects of envenomation are closely related to the volume injected relative to the weight of the animal, few snake bites are capable of killing a horse directly but the secondary effects of clostridial myonecrosis and swelling may have a fatal result.

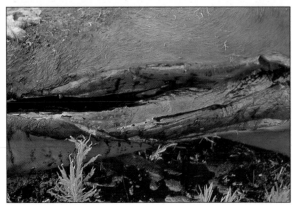

474 Snake bite myonecrosis.

Infectious Disorders

Bacterial Diseases: Necrosis and bacterial infection of muscle masses usually occurs as a result of infected wounds, or from iatrogenic damage following the injection of irritant or caustic drugs (*see* **295**). The injection of antibiotics seldom results in local infection, but quite frequently intramuscular injections result in local myonecrosis and infection subsequently develops (**475**). The injection of other drugs more commonly results in infected sites, and the most serious of these infections are those due to *Clostridia* spp bacteria, in which gas production and extensive myonecrosis produce a life-threatening situation. Local damage of this type within a muscle may have very serious immediate toxic consequences, and affect the function of the specific mass of muscle, adjacent nerves and blood vessels and other structures.

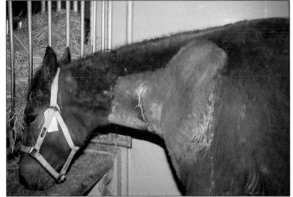

475 Infected intramuscular injection site.

Neoplastic Disorders

Neoplastic conditions involving the muscles of the horse are rare, but possible conditions include **spindle cell tumours** and primary **sarcoma**. Occasionally individual muscles become affected by slow growing defects of structure which may resemble neoplastic changes. The gross proliferation of a normal tissue type in an abnormal site such as this is called a **hamartoma**. Similar lesions may develop in any site in any organ (including the melanotic accumulations in the guttural pouches of grey horses). Their significance is usually in respect of space occupying compression of adjacent structures. A relatively common site for muscle hamartoma formation is the *semimembranosus* and *semitendinosus* muscles, and massive enlargement of these may have secondary effects on bowel and urogenital function **(476)**.

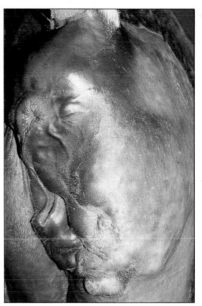

476

476 Hamartoma of muscle (*semimembranosus*).
Note: Physical distortion of perineum.

Further reading

Adams Lameness in Horses (4th Ed) Stashak, T.S. (1985) Lea & Fabiger, Philadelphia, USA

Current Therapy in Equine Medicine (2)
Ed Robinson, N.E. (1987), W B Saunders, Philadelphia, USA

Current Therapy in Equine Medicine (3)
Ed Robinson, N.E. (1992), W B Saunders, Philadelphia, USA

8. The integumentary system

The skin is a large, diverse organ, and diseases and conditions may be primarily of dermatological origin or may be secondary manifestations of disease in other organs. Whilst the clinical signs may be obvious on the surface of the skin some are the result of underlying disorders of metabolism and organ dysfunction. Of all the equine diseases, those of the skin are amongst the most difficult to diagnose and treat.

Developmental Disorders

Heritable disorders of the skin do occur and while some have been well recognised their significance is only now becoming better understood. Mane and tail dystrophy occurs in horses over 3 years of age; affected hairs are brittle and liable to breaking. Horses are presented with shortened, dull manes and significant loss of the long hairs of the tail (**477**); the pathological cause of the condition is unknown.

Linear keratosis is a relatively common disorder in which a focal keratinization defect manifests as one or more linear, usually vertical, bands of crusting and alopecia (**478**). Clinically, this disease closely resembles the aftermath of blister application, when scurf and scale are at their peak, but such cases do not alter over prolonged periods of time and indeed, they may show the same predictable pattern for their entire lives. It is often of benefit to clip the area carefully to establish the extent and linear nature of the lesions. They are most often located on the sides of the neck, or over the buttock (*see* **478**) but may be found elsewhere.

Cutaneous asthenia (dermatosparaxis) is an inherited defect of collagen synthesis caused by a deficiency of procollagen peptidase, which results in abnormal folding of the skin particularly of the shoulders (**479**), body (**480**), and upper limbs. This usually causes considerable, abnormal local folding of the skin which is noticeably thin on palpation. The skin is excessively fragile and is liable to trauma. Healed lesions involving this skin show abnormally prominent scarring.

477

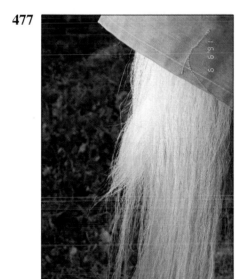

478

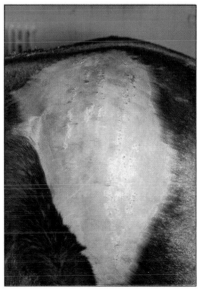

477 Mane and tail dystrophy.
Note: Broken, brittle tail hairs.

478 Linear keratosis.
Note: Linear areas of hyperkeratosis running down the buttock.

479

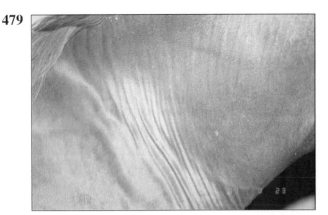

480

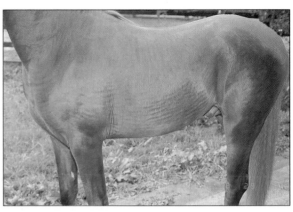

479 Cutaneous asthenia.
Note: Abnormal folding of thin, fragile skin at base of neck

480 Cutaneous asthenia (Body).

481

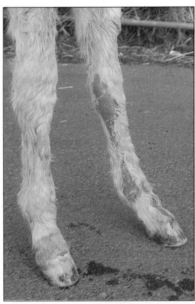

482

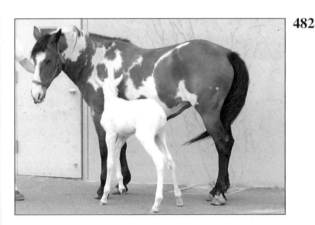

481 Epithelial agenesis (*Aplasia cutis*).

482 Albinism.
Note: Foal of Ovaro-Paint mare. Foal also afflicted by severe gastro-intestinal abnormalities (*see* **87**).

483

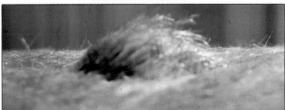

484

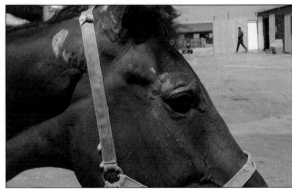

483 Dermoid cyst.
Differential Diagnosis:
i) Larva of *Hypoderma bovis* (warble fly)
ii) Insect bite (localised hypersensitivity)
iii) Nodular sarcoid fibroma

484 Skin sloughing dermatitis.
Note: Subsequent to bruising trauma of skin. Area healed normally with no deficit of hair and no colour changes.

New born foals are occasionally affected by a congenital discontinuity of the squamous epithelium (**epithelial agenesis**) which is supposedly due to a single autosomal recessive gene. Lesions are most common in the limbs (**481**), but have also been reported on the head and tongue; euthanasia is usually recommended as attempts to cover the defective area with grafts or through surgical closure are unrewarding.

Where there is congenital absence of normal pigmentation in the body (hair, skin and eyes), a condition of **albinism** exists (**482**). Full or partial loss of iris pigment (*see* **602**) is, however, much more common than pure albino hair and skin. Palomino and cremello coloured horses are more likely to have albino foals than stronger coloured animals. A more complex loss of pigmentation occurs with **lethal white foal syndrome**, which appears primarily in Ovaro-Paint horses, where there are both hereditary pigment abnormalities and serious (and invariably fatal) developmental abnormalities of the intestinal tract (*see* **87**).

A number of developmental cystic conditions of the skin occur relatively commonly. These include the **epidermoid inclusion cyst (atheroma)** (*see* **180**) found in the subcutaneous connective tissue caudo-dorsal to the caudal limit of the false nostril. Single or multiple **dermoid cysts** (**483**) are found on the skin of the dorsal midline, particularly in Thoroughbred horses between 6 months and 3 – 4 years of age. These contain coiled hair and a cheesy, caseous, sterile material. They are seldom painful unless they burst and become infected, and close examination will establish their origin and differentiate them from the inflammatory, neoplastic and parasitic lesions which sometimes occur in the same vicinity. **Temporal teratoma** and **dentigerous cysts** (*see* **21**) may have open discharging sinuses onto the skin but are usually associated with aberrant dental tissue. The latter may contain no obvious dental structures but a true cystic lining results in a persistent discharging sinus, almost invariably located on the anterior (leading) border of the pinna. While some of these cystic structures are more or less inapparent, many cause obvious disfigurement and may be removed for cosmetic reasons.

Non-Infectious Disorders

The scope for non-infectious disease or damage to the skin of horses is extensive. An almost infinite variety of injuries may occur. In many cases the healing process may be retarded or, in some cases, may fail completely, resulting in persistent, unsightly and unacceptable scars. Trauma to the skin of horses is frequently directly attributable to their lifestyle or to their excitable nature when confronted by unusual events such as storms, transport, strange horses, new paddocks etc. In many cases the more serious consequences of the injury involve underlying structures such as tendons (*see* **442, 489**), ligaments, nerves or blood vessels. Apparently minor skin injuries may have particularly severe consequences when the injury extends into adjacent synovial structures (*see* **432**) or body cavities (**see 244**). Injuries to the skin, including those which do not break the surface, should therefore always be treated with caution and a thorough investigation carried out to establish the full extent of any underlying damage.

Simple injuries which may be a result of self-inflicted trauma or minor abrasions usually only cause superficial skin erosions and inflammation (*see* **150**). Bruising, accompanied by localised swelling, is due to leakage of relatively small quantities of blood or plasma into the local tissues. The natural colour progression of localised skin or subcutaneous bruising is usually not apparent in horses and may only be detected by a careful examination of the clipped or shaven skin. In most cases erosive lesions and bruising of the skin result in scabbing and sloughing of the superficial layers of the dermis (**484**).

Where more extensive vascular damage occurs without breaking the surface, a hematoma may form (**485**). These commonly arise from blunt trauma, such as running into a solid object or from kicks and are therefore most often found on the brisket and sides of the thorax and abdomen. Most hematomas arising in otherwise healthy horses resolve gradually as clot retraction occurs, but some may persist as fluid filled masses or may form dense masses of fibrous tissue which in some cases may even become calcified. Horses suffering from disorders of coagulation (either from hereditary hemophilia or acquired coagulopathies) are more liable to develop large hematomas without obvious cause, or following apparently minor trauma (*see* **311**). The development of persistent or multiple hematomas without any apparent cause, particularly where these are accompanied by joint bleeding (hemarthrosis), should alert the clinician to the possibility of an underlying coagulopathy. Horses so affected often show anemia,

485

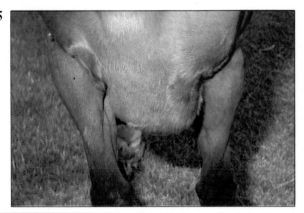

486

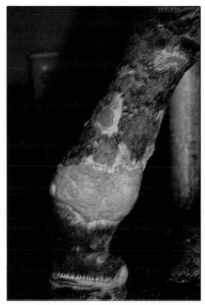

485 Hematoma.
Differential Diagnosis:
i) Abscess
ii) Hernia/rupture
iii) Acquired bursitis

486 Wound healing with exuberant granulation.
Differential Diagnosis:
i) Sarcoid
ii) Infected wound site or foreign body

epistaxis, and bleeding into joints or body cavities. Hematomas developing after venepuncture should be regarded with suspicion, particularly in toxemic or septicemic horses which might be suffering from the advanced stages of a consumptive coagulopathy such as disseminated intravascular coagulopathy (*see* **293**).

Healing of limb wounds is often slow, particularly if injury, such as deep wire cuts, involves deeper tissues. Where the periosteal blood supply is disrupted sequestration of the underlying bone frequently occurs (*see* **418, 419**). Failure of even relatively minor wounds to heal at sites subjected to trauma involving (even minor) periosteal damage should be investigated carefully in case such sequestration has occurred. These wounds invariably completely fail to heal under these circumstances until either the sequestrum has been spontaneously reabsorbed or surgically removed. Other reasons for the failure of wounds to heal include excessive movement at the site, inadequate wound contraction, infection (bacterial and parasitic), poor or interrupted blood supply, foreign bodies, excessive blood loss and underlying systemic disease.

Wounds in some areas such as the thorax and neck often heal rapidly (*see* **466** and **467**), relying on a combination of wound contracture and effective spontaneous drainage of exudates and inflammatory debris. Wounds involving the eyelids, or the margins of the mouth, nose and vulva may heal effectively by second

intention healing but may result in a possibly more serious secondary effect after cicatrization (scarring) has taken place. Eyelid defects, for example, may leave a wiping-defect of the cornea and extensive ulceration and corneal scarring may arise. Alternatively, such a defect may merely result in overflow of lacrimal secretion (epiphora) and while this is usually of little clinical consequence, in some areas of the world where habronemiasis occurs the consequences may become more important.

The healing process of skin wounds in the horse is notoriously different between the various areas of the body. Wounds occurring over large muscle masses (*see* **466**) often heal rapidly by wound contraction and the resultant scar is often remarkably small (*see* **467**). Even very large body wounds which involve the skin only, often heal well and, if vertical, are amenable to suturing with relaxation sutures for support. Failure to adequately relieve the tension on wound edges and eliminate dead space often results in wound breakdown. The consequences of this in some trunk wounds are probably less serious than those occurring on the limbs. Surgical closure of horizontal wounds on the shoulder, hip and thigh is often requested by owners of horses, but experience shows that they rarely heal by primary intention due to pocketing (dead space) and/or excessive suture tension. Many heal rapidly if they are kept clean, and complications from fly activity and self-inflicted trauma are minimised.

487

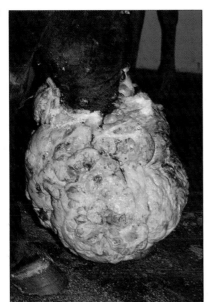

488

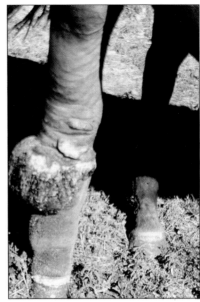

487 Exuberant granulation tissue (neglected case of 2 years duration).
Note: Thirty-five kilograms of granulation tissue was removed from the site which originated from a small wire wound in the pastern region.

488 Cheloid scarring.
Note: Wounds untreated for 18 months. Note thickening of limb distal to scar and excessive fibrous scar formation at sites of wounds.
Differential Diagnosis:
i) Sporadic lymphangitis
ii) Ulcerative lymphangitis
iii) Sarcoid

Where blood supply is less and where there is little or no scope for wound contraction, such as on the lower limb, healing is significantly slower and the extent of scarring correspondingly greater. Where wounds occur at sites overlying limb joints, or where the blood supply is poor (such as in the lower limb), or where foreign matter (including necrotic tissue and bone) is present in the wound, the horse and mule have a marked propensity for the production of large amounts of exuberant granulation tissue. Wounds over the carpus, hock and the limb distal to these joints, often heal particularly poorly (**486**). Scrupulous cleanliness, restriction of movement at the site and careful removal of foreign matter or sequestra may reduce the healing time remarkably. Non-healing wounds of the lower limb (or elsewhere) which produce large accumulations of exuberant granulation tissue (proud flesh) (**487**) create a considerable problem for the clinician. Repeated debridement of the granulation tissue and subsequent skin grafting (usually pinch grafting) is required, but such wounds should first be explored by all possible means (including radiography and ultrasonography) to ensure that there is no obvious reason for the failure to heal. Careful handling of wounds in these areas will ensure that healing when it finally occurs, will contain the minimum amount of unsightly fibrous and/or osseous tissue (**488**). Wounds which fail to heal should also be examined carefully for the possibility that the apparent granulation tissue is in fact sarcoid (*see* **527, 528**).

Where underlying joints (*see* **432**), tendons (*see* **442**), nerves, and/or major blood vessels are involved in skin wounds, a more serious prognosis must be given. An aggressive treatment schedule is essential for although the wound may be relatively minor in extent, recovery may be problematical and performance horses may not recover to meet the demands of their work. Contaminated (infected) or open wounds of synovial structures (**489**) require particularly intensive management and the skin wound is usually of lesser importance. Wounds which, from their anatomic location, might involve underlying synovial structures should always be explored thoroughly, and discharge from such wounds should be examined for the possibility that it contains synovial fluid. Skin wounds contaminated with synovial fluid and open fistulae between a synovial structure, such as a bursa, and the skin, frequently fail to heal (*see* **462**) and often provide a persistent portal of entry for infection into the synovial structure.

489

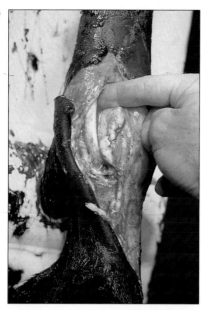

490

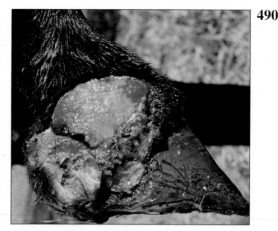

489 Complicated skin wound.
Note: Digital sheath open and extensive disruption of fetlock ligaments. No apparent damage to substance of superficial flexor tendon.

490 Coronet and hoof wound.
Note: Treated by casting

491

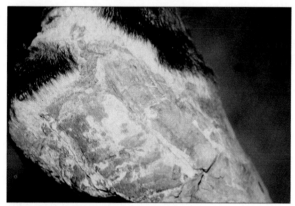

492

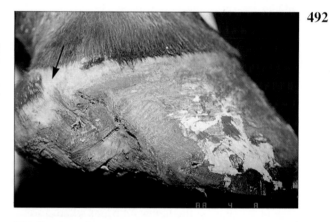

491 Coronet and hoof wound (same case as 490).
Note: Eighteen months later, wound healed but permanent coronet and hoof deformity.

492 Sand crack.
Note: Persistent defect in hoof wall integrity arising from coronet injury (arrow).

Injury to the coronet and coronary band (**490**) may leave a permanent deformity in the coronary band and its related horn (**491**). In some cases the damage to the coronary tissues results in failure to produce horn over a greater or lesser length of coronet, and the resultant defect in the hoof wall extends to the distal border. Such sandcracks create a permanent portal of entry for foreign bodies and infection into the underlying sensitive laminae (**492**).

Foreign bodies which are introduced through skin wounds may lead either to a persistently discharging, non-healing wound or to discharging sinuses in the skin. The latter may discharge a considerable distance from the original site and this may be misleading when such wounds and sinuses are examined. Radiography (using probes and/or contrast media if necessary) ultrasonography and careful exploratory surgery under general anesthetic may be required in order to locate and remove such foreign bodies.

Self-inflicted injury also occurs as a result of irritation from biting insects such as *Stomoxys* spp **(493)**. Skin mutilation can also occur as a result of the self-mutilation syndrome in stallions; horses bite severely at flanks, ribs and pectoral areas (*see* **719**), causing patchy alopecia, leukotrichia and scarring. The use of aluminum muzzles or neck cradles which allow the horse to eat and drink normally but prevent self-molestation, may be necessary in this and in other skin conditions accompanied by self mutilation. It is unusual for horses to chew or lick at open wounds unless they are associated with nerve damage or with foreign bodies, but they do occasionally chew dressings and bandages where these are poorly applied or where there is an excessive exudation.

A more chronic type of skin trauma occurs from poorly applied plaster casts or from localised pressure over bony prominences during prolonged recumbency. Leg casts and bandaging may cause scalding followed by friction rubs which if uncorrected, cause vascular compromises in the skin and lead, occasionally, to damage to underlying structures (*see* **446**). This leads to sloughing of the affected area. These wounds and decubital (pressure) sores are notoriously slow to heal. Residual slow healing occurs only if the pressure is relieved and appropriate treatment applied.

Where skin trauma is prolonged but intermittent, and/or is not severe enough to cause circulation problems, the skin reacts to form a callus. These are common over joints and bony protuberances, especially at the knee, fetlock, elbow, hock and tuber ischia. False or acquired bursae are often encountered where the

pressure is applied such as over the carpus in horses which habitually kneel. Skin thickening and lichenification are common sequels to such injuries. Embedded foreign bodies are also a possible cause of such thickened skin but the history of the lesion is notably different. In all these conditions the lesions are usually cold and non-painful. Prevention of pressure and local irritation may improve the condition but, again, the total resolution is often disappointing.

Thermal injury may occur as a result of either heat loss as in frost bite, cryotherapy or heat excess such as sunburn, photosensitization, thermocautery or accidental fire burns. Skin injury caused by exposure to extremely cold environmental conditions appears to be particularly unusual in horses and where it does occur it primarily affects the tail and ears. Even very low environmental temperatures appear to have little effect upon the limbs. Cryosurgery using liquid nitrogen (at -196°C), or other cryo-agents, initially causes the skin and surrounding area to become erythematous and swollen. This is followed within a day or two by exudation, and progressive necrosis. The necrotic tissue then sloughs out from the underlying healthy bed of granulation tissue which may (or may not) heal in much the same way as other granulating wounds at the same site. A similar sequence of events follows prolonged exposure to very low temperatures or to the focal application of high temperatures. These wounds are initially slow to heal due to the adjacent tissues being marginally affected, thus slowing the healing process. Once healing takes place leukotrichia and scarring occurs. This process is used therapeutically in the treatment of skin neoplasia,

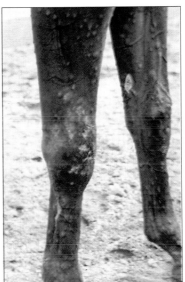

493

493 Self-inflicted injury (as a result of *Stomoxys Calcitrans* (Stable fly) bites.

494

495

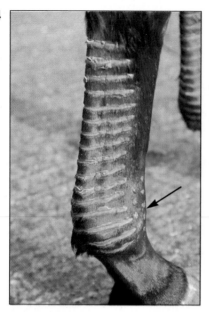

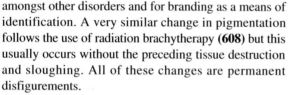

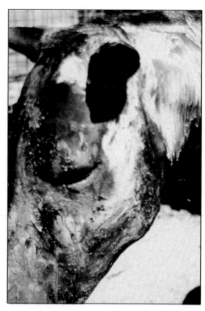

494 Iatrogenic trauma (burn) scars.
Note: 'Line' firing (thermocautery) on plantar and lateral aspects of cannon and 'Pin' firing over dorsal fetlock (arrow). Procedure performed 3 weeks previously.

495 Thermal injury (24 hours after injury).
Note: Second and third degree burns showing edema, serum exudation and sloughing of superficial layers of skin.

amongst other disorders and for branding as a means of identification. A very similar change in pigmentation follows the use of radiation brachytherapy (**608**) but this usually occurs without the preceding tissue destruction and sloughing. All of these changes are permanent disfigurements.

Application of severe heat, such as was historically used in the firing of horses legs in the expectation of a therapeutic effect upon the underlying tendons or bone, causes swelling, exudation and residual scarring (**494**) in much the same order as freezing injuries.

Horses trapped in burning stables, horse transporters or forest fires, may sustain very severe skin damage (**495**). The most common sites for severe burns are around the head and dorsum. Horses with burns which cover more than 50% of the body surface almost invariably die from the secondary circulatory, renal and cardiovascular effects. The extent of involvement of the layers of the skin is used to classify burns into four degrees with the most severe, fourth degree burns involving the entire depth of the skin and underlying tissues. The deeper the skin involvement the more plasma protein is lost in the acute stage and the more severe the consequent scarring. The typical thick, coagulated crusts or sloughs which develop following thermal (or chemical or physical) cauterisation of the skin are called eschars. Severe exudation, loss of body fluids and extremely slow

healing of up to 12 months or more, with extensive hairless scarring commonly follows burns of third or fourth degree. The treatment of extensive or localised burns of any degree should be oriented towards controlling the loss of plasma as well as toward pain relief and the limitation of subsequent sloughing. Skin grafting may be an effective method of speeding the naturally slow healing process. Secondary complications, including severe pneumonia due to inhalation of smoke and/or noxious chemicals released from fires (such as burnt plastic), may result in death during 24–48 hours after the incident.

Endocrine and nutritional diseases with cutaneous manifestations are infrequent in horses. Nutritional diseases are poorly differentiated and have non-specific skin changes more related to general health than specific deficiency. However, specific mineral deficiencies including zinc, iodine and copper may be associated with skin disorders.

Zinc deficiency causes a generalised alopecia and flaking of the superficial skin layers giving a dandruff-like appearance. Young foals born to mares with sub-optimal iodine diets during pregnancy may be born with an obvious **goitre** (*see* **357**) and such foals are often weak and have a very poor coat quality. On occasion they may be almost hairless.

Copper deficiency is particularly unusual in horses, even in areas with a primary copper deficient soil or in

496

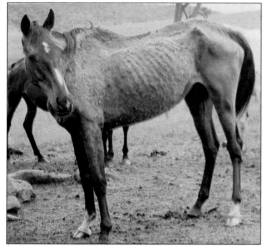

496 Arsenical poisoning (chronic).
Note: Emaciation and exfoliative dermatitis.

497

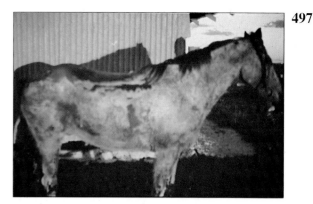

497 Mercurial poisoning (chronic).
Note: Extensive loss of body hair but retention of mane and tail hair.

498

498 Selenium poisoning (acute) (selenosis).
Note: Separation of coronary band with slippering of hoof.
Differential Diagnosis:
i) (Idiopathic and other) laminitis
ii) Arterial occlusion (neuroma)
iii) Infection within hoof

areas with high soil molybdenum concentrations, but in the event that the animal is unable to maintain its copper status, alteration in the colour of the hair (hypochromotrichia) is usually all that is seen. Dark pigmented hair may become obviously russet in colour.

Some toxic plants and heavy metals, if ingested in sufficient quantities, produce skin changes as well as other systemic disturbances. Ingestion of arsenical and mercurial salts usually causes severe loss of condition and an exfoliative dermatitis with patchy or extensive loss of hair (**496**). In some cases of arsenical poisoning an abnormally long hair coat and extensive seborrhoea develop. In all cases however, the hair is brittle and easily pulled from the skin. **Mercurial poisoning**, which is usually the result of ingestion of seed corn treated with organic, mercurial fungicides, causes loss of body hair without as much loss of mane and tail hair (**497**). The differential diagnosis is often difficult but may be assisted by analysis of hair coat for heavy metals. There are often severe accompanying signs including weight loss, diarrhea, icterus and/or central nervous signs which may alert the clinician to the underlying disorder. If such

horses are killed, significant concentrations of either metal can be found in samples of liver and/or kidney.

Selenium also causes toxicity either in metallic base form (usually following over enthusiastic feed supplementation) or from plants which either concentrate selenium, or which have increased selenium levels as a result of seleniferous soils. Loss of mane (*see* **359**) and tail hair (*see* **360**), occurs as well as the prominent signs of laminitis (*see* **409** *et seq.*). In some cases the laminitis may be severe enough to result in separation of the coronary band and sloughing of the hoof (**498**). Long term toxicity or repeated episodes may result in obvious laminitic deformities of the hoof walls with converging growth lines (**499**).

Leucena spp. trees including *Leucena leucocephala* (**500**) and *Leucena glauca*, which are found in Australasia, New Guinea, the Philippines and West Indies, contain a potent depilatory alkaloid and are readily ingested by horses. The toxicity is characterised by patchy alopecia, which particularly affects the mane and tail hair (**501**), and laminitis. Both the hair and hoof disorders may develop within 7–10 days following ingestion.

499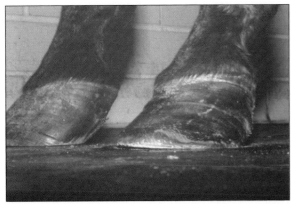

500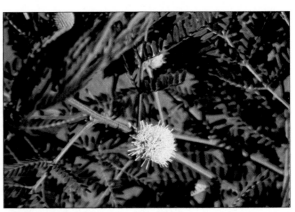

499 Selenium poisoning (chronic) (selenosis).
Note: Severe laminitis with obvious growth bands on hoof wall showing converging growth pattern at toe relative to heel.

500 *Leucena leucocephala* (Mimosa tree) from Australia.
Note: Toxic effects include loss of tail hairs.

501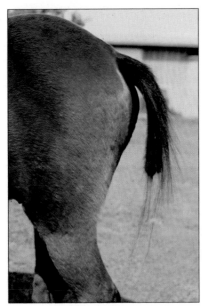

502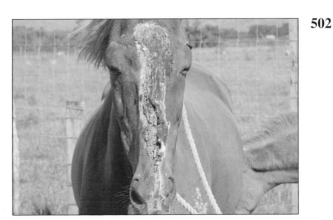

501 *Leucena leucocephala* poisoning.
Note: Loss of tail hairs following sustained ingestion of the plant leaves.

502 Photosensitive dermatitis (ingestion of *Echium lycopsis*).
Note: Extensive skin sloughing restricted strictly to white stripe down face.
Differential Diagnosis:
i) Hepatic failure
ii) Chorioptic dermatitis (only affects lower limb usually)

Other plants, such as *Echium plantagineum, St.John's Wort*, buckwheat, wild carrot and burr trefoil, as well as some drugs, including phenothiazine, sulpha drugs, tetracyclines and methylene blue, have caused photodermatitis on ingestion. This leads to sloughing of white haired, white skin areas **(502)** or acute sunburn. Healed lesions may leave a residual scarred area which may be a significant worry where harness contact induces further injury and so renders the horse unsuitable for further work. The pathogenesis of primary photosensitive (photoactivated) dermatitis is significantly different from secondary hepatogenous form due to hepatic failure. In the primary condition the photodynamic agent(s) is either preformed in the body or is produced within the body during normal metabolism. In hepatic failure the photodynamic substance phylloerythrin (a derivative of plant chlorophyll) which is normally removed by the liver is allowed into the circulation and is then deposited in the skin. In the case of drugs and some plants the photodynamic agent is not affected by normal hepatic function and the substance is deposited in the skin. In either case, however, the effect is the same when the agent is subjected to ultraviolet light which is particularly absorbed through non-pigmented areas of skin. The damage which arises is due to massive release of inflammatory mediators. All horses showing evidence of **photosensitive dermatitis** should, even when they

503

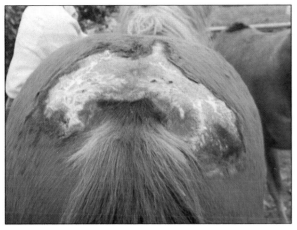

503 Chemical Burn.
Note: Alopecia and excoriation. Due to over strength surgical preparation of abdominal surgery site which remained in contact with the skin for several hours. Healing was very slow and extensive scarring was associated with persistent pain and irritation.

504

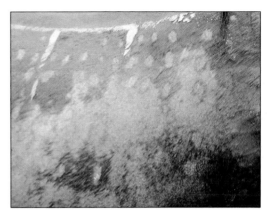

504 Chemical burn.
Note: Ringworm lotion at twice normal strength was applied and caused alopecia and excoriation.

are known to have ingested a photodynamic plant or chemical, be carefully investigated for hepatic failure, whether or not there are other supportive signs. The secondary hepatogenous form is far more common than the primary form. Another interesting form of photoactivated dermatitis has been identified in pale-skinned horses and is often (but not always) associated with cutaneous infection of *Dermatophilus congolense*. Some cases are identifiable histologically as the result of an acute vasculitis **(see 297)** resulting in focal inflammatory lesions only in the white skin of the distal limb and non-pigmented coronary bands. This disorder is apparently related to photosensitive dermatitis but usually only affects the lower limbs and is restricted to the white skinned areas.

A relatively common endocrine disorder with dermatological signs is **equine Cushing's disease** which is most often due to functional pituitary adenomas. Older horses (range 15–30+ years) are more commonly affected with ponies showing a somewhat higher incidence than the larger breeds. A long, thick, curly, hair-coat (hirsutism) is seen with the majority of cases and this hair frequently is not shed (*see* **362** *et seq.*). Other cases show increased density and winter-hair growth with slow moulting, or even non-shedding, in the spring. Other clinical signs which occur are polydipsia and polyuria, hyperglycemia, hyperhidrosis and laminitis. An obvious 'pot-bellied' abdomen occurs in some cases. Differential diagnosis should include renal disease, diabetes insipidus, and laminitis from other causes.

Anhidrosis has skin manifestations with patchy loss of hair and thinning of the hair coat. In the early stages a marked absence of sweating, poor exercise tolerance, polyuria and polydipsia are present with hyperthermia and a characteristic 'puffing' respiration. Long-standing cases show more prominent hair coat abnormalities with a harsh, staring, dry and thin coat quality (*see* **361**).

Physical agents such as chemicals, acaricides, blisters, shampoos, toxins such as snakes, spiders and ticks, cause various clinical signs to develop. Where irritation is mild, there may be only wrinkling of the skin. With more severe irritation, such as occurs with irritants like phenols and wood preservatives, there may be obvious destruction of the skin **(503)**. 'Therapeutic' blistering (counter-irritation) of the skin using mercurial compounds or extracts of cantharides is commonly practiced and results in moderate or severe caustic burns to the skin. Particularly severe reactions may arise if these chemicals are accidentally transferred to the lips and mouth, or eyes. The skin lesions heal particularly slowly at these sites and may even lead to permanent scarring. Milder forms of blister treatment, such as mustard, applied to the skin of horses usually induces swelling and scale formation, without any significant permanent effects.

The ill-judged application of topical therapeutics in the treatment of skin diseases, based upon the philosophy that if the stated concentration is effective, twice must be twice as effective, is commonly undertaken and the consequences of such an approach

505

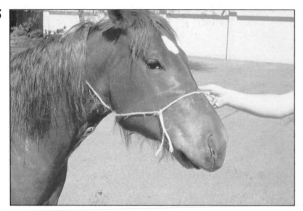

506

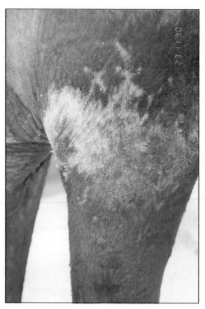

505 Snake bite envenomation.
Note: Site of bite is not always obvious but its character may help to identify the type of snake involved. Secondary effects of myonecrosis, coagulation defects and neurological signs may develop.

506 Leukoderma with leukotrichia.
Note: Lesions appeared some months after repeated episodes of systemic lupus erythematosus-like syndrome (*see* **514** *et seq.*) and were permanent.

are potentially very serious. Some chemicals, such as topical antifungal drugs used to treat dermatomycosis (ringworm) may cause obvious, well defined areas of alopecia and excoriation which corresponds to the area of application (**504**). Others, such as strong tincture of iodine applied to the umbilicus of new born foals, can cause widespread severe excoriation. The use of over-strength acaricides for lice or ticks may cause permanent scarring with alopecia and scaling over the injured areas. Persistent discharges including plasma, serum, urine, diarrheic feces or exudates from abscesses and sinus tracts are also liable to result in hair loss, excoriation of the skin and sloughing of superficial epidermis.

Zootoxicosis is caused by the bite or sting of venomous snakes, arachnids and insects. While in most cases the effects of envenomation remain localised (*see* **474**), some toxins are potentially lethal and have significant effects upon the nervous system or upon blood coagulation, or both. Venoms are also usually highly allergenic and previously sensitised animals may show severe anaphylactic reactions. In the horse the ratio of body weight to the volume of toxin introduced makes systemic effects unusual. In most cases the bites induce localised erythema, edema (**505**), exudation and necrosis of skin and underlying muscle (**474**) and sloughing of the skin. The biting parts of many noxious animals such as snakes are often heavily contaminated with bacteria and localised infections frequently follow such bites. Permanent damage to the blood vessels, veins and lymphatics can also occur particularly from spider bites.

Usually the prevalent dangerous snakes, spiders and scorpions etc. are well known in their respective regions of the world and while most such bites are un-accountably feared beyond their potential toxicity, many are, indeed, extremely dangerous.

Disorders of pigmentation and hair density commonly occur in horses and the ease with which white hairs (**leukotrichia**) occur after an apparently relatively mild skin injury, is frequently a worry to equine surgeons. Freeze-branding for identification purposes, and radiation brachytherapy in the treatment of cutaneous neoplasia, result in obvious leukotrichia (*see* **608**). Often, where injury is more severe, depigmentation of skin also occurs (leukoderma) and may be seen in healed areas after the application of severe 'therapeutic' blisters. In many cases involving deep scarring and leukoderma, the scarred areas are hairless (*see* **503**) or have markedly reduced hair density.

Idiopathic depigmentation or vitiligo is common in horses and may occur as small isolated single or multiple macules which may increase in both size and number over a period of years to form obvious larger patches. The areas of leukotrichia are not always associated exactly with an underlying leukoderma. Close examination of the skin (perhaps even after shaving the · hair) will usually establish the extent of the scarring and often will help to identify the original cause. Any generalised or focal inflammation of the skin may result in **leukoderma,** with or without leukotrichia (**506**), or a change to black pigment (**melanotrichia /melano-**

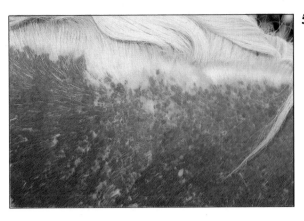

507 Melanoderma and melanotrichia.
Note: Marked pigmentary changes developed over 12 months following repeated insect hypersensitivity in this otherwise pink skin. The changes were restricted to the sides of the neck and the shoulders.

derma) **(507)**. **Idiopathic (spontaneous) leukoderma or melanoderma** is usually accompanied by apparently normal skin with no apparent scarring and is often encountered around the muzzle and over the thorax and abdomen (of older horses).

Variegated or reticulated leukotrichia occurs in Standardbreds and Quarterhorses more commonly than other breeds. Horses usually develop the first signs as yearlings and the eruption is not associated with any evidence of pain or discomfort. The initial crusting, which develops in a characteristic lace-like fashion over the back between the withers and tail, and over the sides of the neck, sheds leaving a transient alopecia which is followed by the permanent growth of white hair in the same pattern. Leukoderma is not usually present. While the cause is unknown, hereditary factors may be involved and therefore affected animals should not be used for breeding. A **spotted leukotrichia** is recognised in Arabian and Arabian cross horses in which a similar course is followed but in which single or multiple spots develop over the rump and sides. An extremely painful idiopathic form of leukotrichia has been recognised in California, in which single or multiple crusting lesions develop along the dorsal midline between the withers and tail. In these cases the lesions are very sensitive to touch during their active phase but gradually subside into discrete areas of leukotrichia which are permanent and non-painful.

Immune mediated skin diseases were once rarely diagnosed in horses because of the difficulty in establishing a diagnosis and the relatively poor differential diagnosis of the more commonly occurring diseases such as dermatophytosis and dermatophilosis, both of which can cause confusion with each other, and with less common diseases such as pemphigus and systemic lupus erythematosus. The use of skin biopsy, special stains and the development of specialist veterinary dermato-histopathologists has greatly increased both our awareness and knowledge of these conditions.

Urticaria and angioedema may have both immunologic and non-immunologic etiology and cause pruritus and edema. It may be transient, prolonged or chronically recurring, and may arise from several possible stimuli. These include stimulation of immune processes, typically involving Type I (immediate/anaphylactic) and Type III (immune complex) hypersensitivities. Non-immunological causes include physical factors such as heat, exercise, sunlight or even rug pressure, as well as various drugs and chemicals either applied locally or ingested. Urticaria has also been associated with a wide range of other disorders including viral, bacterial, fungal and protozoal infections. Insect bites, contact with noxious chemicals such as phenol-based wood preservatives and pour-on insecticides may also induce an urticarial rash. A wide variety of systemic medications including penicillin and/or streptomycin, oxytetracycline, phenothiazine, potentiated sulfona-mides, iron dextrans, various vaccines and sera (Tetanus toxoid and antitoxin, Salmonella vaccine, Strangles and botulism vaccines), have also been blamed for its development. Changes in dietary components including sudden access to fresh hay, green grass or 'new' grain and other noxious animal bites (snakes, spiders, bees), toxic plants such as nettles and inhaled pollens, stable dust and chemicals from fires and sprays may also produce urticaria. The wide variety of possible factors makes the interpretation of the disorder very difficult and an accurate and complete history is vital to the investigation of the condition which appears in all cases, regardless of the specific etiological factor to be clinically the same. A thorough clinical examination will also help to eliminate some of the possible causes.

Urticaria is variously described as 'heat rash', 'hives', 'feed-lumps' and no-doubt many other colloquial names. The clinical signs may be acute or more rarely, chronic and in either case recurrent episodes are relatively common. Urticarial reactions are characterised by localised or more generalised raised

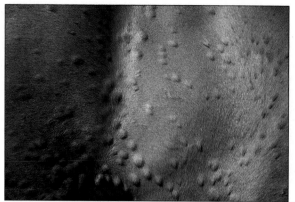

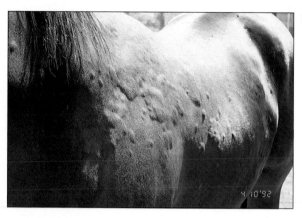

508 Urticaria.
Note: Lesions are well defined edematous plaques without any central depression and developed within 4 hours of a subcutaneous injection of tetanus antitoxin and resolved spontaneously within 12 hours.
Differential Diagnosis:
i) Insect hypersensitivity
ii) Bee/wasp stings
iii) Urticaria
iv) *Purpura haemorrhagica*

509 Urticaria.
Note: Diffuse urticarial (edematous) plaques developed after fresh barley grain was fed to this stallion.
Differential Diagnosis:
i) *Purpura haemorrhagica*
ii) Anaphylaxis
iii) Viral arteritis
iv) Immune mediated vasculitis
v) Systemic lupus erythematosus-like syndrome

skin wheals. There may be multiple small wheals (**508**) or more extensive plaques (**509**) which may occur on the neck, trunk or legs. A less well-defined edema and swelling of the face, eyelids and nose may be present. The lesions themselves pit on pressure and, usually, individual lesions are not long-lasting. In some cases the extent of the local edema is such that serum or even blood exudes through the skin at the site. Conditions in which vasculitis is a presenting feature, such as **immune mediated vasculitis, systemic lupus erythematosus, equine viral arteritis and photoactivated vasculitis,** may produce lesions which are almost identical in clinical appearance but generally have other significant clinical signs.

Although **atopy** has not been confirmed in horses an atopy-like, seasonal disease has been observed in young horses between 1 and 4 years of age. Arabian and Thoroughbred breeds are most often affected. Atopy is an uncommon genetically programmed pruritic disease probably associated with sensitization to inhaled antigens. Specific antigens presumably trigger the release of IgE, possibly IgG, and reaginic antibodies in the production of a Type I (anaphylactic) hyper-sensitivity. Clinical signs are those of intense pruritus, usually with self-mutilation to the face, limbs and body. This can be so intense as to cause actual skin tearing and bleeding. During repeated attacks the horse usually mutilates a different area of the body and therefore scarring or evidence of previous attacks are usually not obvious. Typically the horses do not seem able to stop the frenzied biting and rubbing once an attack begins. Predisposing causes include changes in environmental temperature such as extra rugs or in other instances, increased cold rather than heat. Differential diagnosis is difficult and relies on accurate history and elimination of all other possible causes. Intradermal skin testing and immune specific radio-allergosorbent testing (RAST) of blood are sometimes useful aids towards identifying specific allergens.

Food and contact hypersensitivities are rarely reported. Almost all normal horse feeds have been blamed but definite proof is often difficult. Resolution of the clinical signs following strict withdrawal of the allergen followed by return of identical and typical lesions after re-introduction of the allergen is a protocol which is strongly suggestive of food allergy. Clinical signs include pruritic urticaria (*see* **509**), plaques, generalised pruritus, tail rubbing and occasionally gastrointestinal tract disturbances such as diarrhea or colic. Again, diagnosis can be extremely difficult. Horses suffering from feed allergies create a considerable management problem and a diet of alfalfa hay is regarded as being hypoallergenic to horses. The nature of hypersensitivity disorders makes strict avoidance of the allergen imperative but maintenance of such a state is extremely difficult unless the specific allergen is identified and can be identified in potentially hazardous food.

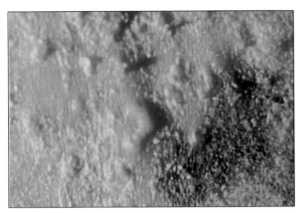

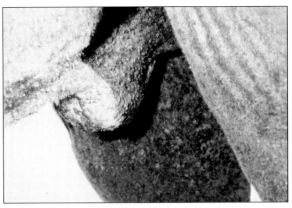

510 Pemphigus (foliaceus and bullous) (Early case).
Note: These intact bullae represent a transient early stage of the condition. The lesions rupture and leave large ulcerative and erosive lesions at the muco-cutaneous junctions in particular.

511 Pemphigus foliaceus.
Note: Lesions of an extensive exfoliative dermatitis, with no perceptible blistering, had been present for six months. Similar lesions were present over the neck and inside the ear.
Differential Diagnosis:
i) Dermatophytosis
ii) Bacterial (staphylococcal) folliculitis
iii) Sarcoidosis
iv) Equine exfoliative eosinophilic dermatitis
v) Systemic lupus erythematosus-like syndrome
vi) Dermatophytosis

Autoimmune skin conditions are a particularly difficult group of rarely occurring exfoliative diseases which require extensive and careful examination as well as multiple biopsies. It is particularly important that biopsies are taken correctly from new lesions. The most common of these disorders is **pemphigus foliaceus**. The condition occurs without sex or age predilection with lesions which initially occur on the face and limbs and then spread over the body. Clinically, very short lived vesicles **(510)** may be seen with epidermal collarettes which progress rapidly to pustule, crusting, seborrhea and skin folding **(511)**. More chronic lesions show heavier crusting. There is concurrent fever, depression and rapid weight loss. Differential diagnosis includes dermatophilosis, dermatophytosis, equine sarcoidosis, exfoliative dermatitis and systemic lupus erythematosus. Definite diagnosis relies on histopathological examination of (multiple) skin biopsies obtained from early lesions and on the application of immune histochemistry.

Bullous pemphigoid is a rare vesiculo-bullous, ulcerative disease of the muco-cutaneous junctions and the skin. It represents a Type II (cytotoxic) hypersensitivity and is characterised histologically by dermo-epidermal vesicle formation and immunologically by auto-antibody at the basement membrane of the skin and mucosa. Clinically, sub-epidermal vesicles and erosions occur around the mouth, eyes, nose **(512)**, tongue and vulva. Chronic lesions in advanced cases show crusting and ulceration with epidermal collarettes. Severely affected horses lose condition, become depressed and may be febrile. Treatment is unrewarding, requiring high doses of corticosteroids and or other immuno-suppressive drugs; ultimately euthanasia is invariably indicated.

Equine sarcoidosis is an exfoliative dermatitis of unknown etiology. It is associated with severe, progressive and often fatal wasting. Multiple internal organ involvement is present and clinically horses show loss of appetite, persistent low grade fever, severe loss of body condition and a generalised exfoliative dermatitis **(513)**. Diagnosis is based on skin biopsy which shows the presence of sarcoidal granulomatous perifollicular and mid-dermal dermatitis. The same type of lesions are also found in mesenteric and thoracic lymph nodes, lung, liver, spleen and throughout the gastro-intestinal tract. The disease may be related to the generalised granulomatous disease of horses (*see* **521**).

Although cases of **systemic lupus erythematosus (SLE)** have not been confirmed in the horse, a syndrome which is clinically very similar, has been described and is referred to as the SLE-like syndrome of horses. It is a multisystemic autoimmune disorder with no obvious or consistent etiology, although some affected animals have

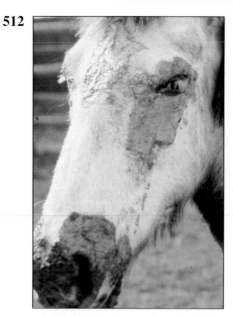

512 Bullous pemphigoid.
Note: Chronic severe lesions involving the (ears), eyes and mouth of a 5 year old Thoroughbred mare.
Differential Diagnosis:
i)   Drug reaction/hypersensitivity
ii) Vesicular stomatitis
iii) Coital exanthema
iv) Horsepox
v) Systemic lupus erythematosus-like syndrome

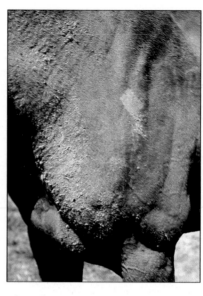

513 Equine sarcoidosis.
Note: Heavy scurf, crust and exfoliative dermatitis with areas of alopecia. Weight loss and epidermal folding were evident.
Differential Diagnosis:
i)   Dermatophilosis
ii) Dermatophytosis
iii) Pemphigus foliaceus
iv) Seborrhea
v) Systemic lupus erythematosus-like syndrome
vi) Exfoliative eosinophilic dermatitis
vii)Arsenic and mercury poisoning

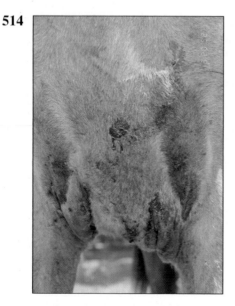

514 Systemic lupus erythematosus-like syndrome of horses.
Note: Vasculitis lesions and edema of subcutaneous tissues of brisket.

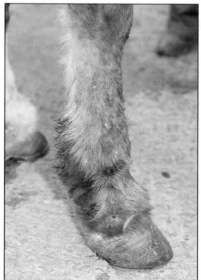

515 Systemic lupus erythematosus-like syndrome of horses.
Note: Vasculitis lesions in lower limb resulting in serum exudation and focal necrosis.

516

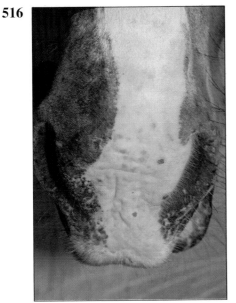

517

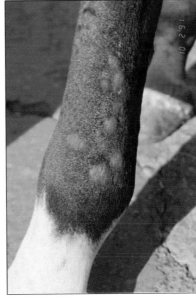

516 Systemic lupus erythematosus-like syndrome of horses.
Note: Fresh and older vasculitis (hemorrhagic) lesions in skin of muzzle.

517 Immune mediated vasculitis.
Note: Exudative lesions developed two weeks after upper respiratory tract infection.
Differential Diagnosis:
i)   Bullous pemphigoid
ii) Systemic lupus erythematosus-like syndrome
iii) Equine viral arteritis
iv) Drug Sensitivity/toxicosis
v)   Purpura haemorrhagica

a history of previous respiratory tract infection. Clinically, affected horses have prominent skin pathology with exudative lymphedema of the legs, ventral abdomen and brisket **(514)**, panniculitis, alopecia and prominent scaling of the legs **(515)**, face and sheath. The multi-organ involvement often includes the eye with marked (if transient) recurrent hypopyon (*see* **642**) and uveitis (*see* **623**). Joint inflammation, with chronic, ill-defined, shifting-leg lameness and joint swelling is often present. A severe thrombocytopenia and vasculitis may be present and these manifest as obvious pin-point (or larger) hemorrhages in the skin **(516)** and mucous membranes **(Plate 8h**, page 179**)**. Mild forms of the disease may show only areas of skin and hair depigmentation over the body and face, which appear to ebb and flow, and are also temporarily responsive to oral corticosteroids. However, the course of the disease is notoriously unpredictable; remissions have been reported, but where general wasting and other systemic abnormalities such as thrombocytopenia, polyarthritis, monoclonal gammopathies and recurrent fever, have occurred, the prognosis is unfavourable. Diagnosis is dependent upon the presence of the typical transient and recurrent, multiple organ clinical signs, and positive multiple

biopsies, which show a characteristic hydropic interface dermatitis. While a positive antinuclear antibody in serum is highly suggestive, this is seldom demonstrated in horses showing all the signs of classical systemic lupus erythematosus. The specific detection of lupus cells has also not been established in these cases.

Immune vasculitis perhaps occurs more commonly as a sequel to streptococcal infections than may be realised. Clinically, it shows as purpura with edema, necrosis and ulceration of the lower limbs and oral mucosa. The changes are typical of a Type I (anaphylactic or immediate) or Type III (immune complex) hypersensitivity reaction. The clinical signs are largely similar to those described for the systemic lupus erythematosus-like syndrome and, indeed the separation of the two may be difficult. Commonly, lesions are found on the coronet and lower limb **(517)**. Early lesions show hair loss and erythema followed by necrosis and sloughing of the skin; wounds are slow to heal and where severe coronary lesions occur, euthanasia may be the only option. Biopsy of the early lesions shows neutrophilic (leukocytoclastic), eosinophilic, lymphocytic or mixed vasculitis. Direct immunofluorescence testing may demonstrate

273

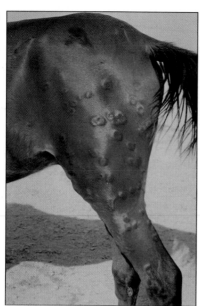

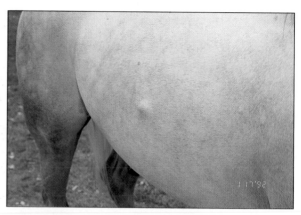

518 Erythema multiforme.
Note: Arciform and serpiginous lesions over the hind quarters of a Thoroughbred mare. Doughnut-like lesions are typical.
Differential Diagnosis:
i)   Urticaria
ii) Amyloidosis
iii) Mastocytoma
iv) Cutaneous histiocytic lymphosarcoma
v) Vesicular dermatoses

519 Equine (axillary) nodular (eosinophilic) necrosis.
Note: Non painful, solid, dermal nodules in the girth area.

immunoglobulin or complement. ***Purpura haemorrhagica***, an acute form of the disease is characterised by hemorrhage in the mucous membranes (**Plate 8g**, **Plate 8h**, page 179) as well as edema of legs and subcutaneous tissues (*see* **296**); sloughing of the skin occurs with extensive serum exudate from the limbs, in particular.

Erythema multiforme, is a rare, acute, self-limiting, urticarial, maculopapular or vesiculo-bullous dermatosis, with characteristic 'doughnut-like' urticarial plaques in the skin (**518**) which develop rapidly. There is no scaling, crusting or alopecia associated with these lesions. Biopsy shows a hydropic interface dermatitis.

Equine axillary nodular necrosis occurs infrequently. As its name implies it is characterised by the development of an irregular number of firm, well-defined skin nodules of varying size which are particularly distributed in the girth and axillary regions. Clusters of lesions are usually encountered and these may, in fact, be found at any location including the withers and the hind quarters. The lesions do not at first involve the loss of overlying hair but latterly they may become larger and usually show a focal area of alopecia (**519**). The lesions themselves are histologically distinctive and are benign in their behaviour.

Equine cutaneous amyloidosis, a rare papulo-nodular disorder of skin and nasal mucosa, clinically shows as nodules (**520**) and plaques in the skin and the mucosa of nasal passages (*see* **203**). The lesions often appear suddenly and are slowly progressive. Epistaxis may be the earliest sign of the condition. Diagnosis is based on the history, which often reveals repeated immune stimulation, underlying neoplasia or a chronic organic infectious process. Histopathology of lesions shows the presence of amyloid.

Generalised granulomatous disease of horses is a recently recognised clinical syndrome with prominent skin lesions and widespread internal organ involvement. The cases are usually presented for the investigation of weight loss and the skin lesions may take two distinct forms, although they may co-exist in the same animal at the same time. The rarer form shows nodules and large tumour-like masses in the skin while the more usual type shows multiple small pustular lesions (**521**) which may extend over a relatively small area at first but which tend to spread and coalesce. The ventral abdomen and the inguinal region are most often involved. There is seldom any lymphadenopathy in the external (palpable) lymph nodes but internal lymph nodes (including iliac and mediastinal nodes), lungs, liver, spleen and gastrointestinal tract contain distinctive (but often microscopic), non-caseating granulomas which histologically resemble the skin lesions.

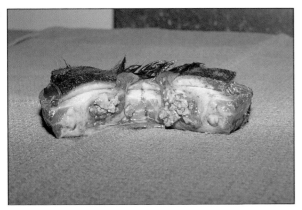

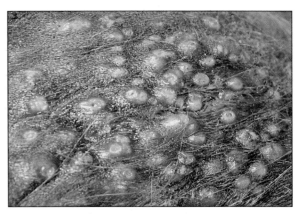

520 Cutaneous amyloidosis.
Note: Multiple, non-painful, non-pruritic, cutaneous nodules and plaques were present over then head, neck and shoulders. Epistaxis (Plate 8e, 8g) and nasal mucosal plaques which bled easily were present (see 203)
Differential Diagnosis:
equine eosinophilic granuloma
ii) Mastocytoma
iii) Infectious granulomas

Evidence of prolonged immune stimulation may be found in serum with gammopathies, hyperfibrinogenemia and neutrophilic leukocytosis. The pathogenesis of the disorder is uncertain. It is thought to be the result of an inordinate

521 Generalised granulomatous disease of horses.
Note: Miliary pustular, nodular and fibrous lesions were present over the entire ventral abdomen of a 5 year old Thoroughbred mare. Iliac lymph nodes were grossly enlarged and an acid-fast organism was identified in sections from the lesions.
Differential Diagnosis:
i) Equine sarcoidosis
ii) Staphylococcal/folicular dermatitis

immune response but, apart from the finding of some acid-fast organisms within the skin lesions of isolated cases, the reason for this response is undetermined. There are some similarities to equine sarcoidosis (*see* **513**).

Infectious Disorders

Important infectious skin disease may be caused by viral, bacterial or fungal agents. Commonly they all cause hair-loss and variable epidermal exfoliation and exudation. In the case of deeper tissue diseases such as pythiosis and other systemic mycoses, excessive fibrous tissue formation and more copious exudation are typically present. Pruritus may be intense or may be absent. Secondary physical damage can occur from self-inflicted trauma, which in turn encourages continued self-mutilation.

Virus Diseases

Equine sarcoid is a locally aggressive, fibroblastic tumour of equine skin with a variable epithelial component, and circumstantial evidence supports the idea that it is caused by a virus (possibly a retrovirus or a virus related or identical to the bovine papovavirus (papilloma) virus). For this reason, the condition is presented here as a primary viral disease rather than as a skin tumour. A wide variety of forms exist and for convenience they are divided into five types.

Type I: Occult sarcoid

Clinically, these are recognised as a well defined alopecic area (**522**). With time, the area of alopecia may increase or it may remain static for months or years, without any tendency to return to normal. The lesion involves only the most superficial layers of the dermis and alopecic areas may have a flaky surface and are often mistaken for ringworm lesions (dermatophytosis). It is quite common for these to develop areas of more warty, grey, hyperkeratinized tissue (**523**) or obvious single or multiple nodules (nodular sarcoid) in and under the skin. Many of these lesions are not progressive and unless traumatized, do not clinically change over long periods. Some, however, gradually develop increased numbers of nodules or hyperkeratinized areas which may become more verrucous (warty), but still remain relatively sessile. These hyperkeratotic nodules may further increase in size and if abraded, may result in the development of a more aggressive fibroblastic form of the tumour.

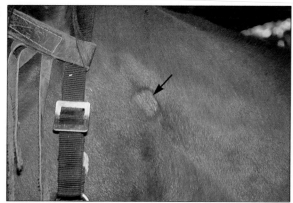

522 Occult sarcoid.
Note: Discrete area of alopecia (arrow).
Differential Diagnosis:
i) Dermatophytosis
ii) Traumatic/ rubbing injury

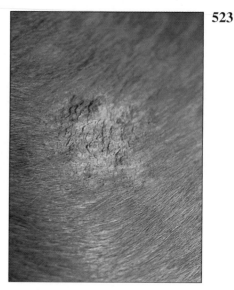

523 Occult sarcoid.
Note: Verrucose surface

Type II: Verrucose (warty) sarcoid

An increased dermal involvement results in the appearance of obvious, irregular flat areas of hyperkeratosis with marked skin thickening. The extent of hyperkeratosis is very variable with those occurring in the periorbital skin often being almost smooth and hairless. They may be sessile, with a broad base (**524**) or pedunculated (**525**). Extensive verrucous sarcoids are sometimes present on the medial thigh and in the axiliary region. Typically, this type is slow growing and seldom become more aggressive until abrasion, injury or surgical interference occurs. They may then become granulomatous and commonly adopt a more aggressive, fibroblastic appearance.

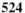

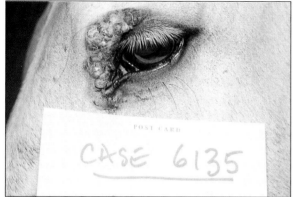

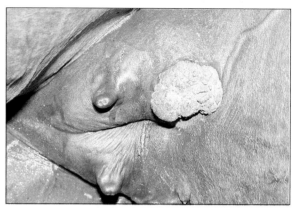

524 Verrucose sarcoid (sessile).
Note: Warty, grey, hyperkeratotic appearance.

525 Verrucose sarcoid (pedunculated).

Type III: Fibroblastic sarcoid

These tumours have both dermal and subdermal components and are much more aggressive in both appearance and character than the previous two types. Lesions are often pedunculated, ulcerated and red in colour (**526**). They may enlarge rapidly, especially those occurring on the lower limbs, and may attain considerable size (**527**) within weeks or months and then may remain static for years, showing variable periods of apparent improvement and deterioration. They are highly vascular and many bleed significantly following minimal trauma (*see* **526**). Some of the largest fibroblastic lesions develop when the other, more superficial, types have been traumatised and others can be associated with wound scars (*see* **527**). A particularly aggressive fibroblastic sarcoid (malevolent form) which spreads along lymphatic vessels creating extensive nodules and multiple, ulcerating fibroblastic masses is occasionally encountered (**528**) and represents an advanced stage with a very poor prognosis. Occasional fibroblastic forms on the lips may erode through to give ulceration on the buccal mucosa. The superficial appearance of fibroblastic sarcoids may belie the extent of dermal and subdermal involvement and surgical excision is often followed by rapid regrowth of an increasingly aggressive fibroblastic tumour-like mass. Multiple lesions are also common at sites of attempted excision or cryosurgery.

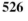

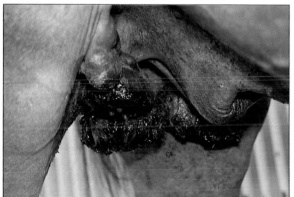

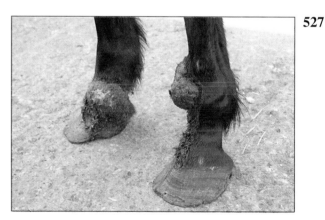

526 Fibroblastic sarcoid (pedunculated and sessile).
Note: Fleshy appearance. Other nodular lesions are present in the groin.

527 Fibroblastic sarcoid (sessile).
Note: Lesions developed at site of traumatic injury on coronet of right foot and on fetlock of left leg.

528

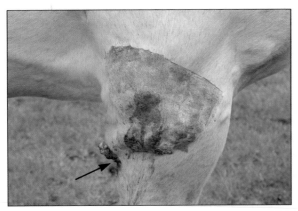

529

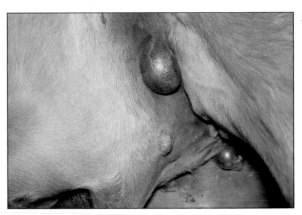

528 Fibroblastic sarcoid (malevolent form).
Note: Primary lesion on caudal aspect of elbow (arrow). Extensive nodular and linear fibroblastic sarcoids in lymphatic vessels of shoulder. Prescapular lymph node enlarged and contained sarcoid tissue.

529 Nodular sarcoid.
Note: Large subcutaneous nodule in flank. Smaller nodule in site of castration wound and in lateral aspect of sheath. These are sometimes recognised as fibromas

Type IV: Nodular sarcoid

This form of sarcoid is entirely sub-cutaneous although occasionally they may erupt through the overlying skin and then have a similar appearance to the fibroblastic form. The more usual appearance is of one or many, dense, often spherical nodules lying below the skin (**529**). Typical sites for the development of this type of lesion are the thin skinned areas of the inguinal region, the sheath, medial thigh and the eyelids (*see* **659**). The overlying skin is most often normal and the nodule may be mobile under it. In some cases, however, nodules which are histologically and clinically identical occur within the skin itself and under these circumstances the nodule moves with the skin. With the exception of those nodular sarcoids occurring in the eyelids, which are often adherent to the overlying skin, this form appears to have a more benign character and is reasonably amenable to surgical excision. On section the nodules show a typical dense appearance (*fibroma durum*) with a well demarcated edge. Biopsy or other trauma to the overlying skin, however, often causes a dramatic change to the fibroplastic form (*see* **526**).

Type V: Mixed verrucose, fibroblastic and nodular sarcoids

A wide variety of mixed sarcoids occurs having areas which are characteristic of the other more easily defined single types (**530**), and they may merely represent a transition from the occult, verrucose or nodular sarcoids to the more aggressive fibroblastic type.

Interference with any of the individual types may

530

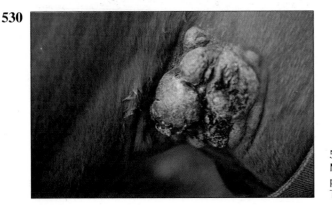

530 Mixed sarcoid.
Note: Nodular, fibroblastic and verrucose elements present in sarcoid in throat region of 5 year old Thoroughbred mare.

result in marked increase in the fibroblastic component of the mass and it is likely then that the mixed forms are the result of minor or major, localised or generalised insults applied to otherwise less aggressive lesions. It is unusual for the verrucose, nodular or occult forms to develop into anything other than the fibroblastic form following interference (including biopsy or accidental damage).

It appears that some areas of the body are more liable to the development of specific forms of sarcoid. Around the eye all forms may be found but within the eyelid the nodular form is by far the most common (*see* **659**). Similarly the nodular form is rarely encountered on the limbs but is particularly common in the skin of the medial thigh, sheath and inguinum (*see* **529**). Limb and brisket sarcoids are most often fibroblastic in character (*see* **527**) while lesions occurring in the axilla are usually of mixed type (*see* **530**). Lesions on the sides of the neck and on the breast are commonly occult (*see* **522**) or verrucose sarcoids. While this distribution pattern is commonly encountered it should be emphasised that it is by no means invariable and that any interference, in particular, and natural progression may result in significant variations in the basic pattern. The recognition of sarcoids is usually simple and does not warrant the risks associated with biopsy, although this is characteristic histologically. Neurofibromas and fibromas are similar in gross appearance but histologically and culturally distinctive.

Equine genital herpes virus (coital exanthema) infections which are due to equine herpes virus-3, occur throughout the world and while transmission is, in most cases, by venereal means during coitus the disease has occurred in sexually naive animals. Spread by inhalation of infected fomites and insect bites has been blamed for these. Following an incubation period of between 7 and 10 days, papules and vesicles develop on the affected skin of the penis and prepuce or vulva. These rapidly develop into pustules in the penile skin (*see* **858**) and vulva (*see* **809**). Infection may extend to the anus and skin of the tail. Spontaneous regression occurs with developing immunity over up to approximately 3 weeks and during this time the affected horse is potentially infective. Recurrence of lesions can occur in both stallions and mares due to lowered resistance such as might be caused by other generalised disease, over work, and parturition.

Horsepox viruses form a loosely related, unclassified group, but are responsible for several well recognised skin disorders. Infection occurs directly through the skin or the respiratory tract. Pox lesions have a typical clinical appearance of macules, papules and vesicles which then develop into pustules with a depressed centre. **Horsepox** occurs relatively commonly in Europe as a benign disease and may present with lesions on the mouth, face and nose (**531**), pastern, fetlock and vulva, which are essentially papules with a darker hemorrhagic centre. While most of the lesions are not painful, horses with leg lesions may show lameness.

Viral papular dermatitis, due to another unclassified pox virus, initially shows papules which develop crusts and after some 10 days the lesions develop an annular alopecia with scaling (**532**).

Equine molluscum contagiosum is caused by another unclassified pox virus, with a clinical appearance of circumscribed, raised, smooth, often umbilicated, papules with a waxy surface (**533**). A caseous plug may be found in the centre of the oldest lesions. The lesions most frequently occur around the genital organs of mares and stallions, and the axilla and muzzle. Diagnosis may be confirmed by biopsy.

531

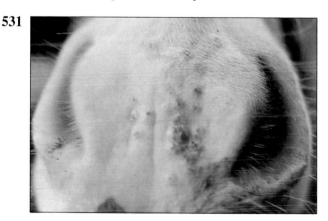

531 Horsepox.
Note: Papules with darker hemorrhagic centres and crusting of the area due to serum exudation.

532

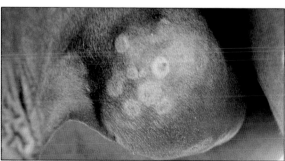

532 Equine viral papular dermatitis (vaccinia).
Note: Typical annular papules with darker hemorrhagic centres.

533

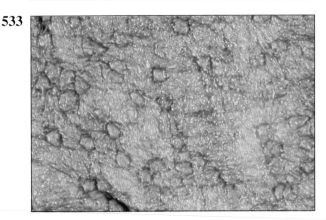

533 Equine molluscum contagiosum.
Note: Small pearly, umbilicated papular epithelial lesions.

534

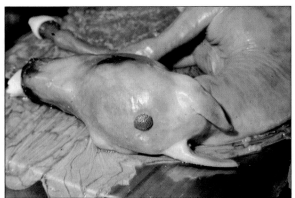

534 Viral papillomatosis (congenital lesion on aborted fetus).
Note: The disorder was not responsible for the abortion.

535

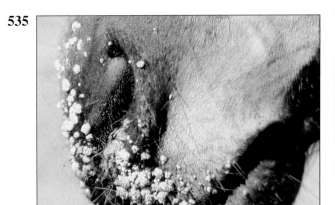

535 Viral papillomatosis.

536

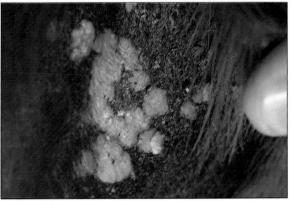

536 Viral papillomatosis (aural plaques).

Papovavirus has been associated with the development of papillomatous skin lesions on new born foals and these show as warty growths on any body location (**534**). In most of these congenital cases the lesion persists, though spontaneous regression may sometimes occur.

Virus warts (papillomata) are one of the most common skin diseases of grazing, yearling horses and are due to papovavirus infection. The condition can occur in older horses which are immunologically naive to the virus. The characteristic lesions show as single or multiple small verrucose tumours, principally around the nose, lips (**535**), and eyes. They may occur singly or form tight groups and may extend over a wide area of the face at an alarming rate. Lesions almost invariably regress spontaneously after 3 – 4 months. The virus appears capable of survival from season to season with each succeeding crop of weanling foals developing the condition at approximately 10-12 months of age each year on affected farms. Old horses (>18 years) may also become affected with large numbers of papillomas (warts) over the nose and genitalia. These do not appear to regress but likewise have no clinical significance but should be differentiated from the verrucose forms of sarcoid which are clinically much more significant. A clinically distinct form of papillomatosis occurs on the inside of the ears of adult horses, recognised as **aural plaques**. These commence as small, smooth depigmented papillae and progress to large, often extensive hyperkeratotic plaques on the inner surface of the pinna (**536**). These lesions seldom regress spontaneously and although they have little or no harmful effect they may become unsightly.

Bacterial Diseases

Normally, horse skin is highly resistant to bacterial infection unless constantly exposed to factors which cause lowering of the natural skin defence mechanisms. This will occur with excessive wetting, friction, physical trauma, biting insects and arthropods, injurious topical treatments and self mutilation. Bacterial skin disease may be primary or secondary to infection elsewhere in the body. Changes to the skin related to systemic infection may not necessarily be suppurative, but may show as vasculitis related to a spontaneous hypersensitivity to the common streptococcal organisms and this reaction may be a major presenting sign of ***purpura haemorrhagica*** (*see* **296; Plate 8h**, page 179).

Diagnosis of (primary) bacterial dermatitis is confirmed by the identification of bacteria obtained by skin scrapings or smears, but must be interpreted in conjunction with the clinical signs, due to the wide variety of organisms present as commensals on normal skin and the rapid secondary infection of wounds. In order to establish the true significance of a bacterial species with respect to its role in skin disease, such smears or samples should be taken from intact pustules, nodules or deep swabs from abscesses, preferably by needle aspiration or by direct culture from biopsy samples.

Dermatophilosis, due to *Dermatophilus congolensis*, is a common, superficial, infectious disorder characterised by a moist exudative dermatitis and pustular crusting of the hair. The condition is often referred to as 'rain scald' and occurs worldwide. It is particularly prevalent during periods of heavy or persistent rainfall and is commoner in the autumn and winter. Prolonged wetting of the *stratum corneum* results in the skin becoming more liable to trauma from rubbing, grooming instruments and ectoparasites. The exudation of even very small amounts of serum onto the skin-surface acts as an ideal environment for the organism. Sweating may also provide conditions which are conducive to the multiplication of *Dermatophilus congolensis*. It is clear that the pathogenesis of the disease is complex and the most severe cases are probably the result of more than one inciting factor. Furthermore, there are probably immunological components associated with the severity and/or duration of the condition. Hereditary factors involving the density and length of the hair-coat may also be important in determining the type and extent of infection in a particular breed or individual. The condition quite frequently affects groups of horses maintained together under unhygienic conditions, but individuals may become affected even when their environment is apparently satisfactory. The distribution of the lesions differs in the different forms but the moist exudative form is frequently restricted to areas of the body which are persistently wet or sweaty. Thus, under damp conditions it tends to affect the back and the sides (**537**), and is seldom found on the ventrum or on the upper, medial aspects of the limbs (areas which would probably never be persistently wet as a result of rain). The clinical appearance of the disease also varies with the hair density and length. Long-haired horses usually develop large plaques of matted hair overlying inflamed skin which tend to become increasingly exudative. Extensive

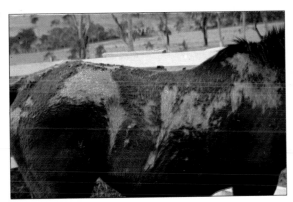

537 Dermatophilosis (winter/long-coat form).
Note: Loss of hair follows water run-off pattern. Remaining hair is matted with exudate, some areas of hypopigmentation over gluteal region.

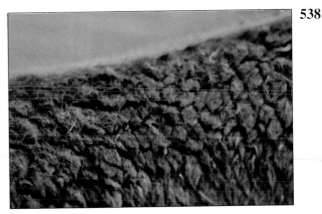

538 Dermatophilosis (winter/long-coat form).
Note: Hair matted in a tesselated pattern.

539

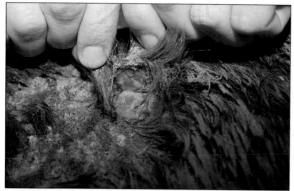

540

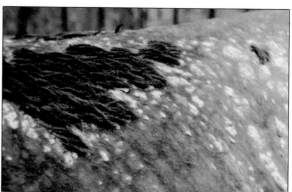

539 Dermatophilosis (winter/long-coat form).
Note: Pale glistening surface with purulent exudate found under matted hair.

540 Dermatophilosis (winter/long-coat form).
Note: Extensive hair loss leaving hyperkeratotic linear scabs and skin denuded of hair.

541

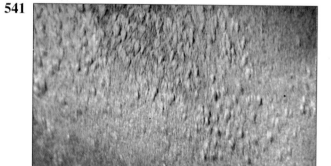

542

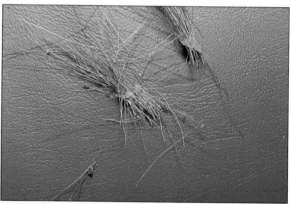

541 Dermatophilosis (summer/short-coat form).
Note: Paint-brush effect with denudation of hair. No purulent exudate, skin surface very dry.

542 Dermatophilosis (summer/short-coat form).
Note: Hair plucked from case shown in **541**, showing 'paint-brush' effect.

crusting and exudation with hair loss, or hair matted with exudate and bare skin areas showing patchy hypopigmentation are common developments (*see* **537**). Early cases of the disease in horses with long winter coats often show a matted, tessellated coat (**538**) over the affected areas, which, on being plucked, reveals a purulent undersurface (**539**). The lesions may be painful but are rarely, if ever, pruritic. As the matted hair is shed, it may leave long, linear, hyperkeratotic scabs (**540**). In short-haired horses (including summer-coated animals), lesions are smaller and occur as multifocal skin 'bumps' covered with crusts or scale. Although the lesions are obvious in severely affected horses (**541**) they are often more apparent by palpation than by visual inspection in mildly affected horses. Examination of tufts of hair plucked from these lesions reveals typical dermatophilosis scabbing at the roots of the hair giving a paint-brush effect (**542**). Denudation of hair is common in this

'summer/short-coat' form (**543**). An extensive, more severe form results from prolonged wetting of the skin. Interestingly, white-skinned areas appear to be particularly sensitive/susceptible to the condition and it is therefore commonly encountered on white areas of the distal limbs, particularly if the horse is maintained in long wet grass. Dermatophilosis on the skin over the metatarsals (hind cannons) is commonly encountered, independently of colour of hair, in racing horses which are exercised on cinders or in long, wet grass. It is likely that persistent wet and the trauma of cinders or grass, on the lower limbs is responsible for abrading the *stratum corneum* and introducing the organism to the deeper skin layers. Affected horses may be lame. Persistently muddy and wet underfoot conditions are associated with a skin disease known as 'Mud Fever' or 'Mud Rash' which occurs, again predominantly on the white areas on the palmar/plantar pastern and bulbs of the heels (**544**). The

543

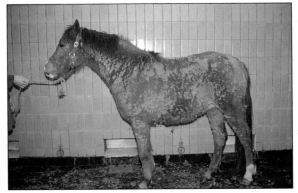

544

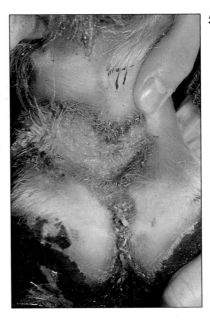

543 Dermatophilosis (generalised) (summer/short-coat form).
Note: Extensive hair loss followed minor grooming effort, leaving denuded skin with minimal scabbing and no apparent exudate.

544 Dermatophilosis (Mud rash, Mud fever).
Note: Extensive deep exudative dermatitis with cracking and thickening of skin on palmar pastern of white foot.

condition is entirely typical of dermatophilosis with moderate or severe dermatitis and exudation. The areas commonly become severely matted and the true extent of the condition is sometimes not appreciated. Persistent neglect of these lesions may result in lameness but more commonly causes thickening, scabbing and cracking of the area as the animal moves. Continued serum exudation provides ideal conditions for replication of the bacterium and other secondary pathogens such as *Staphylococcus* spp. Lesions of dermatophilosis may also occur on the head and again, at this site, white-skinned areas are more susceptible. A diagnosis of dermatophilosis is sometimes difficult as a result of prolonged, heavy, secondary bacterial contamination, but Giemsa, methylene blue or Gram stained smears of the exudate from fresh lesions show typical branching filaments or rows of coccoid bodies having a 'railway-line-like' appearance. In most cases dermatophilosis is a self-limiting condition, provided that all inciting factors such as wetness, skin trauma, sweating and ectoparasites are eliminated and the micro-environment for the organism is thereby altered to preclude its multiplication.

The coagulase-positive *Staphylococcus intermedius* and *Staphylococcus aureus* gain entry to the skin through wounds and abrasions after contact with dirty or contaminated tack such as saddle blankets, saddles, girths, bridles etc. The disorder is commoner at the end of winter when coat shedding is occurring and during periods of increasing ridden work in higher environmental temperatures. Poor grooming method or equipment and poor hygiene with respect to grooming equipment may also be responsible for introduction of the bacteria into relatively innocuous skin abrasions. Infection takes the form of a folliculitis and occurs particularly around the shoulders and in the saddle area **(545)**. Prominent exudation of serum occurs in the affected area and the purulent material often mats the hair producing a heavy scab. Lesions are seldom pruritic but are almost always inordinately painful, causing the horse to bite or kick while the sites are being examined. Some lesions may develop a central ulcer which discharges pus or a serosanguineous fluid and then become encrusted. This often leaves alopecic areas which can be confused with ringworm (dermatophytosis) lesions. Scurfing, leukoderma and leukotrichia can follow. Lesions occurring in the saddle area, girth and the withers often induce marked and permanent leukotrichia, producing the so-called 'saddle marks'.

Botryomycosis is primarily a chronic bacterial (staphylococcal), granulomatous, disease of the skin but may, on occasion, involve internal organs. The most common clinical entity is that which follows contamination of limb or scrotal wounds. The lesions are non-pruritic, non-healing, granulomatous nodules which sometimes develop into larger tumour-like growths **(546)**. Botryomycosis occurring at the site of contaminated castration wounds results in a non-healing, discharging mass of fibrous tissue at the end of the spermatic cord, containing myriads of small septic foci (*see* **842**). These wounds seldom, if ever, heal

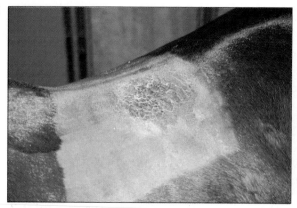

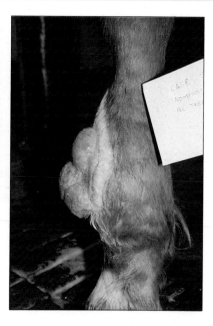

545 Staphylococcal dermatitis/folliculitis.
Note: Lesion restricted to saddle-contact area. Very painful lesion with exudate.

546 Botryomycosis (chronic, possibly staphylococcal dermatitis).
Note: Lesion had been present with little change for several years.
Differential Diagnosis:
i)   Exuberant granulation tissue
ii) Cutaneous habronemiasis
iii) Fungal granuloma/mycetoma
iv) Sarcoid
v) Neoplasia

spontaneously and a chronic discharging sinus is usually present at the scrotal incision which is known as a scirrhous cord (*see* **841**). A diagnosis is only confirmed histologically from surgical sections or biopsy which show a nodular to diffuse dermatitis with tissue granules.

Discrete **abscesses** associated with skin injuries are unusual in the horse unless there are complicating factors such as necrotic tissue or foreign bodies. However cheek abscesses may also occur in relation to sharp teeth causing gum erosion becoming infected with *Staphylococcus* spp. bacteria. This causes hard, hot, painful swellings to arise externally which eventually rupture, discharging thick purulent material.

Streptococcal skin infection occurs widely amongst the horse population and *Streptococcus equi*, *Streptococcus zooepidemicus* and *Streptococcus equisimilis* are probably the commonest secondary bacterial invaders of skin wounds in horses. Skin infection may arise directly from contamination of wounds or as a result of systemic infections such as Strangles (*see* **226** *et seq*). The skin infection usually results in the local development of a furunculosis (**547**), folliculitis, ulcerative lymphangitis and focal abscess.

Ulcerative lymphangitis is an uncommon bacterial infection of the cutaneous lymphatics and is generally attributed to lymphatic infection by *Corynebacterium equi*

or *Corynebacterium paratuberculosis*, as well as some other opportunist pathogenic bacteria. The disease occurs under conditions of poor hygiene and poor management and may be related to dust and insect bites. Lesions are mostly found on the hind limbs of both foals and adults and consist of hard or fluctuant subcutaneous nodules which ulcerate and then burst onto the skin surface. Chronic draining sinus tracts develop (**548**). A condition known as **Pigeon Chest, Wyoming Strangles** or **False Strangles**, in which a large pectoral or ventral abdominal abscess develops (**549**), occurs in the western states of the United States of America and in Brazil. The condition is possibly spread by biting flies and is due to *Corynebacterium pseudotuberculosis*. The abscesses characteristically contain (and discharge) a creamy or caseous white to greenish pus. All these disorders cause various degrees of lameness and debility and there is a high incidence of clinical complications including *purpura hemorrhagica*, abortion, and endocarditis. Diagnosis is therefore very important. However, the organism may be present in very small numbers (even in large abscesses) and only poor serological tests are available at present which are not directly indicative of the extent of infection.

Clostridium species are spore forming, gram-positive rods, whose toxins are associated with neurological diseases such as **tetanus** (*see* **731** *et seq.*) and **botulism**

547

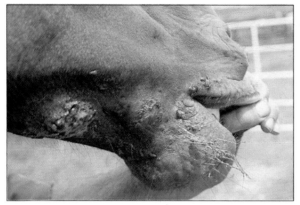

548

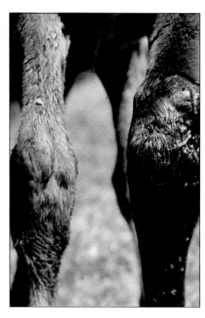

547 Streptococcal furunculosis.
Note: *Streptococcus equi* and *Streptococcus zooepidemicus* were isolated.

548 Ulcerative lymphangitis (*Corynebacterium equi*).
Note: Lesions affecting the lower hind limbs of foal above the hock. It is unusual to find lesions above the hock or on the front limbs.
Differential Diagnosis:
i) Glanders (Farcy)
ii) Equine histoplasmosis
iii) Tuberculosis

(*see* **735**). However, localised infections with organisms such as *Clostridium septicum* and *Clostridium perfringens* are capable of acute and dangerous wound infection at sites of injections, trauma and/or surgery. Cases of clostridial abscess in horses which have received injections of steroid hormones, selenium compounds and ivermectin have been recorded. Abscesses may develop over a period of days and result eventually, in a hot painful swelling and severe lameness (depending on the site of injection). Many require surgical drainage to release their purulent to serosanguineous gassy contents; necrosis of overlying skin and adjacent muscle (*see* **475**) is not uncommon. Injections which are contaminated by *Clostridium chauvoei* may be extremely serious and result in a life-threatening myonecrosis.

Glanders (Farcy) occurs in Eastern Europe, Asia and North Africa, and is caused by *Pseudomonas mallei* Both acute and chronic forms of the infection are encountered which involve the skin and/or the respiratory tract. Cutaneous Glanders (Farcy) occurs as ulcers or nodules anywhere on the body, but most commonly on the medial aspect of the hock (**550**), face and neck (**551**). The lesions begin as subcutaneous nodules which rapidly ulcerate and discharge a honey-like exudate. Corded lymphatics and swollen lymph nodes are common. The accompanying respiratory signs are much more serious in the acute forms, but some horses may show only the cutaneous form (Farcy) with minor nasal involvement for many years, performing reasonably well, until stress or debility reduces their resistance and these then succumb to the pulmonary form. Glanders is almost always directly fatal or results in a severe and debilitating and protracted illness from which few horses recover sufficiently to perform normally. It is an important zoonosis which has been eradicated from large areas of the world, but which still poses a threat to horses everywhere.

Spherophorus (Fusiformis/Fusobacterium) necrophorus has caused liver abscesses in horses but also has a cutaneous manifestation. Affected horses exhibit an extremely painful, exudative dermatitis of the lower limbs, the cannon bone, fetlock and coronet (**552**). In some cases the disease is the result of poor hygiene. Deep, wet bedding or muddy underfoot conditions, such as might be encountered around water troughs, are often associated with the disease. Co-habitation with cattle under the same conditions may also, significantly, increase the incidence of the condition.

549
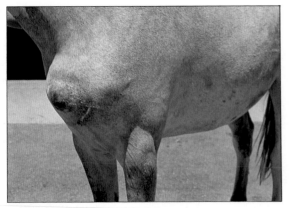

550
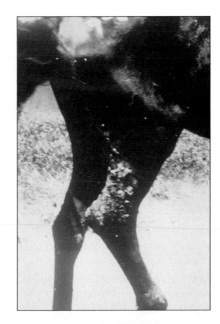

549 Chest abscess (pigeon breast / Wyoming strangles) (*Corynebacterium equi*).

550 Glanders (*Pseudomonas mallei*).
Note: Chains of ulcerated, discharging nodules following lymphatic versals

551
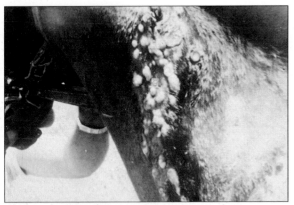

552
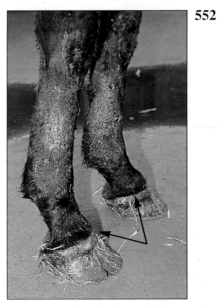

551 Glanders (*Pseudomonas mallei*).
Note: Chains of ulcerated lymphatic nodules.

552 Necrobacillosis
(*Spherophorus/Fusobacterium/Fusiformis necrophorus*).
Note: Highly painful necrotic changes in skin of coronet (arrow). May also affect the skin of the distal limb causing an exudative necrotizing dermatitis.

Fungal Diseases

Fungal dermatoses probably represent the most common skin diseases of working horses. Three separate entities, involving different fungi, are recognised. These include superficial (cutaneous), subcutaneous and systemic mycoses. The subcutaneous forms, including **pythiosis** and **mycetomas** are much less common than the superficial forms, while the systemic or deep mycoses due to **blastomycosis**, **cryptococcosis** and **histoplasmosis** are even rarer. In limited areas of the world the latter diseases are very important while in all areas the superficial mycoses are relatively common.

Superficial mycoses include the diseases known as **ringworm (dermatophytosis, dermatomycosis)** which is a fungal infection of the superficial keratinized layers of the epidermis. Tissue penetration is limited only to actively growing hair follicles. Broadly, only two fungal species affect the skin of horses in this way. These are *Trichophyton* spp. and *Microsporum* spp., but other fungi such as *Candida* spp may occasionally induce skin disease. A wide variety of specific organisms has been identified from cases of superficial dermatophytoses in the horse, although the clinical signs of many of them are largely similar. ***Trichophyton equinum* (var. *equinum* and var. *autotrophicum*)** and ***Trichophyton mentagrophytes*** are the most common pathogens involved in the horse with isolated cases and outbreaks being due to ***Microsporum gypseum***. Transmission of the pathogen is usually through indirect contact (grooming brushes, rugs, saddles, girths etc.), with only occasional cases being acquired through direct contact with other affected horses. A much higher incidence of the disease is encountered in hot humid climates but sunshine appears to have a strong inhibitory effect on most of the species concerned. The spores are notoriously long-lived and may survive for several years in the environment in a viable form. Furthermore, they are highly resistant to many disinfectants and antiseptics. The spores must have access to skin abrasions for the clinical condition to develop and this is the reason for its development in sites where skin friction occurs, such as the girth, saddle and face. Young horses under the age of 4 years are particularly susceptible and show a more prolonged course than older horses. The incubation period varies between 1 and 4 weeks, depending upon the immune status of the host and the ambient temperature and humidity. Clinical signs of each species of pathogen are loosely related to the duration of infection. The most common organisms occurring endemically in racing stables are *Trichophyton equinum* var. *autotrophicum* (TE-vA) and *Trichophyton equinum* var. *equinum* (TE-vE). *Trichophyton equinum* lesions are typically ringworm-like in appearance, initially being well-defined, circular areas of erect, raised or short hair **(553)**. The hair is then lost and the lesions enlarge centrifugally, developing crusts and scabs **(554)**; new hair growth resumes between 35 and 55 days following infection and characteristically starts in the centre of the lesions. Alopecia and scaling are usually associated with

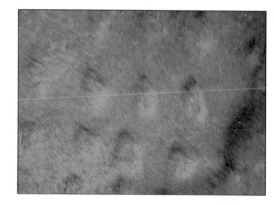

553

553 Dermatomycosis (dermatophytosis / ringworm) (*Trichophyton equinum* var *autotrophicum*). **Note:** Raised hair patches of very early lesions (10 days post infection).

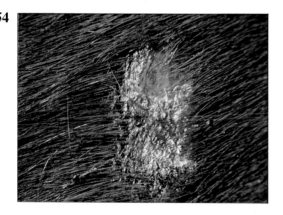

554

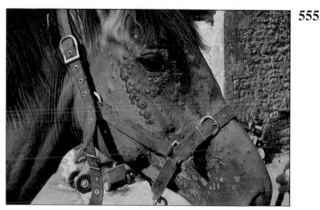

555

554 Dermatomycosis (dermatophytosis / ringworm) (*Trichophyton equinum* var *autotrophicum*). **Note:** Hair loss leaves silvery grey glistening skin which heals within 4 – 5 days. Borders of lesions poorly demarcated. **Differential Diagnosis:** i) Occult sarcoid

555 Dermatomycosis (dermatophytosis / ringworm) (*Trichophyton equinum* var *equinum*). **Note:** Obvious heavy encrustation with minimal exudation.

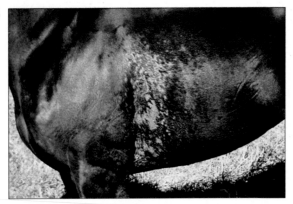

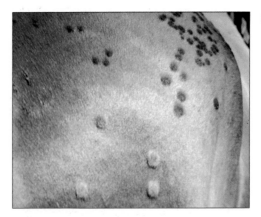

556 Dermatomycosis (dermatophytosis / ringworm) (*Trichophyton equinum* var *autotrophicum*).
Note: Distribution of lesions corresponding with girth position. Several horses sharing saddlery developed an almost identical syndrome over 2 weeks. Lesion approximately 14 days post infection.

557 Dermatomycosis (dermatophytosis / ringworm) (*Microsporum gypseum*).
Note: Location and pattern of lesions (in small groups of two-four) corresponds with biting sites of *Stomoxys calcitrans*. Hair loss not complete and scabs less easily removed than *Trichophyton* spp infection.

limited inflammation. Lesions associated with *Trichophyton equinum* var. *equinum*, which is probably the commonest variety in the northern hemisphere, are inclined to cause more obvious dermatitis (**555**) with severe crusting, exudation and folding of the skin. *Trichophyton equinum* var *autotrophicum*, on the other hand, which is the more common pathogen in the southern hemisphere, produces a more diffuse and scaly appearance (**556**). Plucked hair from areas affected with TEvA reveals underlying gray, glistening skin (*see* **554**), which scales over within one or two days. In both forms the larger, less well-defined areas represent the more protracted lesions. Pruritus is usually only present in earliest stages. As each fresh batch of yearlings enter the contaminated environment, they are soon exposed to rapid and predictable infection. This may take the form of face infection (*see* **555**) from contact with contaminated feeders, or body infection (*see* **556**), usually from contaminated grooming equipment or tack. Should infection not occur during the initial handling period, horses usually become infected during breaking-in or training, usually from contaminated girths, jockey's boots, or from the use of contaminated tack such as rugs. The location of the primary lesions is entirely predictable in areas of physical damage and indirect contact with infective material. Further rapid spread may occur from the initial lesions by the use of contaminated grooming brushes, to the extent that generalised infection is relatively common. Horses can become accidentally infected with **Trichophyton verrucosum** through contact with infected cattle or a contaminated environment where cattle have been stabled. In these cases lesions are more commonly found on the lower limbs, appearing initially

as raised hair with a thick, closely adherent crust. The hair is gradually shed usually leaving a large alopecic area with dense hyperkeratotic scaling.

Horses affected with **Microsporum gypseum** generally have smaller well-defined lesions, usually over the buttocks (**557**) and neck. The hair, in these lesions, plucks noticeably less-readily than that in *Trichophyton* spp. lesions. *Microsporum gypseum* is a soil saprophyte gaining entry to the horse's skin by abrasion and contact, or by biting insects such as *Stomoxys* spp. and mosquitoes, and the siting of the lesions reflects this mode of transmission. Contact with contaminated soil or bedding or horse transporters also spreads the disease; soils from yards containing infected horses yield *Microsporum gypseum* on culture. Other less common organisms which have been isolated include *Microsporum equinum* which produces small annular lesions with light scurf; lesions are usually found on harness pressure areas, and the organism is only weakly infective.

The majority of ringworm infections in horses will ultimately resolve spontaneously if left without treatment but the epidemiological factors involved with such a highly contagious disease makes its early recognition important. Although the clinical features of each species and each type have characteristic clinical signs these are by no means definite and the recognition of the specific organism is often important with respect to control and therapeutic measures. Hairs plucked from the periphery of the lesions should be examined directly under the microscope. The fungal spores and mycelium may be stained to make their recognition easier. Cultures obtained from the infective material are useful and

558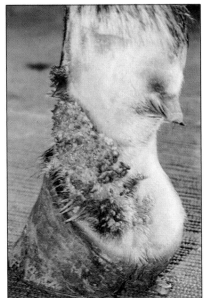

559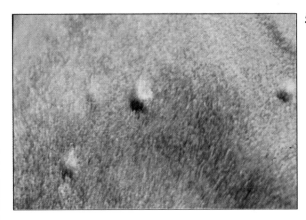

558 Mycetoma (Subcutaneous Mycosis).
Note: Ulceration of skin and development of tissue granules (pyogranulomas).

559 Phaeohypomycosis (*Drechslera specifera*).
Note: Diffuse nodular dermatitis on the neck of a horse , lesions contained dark or pigmented areas with pigmented hyphae. Sometimes with denuded plaques studded with pustules and papules.

provide the only practical means of identifying the species concerned but they usually take a long time to grow in culture. The information is therefore often retrospective, but may provide useful information as to future measures of control. All the species responsible for disease in horses have the potential to infect humans, and, indeed the disease may be transmitted between horses by attendants.

The differential diagnosis of dermatophytosis includes dermatophilosis (*see* **537** *et seq.*), occult sarcoid (*see* **522**), pemphigus foliaceus (*see* **511**) and linear hyperkeratosis (*see* **478**).

Subcutaneous mycoses occur in horses relatively commonly, particularly in tropical environments. They are usually characterised by localised swellings, draining tracts, and the presence of visible granules in the exudate. Clinically, most present as a chronic abscess which is refractory to normal medical treatment. Most of these fungal diseases need to be diagnosed accurately by means of fungal culture and biopsy. The causative agents may occasionally be identified with the help of specific fungal stains on direct microscopic examination of smears from exudates. In the case of sporotrichosis immunological tests can be used.

Eumycetic mycetoma is caused by several different fungi (*Curvularia geniculata, Helminthosporium spiciferum, Pseudoallescharia boydii* and *Madurella* spp.) which invade body tissues following skin injury. The disease may occur at any site where the organism is introduced into traumatised skin. Clinically, the lesions which are usually on the body trunk, external

nares or the legs (**558**) resemble a chronic abscess or pyogranuloma. The purulent discharge usually contains distinct, small granules which are black-brown in colour when associated with *Curvularia geniculata*, and cream-white when the organism is *Pseudoallescharia boydii*. A diagnosis is based on the chronicity and the failure to respond to any normal treatment and may be confirmed by culture and biopsy.

Phaeohypomycosis is a chronic subcutaneous infection caused by several different fungi including *Drechslera speciferum* and *Phialophora verrucosa*). The condition often occurs as solitary, painless nodules (**559**) which exude pus. Diagnosis is based on history, physical examination, biopsy and culture. *Aspergillus* spp. organisms have only rarely been found to cause skin disease in horses, although they have been responsible for invasive and non-invasive lesions in the nasal cavity (*see* **249**) and guttural pouch (*see* **250** *et seq.*). In animals suffering from immune suppression it may however be found associated with skin lesions of a similar type. Diagnostic procedures must include growth of the organism on Sabouraud's agar as well as positive histopathological findings.

Sporotrichosis occurs when skin wounds are contaminated by the soil saprophyte *Sporothrix schenckii*. It is generally regarded as a non-contagious disease. Clinical signs include cording of the lymphatics and enlarged cutaneous nodules on the legs and body (**560**). Ulceration with crusting, and discharge of a thick red/brown pus or serosanguineous fluid is common. Generalised body infection may show as similar crusted

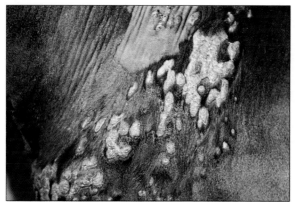

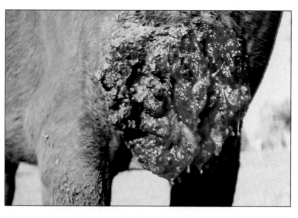

560 Sporotrichosis (*Sporothrix schenckii*).
Note: Multiple nodules and crusted plaques over the shoulder.
Differential Diagnosis:
i)   Bacterial/fungal granulomatous dermatitis
ii) Cutaneous histoplasmosis
iii) Glanders

561 Zygomycosis - Basidiobolomycosis (*Basidiobolus haptosporus*).
Note: Intense pruritus and serosanguineous exudate. Typical circular appearance. Lesions are seldom found on the limbs.

nodules and plaques. Diagnosis is confirmed by appropriate culture, skin biopsy, mouse inoculation, fluorescent antibody tests and indirect immuno-peroxidase staining of biopsy specimens.

Zygomycosis is a chronic fungal disease with cutaneous, subcutaneous, nasal and systemic forms, which is largely restricted to tropical regions. Organisms which may be isolated from horses include *Basidiobolus haptosporus* and *Conidiobolus coronatus*. Basidio-bolomycosis is a pruritic, ulcerative granulomatous disease, occurring characteristically on the chest, trunk, head and neck but very rarely affecting the limbs. Infection probably occurs from contact with contaminated soil. Lesions are ulcerative granulomata which may be extensive, and are often circular and exude a serosanguineous discharge which drips persistently from the lesion (**561**). Pruritus is a common feature. Lesions contain small, coral-like, granular 'kunkers', and diagnosis is based on biopsy and culture. Biopsy shows a pyogranulomatous dermatitis with plasma cell and eosinophil infiltration. Conidio-bolomycosis, caused by *Conidiobolus coronatus*, occurs most commonly as an infection of the external nares or nasal passages, as single or multiple ulcerating nodules on the external mares, nasal septum (*see* **248**), and/or nasal turbinates. The characteristic intermittent serosanguineous nasal discharge becomes persistent and may have a fetid odour. In severe cases respiratory obstruction with dyspnea may occur from the enlarging granulomas.

Pythiosis (phycomycosis, bursatti, swamp cancer, Florida horse leeches, hyphomycosis) is a relatively common disorder of the skin occurring in tropical and subtropical areas and particularly in the Gulf States of America, Australia and South America. It is usually associated with swampy conditions where horses either habitually graze in water, or are flood-bound, standing in water for long periods. The organism is probably not a genuine fungus but both its behaviour and the clinical syndrome it produces are typical of subcutaneous mycosis. The organism induces a severe pyogranulomatous reaction as it spreads throughout the tissues. The expansion of the lesion is extremely rapid due to the formation of granulation tissue and hemorrhage is a common feature of these lesions. Blood loss may be sufficient to cause significant anemia. Most lesions are found on the distal extremities and the ventral abdomen and chest, and are usually single. However, bilateral and multiple lesions may occasionally be encountered. Lesions are often initially relatively small and innocuous-looking, roughly circular, ulcerative granulomas, but they may arise explosively from an area which has previously only appeared to be mildly swollen. However, like a malignancy, the lesions rapidly destroy surrounding tissue and may spread through lymphatic vessels to the regional lymph nodes, and sometimes even into the abdominal cavity. The cutaneous manifestation of the condition is characterised by the copious out-pouring of a stringy, mucopurulent, serosanguineous discharge (**562**). The presence of large 'kunkers' or 'leeches', which are found in the multiple draining tracts represent cores of necrotic tissue

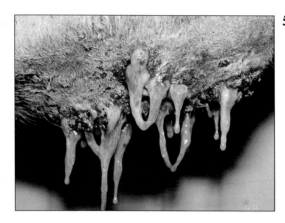

562 Pythiosis (phycomycosis) (Florida horse leeches) (*Pythium* spp.).
Note: Multiple, roughly circular, ulcerative, granulomatous lesions on abdominal wall. Stringy, hemorrhagic, serum exudate forms hanging 'leeches'.

containing the organism. Pruritus may be severe and result in extensive complicating self-inflicted trauma. Old lesions show chronic surrounding fibrosis and there may be long periods of time without the characteristic discharge. Lesions can occur on the lower limbs and frequently then involve tendons and joints or may occur at any other sites where the organism is introduced to wounds. Diagnosis is by biopsy and culture.

Differential diagnosis of all fungal diseases should include bacterial granuloma, habronemiasis, exuberant granulation tissue, foreign body reactions, sarcoid and various neoplasms. It is also possible to encounter mixed infections involving fungi, sarcoid and habronema larvae in a single lesion. A very careful clinical assessment and confirmatory biopsy and culture are then a necessity.

Systemic mycoses which cause fungal infection of internal organs may have secondary skin manifestations. Typically most responsible fungi exist in soil and vegetation and are rare pathogens. Even where organisms occur endemically, exposed animals do not often develop clinical disease.

Infections with *Cryptococcus neoformans*, *Coccidioides immitis*, *Histoplasma capsulatum* var. *farciminosi* and *Blastomyces dermatitidis* have all been reported to cause skin disease in horses. Cryptococcosis is unusual in distribution and is believed to be spread by pigeon droppings. The disease normally affects the respiratory and central nervous systems, bone and rarely the skin where it has been reported to cause granulomas on the lip. Blastomycosis has also been recorded as causing multiple granuloma and abscesses around the mammary gland and perineum. Coccidiomycosis has been associated with severe dust storms, high environmental temperatures and inhalation of organisms. Cutaneous infection may follow skin abrasions, and

appears as cutaneous ulceration, abscesses and multiple draining sinus tracts. Specimens for culture from suspected cases should be submitted to specialist laboratories dealing in fungal diseases, due to the risk of human infection. **Histoplasmosis** (epizootic lymphangitis, pseudoglanders, African Farcy, equine blastomycosis, equine cryptococcosis) due to the dimorphic fungus, *Histoplasma farciminosus*, is a chronic cutaneo-lymphatic infection which is endemic in Africa, Asia and Eastern Europe. It occurs in horses, mules and very rarely donkeys. Biting insects can be vectors of the disease and trauma appears necessary for infection to occur. Clinical signs initially include nodules (15–25 mm diam.) on the skin of the face, head, neck and rarely on the limbs. The nodules soften and eventually rupture, discharging a light-green, blood-tinged exudate. Progressive ulceration occurs with ulcers reaching up to 10cm in diameter. Some cases show nodules and ulceration along lymphatic chains. The lesions are almost indistinguishable from those of Farcy (cutaneous Glanders) (*see* **550, 551**) except that respiratory tract involvement is not common. Ocular histoplasmosis involving the medial canthus of the eye (*see* **669**) and, in particular, the puncta and naso-lacrimal duct (*see* **670**) is relatively common in donkeys in North Africa and the Middle East but is rare in horses. Infections may also involve one or more joints, leading to a purulent synovitis and severe disabling lameness. Diagnosis is based on direct smears, biopsy and culture. Direct impression smears, stained with Giemsa or Wright-Giemsa, typically show macrophages containing 4–6 round, unicellular organisms. Other tests such as intradermal skin tests and fluorescent antibody techniques are also used. The prognosis for affected animals is poor and there is no known, effective treatment.

Ectoparasitic Diseases

Dermatoses caused by ectoparasites form a large proportion of the common skin disorders of horses. As a group they are generally associated with pruritus and hair-loss. Irritability, rubbing of the mane and tail in particular and, in some instances, severe self-mutilation may be presented. Ectoparasites are also important vectors for the transmission of some very serious viral, bacterial, fungal, protozoal and helminth diseases. While the detection of parasites may simplify the diagnosis, a very careful and through examination may still fail to identify the causative agents involved and may necessitate the use of night-light traps, skin scrapings, culture of skin scrapings, biopsy and prolonged environmental studies. Many of the dermatoses due to ectoparasites are geographically restricted as well as seasonal, and this may help significantly in the diagnosis of clinical conditions which can be difficult to differentiate on clinical grounds only.

Pediculosis (louse infestation) is one of the more common causes of skin disease throughout the world. Both biting and sucking lice occur in horses and donkeys and the clinical effect of each is correspondingly different according to the life style of the parasite. Louse infestation is probably the most common form of pruritus in foals. Even small numbers of the biting louse, *Damalinia equi*, cause severe pruritus, scurf and alopecia of the head, the neck (usually under the mane) and the dorso-lateral trunk (**563**). Careful, prolonged examination of the horse is essential as the number of parasites involved is usually small, and skin scrapings from pruritic areas may be necessary to locate them or their eggs; a hand-lens may be a useful aid.

Much greater numbers of sucking lice, *Haematopinus asini*, are usually present. They are most frequently found at the base of the mane and tail, and over the croup and lower limbs. In horses with long (winter) hair coats, the infestation may extend over the entire skin surface giving the animal a 'moth eaten' appearance (**564**). Both the eggs (nits) which attach to the hair and the adult *Haematopinus asini* lice are visible to the naked eye (**565**). Severe tail-rubbing with hair loss and skin damage are usually encountered. These signs are common to *Oxyuris equi* infestation (*see* **150**), culicoides hypersensitivity (*see* **572** *et seq.*), and tail mange due to *Psoroptes cuniculi* or *Chorioptes equi* parasites. All louse infestations may be transmitted by direct contact and groups of horses housed in close proximity are therefore likely to develop the condition. Debilitated, diseased and horses suffering from immune suppression disorders, including pituitary adenoma (*see* **362** *et seq.*), are particularly liable to harbour enormous populations of the parasites. Under these conditions both the physical demands of persistent pruritus and, in the case of the sucking lice, blood loss, may result in further dramatic deterioration in body condition and health status.

Mange mites only occasionally cause significant

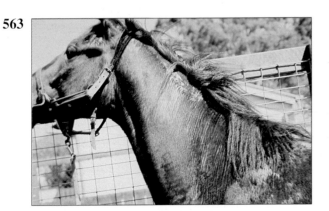

563 Pediculosis (louse infestation) (*Damalinia equi* - the biting louse).
Note: Mites are not usually visible to the naked eye. Typical predilection sites shown include face, base of the mane and over lateral thorax. Severe pruritus resulted in self-inflicted skin excoriation.

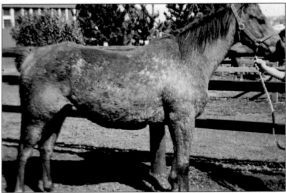

564 Pediculosis (louse infestation) (*Haematopinus asini* - the sucking louse).
Note: Generalised infestation resulting in a 'moth-eaten' appearance of the winter coat.

565

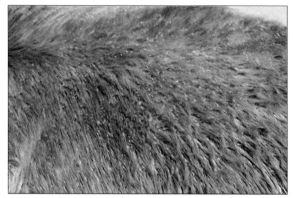

566

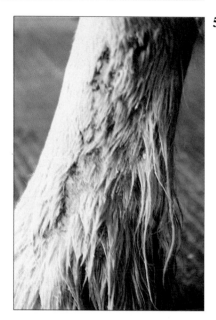

565 Pediculosis (louse infestation) (*Haematopinus asini* - the sucking louse).
Note: Adult lice and eggs (nits) are clearly visible to the naked eye.

566 Chorioptic mange (feather/leg and tail mange) (acute form).
Note: Severe pruritus caused leg-stamping and rubbing with consequent serum exudation and matting over the plantar and lateral aspects of the hind cannons and pasterns.

clinical problems. However, *Psoroptes cuniculi* is a possible cause of head-shaking. *Psoroptes equi* may, cause intense pruritus, crusting and alopecia, especially of the head (ears), mane and tail. It occurs in all ages of horses and particularly those in close contact or those which have common grooming and saddlery equipment. Once introduced into stables, it may infest most of the horses. In particular, yearlings being prepared for sales may display general body pruritus as well as tail rubbing. 'Lop ears' and pruritus with crustiness around the tail base are clinical indicators of this parasite. Skin scrapings obtained from the affected areas usually contain eggs or entire parasites.

Horses with 'feathered' legs can become infected with **chorioptic mange** due to *Chorioptes equi*. The disease is particularly prevalent in winter months and is particularly common in the heavy draught breeds. The parasite burrows into the skin of the pastern, fetlock and cannon (and occasionally the tail head), causing severe pruritus, leg-stamping, self-mutilation and heavy scale and scab formation (**566**). Neglected cases of chorioptic mange in draught horses may eventually lead to a severe, proliferative and exudative dermatitis known as 'Grease' or 'Greasy Heel' (**567**). The diagnosis of the original instigating cause is often impossible in advanced cases due to heavy secondary bacterial infection, myiasis and the dense fibrous reaction in the underlying skin. These factors also make therapy

extremely difficult and the condition carries a very guarded prognosis.

Demodex mites can sometimes be found in the skin of normal horses without the presence of any obvious clinical disease. On occasion, however, facial alopecia and scaling may be encountered. The most common location, even in normal horses, is in the eyelids and the neck from where the parasite may be identified by deep skin scrapings. Clinical disease due to *Demodex caballi* or *Demodex equi* is only probably associated with a reduced immune capacity and this aspect should be seriously considered when a case of serious clinical demodicosis is encountered. The finding in skin scrapings, or more particularly in biopsy samples from several sites is supportive of a diagnosis of demodicosis.

Free-living **trombiculiform mites** including *Trombicula* and *Neotrombicula* spp., forage mites (*Acarus* spp.) and occasionally poultry mites (*Dermanyssus gallinae*) can produce significant and sometimes alarming skin disease in horses. Trombiculid and acarine adults and nymphs are free living, their larvae usually feed on small rodents but may attack horses. Infestations usually occur in late summer and autumn and are mainly seen in pastured animals although preserved hay and bedding straw may harbour significant numbers of parasites inducing clinical disease at other times. Clinical signs include restlessness and leg-stamping with the early skin lesions showing as papules or wheals.

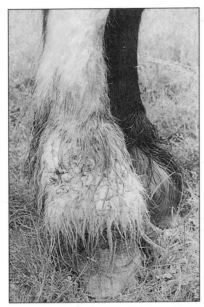

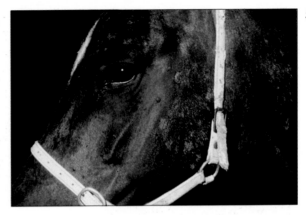

567 Chorioptic mange (grease/greasy heel) (chronic form).
Note: Extensive, foul-smelling, exudative and proliferative, chronic dermatitis which had been present for 4 years. This case was also complicated by heavy screw-worm myiasis. No chorioptic mites could be found but several of its peers had heavy infestations.

568 Trombiculidiasis (*Trombicula autumnalis*).
Note: Head lesion showing small well-defined, circular alopecic lesions.
Differential Diagnosis:
i)   Dermatophytosis (*Trichophyton equinum* var *equinum*)

Extensive numbers of lesions may be present with small alopecic areas developing over the head (**568**), limbs and trunk after the mites fall off. The mites, which may just be visible to the naked eye, are characteristically a yellow-orange colour, but some species are colourless and very difficult to locate. Groomings, scrapings and microscopic examination are necessary to reach a definitive diagnosis. Diagnosis may be particularly difficult as the mites only feed briefly for one or two days and then fall off. The poultry mite *Dermanyssus gallinae*, occasionally affects horses when stabled in or near poultry houses. Infestation occurs at night, causing severe pruritus with papules and crusts forming around the affected skin of the face and lower limb.

Ticks are important seasonal ectoparasites on horses in most tropical and subtropical regions. Skin injury is caused by the local effects of the bites and rarely through consequent self-mutilation. It is unusual for horses to harbour one or two ticks only and their identification usually presents few problems to the clinician. Their major importance lies more in their ability to transmit viral, bacterial and protozoal diseases. Significant blood loss with obvious anemia (**569**) may be an important aspect of massive infestations. Some ticks, even in very small numbers, may induce a

distinctive neurological disorder known as tick paralysis which may be fatal.

Two major families of ticks are known to cause specific clinical entities in horses. The *Argasidae* (soft ticks) includes *Otobius megnini* (the spinous ear tick) which affects a wide range of large animals including horses. Severe otitis externa accompanied by head-shaking, head tilt, behavioural problems and a waxy discharge are typical. The parasite can usually be readily seen in the depths of the external auditory tube.

The *Ixodidae* family of hard ticks include a number of individual species with the ability to transmit disease and induce specific skin disorders in various parts of the world. Tick related dermatoses are seasonal and correspond with the periods of feeding behaviour in the ticks concerned. Some ticks are slower to develop than others and some require more than one host during the life cycle. While most species will feed at any site, most have predilection sites such as the eyelids, ear, perineum (*see* **569**), axillae and groin. The lesions resulting from the bite alone are usually localised swelling and edema (**570**) but in many cases there is little local reaction (*see* **569**), in spite of heavy infestations. Severe anemia and loss of blood proteins resulting in generalised debility and edema are possible in heavily parasitised animals.

569

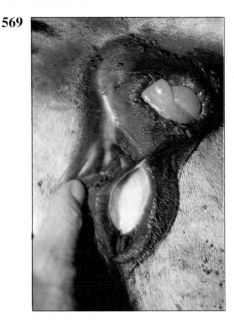

570

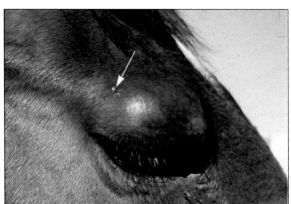

571

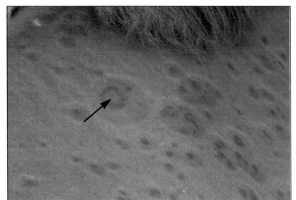

569 Tick infestation (*Rhipicephalus* spp).
Note: Lack of local reaction to presence of ticks. Severe anemia and edema of rectal mucosa. Heavy infestation affected head, ears, inguinum and perineum. No blood parasites were found to explain the anemia which was attributed to internal and external parasitism.

570 Tick infestation (hypersensitivity).
Note: Edema associated with an engorging *Ixodes* spp tick above the upper eyelid (arrow).

571 Insect bite hypersensitivity (*Stomoxys* spp).
Note: Central focus at bite site (arrow) and surrounding plaque of edema. Some bites in this case have subsided to a small central focus only while the more recent show an extensive hypersensitivity reaction.

The complicating factors relating to the transmission of *Babesia* spp parasites (*see* **319**) may exaggerate the clinical effects of these two signs. Any horse carrying ticks, even in low numbers, in areas where protozoal arthropod borne infections are endemic should be carefully assessed for the possibility of these being of pathological significance.

In Australia, hypersensitivity reactions have been recorded in individual horses to the larval stages of *Boophilus microplus*. Affected horses show a rapid onset (within 30 minutes), of multiple papules, principally of lower limbs and muzzle. Pruritus is intense with leg stamping, body rubbing and self mutilation.

A wide range of flies and other biting insects cause immense problems among horses both from local annoyance and the transmission of disease. Diagnosis of skin diseases related to fly damage relies heavily on observation, use of light-traps and careful assessment of the type of damage to the skin. Usually the presence of a

small central scab or focus of inflammation is related to physical bite injury. In some cases there may be almost no superficial evidence of the bites but in most cases there is a surrounding area of edema and occasional animals show marked hypersensitivity reactions to the bites of flies, mosquitoes and midges (**571**). *Stomoxys calcitrans*, the common stable fly, causes local irritation and hypersensitivity and is, furthermore, a potential vector for viral, fungal, protozoal and helminth diseases. These, and other species of flies, are most prevalent in summer and autumn and are particularly active during warm humid periods. They induce severe irritation to horses causing restlessness, stamping, biting and self-mutilation. Clinically the flies cause pruritic, painful papules and wheals (*see* **571**), often with a small central crust or depression.

Tabanus spp., *Chrysops* spp. and *Haematopota* spp, known together as 'Horse Flies', cause more severe bites, great annoyance and are often responsible for

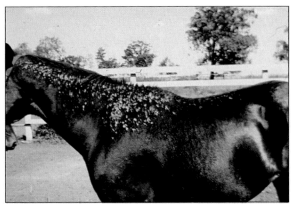

572 *Culicoides* spp. bite lesions.
Note: Typical pattern of lesions due to dorsal-biting species of *Culicoides* over back, withers and dorsal neck.

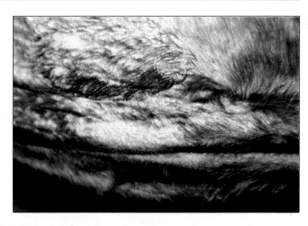

573 Ventral midline dermatitis (*Culicoides* and *Haematobia* spp.).
Note: Distinctive small exudative, granulomatous papules associated with edema, alopecia and severe pruritus. The ventral midline is the predilection site for ventral biting species of *Culicoides* and for *Haematobia* spp. flies.

behavioural problems and significant irritation. Clinically, the bites are the most severe of the fly lesions, causing pruritic papules, wheals, ulceration and even hemorrhage from the bite site. Bites most commonly occur on legs, ventral body, neck and withers. *Haematobia* spp. (horn flies, buffalo flies) also cause skin irritation, although the extent of the local lesion created by the bite is variable between individual horses. Clinically, the flies cause pruritus, painful papules and wheals with a central crust and in the United States of America appear to cause a well recognised ventral midline dermatitis (*see* **573**). Flies aggregate in huge numbers and may cause larger raised nodules and scabs. The bites of these flies usually involve some skin penetration and bleeding and in many cases this is an effective physical means for the transmission of viral, bacterial or protozoal (or other) disease. Flies of the species *Musca* may act as the intermediate host for *Habronema* and *Draschia* spp. helminths which are the cause of non-healing wounds on the legs (*see* **585**), face (*see* **584**), lacrimal sac (*see* **649**) and elsewhere, known as 'Summer Sores' or 'Swamp Sores'.

Culicoides **spp. (gnats, sandflies, biting midges, 'punkies', 'no-see-ums')**, occur throughout the world, and cause severe irritation and hypersensitivity and are important vectors for diseases such as African Horse Sickness and equine viral arteritis. Different species have different preferred biting patterns and regional information, relating to the species and local climate, is useful in assessing their local significance. Adult *Culicoides* gnats are blood-sucking parasites and their bites are immediately painful and annoying for the horse. There is a characteristically rapid onset of pruritus, and the development of local papules and wheals at the site. Individual lesions last for several days, and frequent attacks cause almost continuous irritation. The majority of horses in a group are affected when the populations of *Culicoides* spp. are at their peak. In some enzootic areas in tropical and sub-tropical countries this can be continuous throughout the year. *Culicoides* spp. are most active at dusk and dawn, with little activity during the heat of the day and the cool of night. The preferred sites vary depending on the species, but the neck and back (**572**), the head, and ventral midline (**573**) are commonly affected. They are also responsible for the development of a very common hypersensitivity disorder known as 'sweet itch' and for a ventral midline dermatitis. **Equine ventral midline dermatitis** which affects horses over 4 years of age, is seasonally and geographically related to the presence of biting flies and particularly to *Haematobia irritans* and *Culicoides* spp.. Clearly demarcated areas with punctate ulcers, thickened skin, alopecia, variable pruritus and in severe cases, an eczematous appearance, develop along the ventral midline of the abdomen (*see* **573**), following even limited numbers of bites. Progressively more severe pruritus probably indicates an inordinate hypersensitivity in the affected individual. Leukoderma occurs in long-standing cases. Diagnosis is based on history, the presence of flies and the typical clinical appearance and distribution of the lesions. Skin biopsy shows variable degrees of superficial perivascular dermatitis with numerous eosinophils, indicative of a hypersensitivity reaction.

Equine insect hypersensitivity, as opposed to ventral midline dermatitis, is a seasonal pruritus, related to the presence of *Culicoides* spp., *Simulium* spp, *Stomoxys calcitrans* and/or *Haematobia irritans*. The disorder is attributed to a Type II (cytotoxic) and Type IV (cell mediated or delayed) hypersensitivity to the salivary antigens of these flies. Individual animals may have greater or lesser sensitivities to the individual species of flies but some are sensitive to more than one. Certain breeds, including the Icelandic Pony and the Welsh Pony, appear to be more likely to develop the condition, and there are strong familial associations within breeds, supporting the contention that the sensitivity is of genetic origin. Intradermal skin testing indicates that the *Culicoides* species shown below are the most frequently implicated of the group, but in different countries the species of *Culicoides* involved is often different, suggesting that the sensitivity is not really specific to one or two individual species.

COUNTRY	SPECIES
AUSTRALIA	C. brevitarsis (robertsi)
CANADA	C. obsoletus
GREAT BRITAIN	C. pulicaris
ISRAEL	C.circumscripta, C.imicola, C.lupicaris, C.nebeculosus, C.punctatus
UNITED STATES OF AMERICA	C.insignis, C.spinosus, C. stellifer, C.varipenis

In spite of the geographical and species diversity of the flies involved in the hypersensitivity, the clinical pattern is very similar and is known by various colloquial names including 'Dhobi itch', 'sweet itch', 'kasen', 'Queensland itch', 'summer sores', 'summer eczema', 'allergic dermatitis', 'mange', 'summer dermatitis' and, others. There are three patterns of skin disease associated with the general condition.
- dorsal distribution from the ears to the tail
- ventral midline
- varying combinations of both

The early dorsal form shows as papules and nodules with severe pruritus affecting the head (**574**), ears, neck (**575**), tail (**576**) and back (**577**). As further attacks and further self-mutilation occur, the skin damage becomes progressively more severe (**578**) and, over a period of years, it becomes permanently damaged developing thick, lichenified folds (rugae, (**579**). Tail and mane rubbing result in chronically damaged skin and loss of hair (**580**). A diagnosis of insect hypersensitivity is often difficult to confirm as the flies are virtually uncontrollable. Their small size and vast numbers makes

574

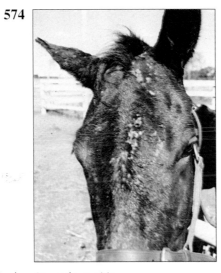

575

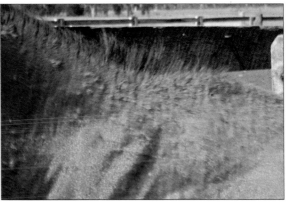

574 *Culicoides brevitarus* dermatitis.
Note: The face and the top of the neck (under the mane) are the predilection sites for this species of midge.

575 Culicoides hypersensitivity (sweet itch, summer eczema, Queensland itch).
Note: Early stage showing papules and nodules associated with the bites of the prevalent *Culicoides* spp insect. Severe pruritus may result in nodules becoming abraded and serum exudation. Note the scrubbed appearance of the mane.

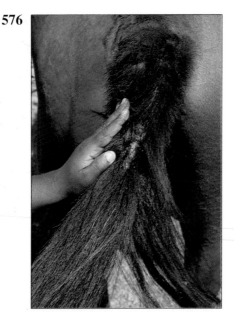

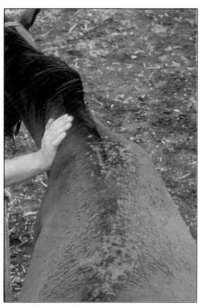

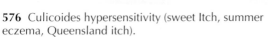

576 Culicoides hypersensitivity (sweet Itch, summer eczema, Queensland itch).
Note: Acute tail base lesions with excoriation from self inflicted trauma and prominent breaking and rubbing-back of the tail hairs at the base of the tail.
Differential Diagnosis:
i)   Pediculosis (louse infestation)
ii) Oxyuriasis (*Oxyuris equi)* infestation
iii) Physical tail trauma (eg over-tight bandaging) (**Note**: non pruritic and very painful)

577 Culicoides hypersensitivity (sweet itch, summer eczema, Queensland itch).
Note: Continuous attacks of *Culicoides* spp insects results in progressive irritation and intense pruritus, rubbing and self-mutilation. Nodules lose their character and extensive dermal ulceration may occur.

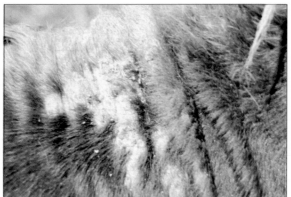

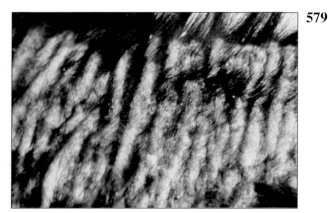

578 Culicoides hypersensitivity (sweet itch, summer eczema, Queensland itch).
Note: Progressive self-inflicted trauma results in skin thickening and continued rubbing and self mutilation.

579 Culicoides hypersensitivity (sweet itch, summer eczema, Queensland itch).
Note: Chronic case showing lichenification and rugae formation with poor hair growth resulting from permanently damaged skin.

580

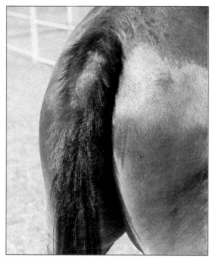

580 Culicoides hypersensitivity (sweet itch, summer eczema, Queensland itch).
Note: Chronic mild challenge by *Culicoides* spp. insects caused persistent tail rubbing with loss of hair and damage to the tail base and the formation of nodules of hyperkeratinized skin giving a 'rat-tail' effect.

581

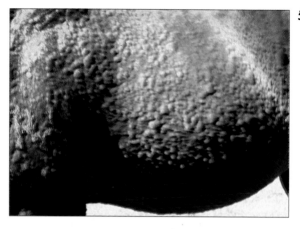

581 Wasp stings.
Note: Multiple bites from wasps caused this severe reaction. Wasps are seldom found in swarms and individual wasps may sting several times, they are therefore seldom as numerous and the stings are often distributed in small groups. In contrast to bee stings they do not leave the sting in the skin. In both cases the horse often shows edema of the face and in some cases anaphylactic reactions.
Differential Diagnosis:
i)   Feed (or other allergy)
ii) Equine viral arteritis
iii) *Purpura haemorrhagica*

prevention of contact difficult and eradication virtually impossible. Circumstantial evidence is often sufficient however, to make a presumptive diagnosis with seasonality and the typical appearance being useful indicators. Horses suffering from this disorder which are proven to be sensitive to *Culicoides* spp. gnats are invariably permanently sensitive and an anual treatment and control programme, involving fly repellents and grazing controls, create almost impossible demands upon the owner of these unfortunate horses. Movement to areas where the parasites are not present such as windy hill-sides or dry, inhospitable climatic conditions may be an alternative, if less practical, solution to some cases.

Simulium spp. (black flies, sandflies, buffalo gnats) also cause severe irritation and tend to occur in vast numbers following rain in spring and early summer. The clinical signs associated with their presence are painful papules and wheals. With huge numbers of flies, lesions may become vesicular, haemorrhagic and necrotic. The bites may also cause aural plaque (*see* **536**) formation

and are also be responsible for hypersensitivity reactions which are indistinguishable from that produced by *Culicoides* spp.. Absorption of toxin from the bites has been recorded as causing cardiorespiratory dysfunction when depression, weakness, staggers, tachycardia, tachypnea, shock and death may be encountered. Diagnosis is made by confirmation of the presence of flies in large numbers, although the number of bites need not be great to have a serious clinical effect. The Icelandic pony is particularly susceptible to its effect.

Mosquitoes (*Aedes* spp., *Anopheles* spp., and *Culex* spp.) are locally annoying as well being vectors for viral and protozoal disease. Multiple bites cause papules and small wheals. Contact scabs are difficult to see or may be absent. The presence of large numbers may cause irritation and weight loss in horses.

Horses attacked by bee swarms often have obvious stings in the skin and a surrounding area of edema and pain. The head and neck are most often attacked and show edema of the eyelids and muzzle. Papules with edema occur wherever stings have occurred. The

582

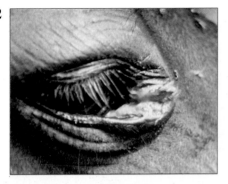

582 Fly damage (*Musca* spp).
Note: Massive numbers of flies aggregating in the corner of the eye commonly cause this physical damage, but in the early stages swelling and some local inflammation may be all that is present. Note similarity to **649**
Differential Diagnosis:
i)   Habronemiasis
ii) Ocular histoplasmosis
iii) Squamous cell carcinoma

583

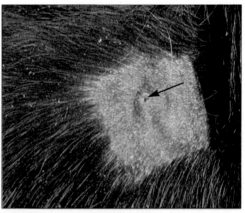

583 Hypodermiasis (*Hypoderma* spp) (warble fly).
Note: Subcutaneous nodule (or cyst) located over the withers, shows typical breathing pore of third stage larva (arrow).

Differential Diagnosis:
i)   Epidermoid/dermoid cysts
ii) Parafilariasis
iii) Infected granuloma, foreign body
iv) Neoplasia (mast cell tumour, sarcoid)
v)   Eosinophilic granuloma

identification of the sting lodged in the skin at the site of these lesions confirms the diagnosis but it may be particularly difficult to find them. An occasional horse suffers from an anaphylactoid reaction following even single (or few) bee stings. Severe respiratory embarrassment and gross urticaria with extensive edema are typical. Wasp stings are more often single but may be multiple (**581**) from one or more wasps and the stings lead to the formation of painful papules and plaques over the body which closely resemble bee stings but which have no residual sting remnants. Edema of the head and muzzle, and anaphylactoid reactions may occur, however, and cases must be carefully assessed to eliminate the possibility of allergic diseases such as urticaria and angioedema.

Non-biting flies such as *Musca* spp. flies are surface feeders but often, due to high populations, can cause ulceration of moist skin, eyes, nostrils and prepucial areas. *Musca autumnalis* (face fly of North America) and *Musca domestica* (domestic house fly) and *Musca vetustissima* (bush fly of Australia), have a tendency to congregate around the eye and cause physical ulceration damage through sheer numbers in the periocular skin (**582**). These wounds are characteristically slow to heal and often become complicated by the presence of *Habronema* spp. larvae in the wounds, conjunctiva or in the nasolacrimal duct (*see* **648, 649**).

Hypodermiasis due to the tissue migrating larval stages of *Hypoderma lineatum* and *Hypoderma bovis*

occasionally affects horses, particularly those in contact with cattle over the warmer summer months. Younger horses in poor body condition are more likely to be affected. Small numbers of subcutaneous nodules and cysts appear in the skin along the dorsal midline between the withers and the tail head, in the early spring months in the year following infection. While most of these develop a breathing-pore in the overlying skin (**583**), some are more swollen and painful and produce no breathing aperture. Furthermore anaphylactoid type reactions may occur following the rupture or death of third stage larvae in the skin during accidental injury or attempts to squeeze the larvae out, or during their migration through the body tissues. A particularly serious complication may arise if the larvae penetrate the spinal cord and then die. A diagnosis may be difficult to establish unless the larva can be identified after removal.

Flies of the genera *Calliphora*, *Chrysomyia*, *Lucilia*, *Phormia*, *Sarcophagi* and some other species may be involved with **fly strike** (**calliphorine myiasis**) in horses. This mostly occurs in contaminated, infected wounds, under badly managed plaster casts and occasionally in fresh surgical wounds such as castrations (*see* **843**). The presence of the fly larvae is usually very obvious and the horse often bites or chews at the malodorous area. Bacterial cultures from wounds affected by myiasis are often surprisingly unrewarding and the wound is often remarkably free from tissue

584

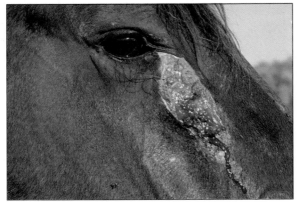

585

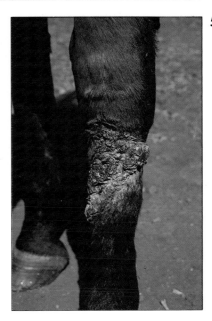

584 Habronemiasis (*Habronema* spp).
Note: Lesion of 28 days duration.
Differential Diagnosis:
i) Cutaneous histoplasmosis

585 Habronemiasis (*Habronema* spp) (swamp sore, summer sore).
Note: Non-healing wound infested with *Habronema* spp. larvae. Wound healed during winter but required control of granulation tissue.
Differential Diagnosis:
i) Exuberant (proud) granulation tissue
ii) Fibroblastic sarcoid
iii) Pythiosis

detritus. Removal of the larvae and normal wound management results in rapid healing in most cases although the tendency towards exuberant granulation tissue may still be a problem in some sites.

Screw worm presents a serious problem in tropical areas. The adult flies (*Callitroga hominivorax* and *Callitroga macellaria* in the Americas and *Chrysomyia bezziana* in Africa and Asia) lay their eggs on open wounds, the umbilicus of neonates, body orifices and even onto moist intact skin. The larvae hatch within 12-24 hours and burrow into the underlying tissue causing intense pruritus and a severe malodour, which serves to attract more flies. The larvae leave the wound after 3-6 days but usually successive waves of maggots result in extensive tissue destruction. The presence of the maggots is usually very obvious but on occasion the extent of the invasion is not apparent until the area is clipped and examined closely.

Cutaneous habronemiasis causes chronic ulcerative granulomata which are known variously as 'summer sores', 'bursautee', 'bursatti', 'swamp sore', 'kunkers', 'esponja', 'granular dermatitis'. The condition occurs commonly, particularly in the tropics and sub-tropics. Three adult nematodes *Habronema muscae*, *Habronema majus* and *Draschia megastoma* inhabit horses stomachs, eggs or larvae being passed in feces. The resultant larvae are ingested by the larvae of the intermediate host *Musca domestica* (the house/domestic fly) or *Stomoxys calcitrans* (the stable fly). These larvae are released from the adult flies while they feed on exudates or body secretions (such as in open wounds, facial skin moistened by lacrimation, the urethral process and the conjunctiva). The larvae penetrate intact skin or infest the surface of wounds or, if they are deposited near the mouth they are swallowed to continue their life cycle in the horse's stomach. It is believed that hypersensitivity by some horses, to the larvae, causes the appearance of clinical disease. The disease has a strong seasonal nature with spontaneous remission over the winter. Although horses may be congregated, single individuals may be affected. Often, the same horse is reinfected in the succeeding summers, indicating that there is little or no immunological or cellular resistance. Lesions commonly occur around the medial canthus of the eyes (*see* **649**), face (**584**), urethral process (*see* **862**), prepuce, ventral abdomen and legs. In the absence of an open skin wound progress of the disease is usually rapid with small papules on intact skin quickly enlarging and ulcerating. This is particularly obvious on the face especially around the medial canthus, where the lesion can progress to large granulomatous sores within four weeks (*see* **584**). Wounds which become infected with

586

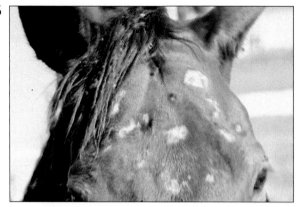

586 Cutaneous onchocerciasis (*Onchocerca cervicalis*). **Note:** Annular lesions on head showing alopecia, scaling and crusting (3 months duration) Initially the lesions were poorly demarcated areas of acute dermatitis with prominent pruritus.
Differential Diagnosis:
i) Dermatophytosis
ii) *Culicoides* spp. hypersensitivity
iii) Forage mite sensitivity
iv) Psoroptic mange

Habronema larvae, develop granulation tissue particularly rapidly (**585**), and often show a saucer-like configuration and heal extremely slowly unless treated specifically for the habronemiasis. Untreated habronema lesions on the urethral process (*see* **862**) cause great enlargement which can lead to bleeding during coitus, thus causing a lowered fertility and reduced libido.

Cutaneous onchocerciasis occurs as an unusual clinical syndrome and many horses may harbour larvae (microfilaria) without any clinical signs, with some parasites being regarded as a normal occurrence. Four species of *Onchocerca* have been found in horses *Onchocerca gibsoni*, *Onchocerca gutturosa*, *Onchocerca reticulata*, and *Onchocerca cervicalis*. Adult *Onchocerca reticulata* live in the connective tissue of the flexor tendons and suspensory ligament while those of *Onchocerca gutturosa* and *Onchocerca cervicalis* primarily inhabit the ligamentum nuchae. Microfilaria are most numerous in the dermis of the legs and ventral midline (*Onchocerca reticulata*) or ventral midline, face and neck (*Onchocerca cervicalis*). Many horses (25 – 100%) are infected with *Onchocerca cervicalis*, but only a very few show clinical signs. The cutaneous form of the disease is thought to represent a hypersensitivity reaction. Affected horses are commonly older than 4 years, with horses under 2 years of age being particularly rarely affected. Clinical lesions may appear during any time of the year, but are usually more severe in warmer weather. This may also be related to increased activity of the insect vectors, such as *Culicoides* spp. The lesions, which are commonly located on the head (**586**), neck, ventral midline and palmar/plantar aspects of the limbs, are initially localised, poorly demarcated and intensely pruritic. Rubbing and biting at the sites abates after some days and the lesions develop into circular patches of scaling and crusting (*see* **586**). Long-standing Onchocerca

lesions show leukotrichia and leukoderma which is usually irreversible. Diagnosis is aided by biopsy and examination of minced skin for microfilaria. It is important to realise that microfilaria may be present in normal blood and in normal skin without any pathological effect. The use of ivermectin as an anthelmintic has resulted in a dramatic reduction in the incidence of this parasite in some parts of the world but the initial use of this drug may cause severe localised allergic-type reactions when the microfilaria are killed in the capillary beds of the skin.

Parafilariasis is a seasonal hemorrhagic nodular skin disease of horses which occurs in Eastern Europe and Great Britain. *Parafilaria multipapillosa* adult worms live coiled up in subcutaneous nodules which open to the skin surface, discharging a bloody exudate. *Haematobia atripalpis* serve as a vector for the parasite. The clinical disease appears in spring and summer with papules and nodules suddenly appearing, principally on the neck, shoulders and trunk. Lesions are not usually painful or pruritic. New lesions develop as the old regress. The differential diagnoses of the condition include fungal, bacterial and other parasitic granuloma and hypodermiasis. The diagnosis may be confirmed by direct smears from the bloody exudate when larvae, rectangular embryonated eggs and numerous eosinophils will be visible, and by biopsy when nodular to diffuse dermatitis with coiled nematodes is present.

Oxyuriasis, infestation with *Oxyuris equi*, the pin worm, may cause pruritus of the anus and rubbing of the tail (*see* **150**). The adult female worms deposit their eggs in a gelatinous mass around the perianal area. Clinical signs include tail-rubbing and a rat-tail appearance develops with increasing self depilation. Diagnosis is confirmed by finding characteristic triangular eggs around the perineum. A strip of adhesive cellulose tape is a useful way of harvesting the eggs for examination.

Neoplastic Disorders

Skin tumours are one of the most common neoplasms seen in horses. While any unusual tissue change which involves invasion of the surrounding normal tissue may be loosely described as a tumour, those changes related to infective agents are dealt with in their own section, leaving only those tumours which represent abnormal cellular growth and have been designated neoplastic through their pathological features. As an added challenge, it must be remembered that neoplasms can also become infected by bacterial, fungal, viral and parasitic disease. Also, the horse has a great propensity to produce excessive granulation tissue, especially on the lower limbs which further complicates clinical diagnosis, and forces the clinician to resort to biopsy and histopathological studies on all tissues which are considered to be abnormal. For this reason, all tumours which are removed should be carefully recorded and accurately diagnosed by laboratory means to establish an individual prognosis which may vary from good to very guarded, depending on the type, location and duration of the tumour.

Squamous cell carcinoma is one of the most common skin tumours. Some seem related to poor skin pigmentation and exposure to ultraviolet radiation from the sun but others may have no such obvious origin. The most common forms occur at muco-cutaneous junctions. Most are malignant, locally invasive and some metastasize. Some are highly active and require immediate aggressive treatment and carry a poor or guarded prognosis while others are less aggressive and surgical removal has a good prognosis. The tumours occur most commonly around the head, eyes and adnexa, muco-cutaneous junctions and the external genitalia of both sexes. The ocular forms of squamous cell carcinoma (*see* **650** *et seq.*) represent by far the commonest site for this neoplasm. The lesions occurring on the upper or lower eyelids are more serious but less common and have a greater tendency to invade the orbit and to metastasise both to the regional lymph nodes (usually the parotid) and more extensively by hematogenous spread. Squamous cell carcinoma of the nose and lips appears as raised and granulomatous or flattened ulcerated depressed lesions, or both (**587**). The Clydesdale breed appears to be prone to this condition especially in regions of high sunlight exposure. Surgical ablation, in this site, may not be successful, and the tumour frequently metastasizes both locally and to remote sites. Tumours occurring on the penis (glans, body) or preputial skin are a common occurrence (*see* **863** *et seq.*), while lesions on the lips of the vulva (*see* **812**) are somewhat less common.

Melanoma and melanosarcoma may occur in horses of any colour but are much more frequently observed in grey horses. While they may occur as isolated tumours in the skin, on the nictitating membrane (third eyelid) (*see* **657**), within the iris, and within the guttural pouches (*see* **275**), they are most frequently found around the anus, vulva and tail (*see* **813**) and either in the lymphatic tissue or the salivary glands in parotid region (*see* **58**). Melanosarcoma may be found in the same locations but is more aggressively invasive. Cut lesions show characteristic dense black tissue (**588**) and needle biopsy is readily indicative of melanoma.

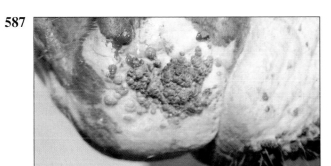

587 Squamous cell carcinoma.
Note: Lesion of several weeks duration, restricted to non-pigmented skin, showing papillomatous area with a small non-healing, granulomatous sore.

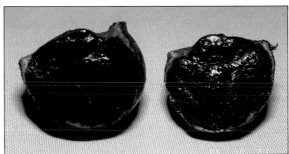

588 Cutaneous melanoma.
Note: Lesion removed from the peri-vulval skin of the horse illustrated in **813**.

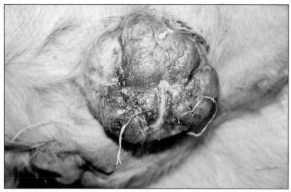

589 Fibroma (ulcerated).

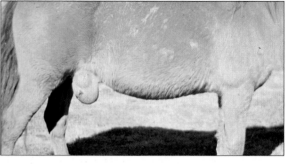

590 Subcutaneous lipoma.

Neurofibroma (Schwannoma, neurilemomas, neurinomas) and the less common neurofibrosarcoma arise from dermal or subcutaneous Schwann's (nerve sheath) cells, without any known predisposing factor. They occur initially in horses between 3 and 6 years of age and, while some remain relatively dormant for long periods, most become very aggressive when subjected to attempted surgical excision. The most common site is in the upper eyelid and periorbital subcutaneous tissue (*see* **660** and **745**). The tumours are frequently hard shot-size nodules (2 – 3mm) in the upper eyelids which gradually enlarge and finally, if untreated, erode through the epidermis. Surgical intervention often locates small 'seed' tumours adjacent to the main tumour. Recurrence following surgery may take months to years and frequently occurs adjacent to the previous surgical site.

Fibromas and **fibrosarcomas** are uncommon tumours of dermal or subcutaneous origin. They are reported to occur in older horses, usually as a solitary tumour. Fibromas may be firm (*fibroma durum*) or soft (*fibroma molle*) (**589**), well-circumscribed nodules in dermis or subcutaneous tissue. Fibromas also in the foot occur as firm fleshy growths of the frog and like the more usual dermal lesions, surgical ablation is usually successful. Fibrosarcomas tend to be poorly demarcated, firm infiltrating subcutaneous tumours. The surface of the tumours may ulcerate, but more commonly, fibrosarcomas may clinically resemble the fibroblastic form of the equine sarcoid (*see* **527**). Histopathological examination is required to confirm the diagnosis.

Lipomas are benign tumours arising from subcutaneous fat. They are soft to flabby, well circumscribed, and occur about the neck, lower chest, abdomen (**590**) and, occasionally, the limbs. Biopsy easily defines this tumour. Surgical removal effects full recovery.

Cutaneous histiocytic lymphosarcoma is rare, occurring almost exclusively in older horses. More usually, lymphosarcoma is found as a systemic disease without cutaneous manifestation. The cutaneous form shows as multiple dermoepidermal or subcutaneous papules and nodules (**591**) anywhere on the body including the nasal mucosa and the pharyngeal wall (**592**). The lesions are usually firm and discrete (**593**) or may be more fluctuant, or may resemble urticarial wheals (*see* **591**). Significant immune suppression may be present in affected horses and secondary infections, resulting in cutaneous, oral and internal abscesses and pulmonary diseases, and infestations of internal and external parasites, are relatively common. Where internal organs are involved, the outcome is invariably fatal, but cases in which only the skin is affected have a somewhat more favourable short term prognosis. The ultimate outcome is inevitably fatal, however. Single lymphomas occurring in the skin usually have an ulcerated surface (**594**) and these have occasionally been successfully surgically removed. Diagnosis in all these tumours is confirmed by biopsy or by aspiration, both of which show infiltration with characteristic malignant lymphocytes. Early cases can, however, be difficult to confirm.

591

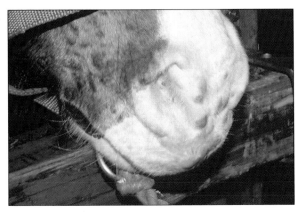

592

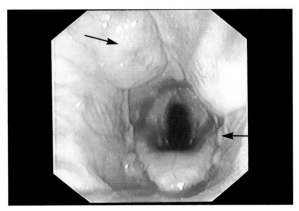

591 Cutaneous histiocytic lymphosarcoma.
Note: Multiple nodules and plaque-like lesions over muzzle and side of face.
Differential Diagnosis:
i)   Allergic urticaria (transient)
ii) Insect bites
iii) Systemic lupus erythematosus-like syndrome.

592 Cutaneous histiocytic lymphosarcoma (endoscopic view of pharynx).
Note: Plaques of tumour tissue on wall of pharynx (arrows).

593

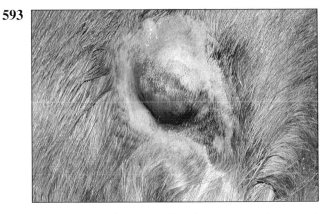

594

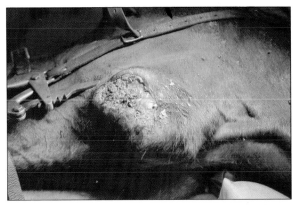

593 Cutaneous histiocytic lymphosarcoma (close-up of single lesion).

594 Lymphoma.
Note: Depressed ulcerative, granulating, non-healing lesion with subcutaneous spread. Little discharge.

Mastocytomas (mast cell tumours) are rare and are most commonly found in male horses. They have a variable clinical appearance, but are usually nodular. The head **(595)**, neck and limbs are the predilection sites for these solitary tumours which may vary from 2 – 20cm diameter. They may be firm or fluctuant, and the overlying skin may or may not be alopecic, ulcerated or hyperpigmented. Remission can be spontaneous, and there are no reports of metastasis. Incomplete excision does not usually exacerbate the tumour. Diagnosis is based on history, clinical examination, cytology and histopathological examination of biopsy specimens.

Keratomas are uncommon benign tumours of keratin of the horn layer of the hoof (*see* **435, 436**). The cause is unknown but may be related to chronic irritation of horn cells at the coronary band. The tumour may extend down the wall to the white line and be visible as a bulge in the wall (*see* **435**) and a deformity of the white line (*see* **436**). Lameness and draining tracts may also be present. Diagnosis is based on radiography and by horn biopsy. Complete stripping of the tumour from the underlying sensitive laminae over the full length of the mass is indicated and is usually curative.

595

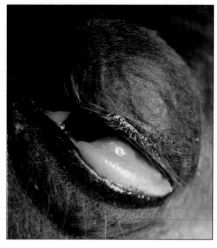

595 Mastocytoma.
Note: Unusual form of mastocytoma involving the orbit resulting in exophthalmos and chemosis. More usually they are found on the skin of the head or neck as solitary, hard subcutaneous tumours.

Further reading

A Colour Atlas of Equine Dermatology
R.R.Pascoe (1990) Wolfe, London UK

Current Therapy in Equine Medicine 2
Ed. N.E.Robinson (1987) W.B.Saunders, Philadelphia, USA

Current Therapy in Equine Medicine 3
Ed. N.E.Robinson (1992) W.B.Saunders, Philadelphia, USA

Equine Wound Management
T.S.Stashak (1991) Lea & Febiger, Philadelphia, USA

Large Animal Dermatology
D.W.Scott (1988) W.B.Saunders Philadelphia, USA

Manual of Equine Practice
Rose & Hodgson 1993

9. Disorders of the eye

The recognition of significant eye disorders is clearly important. Many apparently dramatic lesions involving structures of the eye appear to have little or no effect upon vision, but it is almost impossible to assess, clinically, whether there are minor visual deficits in the horse. Partially sighted horses are probably capable of rapid and effective compensation and may show no detectable impairment of function. The examination of the eye and the detection of abnormalities requires considerable experience and the extent to which obvious (or sometimes less obvious) defects influence vision is left in many cases to the judgement of the clinician. Where there is an obvious field deficit the animal may be patently blind in the affected eye(s), but partial blindness is almost always impossible to assess. The clinician should therefore always consider the possible implications of any deficit of sight upon the rider or other attending personnel, or the horse itself.

Developmental disorders

While there is a wide variety of possible congenital defects and deformities of the eye and adnexa, some are more common than others. Some ocular disorders are suspected as being of hereditary origin but most are likely to be idiopathic and sporadic.

Congenital colour dilution of the skin of the eyelids is particularly prevalent in Appaloosa, Pinto and albino (cream) horses with partial depigmentation being relatively common. Typical depigmentation is however, sometimes, also encountered in horses of all colours. Where the lack of pigment extends into the eyelids themselves rather than the adjacent peri-palpebral skin the eyelids may be considerably more sensitive to environmental factors such as ultra violet (sun) light, dust and wind. The implications of this are usually only apparent in later years when neoplastic conditions (squamous cell and basal cell carcinomas and melanoma) may develop in either the eyelids or the third eyelid in particular.

Congenital eyelid deformities are usually part of a complex of malformations including **anophthalmia (596)** and **microphthalmia (597)**. **Multiple congenital abnormalities** including combinations of defects (*see* **597**) may be encountered and may include defects of eyelid shape and structure, globe size and integrity, and distortions of the structure of individual components of the eye. Examination and accurate assessment of the extent of such defect may be very difficult even with the help of ultrasonography, and cases presented with more than one congenital defect should be regarded with suspicion even if the internal structures cannot be examined in detail.

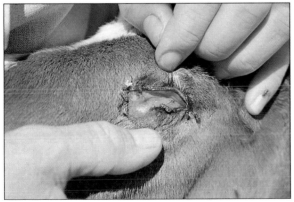

596 Congenital anophthalmia.
Note: No eye tissues present in the orbit. The contralateral eye was normal.

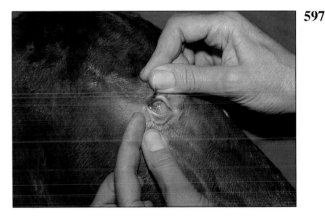

597 Microphthalmia with severe multiple eye defects.
Note: Staphyloma (bulging defect of the cornea lined with uveal tissue). Both eyes equally affected.

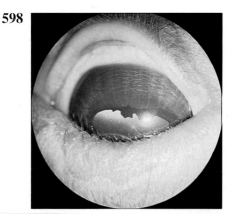

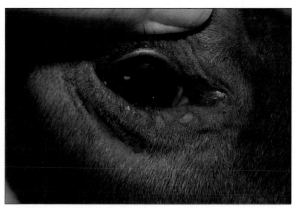

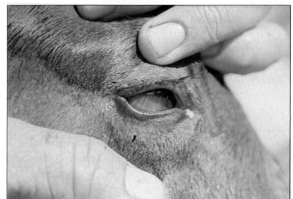

598 Congenital entropion.
Note: Little apparent discomfort. Minimal corneal damage.

599 Entropion.
Note: Blepharitis and excoriation of the lower lid. A shallow corneal ulcer was detected

600 Entropion.
Note: Marked keratitis and slight purulent ocular discharge. Corneal ulceration was present.

Foals are often born with in-turned lower eyelids (**entropion**) (**598**). The condition generally only affects the lower eyelid. In the Thoroughbred, it is considered to be an hereditary disorder. Entropion is easily recognised by simple examination which will reveal the inward rolling of the eyelid. While some foals are apparently almost unaffected by the disorder (*see* **598**), showing little discomfort or clinical effects, others show marked secondary changes resulting from the contact of the facial hair and eyelashes with the cornea and conjunctiva. Lacrimation, blepharitis (**599**), conjunctivitis and corneal ulceration with corneal fibrosis (**600**) are common secondary effects. Some cases of entropion are the consequence of globe retraction; withdrawal of the globe into the socket will result in a passive prolapse of the third eyelid, and also provides a further opportunity for entropion to develop. Enophthalmos as a result of dehydration, pain or neurological disorders such as tetanus (**see 731** *et seq.*), or the loss of retrobulbar fat in horses which have lost weight, may all result in passive prolapse of the third eyelid (*membrana nictitans*) and entropion in both foals and adult horses.

The eyelids of foals (and adult horses) which show persistent corneal opacity without any evidence of entropion should be closely examined, preferably with a magnifying lens, for the presence of extra eyelashes (**distichiasis**) arising from the tarsal (meibomian) gland orifices.

Linear (band) opacities crossing the cornea, which appear as faint, grey or cloudy, well-defined lines within the cornea, are a frequent incidental finding in all types and ages of horse. They are, in most cases, due to a developmental thinning of Descemet's membrane which lies under the corneal endothelium on the inner surface of the cornea. They are best observed against the closed pupil. Most frequently they extend across the meridian of the cornea extending from limbus to limbus and may branch one or more times. They almost certainly have no effect upon the vision of the horse and seldom show any change from year to year.

Dermoids are a relatively common congenital anomaly in foals. The most obvious lesions are usually found at the limbus and have hairs growing from them which persistently irritate the cornea and conjunctiva, resulting in corneal opacity and lacrimation. Others are not haired and have a fleshy appearance (**601**). The consequences of these lesions vary with their extent and location. Large dermoids may cause significant irritation while smaller ones appear to have no significant harmful

601

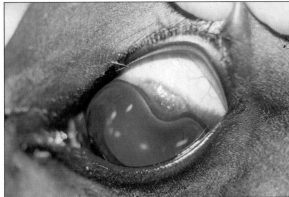

602

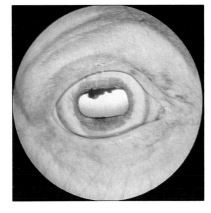

601 (Hairless) Dermoid.
Note: No apparent discomfort or effect on vision.
Differential Diagnosis:
i)   Squamous cell carcinoma

602 Non-pigmented iris and retina.
Note: Cream (albino) pony. Normal sight but some resentment of full sunlight.

effect and remain static for years. Occasional lesions become larger and are cosmetically unacceptable or become significant causes of conjunctival and corneal inflammation.

A number of non-pathological congenital conditions are associated with the iris. The appearance of these may vary markedly, particularly with respect to the colour of the iris. Iris colour is usually of no significance although a totally non-pigmented (albino) iris (**602**) may render the horse photophobic. Such eye colours are usually associated with pigmentary changes in the skin and eyelids. The retina of pale skinned horses including albino (cream) animals, is usually poorly pigmented (*see* **602**). In spite of apparently profound depigmentation in some cases, there is usually no apparent detrimental effect upon vision. In some of these cases the retinal blood vessels, which are not normally visible except where they run across the margin of the optic disc, become very obvious and their prominence may be alarming for the inexperienced examiner. Where the eye is truly albinotic the animal may be photophobic to particularly bright light.

Iris stromal cysts are most often associated with the heterochromia or 'wall-eye' pale blue iris. They appear as protruding iris swellings in the superior mid-iris region (**603**) where they may be mistaken for an iris tumour. The latter are particularly uncommon, while stromal iris cysts are much more frequently encountered. Pale, almost translucent cysts within the iris stroma may be associated with a pale blue eye having a particularly thin iris (**604**). These may be seen to vary in size with the size of the pupil, being largest and palest when the pupil is fully constricted and smallest and densest when fully dilated. They usually create a more or less obvious

defect of iris shape (*see* **605**). Careful examination shows the membrane on either side of the cyst to be intact and the cyst usually contains a clear fluid, through which the posterior chamber can be seen. These may rupture and create an **acquired coloboma** (discontinuity or defect) of the iris. **Iris colobomata** are defects in the iris (**605**) and are more usually of congenital origin. They appear to have no pathological significance in most cases being seen incidentally in normally sighted horses. **Pupillary or anterior chamber cysts**, which originate from the pigmented epithelium of the posterior iris, are commonly encountered in brown-eyed horses. These are spherical, black or very dark brown and, while they may hang over the pupillary margin at any point, most are located along the inferior pupillary margin (**606**). Where they derive from the upper pupillary margin they may be associated with the normal *corpora nigra* (*granula iridica*) and in these cases the cysts may be observed to enlarge in the first six months of life, whereas the *corpora nigra* do not. **Hypertrophy of the granula iridica** or cystic changes within them are perhaps more common in the superior margin of the pupil. Iris cysts are almost translucent in appearance, and are occasionally to be seen floating freely within the anterior chamber. Occasionally these free-floating, cystic structures adhere to the anterior surface of the lens, or to the cornea or iris. Even when these cysts are very large, or when the granula iridica are grossly hypertrophied or cystic there is usually no apparent deleterious effects on vision. Where the pupil is grossly occluded the horse may exhibit field deficits, particularly in bright light conditions.

Hereditary cataracts have been recorded in Arabian, Morgan, Belgian, Thoroughbred and Quarterhorse

603

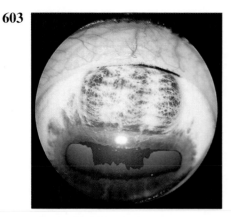

604

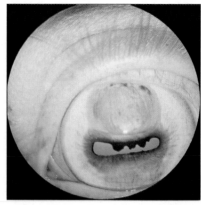

603 Congenital iris stromal cyst.
Note: Heterochromic iris.

604 (Thin-walled) uveal (stromal) cyst.
Note: Cyst varied in size with iris movement.

605

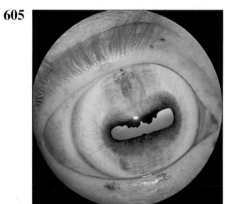

606

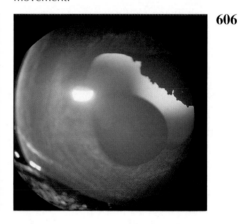

607

605 Iris coloboma.
Note: Distortion in dorsal margin of iris.

606 Congenital iris cyst.
Note: Arising from the posterior pigmented epithelium of the iris and suspended by the stalk of origin over the inferior pupillary margin within the anterior chamber.
Differential Diagnosis:
i)   Iris stromal cyst
ii) Iris melanoma
iii) (Normal) granula iridica

607 Congenital/hereditary nuclear cataract.
Note: Two-month-old Arabian filly.

breeds. Congenital cataracts, which are not necessarily hereditary, may be observed to be present in new born foals (**607**) but may, more rarely, appear at a later age. It is likely that they reflect insults to the developing lens during gestation and the siting of the cataract may indicate the timing and the extent of the insult. Thus, nuclear cataracts may reflect early developmental insults, while lesions limited to small areas of the nucleus may reflect more minor or transient insults occurring during embryonic development. They seldom appear to progress after birth and, indeed, both the physical appearance and sight may in some cases improve significantly as the lens matures.

Non-Infectious Disorders

Damage to the skin of the eyelids themselves, as a result of trauma or surgical interference, characteristically induces a change in the colour of the local skin and hair growth. This is particularly noticeable following the use of cryosurgery or radiation brachytherapy for the treatment of periocular neoplasia **(608)**.

Traumatic damage to the eyelids of the horse is unusual but is commoner in foals which appear to have a less enthusiastic withdrawal (menace) reflex than adult horses. The long-term significance of eyelid trauma depends largely upon the action which is taken to repair the defect. Lesions affecting the lower lid at or around the medial canthus may affect drainage into the nasolacrimal duct. Wounds which are left to heal naturally often leave a significant eyelid deformity which may result in persistent epiphora (overflow of tears) with tear-staining and excoriation of the face below the medial canthus. The consequences of a defective eyelid upon the eye itself may be more serious, when the eyelid function is impaired and the lubrication/wiping of the eye is less than ideal. In these circumstances an area of corneal drying and excoriation may develop leading to significant and painful ulceration and to corneal scarring (fibrosis). Horses with neurological deficits affecting eyelid function, such as Horner's Syndrome (*see* **695**), trigeminal disorders and facial nerve paralysis (*see* **689**), may also have secondary lesions on the cornea which may be very obvious or may be almost inapparent. Interference with sensation may result in failure to respond to foreign bodies or other trauma while impaired motor function to the eyelids may render the menace reflex ineffective. Failure of the sympathetic inervation of the lacrimal glands (such as occurs in Horner's Syndrome) results in impairment of lubrication and drying of the surface of the eye. In these cases however, the defect is usually crescentic in shape and horizontal, reflecting the failure of the eyelid to reach the meridian of the eye and make effective apposition with the opposite lid. Failure of lacrimation results in *keratoconjunctivitis sicca* or dry-eye and although the disorder is rarely a result of organic failure of the tear glands certain neurological and poisoning disorders including Horner's Syndrome and Locoweed (*Astragalus* spp) are known to result in a reduction of tear production. During anesthesia with halothane, tear production is reduced but this is transient and of little significance. The affected horse will show marked pain and blepharospasm (where this is possible) and there will almost invariably be a greenish, sticky mucopurulent ocular discharge. A diffuse keratitis with corneal edema and neovascularization is often present.

Edema of the bulbar conjunctiva (**chemosis**) is often severe in the horse **(609)** and may arise from local trauma or from irritant chemicals and/or dust. Occasionally hypersensitivity (allergic) reactions are responsible and are usually, then, due to pollen or other protein substances. The lacrimal secretions are frequently blood-stained (*see* **609**). A number of virus infections including equine herpes virus-1 and 4, equine viral arteritis (*see* **299**) and African Horse Sickness, show degrees of conjunctival inflammation and edema (*see* **218**). Some local secondary irritation may arise from exposure to excessive sunlight, particularly when the eyelids and third eyelid are non pigmented. Failure of normal conjunctival lubrication and protection, in severe cases, may result in marked desiccation of the protruding and inflamed conjunctiva.

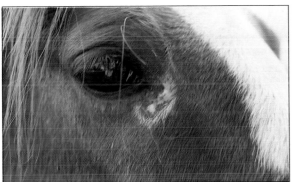

608 Periorbital vitiligo (leukoderma/leukotrichia).
Note: Changes followed radiation brachytherapy for a periorbital sarcoid.

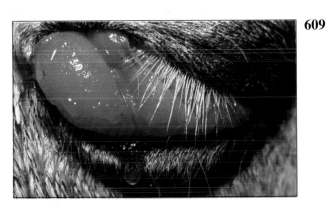

609 Chemosis (edema of the bulbar conjunctiva).
Note: Epiphora and blood staining of the lacrimal secretion and drying of the exposed mucosa.

610

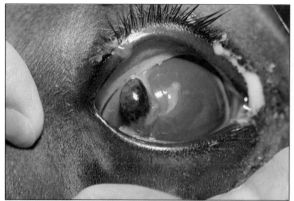

611

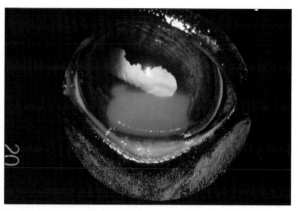

610 Corneal laceration with iris prolapse.
Note: Iridocyclitis and miotic pupil, partial collapse of anterior chamber and hyphema (blood in anterior chamber). Corneal edema along the margin of the corneal wound.

611 Corneal ulceration.
Note: Extensive, shallow corneal ulceration. Obvious but not strong staining with fluorescein. Damage probably limited to superficial loss of corneal epithelium.

Facial trauma often induces hemorrhage or bruising within the conjunctiva or the sclera. Quite prominent **subconjunctival hemorrhages** are often observed in new-born foals and are of no significance in most cases. It is probably the result of trauma during parturition.

Traumatic injury to the cornea may be superficial or deep enough to cause lacerations of the epithelium and/or stroma and in some cases to the deeper structures in the eye. **Lacerations** which do not involve the full thickness of the cornea are painful and induce strong blepharospasm and lacrimation. Such lesions heal rapidly in the absence of complications. Lesions involving the full depth of the cornea are complicated by the collapse of the anterior chamber due to aqueous leakage and more extensive damage to the deeper structures of the eye. Damage to the cornea itself is not accompanied by significant bleeding, but deeper damage involving the iris may induce severe hemorrhage which is apparent both externally and into the collapsed anterior chamber (**hyphema**). **Prolapse of the iris** into a defect in the cornea with attendant corneal edema (**610**) and subsequent healing and fibrosis (**iris staphyloma**), occurs frequently in these cases, and usually limits the immediate loss of aqueous humor and anterior chamber pressure, but nevertheless represents a serious complication. In some cases the corneal wound and the anterior chamber become infected rapidly and the adjacent corneal tissue becomes edematous and ulcerated. Infection of such a wound with bacteria such as *Bacillus cereus* or *Proteus* spp. results in dramatic deterioration (*see* **617**) and frequently leads to an irretrievable **panophthalmitis**.

Foreign bodies are often responsible for the development of corneal and conjunctival inflammation and are frequently encountered. Affected horses are usually in severe pain and are determinedly reluctant to allow examination of the eye. It is frequently necessary to resort to regional analgesia using an auriculo-palpebral nerve block before examination can be effectively carried out. Marked blepharospasm and lacrimation with secondary infection are common, if non-specific, signs of eye pain. All horses with an acute onset of lacrimation, blepharospasm and ocular pain or discomfort should be carefully examined for the possibility of a foreign body which may be obvious, lying on the surface of the eye or may be lodged deep in the conjunctival sac. It may even be necessary to resort to short duration general anesthesia to effectively examine the full extent of the conjunctival sac.

Superficial damage to the corneal epithelium results in the rapid development of a **corneal ulcer** surrounded by an area of corneal edema, resulting from disruption of the epithelial layer and hydration of the normally desiccated corneal stroma. In the absence of any complicating factors such as infection or self-inflicted trauma, superficial ulcers of this type often heal rapidly within a few days leaving a well defined area of corneal scarring which may be much slower to resolve.

While some **corneal ulcers** are obvious, others are much less so, and all may be demonstrated with the help of fluorescein dye applied to the surface of the eye. Ulcerated areas stain very clearly in most cases. Superficial damage to the corneal epithelium resulting from desiccation or from wiping injuries induces shallow, but often extensive, superficial ulceration of the cornea (**611**). Where damage has been slightly deeper (a

612

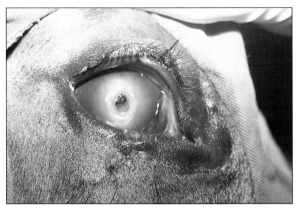

612 Corneal ulceration (chronic, localised, deep).
Note: Corneal edema and extensive accumulation of debris. Inflammatory reaction and neo-vascularisation surrounding the ulcer.

613

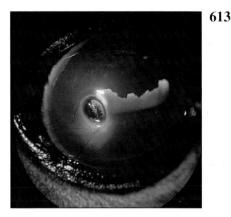

613 (Indolent) corneal ulceration.
Note: Present for 8 months without showing any evidence of healing, vascularisation, significant edema or any detectable progression. Lesion was non-painful.

614

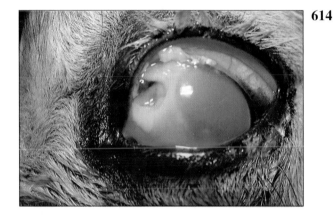

614 Corneal ulceration (melting ulcer) (keratomalacia).
Note: Bacterial contamination with collagenase/protease-producing *Pseudomonas* spp. produced an alarming progression of the ulceration and stromal destruction within 12 hours.

common sequel to foreign bodies, for example) and of several days duration, the corneal stroma, which is normally very anhydrous, becomes contaminated with imbibed water and takes on a cloudy appearance **(612)**. Whilst under normal circumstances corneal repair is rapid, in some cases which may or may not be infected, the damaged cornea fails to heal. Cellular debris can be seen building up around the periphery of the ulcerated area (*see* **612**) and, in spite of extensive neovascularization from the limbus, these lesions often stubbornly fail to resolve. A static state may be present for months or even years. Although in most cases a blood supply will develop, even if this only reaches the edges of the lesion, others show neither a tendency to heal nor significant vascularisation of the affected area **(613)**. These may be a consequence of an epithelial dysplasia, defective basement membrane structure or failure of the epithelium to adhere adequately to the basement membrane. Significantly, in these cases the animals are often not in any apparent discomfort nor do they develop any significant corneal edema around such lesions. In many cases the ulcer is not obvious and in spite of the clinical severity of the lesion, the disorder may pass unnoticed for prolonged periods. Long-standing, shallow ulcers associated with adjacent corneal fibrosis and edema should alert the clinician to the possibility of a sub-palpebral foreign body (such as a grass seed).

The healing process within the cornea is considerably modified by its unique, relatively desiccated and non-vascular nature. Inordinate or inappropriate response to corneal injury by these repair mechanisms may result in local production of collagenase enzymes which result in further **corneal stromal damage**. Superimposed infections, particularly where these are due to *Pseudomonas* spp or *Bacillus cereus*, are a serious complication of corneal ulcerations and lacerations. Proteolytic enzymes with a high collagenase activity and exotoxins, derived from dead and decaying bacteria, are produced, and the severity of corneal ulceration both in depth and extent, may deteriorate alarmingly within hours, to the extent of complete erosion of the cornea

313

615

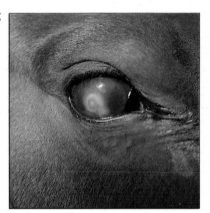

616

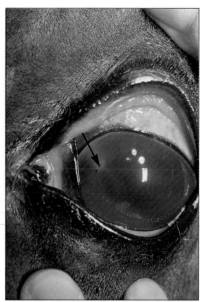

615 Corneal ulceration (healed focal ulceration).
Note: Well vascularized fibrosing scar.

616 Hyphema (blood in anterior chamber).
Note: Site of foreign body penetration (faint, milky-white mark in cornea in upper nasal quadrant (arrow). Intense miosis.

(614) and prolapse of Descemet's membrane (**descemetocele**). In other cases the resulting **diffuse keratomalacia** is accompanied by the development of extensive corneal edema (*see* **614**). Complete **perforation of the cornea and collapse of the eye** (*see* **627**) is a common sequel to neglected or unresponsive keratomalacia.

The eventual, expected, outcome of corneal damage, whether caused by trauma or by other pathological processes, is **corneal scarring/fibrosis**. Although the cornea has a rapid normal propensity for healing the return of a normal clear cornea is often delayed by the persistence of invading blood vessels and the dense white corneal fibrosis (**615**) which represents the healing stage of the lesion. Ultimately, however, most corneal ulcers and wounds heal, leaving a permanent or semipermanent, obvious or faint white scar of corneal fibrosis. Over extended periods of time (often years) the size and density of the scar may reduce but others remain constant. They seldom affect vision unless they are extensive and very dense.

Complications arising from relatively minor corneal trauma may be far more serious than is initially apparent. Penetrations of the cornea by small foreign bodies (such as thorns) may appear to induce relatively small corneal lesions with corneal edema over a very limited area surrounding the penetration site (**616**), but may result in extremely serious complications. **Uveal hemorrhage** may also follow blunt trauma to the eye. In the acute stages of such an injury, bleeding into the anterior chamber (hyphema) (*see* **616**) may be encountered, where either the iris itself or the entire uveal tract has been traumatised. The iris is a highly vascular structure and, while hemorrhage may be very

severe, its extent would, normally, eventually be limited or controlled by increasing intraocular pressure. In these cases, and occasionally independently, the uveal tract may respond with profound and dramatic inflammatory changes. In many cases the extent of intraocular hemorrhage is less dramatic but the associated inflammatory response is almost always considerable. A **panuveitis** in which the entire uveal tract is inflamed may result and the eye is, at first, usually extremely painful (*see* **621**) and the iris is typically intensely miotic with a very small pupil (**616**). The iris may be seen to have a characteristic burnt-leaf appearance, indicative of acute inflammation, but the development of a diffuse opacity in the aqueous humour (**aqueous flare**) may prevent such detailed observation (**617**). The development of secondary infection and the accumulation of cellular debris within the anterior chamber of the eye may be seen as an obvious yellow accumulation (**hypopyon**) in the inferior segment of the anterior chamber (**618**).

While the complications of eye trauma may be immediate and obvious, they may also be slower to develop and may, in some cases be less dramatic, though no less serious. Even minor trauma to the eye sometimes induces **changes within the lens** or **alterations of lens position** within the globe. **Blunt trauma** to the eye sometimes results in **tearing of the anterior or posterior capsule of the lens** (or both). The consequences of the tearing depend upon the extent of the damage and range from **partial or complete dislocations** of the lens to relatively minor **capsular cataract** development subsequent to capsular tearing/rupture. **Lens dislocations** in the horse are rarely

617

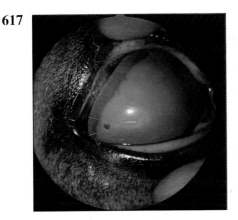

618

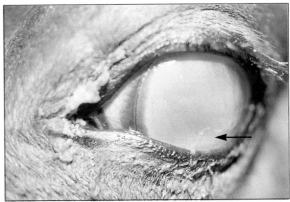

617 Panuveitis.
Note: Penetrating foreign body 48 hours previously. Deep vascularisation (showing as a perilimbal brush border). The site of corneal penetration is visible. Intense miosis with 'burnt-leaf' appearance of iris.

618 Hypopyon and corneal edema.
Note: Intense panuveitis/ iridocyclitis with miosis. Distinct deposit of inflammatory debris in the anterior chamber (arrow).

619

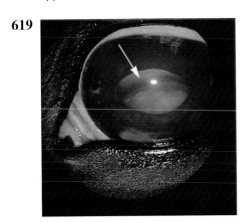

620

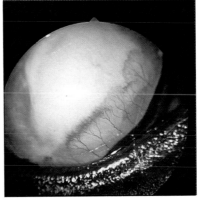

619 Lens luxation (posterior).
Note: Cataractous lens in posterior chamber with aphakic crescent (arrow).

620 Lens luxation (anterior).
Note: Lens material creates poorly defined shape due to rupture of lens capsule. Perilimbal neovascularization due to contact of lens material with endothelium of cornea.

spontaneous, most cases being the result of trauma or chronic uveitis and iridocyclitis. Lens luxations are most often posterior displacement within the anterior chamber **(619)**. More rarely, anterior luxation occurs and this is often accompanied by a marked inflammatory response in the cornea over the contact area **(620)**. Secondary glaucoma is unusual but may be encountered when the aqueous drainage is impaired either at the iris or more often at the drainage angle in the anterior chamber. Following trauma to the eye lens luxation may not be immediately apparent. Any tearing of the attachments of the lens resulting in even minor displacements in either an anterior or posterior direction may result in anterior vitreous prolapse. Where trauma induces direct

lens dislocation, the extent of obvious ocular trauma is extensive in most cases. Almost every lens which is dislocated, including those which are completely or partially displaced, becomes cataractous eventually (*see* **620**). An aphakic crescent may be observed where the lens is displaced sufficiently to allow the posterior chamber and fundus to be examined beyond the limits of the lens (*see* **619**).

One of the most important disorders of the equine eye is **equine recurrent uveitis** which is also known as 'Periodic Ophthalmia' and 'Moon Blindness'. The disorder is of world wide significance and horses of all breeds and all ages are subject to the disease. While many etiological factors have been suggested, it is clear

621

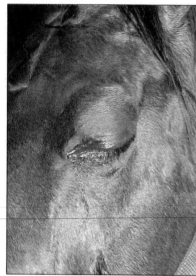

622

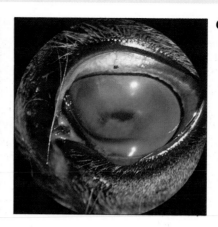

623

621 Equine recurrent uveitis syndrome ('moon blindness', 'periodic ophthalmia').
Note: Blepharospasm and epiphora/lacrimation.
Differential Diagnosis:
i)   Foreign body
ii) Corneal ulceration
iii) Trauma

622 Equine recurrent uveitis syndrome ('moon blindness', 'periodic ophthalmia') (acute).
Note: Diffuse fibrinous accumulation in anterior chamber (aqueous flare), intense miosis and iritis.
Differential Diagnosis:
i) Traumatic anterior uveitis
ii) Traumatic posterior uveitis

623 Equine recurrent uveitis syndrome (acute).
Note: Iris inflammation, miosis (pupil constriction), aqueous flare (diffuse, 'smoky' opacity of aqueous humor resulting from fibrinous and inflammatory proteins), hypopyon (inflammatory debris in the anterior chamber) and diffuse corneal edema.

that the clinical syndrome represents a response of the uveal tract to traumatic and immune mediated inflammation. It is usually defined as an acute, nongranulomatous inflammation of the uveal tract. One or both eyes may be affected and there is a marked tendency to recur with irregular severity at indeterminate/irregular intervals in the same eye or in alternate eyes or in both eyes. Single episodes of uveitis involving one eye (or rarely both) are more commonly associated with trauma-induced uveitis while recurrent episodes involving alternate eyes or both simultaneously or only one eye are more often associated with the endogenous, immune-mediated forms of the disorder. The recognition of the two distinct possibilities is of major importance with respect to prognosis. A single incident of trauma-induced uveitis may have no further consequences beyond those which become evident immediately or shortly after the episode. Horses affected with the immune-mediated (endogenous) form have a much poorer prognosis in view of the unpredictable recurrences which are

characteristic. Repeated episodes, furthermore, also result in progressively increasing severity and complexity of the secondary effects. The secondary effects of uveitis are usually marked and may affect any or all of the other structures of the eye including the retina, lens and cornea. Typically, the disease, however caused, has an acute onset with marked pain, blepharospasm, lacrimation **(621)** and photophobia, usually in one eye (but sometimes in both). Affected horses will, generally, not allow examination of the eye without systemic analgesics, topical analgesia and/or palpebral nerve block. Unusually a mild ocular inflammation with limited blepharospasm and a short course may be all that is seen. In the acute stage the iris is inflamed, becoming turgid and thick and losing its normal appearance. The pupil is invariably intensely miotic (constricted) **(622)**. The accumulation of inflammatory debris in the aqueous humor creates a more or less diffuse milky opacity **(aqueous flare)**. This inflammatory debris precipitates into the inferior angle of the anterior chamber, producing

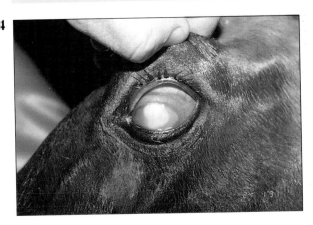

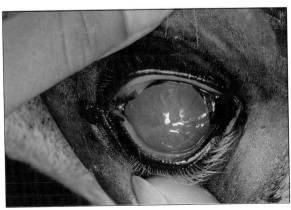

624 Equine recurrent uveitis syndrome (severe, acute). **Note:** Prominent limbal vascularising keratitis, corneal edema and corneal ulceration. Impossible to examine internal structures visually.

625 Equine recurrent uveitis syndrome (later stages). **Note:** Extensive vascularisation of the cornea without ulceration. Direct examination of the internal structures of the eye impossible.

626

627

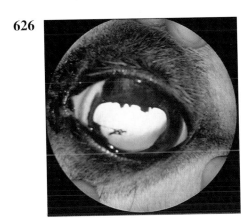

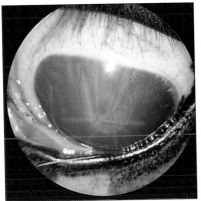

626 Equine recurrent uveitis syndrome (quiescent stage). **Note:** Adhesions between iris and anterior lens capsule (posterior synechiae) and irregular shaped pupil. Limited movement of the iris was possible. **Differential Diagnosis:** i) Traumatic iritis

627 Equine recurrent uveitis syndrome - phthisis bulbi (collapse/shrinkage of globe). **Note:** Linear corneal opacities from folding of Descemet's membrane, and superficial vascularisation. Acquired heterochromic iris.

a distinctive but seldom extensive hypopyon (**623**).

Persistent cases of uveitis with corneal involvement or those having a particularly rapid progression develop severe **ulcerative keratitis (624)** and/or extensive **deep and superficial episcleral and corneal neovascularisation (625)**. In such cases examination of the interior components of the eye is obviously impossible, but the history, taken in conjunction with the absence of conjunctival or corneal foreign bodies, is often enough to support a diagnosis of acute uveitis. There is considerable benefit to be gained from ultrasonographic examination of the eye under these circumstances and a 7.5 MHz (or higher) linear or sector probe will establish the presence of a thickened iris and possibly the earliest complications of the disorder.

The quiescent stage of the periodic disease, which may last for hours, days, months or years, may be detected between the acute episodes, and is particularly apparent immediately following an acute episode. A turgid iris is visible with a 'bound-down' pupil which does not respond normally to light. This is due to the development of adhesions between the posterior aspect of the iris and the anterior capsule of the lens (**posterior synechiae**). These limit the mobility of the iris in most cases but may occasionally rupture, leaving thin strands of iris tissue adherent to the lens capsule (**626**). These often result in gross distortions of the iris. The recognition of iris distortions and irregularity in otherwise apparently normal horses should alert the

628

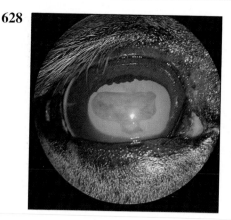

629

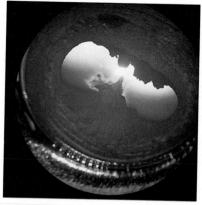

628 Anterior capsular cataract.
Note: No previous history of eye disease or trauma. No apparent visual deficit.

629 Anterior capsular cataract.
Note: Posterior synechiae and iris tags.
Differential Diagnosis:
i) Equine recurrent uveitis syndrome
ii) Trauma-induced uveitis
iii) Penetrating foreign body
iv) (Partial) lens luxation

630

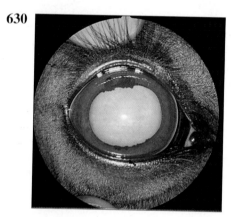

6

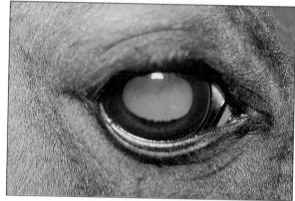

630 (Mature) cortical cataract.
Note: Typical ground-glass appearance indicative of cataract maturity.

631 Cortical cataract.
Note: Diffuse ground-glass appearance with prominent 'Y'-suture and localised areas of increased cataract density.

clinician to the possibility of previous (and therefore future) episodes of uveitis. Extensive adhesions between the lens and the posterior surface of the iris may result in a dramatic increase in pressure in the posterior portion of the anterior chamber and result in an obvious bulging of the iris into the anterior chamber (**iris bombé**). In some cases, retinal defects including scarring (*see* **637**) and detachments which may be complete (*see* **632**) or, more usually, focal or partial may be detected by funduscopic examination in the quiescent phase of uveitis. The long-term consequences of untreated or refractory cases of recurrent uveitis may be severe and a wide variety of intra-ocular abnormalities have been described. Associated defects within the lens, including sub-capsular and cortical cataracts may also be encountered. The appearance of capsular cataracts which are the result of periodic uveitis (*see* **628**) is often distinctly different from those caused by single traumatic episodes (*see* **629**). However, as is the case with most of the serious disorders of the globe, most affected eyes eventually become contracted (**phthisis bulbi**) (**627**) and are then usually unsighted. In some cases the globe is severely shrunken and prolapse of the third eyelid (*membrana nictitans*) covers what remains of the eye and various catarrhal and purulent ocular discharges are persistently present at the medial canthus. The recognition of the less dramatic chronic changes encountered in cases of equine periodic uveitis is vitally

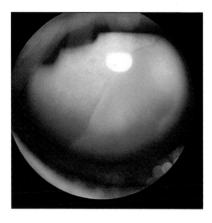

632 Retinal detachment.
Note: Retina can be seen floating in the posterior chamber of the eye and the optic disc is only vaguely visible. Eye totally unsighted.

important as, during the quiescent phases of the disease, the eye may otherwise appear normal and there may be no obvious defect of vision. No case can be considered to have recovered from the disease and every horse which has a history of equine periodic uveitis is best regarded as being in the quiescent phase, no matter what the interval between the acute episodes. There are almost no predictable features of the disease with respect to either its epidemiology or its clinical features in a particular horse. The trauma-induced form of uveitis, however, carries a good prognosis and these seldom, if ever, recur and the secondary changes are often static (even although, on occasion, they may be dramatic).

Disorders of the lens represent an important diagnostic challenge. Secondary changes in the lens structure arise following a wide variety of ocular insults including, most commonly, trauma and uveitis. While some, such as the **congenital cataract** (lens opacity) (*see* **607**), may be non-progressive and indeed may improve with time, lens opacities occurring in adult horses, as a result of primary ocular disease, carry a much less favourable prognosis.

Anterior capsular cataracts (628) are usually secondary, either to blunt ocular trauma or develop as a result of anterior uveitis. There may be no involvement of the iris or other structures but in some cases, particularly where trauma is responsible, posterior synechiae are commonly present in addition and may actually adhere to the lens in the region of the cataract **(629)**. They may be progressive and many eventually have a deleterious effect upon vision.

Extensive cataract development in the cortex of the lens is a serious disorder carrying a poor prognosis. They may arise subsequent to trauma or uveal tract inflammation and some develop without any evidence of either of these. **Mature cataracts** present at birth are usually non-progressive but acquired forms occurring in older horses often progress (either slowly or more

rapidly) and ultimately result in blindness. They may be unilateral or bilateral. Affected horses are usually 'light hungry' with a widely dilated pupil. The lens usually has a milky appearance which may be obvious, even from a distance **(630)**. Long-standing (mature) cataracts are usually very crystalline in appearance and suture lines are often obvious **(631)**. Suture lines having a distinctive 'Y'-shape are the most visible. The suture lines on the anterior capsule are usually the most visible because they are emphasised against the background of the cortical cataract (*see* **631**).

Many normal horses have faint speckles or single highly refractile particles within the lens which may easily be recognised ophthalmoscopically but which are not cataracts and which have no clinical significance. Old horses often show curvilinear patterning within the lens structure which are normal age-related changes and give the appearance of concentric alterations in lens refractivity (onion rings). They appear to have no effect on vision and do not seem to act as a focus for subsequent cataract development.

Retinal disorders of the horse are rare but their recognition is of great importance in the clinical assessment of sight and visual acuity (sharpness, distinctness), particularly when animals are to be ridden. Many of the retinal disorders recognised in the equine fundus have equivocal effects upon vision and although the lesions may be dramatic in appearance almost all such horses have normal sight. The assessment of visual acuity in the horse is extremely difficult but some useful information may be gained from obstacle tests in bright and subdued light conditions. It is often, however, left to the clinician to make an informed guess as to the effect of any retinal lesion upon the visual acuity.

Detachments of the retina over small or, occasionally more extensive **(632)** areas are encountered in the horse. The causes of such detachments are probably varied but they are usually considered to be the

633

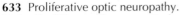

634

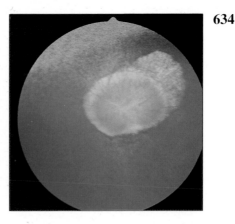

633 Proliferative optic neuropathy.
Note: Cauliflower-like mass attached to border of optic disc. No effect on sight and no changes in shape or position over years.
Differential Diagnosis:
i)   Neoplasia
ii) Exudative optic neuritis
iii) Peripapillary coloboma

634 Atypical coloboma (of the retinal pigmented epithelium).
Note: Discontinuity of the epithelium beyond the embryonic fissure.
Differential Diagnosis:
i)   Exudative optic neuritis
ii) Proliferative optic neuropathy
ii) Neoplasia

result of inflammatory responses within the choroid sufficient to separate the neuro-sensory retina from the underlying retinal pigmentary epithelium. Secondary inflammatory detritus, usually as a result of posterior uveitis, may result in the development of vitreo-retinal adhesions which have been suggested as a cause of localised or extensive retinal detachment. Contraction of these adhesions is possibly responsible for the tearing of the retina from the underlying retinal pigmented epithelium. Any condition which results in a retinal defect which allows vitreous to leak below the retina might also lift it, resulting in more or less complete detachment (*see* **632**). The commonest causes of such inflammatory processes are equine recurrent uveitis or ocular infections resulting in suppurative or exudative optic neuritis (*see* **643**) or blunt (or sharp) ocular trauma (*see* **610**). Where there is significant detachment of the retina, there will always be a visual defect. Horses with bilateral retinal detachment will be totally blind and show marked 'light-hunger' with a widely dilated pupil and the eyelids will be held widely open giving the horses an apprehensive expression. These horses are almost always hyper-reactive to touch or sound. Examination of the fundus will show a thin/delicate veil-like structure floating in the posterior chamber (*see* **632**). Confirmation of such detachments, even in severely inflamed eyes which preclude or severely limit the diagnostic value of visual inspection, may be obtained from ultrasonographic examination of the eye using a 7.5 – 10 Mhz sector, or linear array, probe. An obvious, echogenic structure will be identified, floating freely in the vitreous. Movement of the head during this procedure will establish the floating nature of the lesion and demonstrate the sites of attachment.

A wide variety of retinal or choroidal abnormalities has been recognised. Defects in fundic appearance may be significant or may be incidental. It is therefore important to recognise the significant disorders, in particular. In the horse the thick and fibrous tapetum tends to mask the effects of inflammation arising in the choroid and so most visible chorioretinal abnormalities appear in the non-tapetal retina. Most of the common conditions are unilateral and have little apparent effect on the appearance of the eye itself. Diagnosis is therefore reliant upon careful ophthalmoscopic (funduscopic) examination in suitable, darkened surroundings.

Proliferative optic neuropathy is a poorly understood condition, usually affecting only one eye, which has a typical appearance and which seldom, if ever, has a detectable effect on vision. Usually a cauliflower-like mass can be seen attached to the margin of the optic disc and projecting into the vitreous (**633**). The cardinal features of this distinctive lesion are its apparently non-progressive character and its constant shape. These enable it to be differentiated from other benign, neoplastic or infective lesions involving the optic disc.

The more common, benign, **atypical peripapillary coloboma of the retinal pigmentary epithelium (634)** has a somewhat similar appearance. A range of visible abnormalities of the choroid and retinal pigmentary

635

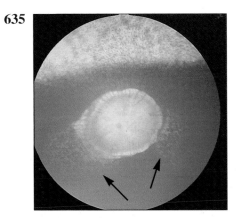

636

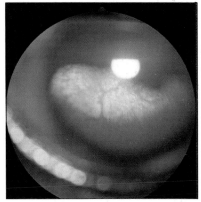

635 Peripapillary chorioretinal degeneration ('butterfly lesion') (arrows).
Note: Obvious attenuation of the contiguous retinal blood vessels. Probably an insignificant lesion. Not usually associated with equine recurrent uveitis syndrome.

636 Peripapillary chorioretinopathy.
Note: Focal areas of hyper and hypo-pigmentation of non-tapetal retina. No effect on vision but suspicion of previous equine recurrent uveitis syndrome.

637

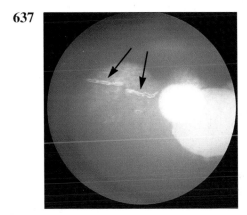

638

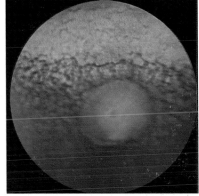

637 Chorioretinitis.
Note: Hyper-reflective scarred areas of tapetal retina (arrows). Causes no apparent visual deficit unless very extensive and accompanied by optic nerve atrophy.

638 Generalised retinal degeneration.
Note: Extensive disruption of retinal pigmentary epithelium and degeneration of neurosensory retina in tapetal fundus. Vision apparently unaffected.

epithelium can be recognised immediately adjacent to the optic disc. The lesions are most often unilateral and in most cases show as discrete areas of depigmentation with focal hyperpigmentation. The so-called '**Butterfly**' lesions of **peripapillary chorioretinopathy** occur medially and laterally to the margin of the optic disc (**635**) and represent areas of retinal degeneration. Their significance is equivocal in view of their generally non-progressive character and the relatively high incidence without any apparent effects upon vision, but some visual deficit may be expected where they are extensive.

Active areas of inflammation and healed areas of **retinitis** (however caused) frequently involve varying degrees of peripapillary and non-tapetal depigmentation with focal hyperpigmentation. These appear as black-pigmented areas in a pale or non-uniform, non tapetal fundus (**636**). The discrete lesions of focal retinal inflammation (**637**) may be observed incidentally in many horses and are particularly commonly encountered in horses suffering from active respiratory tract virus infections. While the lesions heal well in most cases, leaving no apparent visual defect, obvious scars are usually present in the non-tapetum as so-called 'bullet hole lesions', which may be circular or linear in appearance (*see* **637**). Scarring of the choroid and/or the retinal pigmentary epithelium, as a result of even relatively minor incidents of infection or other inflammation, results in abnormal appearance of the retina but are seldom, if ever, associated with disturbances of vision.

Extensive or generalised disruptive degeneration of the retinal pigmented epithelium in the tapetal fundus (**638**) may involve both eyes and, in spite of an alarming appearance, little or no visual impairment is generally present. It seems likely, however, that, with such a severely abnormal retinal appearance, some deficit of retinal function must be present in these cases and if this is so the animal may adapt to such visual deficit.

Infectious disorders

Viral Diseases: Viral infections affecting only the eye are unusual but an unknown (possibly Herpetiform) virus, is known to cause a **primary (viral) keratitis** which presents with a distinctive clinical appearance. Multiple superficial punctate and often microscopic ulcerative lesions which impart a granular appearance to the cornea (**639**), which generally stain with fluorescein are typical. The lesions are hard to visualise directly and oblique illumination is helpful. There is usually minimal intra-ocular or corneal inflammation in spite of extensive corneal involvement (*see* **639**). Corneal edema may also be extensive, but is usually localised and is seldom severe (*see* **639**). The disorder is accompanied by moderate or severe pain, blepharospasm and lacrimation. Healing may be protracted. A definitive diagnosis of viral keratitis relies upon the identification of the virus in swabs taken from the surface of the cornea, but a presumptive diagnosis may be made by testing the response of the condition to the application of specific anti-viral medication. While this disorder is relatively well recognised it is possible that other viruses are involved in the development of similar ulcerative lesions. A catarrhal or muco-purulent ocular discharge is a sign that there may be secondary bacterial infection. Ocular lesions (including keratitis and conjunctivitis) are also a common secondary (or primary) feature of other diseases and, in particular, those affecting the upper respiratory tract. Virus infections, including equine herpes virus (EHV-1, EHV-2 and EHV-4), equine influenza virus, African Horse Sickness, and viral arteritis may show non-specific keratitis lesions and horse pox (Variola) may produce corneal vesicles. In these cases a keratitis and conjunctivitis are present, usually without detectable corneal ulceration and, although the presence of a keratitis may help in the diagnostic process, the major clinical signs of the diseases are usually prominent.

Another viral disease associated with lesions on the eyelids is due to **papovavirus** and may occur seasonally in young horses. Pinkish, grey wart-like lesions develop around the eyelids. Lesions are also often to be found around the muzzle, face and limbs (*see* **535**). Corneal or conjunctival involvement is usually minimal but viral papillomata have been encountered in the conjunctival sac.

A number of virus disorders have profound effects upon the function of the eye, even if not obviously upon the eye itself. Thus horses suffering from the viral encephalitides including Venezuelan equine encephalitis (*see* **724**) and the European arthropod-borne virus encephalitis (Borna Disease) may be rendered blind by their effects upon the central nervous system. There are usually other (sometimes more dramatic) supporting signs which may be used to identify these.

Bacterial infections of the eye are common and may be primary diseases or develop secondarily to viral infections or to traumatic damage to the cornea or other ocular structures. A number of systemic bacterial

639

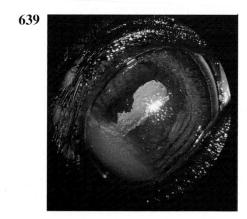

639 Viral keratitis.
Note: Focal pinpoint irregular areas of fluorescein uptake within the affected areas of the cornea. The eye was acutely painful. Cornea shows a faint, lace-like, superficial opacity (corneal edema) which is very difficult to visualise in most cases.

640

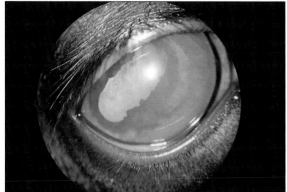

642

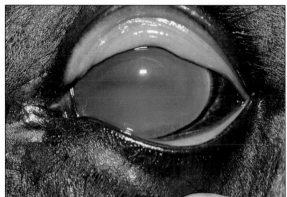

641

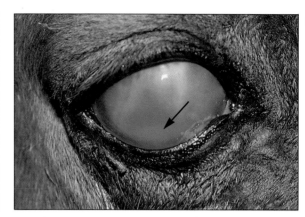

640 Acute bacterial uveitis.
Note: Five-day-old foal with signs of neonatal septicemia due to *Actinobacillus equuli*. Aqueous flare (due to inflammatory debris in aqueous humor), hyphema (blood in anterior chamber). 'Muddy' appearance of iris and miosis.

641 Hypopyon (with keratitis).
Note: Accumulation of inflammatory (purulent) debris in the anterior chamber (arrow).

642 Hypopyon (with minimal corneal involvement).
Note: Horse suffering from severe septicemic *Streptococcus equi* infection (Bastard strangles).
Differential Diagnosis:
i) Systemic lupus erythematosus-like syndrome
ii) Rhodococcus equi

infections including *Streptococcus equi*, *Rhodococcus equi* and *Actinobacillus equuli* may cause severe intraocular pathology, particularly in foals. Septicemia in neonatal foals often involves intercurrent septic uveitis (**640**). A marked aqueous flare, associated with the accumulation of fibrin and inflammatory proteins in the anterior chamber (hypopyon), and varying degrees of hemorrhage (hyphema) are typically encountered (*see* **640**). Generally, as would be expected in such cases, the eye lesions may not be the most obvious presenting signs, but the presence of intra-ocular inflammation in young foals is strongly suggestive of septicemia.

Secondary bacterial infections involving the eye have particularly serious consequences. Certain bacteria such as *Pseudomonas* and several other Gram-negative bacteria are known to produce proteolytic enzymes which may possess strong collagenase activity and once these gain access to the corneal stroma would result in a severe and rapidly progressive 'melting ulceration' (*see* **614**). Horses with bacterial infection within the conjunctival sac exhibit a variable, purulent, ocular discharge. Where this is seen further investigation is imperative to establish the extent and character of the bacteria involved and whether this is secondary to a foreign body or other ocular pathology. *Streptococcus*

equi and *Streptococcus zooepidemicus* often produce a catarrhal or purulent ocular discharge associated with infections within the conjunctival sac. Bacterial infections within the eye arising as a primary event following penetrations of the cornea, or secondarily in cases of intraocular inflammation or primary viral disease, usually exhibit a marked hypopyon (**641**). The presence of inflammatory cells in the anterior chamber, even where this is not accompanied by other evidence of ophthalmic pathology (**642**) should always alert the clinician to the possibility of anterior uveitis (whether this is a result of equine recurrent uveitis or not). Horses suffering from the systemic lupus erythematosus-like syndrome (*see* **514** *et seq.*) present a very similar occular sign but the hypopyon ebbs and flows remarkably quickly.

Suppurative optic neuritis may arise from infectious or non-infectious inflammation in the optic stalk or in the posterior parts of the orbit. Extension of sepsis from the nasal cavity and the sinuses is one of the commoner causes of this condition. The affected eye is usually unsighted and while in the early stages there may be no obvious effect upon the contents of the globe the rapidly expanding, finger-like projections which can be seen over the surface of the optic disc (**643**) and which may

643

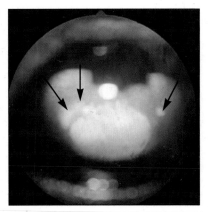

644

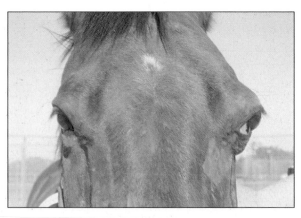

643 Suppurative optic neuritis.
Note: Contents of vitreous and fundus not clearly visible due to diffuse vitreous opacity caused by inflammatory debris. Finger-like projections from optic disc and floating purulent material in posterior chamber (arrows).

644 Orbital abscess.
Note: Unilateral exophthalmos, swelling at supraorbital fossa. Globe normal. Retrobulbar abscess identified by ultrasonographic examination and aspiration.

break off and float away in the liquefying vitreous become progressively more extensive. Small fragments of the inflammatory debris are easily seen in the vitreous (*see* **643**). The appearance of the optic disc, blindness and an intercurrent pathology (either infective or neoplastic processes) in the orbit are however, characteristic of suppurative optic neuritis.

Panophthalmitis or endophthalmitis and orbital abscesses, in which gross and extensive infections are present in the orbital and peri-orbital tissues respectively, represent severe progression of infectious processes in these locations. Horses affected by panophthalmitis show severe pain initially but this may subside to the level where it is possible to examine the eye relatively easily. All the internal structures of the eye are invariably involved in the process although it is unusual to be able to establish the extent purely by visual or ophthalmoscopic inspection. Where these eyes are left to their own devices the eye itself generally becomes phthisic, shrinking into the socket and then has no further function (*see* **627**). Periorbital or orbital infections may extend into the meninges and result in central nervous disorders or suppurative optic neuritis (*see* **643**).

Retro-bulbar abscesses developing within the bony orbit but not directly involving the eye itself usually present a normal eye with a marked and progressive exophthalmos (**644**), often with obvious swelling of the infraorbital fossa (*see* **644**). Pain and varying degrees of ocular discharge are usually present. Aspiration from the retrobulbar tissues may be used to confirm the presence of these lesions within the bony orbit. Ultrasonographic examination, which is possible in the conscious, sedated horse, is a most useful technique in these cases, enabling both the nature and the extent of the lesion to be appreciated. Radiographic examination is usually unrewarding.

Parasitic Diseases: Infection with *Onchocerca cervicalis* is sometimes responsible for a focal keratitis which characteristically, but not invariably, develops in the temporal limbal region of the cornea. It appears as a white, fluffy, poorly defined area on the cornea with varying degrees of neovascularisation and inflammation (**645**). Perhaps the commonest sign of *Onchocerca cervicalis* infection in the eye is, however, a more benign conjunctival depigmentation at the temporal limbus with a chronic keratitis associated with neovascularisation. Linear corneal opacities which are similar in appearance to the congenital opacities arising as a result of hypoplasia of the Descemet's membrane may also be due to the migration of the microfilaria of *Onchocerca cervicalis* through the cornea. Whilst any reaction within the cornea is uncommon, there may be an intercurrent conjunctivitis with chemosis, corneal edema and the parasite is also possibly associated with some cases of acute uveitis. The appearance of the larger more aggressive lesions is very similar to those of early corneal squamous cell carcinoma. Differentiation is of paramount importance - diagnosis having a marked bearing on the prognosis and choice of treatment regime, and may be made on biopsy (including impression smears or sections) and response to appropriate therapy.

Verminous ophthalmia due to *Setaria digitata* is most often encountered in the Indian sub-continent where it produces a disease affecting both the eye and the central nervous system known as "kumri". An

645

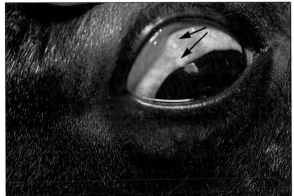

646

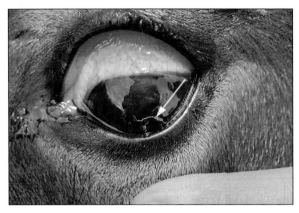

647

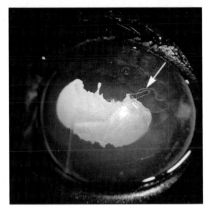

645 Equine ocular onchocerciasis.
Note: Focal inflammatory lesion at superior limbus (arrow) and causing conjunctivitis and chemosis. Small margin of localised interstitial keratitis.

646 *Setaria digitata.*
Note: Fine grey-white parasite in anterior chamber (arrow), size of parasite magnified by cornea.

647 *Thelazia lacrimalis.*
Note: Adult parasites, appearing singly and in groups, on surface of cornea (arrow). Parasites are easier to see when mobile.

immature form of *Setaria equina*, which normally inhabits the abdominal cavity of horses in many parts of the world with little or no pathogenic effect in this site, may also be found in the anterior chamber of the eye. The parasites are transmitted by mosquitoes and possibly by other biting insects. Affected horses are usually only affected in one eye and while most cases show prominent lacrimation, blepharospasm and corneal edema, others are apparently little affected. Horses with live parasites in the anterior chamber make persistent attempts to rub the eye and this often results in considerable self-inflicted trauma to the eyelids and sometimes leads to extensive secondary corneal ulceration. Examination of the anterior chamber will reveal the presence of one to three (or more) fine white hair-like larvae, about 10–20 mm long, which are often usefully magnified by the cornea (**646**), giving an impression of a much larger parasite. Long-standing infestation may result in a severe and disabling keratitis. The parasites may be removed from the aqueous humor by needle aspiration. Both the larval and adult forms of the worm are highly susceptible to ivermectin, although parasites which are killed in the anterior chamber by this

drug may induce a considerable inflammatory response and, possibly, uveitis.

Infestation of the conjunctival sac with **Thelazia lacrymalis** occurs over wide areas of the world and is transmitted by *Musca autumnalis* (the face fly). The condition is most often encountered in horses less than 3 years old. The parasites are often found incidentally, during ophthalmic examinations and it is sometimes regarded as a commensal of the conjunctival fornix. Some cases show significant photophobia, lacrimation, a chronic conjunctivitis and a persistent sero-mucoid ocular discharge. Most infested horses are asymptomatic. Some long-standing cases show a marked superficial keratitis and may even be blind as a result of heavy infestation. The adult parasite is about 10mm long and is quite active and can be seen moving across the conjunctiva or over the surface of the cornea (*see* **647**). Instillation of local anesthetic agents into the eye immobilises the parasites and makes them more difficult to identify. Sudden movement of the parasites within the conjunctival sac has been blamed for sudden, violent eye irritation in some horses. Adult parasites may be removed from the conjunctiva relatively easily but some may be present within the nasolacrimal duct or deep in the fornices of the conjunctival sac.

The larvae of ***Habronema muscae, Habronema microstoma*** and ***Draschia megastoma*** deposited in the conjunctival sac and/or on the skin at the medial canthus of the eye, by the house fly (*Musca domestica*) or the stable fly (*Stomoxys calcitrans*), may produce ocular or conjunctival habronemiasis. Larval deposition on the skin of the face below the medial canthus and on open wounds results in persistent, non-healing granulating wounds (*see* **584**) known as summer sores, kunkers, swamp cancer, bursatti, and by other colloquial names. Initially conjunctival infection results in a markedly pruritic eye with rubbing and lacrimation. Pain may be significant and severe epiphora due to both increased tear flow and to obstructions of the naso-lacrimal duct is a common symptom. A characteristic non-healing granulating wound develops at the medial canthus (*see* **584**) and an ocular discharge which usually has a yellow granular appearance is seen (**648**). Small granular yellow lesions occurring in the medial canthus and on the surface of the membrana nictitans, or more rarely on the eyelid itself, are also typical of **conjunctival habronemiasis**. *Habronema spp.* larvae which gain access to the naso-lacrimal sac induce a severe but very localised granulating, non-healing wound over the site (**649**). In all cases of ocular habronemiasis corneal ulceration may develop and would then probably be a consequence of local surface trauma from conjunctival granulomas, or from self-inflicted rubbing of the corneal surface. The extensive epiphora which is characteristic of the disease serves to provide an excoriated area of the face below the medial canthus in which further infestation may arise (*see* **548**). The disorder resolves over the winter months, leaving varying degrees of facial scarring but there is usually little residual effect from the conjunctival form apart from some corneal fibrosis at the site of old, healed ulcers. More rarely the naso-lacrimal duct may be damaged sufficiently to result in a permanent epiphora.

648

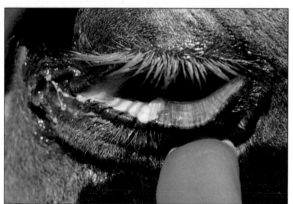

648 Conjunctival habronemiasis (*Habronema musca* and/or *Draschia megastoma*).
Note: Characteristic chronic, yellow, granular, ocular discharge.

649

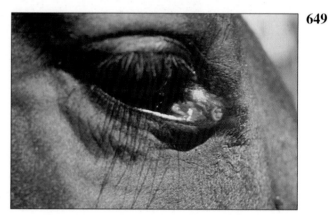

649 Habronemiasis (of nasolacrimal sac). (*Habronema musca* and/or *Draschia megastoma*).
Differential Diagnosis:
i) Squamous cell carcinoma
ii) Ocular histoplasmosis
iii) Sarcoid
iv) Fly damage

Neoplastic Disorders

Squamous cell carcinoma of the lower eyelid, the third eyelid, the sclera or the cornea (or combinations of these) probably represents the commonest carcinoma of the horse. Squamous cell carcinoma also occurs around the anus, on the penis and prepuce of middle aged or old geldings, on the vulva of mares and in other sites around the head and neck. The eye lesions are most prevalent in horses between 6 and 12 years of age in geographical areas where high levels of ultraviolet light are encountered. However, older horses and those living in temperate climates are also affected. The eyelids and third eyelids are common sites for their development. They are usually unilateral but bilateral lesions may be present. Whilst they seldom metastasise from this site they may extend into the bone of the orbital rin. or into the orbit itself and even extend, in rare cases, as far as the nasolacrimal sac/duct and the brain. Their significance should not be underestimated. A diagnosis of squamous cell carcinoma is not usually difficult with the colour, appearance and site giving sufficient

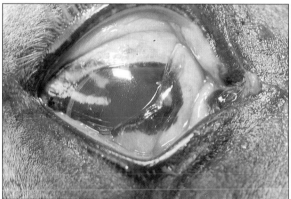

650 Squamous cell carcinoma (precancerous stage). **Note:** Blood- stained lacrimal secretion and slight thickening of *membrana nictitans* (third eyelid).
Differential Diagnosis:
i)   Conjunctival habronemiasis
ii) Hemorrhagic diatheses
iii) Thelaziasis
iv) Chemosis (conjunctival edema)

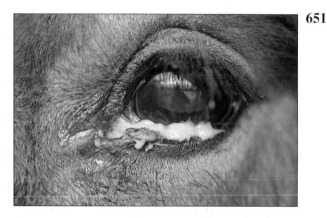

651 Squamous cell carcinoma (chronic, non-invasive, palpebral form).
Note: Lesion present for two years without apparent change. Persistent mucopurulent ocular discharge.
Differential Diagnosis:
i)   Sarcoid
ii)   Histoplasmosis
iii) Fly irritation
iv) Habronemiasis
v)   Papilloma
vi) Mast cell tumour
vii) Neurofibroma
viii) Local infections

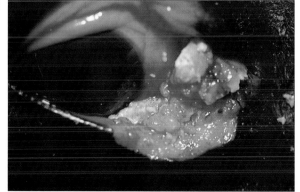

652 Squamous cell carcinoma (ulcerative, invasive, palpebral type).
Note: Extension to, or separate lesion in, third eyelid (*Membrana nictitans*). Aggressive ulcerative and invasive appearance.
Differential Diagnosis:
i)   Ocular habronemiasis
ii) Histoplasmosis

653

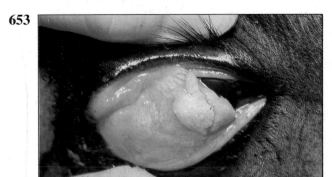

654

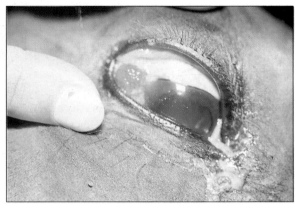

653 Squamous cell carcinoma (papillomatous type).
Note: Slow growth and non-invasive appearance.
Differential Diagnosis:
i) Papilloma
ii) Basal cell carcinoma

654 Squamous cell carcinoma (corneo-limbo-conjunctival form).
Note: Characteristic site at lateral limbus, may also be found on the bulbar conjunctiva.
Differential Diagnosis:
i) Ocular onchocerciasis
ii) Foreign body
iii) Histoplasmosis

655

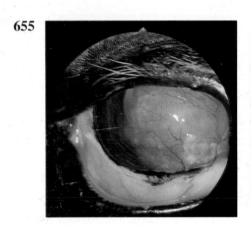

656

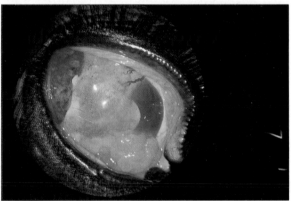

655 Squamous cell carcinoma (carcinoma *in situ*, corneal form).
Note: Proliferative vesicular lesion in upper nasal quadrant of cornea and white, 'fluffy'-looking lesion in cornea of inferior nasal quadrant. Marked neovascularisation.
Differential Diagnosis:
i) Ocular onchocerciasis
ii) Viral (herpetic) keratitis
iii) Corneal edema
iv) Corneal fibrosis

656 Squamous cell carcinoma (Invasive corneo-limbal form).
Note: Extensive corneal involvement and lateral limbal ulceration. Lesion in lower nasal quadrant more superficial than larger lateral lesion.

indication in most cases. One of the earliest signs of the neoplasm is slight hemorrhage within the conjunctival sac giving a serous or sero-mucoid ocular discharge which is visibly hemorrhagic (**650**). Lesions at the muco-cutaneous margin of (more usually) the lower lid may be small and ulcerative (**651**). Such lesions may be relatively quiescent, remaining static for months or years without apparent alteration. However, local invasion and progression to extensive areas of the lid with wide erosive, ulcerative and proliferative lesions are common (**652**). Squamous cell carcinoma lesions developing on the *membrana nictitans* (third eyelid) follow a similar progressive development but extensive ulceration is less usual. Proliferative, papilloma-like masses are more

657

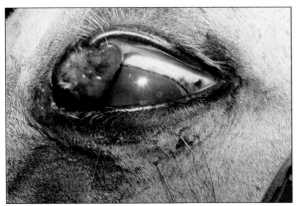

658

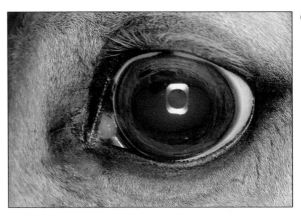

657 Melanoma.
Note: Very slow-growing lesion on third eyelid (*membrana nictitans*) of grey mare. May be other, possibly larger and more significant lesions elsewhere.
Differential Diagnosis:
i) Conjunctival hemangioma

658 Basal Cell Carcinoma.
Note: Very slow-growing, non-ulcerative proliferative mass.
Differential Diagnosis:
i) Squamous cell carcinoma
ii) Fibropapilloma
iii) Neurofibroma
iv) Sarcoid

common in this site **(653)** but extensive, erosive and invasive lesions are possible. Lesions may also develop on the sclera or on the corneal surface. The former are most commonly sited at the lateral limbus **(654)** and may be easily detected. Such cases usually show a mucoid ocular discharge (*see* **654**), which is occasionally hemorrhagic (*see* **650**). Lesions occurring on the cornea may be thin, fluffy, white or pink areas of tissue occupying limited or extensive areas of the cornea – and are referred to as carcinoma in situ **(655)**. They may be much more extensive extending into the corneal stroma, over more or less all of its extent **(656)**. This type often ulcerates and where this occurs has a granular, fleshy, red appearance (*see* **656**). Complicated cases involving one or more of the types described above are relatively common (*see* **656**) and the presence of one type of lesion in no way precludes the presence of others in the same or contralateral eye. Extensive proliferation or invasion of the subconjunctival or bony orbital tissues or, in rare cases, extension to the brain, are extremely serious complications and represent the advanced stage of any (or all) of the above types. In areas with particularly high ultraviolet light levels the growth of these tumours may be particularly rapid with lesions 1–2 mm in size growing to 8–10 mm within 2–3 months. The condition is therefore most often detected during the summer months in temperate climates but in tropical countries it is encountered all year round. The invasive palpebral squamous cell carcinoma lesions are similar in some cases to Habronema lesions and differentiation may be made by biopsy but the latter are seasonal and respond

rapidly to treatment while the neoplastic lesions do not, running an inexorable, if slow, course.

Grey horses are frequently affected by **melanomata** within the eyelid margins and at the medial canthus **(657)**. They are usually slow growing at this site and other lesions are commonly present at other locations (*see* **813**) (*see* **275**). Melanomas developing within the globe are usually located in the iris or the ciliary body and may be mistaken for iris cysts. Amelanotic melanomas may be particularly difficult to identify definitively but their early recognition is important because in their earliest stages they are amenable to surgical excision.

Basal cell carcinomas also occurs within the orbit and most regularly on the third eyelid (*membrana nictitans*). These are much less common than any of the forms of squamous cell carcinoma and may appear at first to closely resemble these. However, they have a more benign appearance and are almost never papillomatous in appearance, being rounded, non-ulcerating **(658)** and very slow growing.

The **equine sarcoid** represents, by far, the commonest neoplasm of the horse. Eyelid lesions are particularly common and may take several different forms. The verrucose form is usually limited to the most superficial layers of the periorbital skin and presents a grey wart-like appearance (*see* **524**). Fibroblastic sarcoids, which may be particularly difficult to differentiate from ulcerated neurofibromas and neurofibrosarcomas, have an ulcerated, proliferative and fleshy appearance. They may have a wide base or be

659

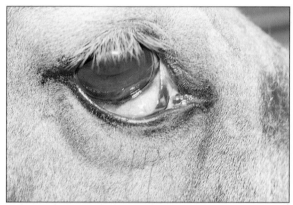

660

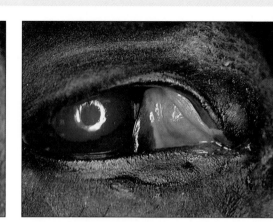

659 Equine sarcoid (nodular, palpebral form).
Note: Multilobed subcutaneous lesion and single very small nodular lesion in lower lid laterally (arrow).
Differential Diagnosis:
i) Neurofibroma
ii) Fibroma

660 Neurofibrosarcoma (sub conjunctival/palpebral form).
Note: Skin of eyelid and conjunctiva apparently uninvolved.
Differential Diagnosis:
i) Equine sarcoid (nodular form)
ii) Prolapse of retrobulbar fat

661

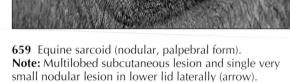

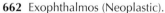

662

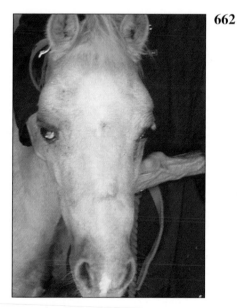

661 Prolapsed retrobulbar fat
Differential Diagnosis:
i)   Squamous cell carcinoma
ii)   Neurofibroma (-sarcoma)
iii) Lymphosarcoma
iv)   Mastocytoma
v)   Chemosis
vi)   Retrobulbar mass or abscess

662 Exophthalmos (Neoplastic).
Note: Prominent swelling of supra orbital fossa. Ultrasonographic examination and radiographs showed a large dense infiltrative mass in the maxillary sinus and orbit (malignant, undifferentiated carcinoma of the maxillary sinus).
Differential Diagnosis:
i) Orbital abscess
ii) Lymphosarcoma

more pedunculated and in the latter case are clearly different from neurofibromas (*see* **745**). Within the eyelid margins the nodular form of sarcoid is frequently encountered. These are firm well defined, often slow growing or static masses within the eyelid itself (**659**) or in the immediate periorbital skin.. The larger masses often produce some eyelid deformity which may be sufficient to cause epiphora and/or corneal ulceration. Mixed forms of these types of sarcoid are encountered. Most eyelid lesions of the sarcoid type are not amenable to surgical excision and cryosurgery, hyperthermia, local (intralesional) injection of BCG and radiation brachytherapy have been found to be effective in some cases.

Neurofibromas and neurofibrosarcomas are nerve sheath tumours and are relatively common in 3 – 6 year old horses. They are often classified with sarcoids which also occur in this location and, indeed, they cannot be differentiated from the equine sarcoid except by histological examination. They are not often identified at sites other than the eyelids and periorbital tissues. In the early stages the masses are very small, dense, shot-like lumps in the periorbital skin, which enlarge slowly or sometimes more rapidly to become larger and possibly ulcerate onto the surface. The lesions are usually well defined solid masses (**660**), and may become very large. They sometimes ulcerate in the periorbital skin and the upper eyelid (*see* **745**) and under these circumstances they are particularly difficult to differentiate clinically from sarcoids.

Prolapse of the orbital fat pad into the sub-conjunctival tissues presents an alarming appearance (**661**) which resembles neoplasia. The condition is probably benign and may disappear spontaneously but may persist and require cosmetic treatment.

Retrobulbar tumours including melanomas, lipomas, adenocarcinomas and tear gland adenomas developing in the retro-bulbar tissues will usually be manifest first by a progressive, usually non-painful exophthalmos (**662**). The function of the eye is usually normal until the later stages of development when an obvious (physical) strabismus may develop (*see* **662**). Gross displacement of the eye may be present particularly where the tumour is slow growing and discrete, such as is the case with retrobulbar melanoma. Swelling of the supraorbital fossa, strabismus and ptosis (drooping of the upper eyelid) which develop rapidly represent a more sinister type of change associated with malignancy or orbital sepsis (*see* **644**).

The Nasolacrimal Apparatus

Atresia of the eyelid puncta of the nasolacrimal duct is a rare developmental, non-hereditary disorder. Atresia of one of the two puncta in the eyelids of one side is unlikely to be detectable with normal tear drainage being possible. Atresia of the nasal puncta of one (or both) lacrimal duct is much more common, possibly because it presents a clinically easily recognisable and treatable syndrome. This is also probably not an inheritable defect. Variable lengths of the distal portion of the nasolacrimal duct may be absent but in most cases it is merely the puncta which is missing. Although one might expect the defect to result in immediate epiphora in the new-born foal, the onset of significant epiphora is often delayed for up to several months or even, in some cases years. Epiphora is often complicated by a mucopurulent ocular discharge (**663**). Fluorescein dye instilled into the conjunctiva fails to appear at the nostril and examination of the normal site of the nasal puncta shows it to be absent. The disorder may be confirmed by the introduction of a fine catheter from the ocular puncti and observing or palpating the catheter in the nasal vestibule (**664**). Obstructions occurring in the more proximal duct may be confirmed with the aid of contrast dacryocystography performed by cannulating both ends of the duct independently. Dermoids affecting the eyelids or third eyelid may be found in association with atretic naso-lacrimal ducts.

Acquired **obstructive lesions affecting one or both nasolacrimal ducts** are commonly encountered as a result of either infection (usually associated with upper respiratory tract or ophthalmic infection) or from traumatic disruption or occlusion as a result of external factors affecting the duct or its openings at either end. Affected horses show epiphora, which is often complicated by secondary infection (*see* **663**) due to failure of duct patency or to obstructions within the duct such as foreign bodies or from external pressure or damage to the duct. Traumatic injuries to the nasal, maxillary, lacrimal and frontal bones (**665**) may have profound effects upon nasolacrimal duct efficiency. Iatrogenic damage to the duct may follow misdirected dental surgery. In most of these cases rupture of the duct into the maxillary sinus will have little or no outward effect, drainage from the eye being normal but

663

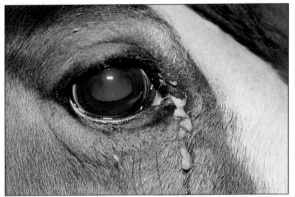

663 Dacryocystitis (chronic, with nasolacrimal duct occlusion).
Note: Mucopurulent ocular discharge at medial canthus above third eyelid (*membrana nictitans*). Minimal conjunctival involvement.

664

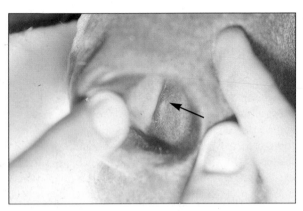

664 Atresia of nasal punctum of the nasolacrimal duct.
Note: Arrow points to the end of a catheter inserted from palpebral punctum.

665

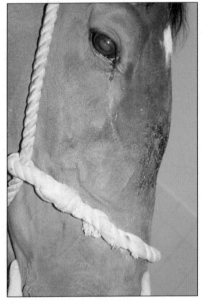

665 Nasoacrimal duct occlusion (facial trauma).
Note: Fracture of maxillary and lacrimal bones. Retrograde flushing not possible. Fluorescein instilled into conjunctival sac failed to appear at nostril.
Differential Diagnosis:
i)   Dacryocystitis
ii) Atresia of nasolacrimal duct
iii) Fronto-naso-maxillary suturitis

666

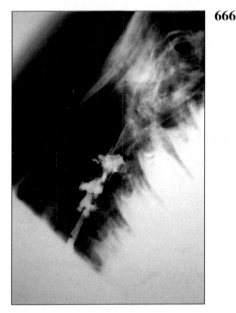

666 Naso-lacrimal duct occlusion (Facial trauma) (Contrast dacryocystogram).
Note: Contrast medium introduced into nasal punctum appears in nasal cavity. Contrast introduced from palpebral punctum appeared in caudal maxillary sinus.

discharging into the maxillary sinus (**666**). Space occupying lesions within the nasal cavity such as nasal polyps (*see* **255**) or large progressive ethmoidal hematomas (*see* **262**) which occlude the nasal opening and invasive lesions such as squamous cell carcinoma affecting the palpebral puncta (*see* **652**) have a physical obstructing effect. Acute onset of complete nasolacrimal obstruction is not usually accompanied by severe epiphora unless there is concurrent irritation or inflammation of the conjunctiva and an excess of lacrimation. The amount of tears naturally produced by a horse is small and some may be reabsorbed or evaporate from the surface of the eye. Thus, in the early stages of obstruction, such as that which follows facial trauma in which the duct is physically damaged the amount of epiphora may belie the severity of the damage

667

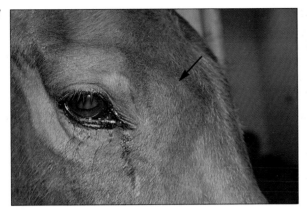

668

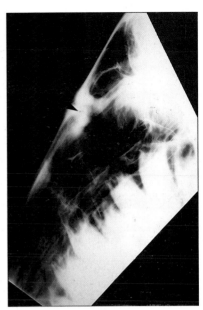

667 Naso-frontal-lacrimal-maxillary suturitis.
Note: Obvious swelling of fronto-nasal and fronto-lacrimal sutures (arrow). Slight but persistent epiphora, no excess of lacrimation. Contrast dacryocystogram showed occlusion of bony component of nasolacrimal duct.

668 Fronto-naso-maxillary suturitis (radiograph).
Note: Same horse as shown in **667**. Obvious thickening at fronto-nasal suture in particular (arrow).

(*see* **665**). Horses with longer standing obstructions which are not complicated by ocular inflammation, may have a mucopurulent ocular discharge (*see* **663**) which may also be apparent at the nasal puncta of the duct. Careful examination of such cases shows the eye to be normal, and the discharge to originate from the medial canthus above the third eyelid (*see* **663**). Infection seldom spreads from this site into the conjunctival sac.

A common cause of obstruction encountered in horses between 3 and 9 years of age involves narrowing of the bony canal which surrounds the caudal portion of the nasolacrimal duct. Thickening of the sutures between the lacrimal, nasal, maxillary and frontal bones results in a significant narrowing of the bony canal carrying the duct, particularly at the orbital end of the bony canal just rostral to the lacrimal sac, and therefore obstructs the nasolacrimal duct. The reason for this active thickening or inflammatory response in the sutures is unknown but some cases are thought to arise from trauma while others are possibly a consequence of metabolic or growth related dysfunction. Cases develop an obvious facial deformity which is usually most apparent along the **fronto-nasal suture** (**667**). Chronic epiphora (*see* **667**), often with facial excoriation, is usually present but its extent will depend upon the extent of the obstruction and the presence or absence of excessive lacrimation and any inflammation within the duct itself. Typically the amount of epiphora in the absence of ocular inflammation is small and often almost insignificant (*see* **667**). Lateral radiographs may be used to identify the thickening of the fronto-nasal suture in particular (**668**)

but contrast dacryocystography will usually be required to confirm the extent and site of the duct obstruction. In most horses with apparent nasolacrimal duct occlusion, retrograde catheterisation and flushing from the nasal puncta is entirely feasible in the conscious animal. Flushing and catheterisation from the palpebral puncta is more difficult and may require general anaesthesia. The combined results of both procedures will often establish the site and extent of the obstruction and may also identify whether the duct is draining into the maxillary sinuses (*see* **666**).

Upper respiratory tract infections and conjunctival infections may be accompanied by an inflammation of the nasolacrimal duct and /or its cyst. Such **dacryocystitis** presents clinical signs which relate to obstruction of the duct itself i.e. epiphora and non-transmission of fluorescein down the duct when placed into the conjunctival sac. Retrograde flushing of the duct from the nasal opening will usually clear the duct and a large catarrhal accumulation will frequently be washed out.

The ocular lesions of *Histoplasma farciminosus* are well recognised in donkeys, and to a somewhat lesser extent in horses, in areas of the world where the disorder is endemic such as Egypt and the Middle East. The organism is transmitted by flies or may be introduced directly from soil or dust. Initially only lacrimation and epiphora are seen, but the infection rapidly progresses to a moderate or severe inflammation of the eyelids, with the lower lid becoming particularly affected (**669**). Facial excoriation and inflammation (tear eczema) develops and photophobia and blepharospasm are

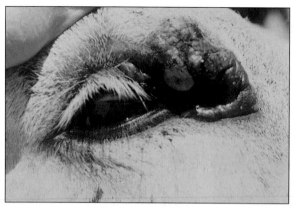

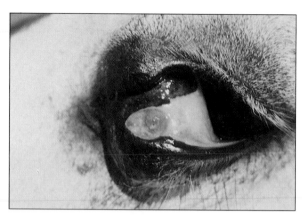

669 Ocular histoplasmosis (*Histoplasma farciminosus*) (epizootic lymphangitis).
Note: A mild, self-limiting conjunctivitis with marked epiphora was present in this case with the typically more severe lesions characteristic of the disease on the eyelids and within the naso lacrimal apparatus. Marked tear dermatitis is often present down the sides of the face. Blepharospasm , blepharitis, chemosis and photophobia are later signs in the course of this disease.
Differential Diagnosis:
i) Squamous cell carcinoma
ii) Habronemiasis
iii) Bacterial/viral conjunctivitis

670 (Granulomatous) histoplasmosis.
Note: Lesions on third eyelid (*membrana nictitans*) and/or at the lacrimal puncta often have an aggressive neoplastic appearance.
Differential Diagnosis:
i) Squamous cell carcinoma
ii) Habronemiasis

present. The discharge from the eye becomes catarrhal or purulent. A fleshy granulomatous lesion sometimes develops on the third eyelid (**670**) or over the lacrimal puncti. The latter lesions may be very similar to lacrimal sac habronemiasis (*see* **649**) or the invasive palpebral form of squamous cell carcinoma (*see* **652**). The lesions are characteristically necrotic and removal of the tissue results in minimal bleeding. Post mortem examination shows the granulating/necrotic tissue to extend into the nasolacrimal duct.

Further reading

A Colour Atlas of Veterinary Ophthalmology
K.C.Barnett (1990) Wolfe, London UK

A Colour Atlas of Equine Opthalmology
Crispin, Matthews, and Barnett (1994) Mosby–Year Book Europe Ltd

Equine Ophthalmology
Ed. K.C.Barnett, P.D.Rossdale and J.F.Wade (1983) Supplement to Equine Veterinary Journal Number 2, British Equine Veterinary Association, Newmarket, UK

Equine Ophthalmology II
Ed. K.C.Barnett, P.D.Rossdale and J.F.Wade (1983) Supplement to Equine Veterinary Journal Number 2, British Equine Veterinary Association, Newmarket, UK

Large Animal Ophthalmology (Volume 1)
J.D.Lavach (1990)   C.V.Mosby St Louis, USA

Current Therapy in Equine Medicine 2
Ed. N.E.Robinson (1987) W.B.Saunders, Philadelphia, USA

Current Therapy in Equine Medicine 3
Ed. N.E.Robinson (1992) W.B.Saunders, Philadelphia, USA

Manual of Equine Practice
Rose R.J. and Hodgson D.R.(1993) W.B.Saunders, Philadelphia, USA

10. Disorders of the nervous system

Developmental Disorders

The developmental disorders of the nervous system of the horses are usually manifest by disturbances of function evident at, or shortly after, birth. Most of these are the result of bizarre genetic defects or insults which have affected the foal during gestation. These include a variety of virus or toxemic disorders affecting the mare. The clinical manifestations depend largely upon the stage of development at which the insult is applied and the extent of the consequent deficit. Thus, virus infections affecting a pregnant mare at the time of neurological development (early in gestation) might produce severe effects on the neurological development of the foal. In many cases the effects are life-threatening to the fetus and intrauterine death is common. Disorders affecting other organs may also affect the neurological function of the foal. For example the **cervical vertebral instability (Wobbler) syndrome** (*see* **371**) is a neurological manifestation of a skeletal abnormality. Defects of circulation such as the development of **porto-caval shunts** also influence the neurological function of young foals. Foals affected by severe neurological developmental defects will be non-viable while others might have obvious immediate or delayed neurological effects but still be consistent with life. The instigating organ or system may not, therefore be immediately obvious. While in some cases the clinical effects of minor neurological problems in foals may be dramatic, in others even apparently gross abnormalities might have surprisingly little effect.

Hydrocephalus is usually an easily recognised, isolated, developmental abnormality which is not often consistent with life. Affected foals are usually born dead or die during parturition, as a result of massive increases in intracranial pressure. They are often premature, with an obvious cranial deformity (**671**). However, cranial deformity is not invariably present in hydrocephalic foals and in such cases a diagnosis may be difficult without radiographic assistance. Some foals born with apparently domed skulls may not be suffering from hydrocephalus. A sagittal section of the head of an affected foal shows the gross distension of the lateral ventricles with generalised compression of the cerebral hemispheres (**672**). The disorder may be secondary to abnormalities of the bone of the calvarium, but the presence or absence of such deformities is of academic interest only. Foals born alive with hydrocephalus die within a few hours at most and the prognosis of all live cases is hopeless.

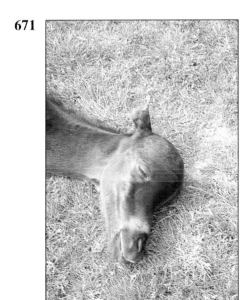

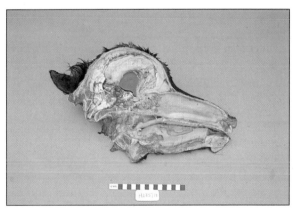

671 Hydrocephalus.
Note: Aborted fetus. Several other developmental abnormalities were also present including palatoschisis (cleft palate) and a complex cardio-vascular abnormality.

672 Hydrocephalus (saggital section of head).
Note: Prominent fluid filled distension of the ventricles.

673

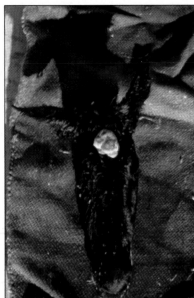

674

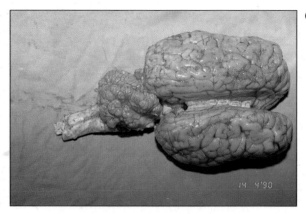

673 Encephalocele.
Note: Foal born alive but unable to rise. Killed at birth.

674 Unilateral Cerebral Hypoplasia.
Note: Yearling Throroughbred colt. The animal had
been dull and blind in one eye since birth.

Failure of the cranium and overlying skin to close during development, with prolapse of either the meninges (**meningocele**) or the meninges with parts of the brain (**encephalocele**) is occasionally seen in neonatal foals (**673**). The development of this defect involves bone and skin growth but is more likely to be a complex of abnormalities relating to the separation of the neural tube from the embryonic ectoderm. The condition which is almost exclusively in the midline may be very small, or involve almost the entire cranium, and may be accompanied by other developmental disturbances including spina bifida. Affected foals are usually either aborted or are born dead or die soon after birth.

Cerebral hypoplasia is not a common clinical disorder of the horse although severe hypoplasia as part of a wider complex of congenital developmental disorders may be responsible for the development of severe epileptiform convulsions in neonatal foals. Affected foals are recumbent and convulsive from birth, and other defects such as cataracts, limb deformities, hydrocephalus and myopathy, are usually present. Unilateral hypoplasia of one cerebral hemisphere (**674**) may be responsible for unilateral central blindness, epileptiform convulsions and ataxia but may also be asymptomatic.

Cerebellar abiotrophy particularly affects the Arabian breed and, while it is rare, there is strong evidence to suggest that it is an inherited abnormality. It has also been encountered in other breeds such as the Gotland pony and the Oldenburgh light horse. Foals of either sex may be affected and the foal is usually of

normal size and is bright and alert. The clinical signs are noticed soon after birth, when an obvious intention tremor becomes apparent and the gait becomes dysmetric. In view of the apparently incoordinated behaviour of normal young foals the condition may only become noticeable after some weeks, when it is noted that the foal has not become normal. The stance is characteristically base-wide and obvious head nodding is present which becomes markedly worse just prior to movement such as when about to suckle (intention tremor). The clinical signs are strongly suggestive of cerebellar dysfunction but the disorder can often only be confirmed by histopathological examination of the cerebellar tissues. In some cases transverse cerebellar sections show an obvious loss of white matter (**675**).

Arab foals born with **occipito-atlanto-axial malformation** (*see* **369**) may be born dead but some are neurologically normal at birth. A rapid onset of tetraparesis and ataxia associated with upper neck deformity or instability may indicate the presence of the malformation. In spite of severe (physical and radiographic) malformations some cases show little or no neurological deficit until a gross displacement occurs, when a severe compromise of the neurological function will be evident immediately. In common with many of the developmental neurological disorders there may be other defects associated with other systems or other gross spinal deviations.

A congenital and possibly hereditary **instability of the cervical vertebrae** occurs in foals and, while the underlying disorder is probably present from birth, the onset of typical clinical signs may be delayed for months

675

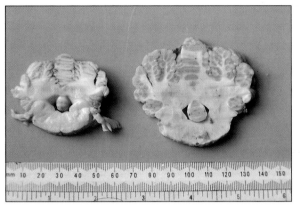

675 Cerebellar abiotrophy.
Note: 2 month old Arabian colt foal showed marked intention tremors and postural and locomotory incoordination. The sections show a marked loss of grey matter and the cerebellum was smaller than normal for a foal of this size and age.

676

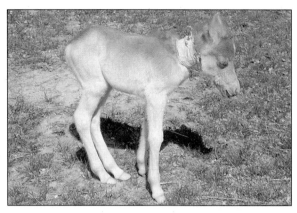

676 Neonatal maladjustment syndrome (NMS).
Note: Dull, 'dummy-like' appearance. Postural deficits. Foal showed seizures begining at 24 hours of age and was depressed. It would wander aimlessly to the left and lost any recognition of its dam. Occasional barking vocalisations were made.

677

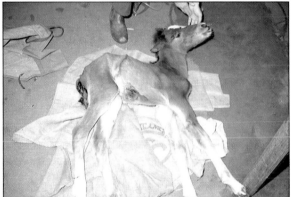

677 Neonatal maladjustment syndrome (convulsive form).
Note: Convulsions started 3 hours after birth. The foal was unable to rise and paddled and galloped while in lateral recumbency. The head was often held in abnormal positions such as over the back or twisted tightly to one side. Eventual total recovery.

678

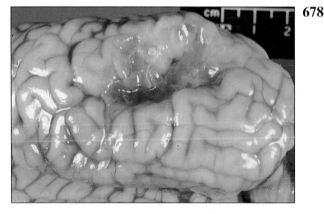

678 Neonatal maladjustment syndrome.
Note: Specimen obtained from an apparently normal foal aged 5 months which had a history of having neonatal maladjustment syndrome. Large cavity on the right parieto-occipital cortex was considered to be the result of a previous vascular injury. This is an unusual example of the syndrome in which the circling had been reported to be to the left. The lesions associated with the disorder are usually much less prominent than the one shown here but foals which die immediately often have obvious, fresh cerebral hemorrhages.

or years. The clinical signs include hypermetria or hypometria and ataxia which usually affects the hind more than the fore limbs and which is exacerbated by neck flexion or extension (*see* **371** *et seq.*). The signs are often clinically indistinguishable from other spinal disorders affecting young horses, including cervical articular process physitis and synovial cysts.

Neonatal maladjustment syndrome is a non-infectious, neurological disorder of new-born foals, associated with gross disturbances of behaviour. It is believed to arise subsequent to either cerebral bleeding or cerebral anoxia (or both), arising during prolonged or difficult parturition but may sometimes develop in the absence of these. In some cases, where the clinical signs are typical, however, parturition may be noted to be swift and apparently normal. Most affected foals are full-term and of normal weight and size. The foals usually show a variety of signs which indicate their

337

failure to adapt effectively to the extra-uterine environment. Most signs are initially vague and not pathognomonic of the disorder, but disorientation, loss of suckle reflex and dam recognition are commonly present in the early stages. Affected foals often wander aimlessly, appearing to be blind, while others adopt abnormal postures and stand in an apparent stupor (**676**). Recumbency and seizures with opisthotonus (**677**) which are typical of the convulsive-foal form of the condition, are interspersed with periods of over-activity, with paddling/galloping, rolling and compulsive walking and circling. Foals are often reported to have a characteristic abnormal vocalisation, the so-called 'barkers', and persistently grind their teeth. Abnormal head postures are frequently present. Concurrent gastric ulceration is often found in the glandular portion of the stomach, although this is probably a secondary disorder (*see* **93**). Post mortem examination usually identifies few systemic features of note but secondary head or limb trauma may be present. Examination of the brain may reveal areas of subdural hemorrhage or more severe ischemic necrosis of the cerebral cortex (**678**). The severity of the cerebral damage is not always proportional to the extent of the clinical signs, with individual cases showing severe neurological signs with minor or even inapparent cerebral damage. Conversely, some individuals with extensive cerebral lesions may show limited signs and subsequently recover and behave in a normal manner, with no obvious neurological or other deficits (*see* **678**).

Non Infectious Disorders

Traumatic injuries to the nervous system of the horse are a relatively frequent occurrence and affect the central nervous system as well as the peripheral nerves.

Cranial and Cord Trauma: Cranial trauma affecting the neurological status of a horse does not always have to be severe enough to cause outward evidence of the damage although this is common. **Fractures of the forehead** are often compound (open) and involve direct cerebral laceration and hemorrhage. These injuries are most commonly the result of kicks from other horses, from impact with solid objects or from rearing over and falling backwards onto the back of the head. In some cases even merely a sudden powerful rearing or pulling back from a firmly fastened head collar or halter, may be responsible for significant trauma, particularly in young horses. The consequent neurological signs are very variable depending on the site of the trauma and its relationship to underlying structures, and the extent of any intracranial bleeding and/or physical disruption.

Closed head injuries (those in which there are no skull fractures) often result in brainstem damage with localised bleeding and, often quite extensive sub-arachnoid bleeding (**679**), which can be detected by cisternal puncture and aspiration of blood stained cerebrospinal fluid (**680**). **Blows to the head of young foals** often cause sudden blindness, depression and circling in a previously normal animal. **Fractures of the basisphenoid and basioccipital bones** most commonly occur after rearing accidents or head collar injuries. While the fracture may be difficult to appreciate radiographically, examination of the roof of the medial compartment of the guttural pouches will often identify either bruising or even the presence of a hematoma over the site of the fracture. Concurrent or incidental complications involving fractures of the hyoid bone may also be present and possibly detectable radiographically and by internal examination of the guttural pouch(es). Typically, the neurological signs associated with this type of trauma are

679

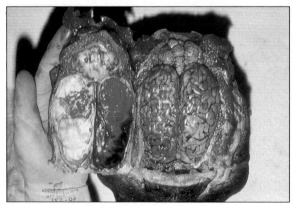

679 Intracranial (cerebral) hemorrhage (traumatic). **Note:** The animal was comatose and showed nystagmus, strabismus and dramatic cardiac irregularities attributed to the brain-heart syndrome.

680

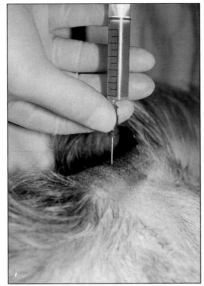

681

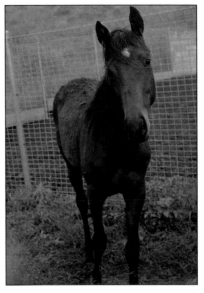

680 Intracranial (cerebral) hemorrhage (traumatic). **Note:** Hemorrhagic cerebrospinal fluid.

681 Cranial trauma (head tilt). **Note:** Rearing injury with blow to right side of the head.

very variable. Individual cases may be comatose but others may show subtle neurological deficits, which may be limited to the individual cranial nerves in the region of the fracture. Under the latter circumstances the signs may be unilateral and may be almost undetectable. **Fractures involving the base of the cranium** will frequently involve one or more of the cranial nerves, and the clinical signs of this damage may be difficult to identify in conjunction with the more severe effects of cerebral, cerebellar or brain stem disruption. Commonly, however, the signs include depression and/or dementia. **Fractures which affect the optic or vestibulo-cochlear nerves** or the central nuclei controlling these organs, will have dramatic and easily recognised signs. In the former case, blindness and pupil-light-reflex deficiencies or discrepancies between the two eyes will be present. Concurrent retinal damage (including detachment) (*see* **632**) and/or lens dislocation may be found. Bleeding from the ear following head trauma (*see* **692**), is indicative of damage to the petrous temporal bone and the vestibular nerve, and/or its nucleus. Affected horses have a marked head tilt towards the affected side (**681**), and are obviously disoriented with circling and nystagmus in which the fast phase is away from the side affected. Usually there is complicating concurrent damage in the base of the brain and weakness, depression and ataxia, amongst other signs are present.

Complicated combinations of neurological deficits can arise from even relatively minor trauma and, furthermore, may take some hours or days to produce their full neurological effect. Horses suffering from

neurological damage as a result of direct trauma may consequently be very difficult to assess accurately and considerable skill must be employed to definitively identify the site and extent of the lesion. The most accurate prognosis is based on repeated detailed neurological examinations with assessment of the rate of progression or resolution and the responses to specific therapeutic measures. Nursing and management procedures have a strong bearing on the prognosis of some cases with dramatic improvements being possible. Failure to appreciate the nursing requirements for neuological cases has a marked deleterious effect on the prognosis. Cerebral and cerebellar lesions usually carry a better prognosis than brain stem lesions and therefore those injuries which are accompanied by bleeding from the ear but few other outward signs, are possibly more serious than the more dramatic injuries to the frontal and facial bones. The use of computed tomography would clarify the extent and type of injury but is not currently accessible to most veterinarians.

Horses suffering from significant **head trauma with neurological signs** may at post mortem examination, show marked hemorrhage within the cranium (*see* **679**). However, brain damage may be more subtle and there may be minimal or very limited bleeding and no grossly visible tissue damage in some severely affected animals.

Trauma to the cervical vertebrae is also a relatively common occurrence, often following severe falls at speed. The extent of the neurological deficit depends heavily upon the extent of the damage to the cord or to

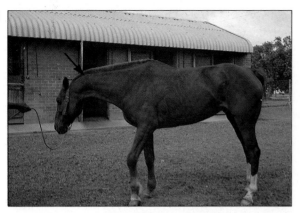

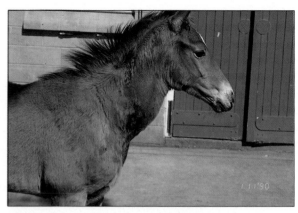

682 Cervical vertebral dislocation (between second and third cervical vertebrae).
Note: Marked deviation of cervical spine (arrow). Concurrent postural deficits in fore and hind limbs. Gradual resolution over 2 years but residual deficits of proprioception.

683 Cervical vertebral fracture (compression fracture of fifth cervical vertebra).
Note: Neck deviation in sagittal plane. No neurological deficits present but guarded when turning. Survived as brood mare.

the meninges or to the peripheral nerves as they pass through the intervertebral foramina. Gross displacement of adjacent vertebrae which results in severance of the cord is accompanied by immediate loss of all conscious proprioception and voluntary motor function distal to the site of the lesion. In some cases, however, the extent of the apparent bony damage may not necessarily correspond to the extent of the neurological deficits. Dislocations of the cervical vertebrae **(682)** often have more serious neurological consequences than many of the fractures **(683)**. Relatively minor physical deformity may be accompanied by severe neurological deficits, while in some cases, even gross deformity appears to have little consequence. Spinal reflexes may be present but are usually either exaggerated or depressed. **Cervical lesions which result in cord compression or disruption (684)** have the most widespread immediate effect on neurological function (*see* **682**), but the consequences of thoracic or thoraco-lumbar fractures, or dislocations (or other lesions affecting the cord at these sites) are equally serious in terms of the prognosis. **Collapse of one or more intervertebral discs** which more frequent in the cervical and cervico-thoracic areas results in a similarly wide range of clinical signs. Again, these are dependent upon the extent of the collapse and the consequent effect on the cord. **Prolapse of lumbar discs**, with associated cord compression, is very rare.

Fractures or dislocations (or both) occurring in the thoraco-lumbar spine are unusual but present with dramatic posterior paralysis **(685)**. A similar clinical condition may be presented as a result of spinal bleeding or any other condition which results in a focal ablation of the cord at a particular site. Mild damage in the thoraco-lumbar region is particularly unusual; disruption requires considerable force and consequently when damage occurs it is often catastrophic. Young heavy horses (and Shire horses in particular) are prone to a severe posterior paraplegia following general anesthesia and dorsal recumbency, which results in a condition which is clinically indistinguishable from fracture or dislocation in the mid-distal thoracic region. Distal spinal reflexes in all such injuries are often intact, but may be reduced (hyporeflexia) or exaggerated (hyperreflexia). Loss of deep pain perception and complete paraplegia distal to the lesion represent the common finding and all horses in which these and loss of anal reflexes are present carry a poor prognosis. **Thoraco-lumbar lesions** which are associated with posterior paralysis and fore-limb extensor rigidity (Schiff-Sherrington reaction) and which gradually ascend are most serious. The site of the damage can be ascertained by identifying the loss of skin (panniculus) reflexes which characteristically occurs abruptly at or just behind the site of the damage.

Horses which suffer from spinal pain and/or posterior paralysis often show extremes of panic and their management is most difficult. Remarkable improvements are possible in cases of cervical vertebral damage, even in some cases which appear clinically and radiologically disastrous. The prognosis for horses suffering from spinal trauma is generally poor, for, although some may recover with time, the intensity of nursing required and the consequences of incoordinated attempts to rise, are often most distressing both for the horse and the attendants.

684

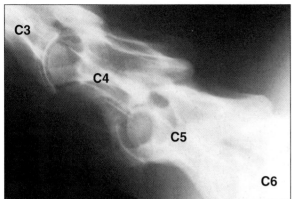

685

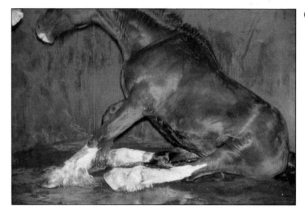

684 Cervical vertebral fracture (compression fracture of fifth cervical vertebra) (standing lateral radiograph).

685 Thoracic vertebral fracture (fracture dislocation between thirteenth and fourteenth thoracic veterbrae). **Note:** Dog sitting position with hind limbs extended. No conscious proprioception in hind quarters. No anal reflex. Sharp 'cut-off' of skin twitch (panniculus) reflex at level of damage.

Sacral fractures may result in fecal (*see* **709**) and urinary incontinence (*see* **714**) and gait abnormalities with subsequent atrophy of pelvic (*see* **711**) and hind limb musculature. These fractures commonly result in loss of motor action of the tail and hypoalgesia of the perineum (*see* **710**).

Peripheral Nerve Disorders: Damage to peripheral nerves occurs relatively frequently as a result of direct trauma to superficial nerves or as result of excessive distraction of nerve roots and plexuses. The damage may be mild and result in a temporary or partial loss of function (neurapraxia) or more severe, causing permanent loss of function (neurotmesis). The extent of the damage is important when assessing the prognosis of peripheral nerve lesions, for, although some regeneration of peripheral nerves is possible this is extremely slow and where nerves are severely damaged resolution may take an unrealistic time. Section or other damage involving the sensory nerves is often accompanied by no detectable clinical effect (such as those in the distal limb), but loss of sensation in other areas, such as the face, may cause severe distress, and result in self trauma.

Trauma to, or degeneration of, cranial nerve trunks results in well-defined clinical syndromes which are, of course, primarily related to the head. Some nerves are more likely to become damaged or be subject to degeneration than others, and these present the best defined clinical syndromes. Complex combinations of cranial nerve damage occur relatively commonly as a result of trauma, particularly associated with fractures of the base of the cranium where the damage involves the *foramen lacerum* and the adjacent outflow foramina

of the cranial nerves. **Degenerative or traumatic disruption within the cranium** may have widespread consequences upon cranial nerve function as a result of damage to their controlling nuclei. The clinical syndromes might individually be indistinguishable from more peripheral lesions. However, careful assessment of the full range of cranial nerves might enable a rational assessment of the extent of the damage and enable a conclusion as to the site and extent of the damage to be made.

Damage to the olfactory nerve (CN-I) is unusual and very difficult to assess, and, in any case, is unlikely to be of any clinical importance on its own.

Damage to the optic nerve (CN-II) as result of trauma, or secondary degeneration as a result of adjacent space occupying lesions within the orbit or in the brainstem (such as pituitary adenomas, (*see* **365**), will have serious consequences on vision. Damage to one side only results in a unilateral blindness which in some cases may be difficult to identify without a specific investigation of the visual acuity of the patient.

Degrees of pupillary constriction (miosis), dilatation (mydriasis) and discrepancies in size between the two pupils (anisocoria) may be indicative of ocular or cranial disorders. **Disorders of the optic and oculomotor nerves and the sympathetic supply to the eye** result in defects of relative and absolute pupil size. Horses affected with **Horner's Syndrome** commonly show anisocoria (inequality of pupil size) as part of the clinical signs. The position of the eye relative to the visual horizon is controlled by complex interactions between the oculomotor (CN-III), trochlear (CN-IV) and abducens (CN-VI) nerves, with further interaction with

686

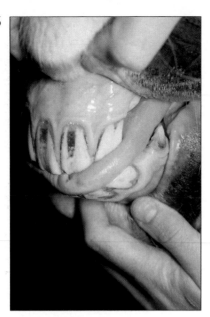

687

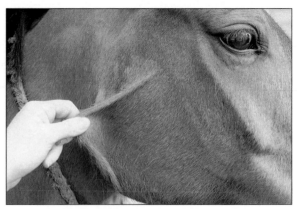

687 Idiopathic trigeminal neuritis (masseter atrophy). **Note:** Bilateral atrophy developed slowly. Inability to masticate effectively. The mouth was hypoalgesic and while a definitive diagnosis was not made even after post mortem examination, the condition was attributed to a bilateral central trigeminal nucleus lesion.
Differential Diagnosis:
i) Equine protozoal myeloencephalopathy
ii) Equine cauda equine neuritis (polyneuritis equi) syndrome
iii) Idioathic masseter myopathy (chronic stage)

686 Bilateral trigeminal neuritis (central).
Note: Lower jaw unable to close fully, unable to chew. Tongue resting between the teeth, had normal tone and resistance to traction. Sensation in the mouth and over the face was normal.

the vestibulocochlear nerve (**CN-VIII**). It is probably only of academic concern to identify specifically which nerve(s) are affected when a manifest lack of parallelism of the visual axes of the eyes (strabismus) exists. Cranial trauma however, commonly results in damage to one or more of the controlling nerves or their nuclei. The persistence of the deviation when the head is moved is an indication of the involvement of the major controlling nerves, while in cases of vestibular-nerve-strabismus, the eye will move away from the apparently fixed and abnormal position during such movement.

   The trigeminal nerve (CN-V) is the largest cranial nerve and has both motor and sensory functions. Motor functions include aspects of prehension, mastication and swallowing while the sensory components control mouth and eye sensation and sensation in the skin of the head. Bilateral loss of motor activity results in a dropped jaw and an inability to chew. The tongue may protrude slightly (**686**) or, in some cases, more obviously. The tongue is often traumatised through concurrent loss of oral sensation but maintenance of sensory function precludes such damage. Drooling of saliva occurs because of the lack of jaw movement and the failure of the mouth to close fully (*see* **686**). Prehension may be possible in some cases where the sensory function is maintained and where the facial nerve (CN-VII) is unaffected, but chewing is almost always severely

affected. Atrophy of the temporal, masseter (**687**) and the distal part of the *digastricus* muscles develops over the ensuing two to three weeks. Where the lesion is peripheral, such as might follow fractures of the hyoid bone for example, the atrophy is generally unilateral, and in these cases, there may be little difficulty with mastication or prehension. A loss of sensory function in the trigeminal nerve, either with motor deficits or on its own, may be difficult to identify, but food material being pouched between the molar teeth and the cheek may be indicative of a loss of oral sensation. Repeated, unconscious biting of the cheeks and tongue during mastication may result in severe damage which may be unilateral or bilateral, and is most often indicative of a trigeminal sensory deficit. Conditions such as **equine protozoal myeloencephalitis**, which affect the controlling nucleus of the trigeminal nerve, exert a dramatic effect which is particularly severe upon the motor functions of the nerve producing a pronounced atrophy (*see* **737**) and dysphagia (**Plate 6r**, page 123). Central multifocal disorders of this type are usually responsible for apparently unilateral lesions appearing with other neurological deficits. Jaw weakness and tongue flaccidity is also a characteristic of **botulism** (*see* **735**) and is, in part, due to the action of the neurotoxin on the nucleus of the controlling cranial nerves. Some cases of damage to the trigeminal nerve are due to a degenerative

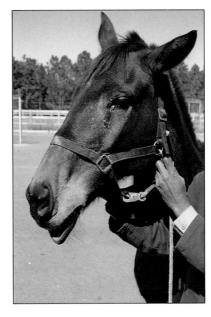

688

688 Facial paralysis (neurapraxia) (left side. central or root lesion).
Note: Paralysis of left lip (upper and lower), drooping left ear and paralysis of upper eyelid. Deep crescentic corneal ulcer was also present (a result of poor blink-efficiency and a consequent area of *keratoconjunctivitis sicca* (dry eye).
Differential Diagnosis:
i)   Equine protozoal myeloencephalopathy
ii) Cauda equina neuritis (*polyneuritis equi*) syndrome
iii) Guttural pouch mycosis
iv) Fracture of basisphenoid or hyoid bone (or both)
v)   Central neoplasia

disorder of the peripheral nerve fibres. Idiopathic trigeminal neuritis is a disorder which results in all the expected signs of peripheral (unilateral or bilateral) damage to the nerve, with loss of motor and/or sensory function to one or both sides of the face. Furthermore, horses affected with the **cauda equina neuritis (equine polyneuritis syndrome)** (*see* **709** *et seq.*) may show cranial nerve signs, including involvement of the trigeminal and facial nerves, in conjunction with the more common lower motor neurone deficits affecting the perineum and hind-quarters. The diagnosis of trigeminal nerve disorders relies heavily upon a detailed assessment of motor and sensory functions and unilateral disorders are particularly difficult to assess in the early stages. Loss of sensation in the muzzle and medial wall of the nasal cavity are supportive findings but central lesions often only affect the motor function. Once atrophy of individual and definable muscle blocks occurs the diagnosis becomes simpler but therapeutic opportunities are correspondingly reduced.

Perhaps the most common cranial nerve injury in the horse occurs to the **facial nerve (CN-VII)**. The nerve is liable to be traumatised in view of its very superficial path. The nerve is closely related at its root to the styloid process of the hyoid bone and to the guttural pouches. The most superficial portions of the nerve pass round the caudal border of the vertical ramus of the mandible and cross the side of the face, lying subcutaneously. It may be damaged at any point along its length from the cranial outflow to the more distal branches. As the nerve is responsible for the motor activity of the muscles of facial expression, the consequence of damage (whether

mild and temporary or more permanent) is an abnormality of facial expression. The facial nerve also forms part of the reflex pathway originating in the sensory components of the trigeminal nerve. Lesions occurring at the base of the brain, including **fractures of the hyoid bone**, **fractures of the cranial floor** and **guttural pouch mycosis** (*see* **251**) and **diverticulitis** (*see* **235**) would probably affect all three major branches of the nerve (i.e. the auricular, palpebral and buccal branches), exerting a more extensive effect than more peripheral lesions. The former cases are presented with a flaccidity of the ipsilateral upper and lower lips, a drooping of the ipsilateral ear and often a ptosis of the upper eyelid (**688**). The consequences of this deficit include a drooling of saliva from the flaccid side and a pulling of the muzzle and lower lip over to the unaffected side (**689**). Superficial lesions occurring more in the buccal branches distal to the caudal border of the vertical ramus of the mandible will exert little or no effect upon the lower lip, and the more distal the lesion, the more limited will be the effect on facial expression. The most common sites for damage to the nerve coincide with the siting of the metal buckles on head collars and halters. Sudden snatching of the head against the head collar, or direct trauma, particularly when the animal falls onto the side of the face (such as sometimes occurs during the induction of anesthesia) might result in damage at, or beyond, the caudal edge of the vertical ramus of the mandible. Damage occurring over the side of the face rostral to the end of the facial crest will result in limited deviation of the upper lip only (**690**). Bilateral lesions involving the peripheral (or central) pathway of

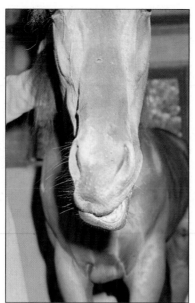

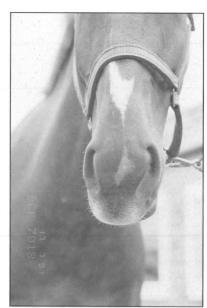

689 Facial paralysis (neurapraxia) (left side, peripheral lesion).
Note: Both upper and lower lip affected. Ear and eyelid were not affected. Lesion probably at vertical ramus of mandible.

690 Facial paralysis (neurapraxia) (Left side, affecting upper lip only).
Note: Lesion probably on side of face in one or more localised branches. Lesion present after recovery from anesthesia.

the nerve results in a symmetrical drooping of the upper and lower lips with profound effects on prehension and obvious saliva drooling may be present (*see* **691**). Jaw tone and mastication are normal however, in contrast to trigeminal nerve lesions, when prehension and facial expression may be normal, but there is a loss of masticatory muscle tone and facial and oral sensation. Most cases of traumatically induced facial nerve damage are temporary and mild, but irreparable damage (**neurotmesis**) results in a permanent distortion of facial expression. However, some return of function may occur gradually over many years even in severed nerves where the damage occurred in the more distal reaches of the nerve. Central, facial nerve lesions are unusual, but may be a sign of generalised degenerative disorders such as cauda equina neuritis syndrome (*polyneuritis equi*) (*see*

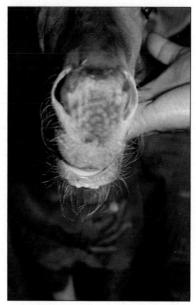

691 Facial paralysis (bilateral, central lesion).
Note: Bilaterally symmetrical paralysis resulting in drooping of upper and lower lips. Both ears and upper eyelids also affected. Mouth closure and chewing normal.
Differential Diagnosis:
i)   Bilateral (peripheral) facial paralysis
ii) Equine protozoal myeloencephalitis
iii) Cauda equina neuritis (polyneuritis equi)
iv) Meningitis
v) Viral or bacterial encephalitis

692

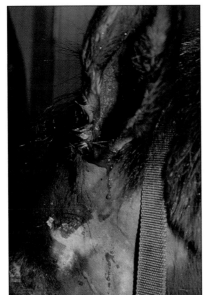

693

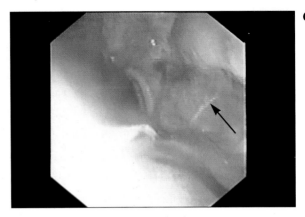

692 Cranial trauma with vestibular damage.
Note: Head tilt to ipsilateral side and hemorrhage from ear.

693 Unilateral pharyngeal paralysis.
Note: Right ostium of auditive tube opened during swallowing (normal) but left remains closed (arrow). Food material, in pharynx.

709 *et seq.*). **Secondary consequences of facial nerve paralysis** include an inability to prehend effectively, epiphora and corneal ulceration. Permanent or fixed grimacing results from over or abnormal activity of the facial nerve and is most likely to be the result of focal forebrain lesions, rather than neuritis or inflammation of the peripheral pathway of the nerve.

Damage to the auditory component of the vestibulocochlear nerve (CN-VIII) is almost impossible to assess, particularly when this is unilateral. Deafness, or more particularly partial deafness, cannot be easily assessed in the horse, although some conclusions may be drawn from the environmental awareness of the patient. **Damage to the vestibular branch of the nerve**, however, has serious consequences. Damage is most often of traumatic origin, including temporo-hyoid region fractures, and may be accompanied by **bleeding from the ear (692)**, or in more severe cases, leakage of cerebrospinal fluid with bleeding. Infective disorders of the outer, middle or inner ear which may be accompanied by aural or nasal discharges, are rarely encountered in horses but, where present, may result in severe vestibular signs. The short pathway of the nerve means that dysfunction is associated with lesions in the immediate vicinity in the base of the brain. These include either the petrous temporal bone or the nucleus of the nerve within the brain stem. The complex inter-relationship between this nerve, those controlling the eyes and the input to the postural controlling centres of the cerebellum, means that damage is accompanied by obvious, often easily recognised clinical signs. **Nystagmus** (rhythmical oscillations of the eyeball) is a consistent feature of vestibular nerve damage. The clinical effects of damage to the nerve, however, may be buffered by optic or postural inputs. Thus, damage to the vestibular nerves may be less obvious if sight is normal and mild damage may be exaggerated by concurrent blindness. Therefore, horses with vestibular nerve damage which are normally sighted often show a marked head tilt, with the axis of tilt about the poll (*see* **681**) which can be dramatically exaggerated by blindfolding. The proximity of the facial nerve makes it relatively common for facial nerve deficits to accompany traumatic or infective vestibular damage. **Otitis media** is rare in horses but ascending infections from guttural pouch infections and foreign bodies in the external auditory meatus (with concurrent otitis externa) are encountered occasionally. The clinical signs are usually somewhat less dramatic than in traumatic disruption of the vestibular nerve pathways. Aural discharges and systemic illness are often present.

Significant **damage to the glossopharyngeal (CN-IX), the vagus (CN-X) and the hypoglossal (CN-XII)** nerves are difficult to separate clinically. The **accessory nerve (CN-XI)** is seldom involved in pathological processes and is in any case very difficult to assess. The most significant lesions involving these nerves, as a group, are those which result in damage to their peripheral pathways and the clinical effects of damage to the glossopharyngeal and vagus nerves are the best recognised. This complex of cranial nerves controls the function and coordination of the pharynx and larynx,

694

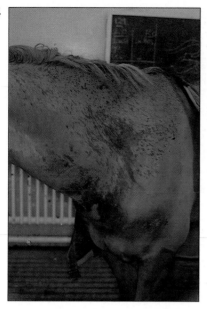

695

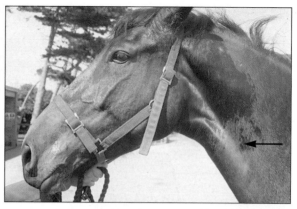

694 Horner's syndrome (intrathoracic or cord lesion). **Note:** Sweating of side of neck. Other signs of Horner's syndrome were present. Large lymphosarcoma lesion found in anterior thorax at post mortem examination.

695 Horner's syndrome (cervical lesion). **Note:** Sweating on neck above site of injection (arrow) and ipsilateral face. Ptosis (upper eyelid paralysis).

with both sensory and motor components, and is integrally related to the sensory components of the trigeminal nerve in particular. Thus the most important signs associated with damage are to be found in disturbances of swallowing and of intrinsic laryngeal muscle movement. The specific effect of injury to the nerves will depend largely on whether the condition is bilateral or unilateral. Bilateral or central involvement of the nerve trunks results in dysphagia (**Plate 6r**, page 123) and/or stertorous breathing due to complete pharyngeal and laryngeal paralysis. Unilateral lesions, which are more common, create significant impairment of pharyngeal (**693**) or laryngeal function (**Plate 5v**, page 116), with inspiratory dyspnea or abnormal inspiratory noises (or both) evident during exercise. The cervical vagus trunks which run in the jugular grooves on either side of the neck are the commonest site of peripheral and focal damage. The superficial position of the vagus nerve within the guttural pouch makes this another common site for damage. Most guttural pouch problems likely to cause interference with function of the vagus and the hypoglossal nerves, including guttural pouch mycosis (*see* **252**) and diverticulitis (*see* **235**), are unilateral and the consequences will usually be a unilateral pharyngeal (*see* **693**) and/or laryngeal (**Plate 5v**, page 116) paralysis. Whilst the idiopathic damage encountered in large breeds of horse and in Thoroughbred and Quarter horses, represents, probably, the commonest type of degeneration of the peripheral components of the vagus nerve and its branches (**Plate 5u** *et seq.*, page 115), damage is commonly due to localised, accidental extravascular

injections in the jugular groove. The extent of the damage is typically variable depending upon the specific drug involved, its volume and its tissue toxicity. Thus, mildly irritant substances may cause a temporary neurapraxia with return of normal function after some time. The consequences are therefore temporary and may even pass unnoticed. More irritant chemicals causing localised abscesses (*see* **294**) or more extensive necrosis of the tissues of the jugular groove (*see* **295**) create more serious, and often permanent, damage to the nerve, effectively creating a severance of the nerve (neurotmesis) at the site. Regeneration of a severely damaged recurrent laryngeal nerve and vagal trunk is virtually impossible, and any consequent effects will, most likely, be permanent.

Severe brain disorders including some infections such as **African Horse Sickness, equine viral encephalomyelitis, rabies and botulism** are also likely to interfere with the central nuclei of these nerves and, in these diseases, pharyngeal paralysis (*see* **693**) is a major presenting sign. In some of these diseases the neurological signs may be the most obvious evidence of the condition but in others the changes may be subtle and their importance may easily be overlooked.

Inflammation within the guttural pouch or in the jugular groove may also result in damage to the cervical sympathetic trunk. The trunk runs in the jugular groove, in close proximity to the vagus, and the cranial sympathetic ganglion lies in the guttural pouch, again close to the major roots of the glossopharyngeal, vagus, and accessory nerves, and the internal carotid artery.

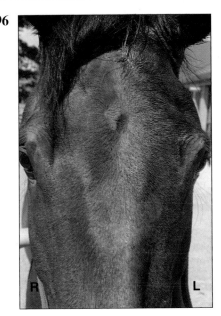

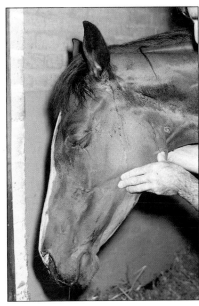

696 Horner's syndrome.
Note: Sweating restricted to left side of face. Ptosis (drooping) of left upper eyelid.

697 Horner's syndrome (guttural pouch lesion).
Note: Sweating restricted to below left ear (lesion situated distal to cranial sympathetic ganglion). Epistaxis from damage to blood vessels in the guttural pouch. Ptosis very obvious.

Disorders such as **guttural pouch mycosis** (*see* **252**) and the **extravascular injection of irritant substances** (*see* **294**) might also, therefore, be expected to affect the sympathetic supply to the ipsilateral side of the head and (in the case of cervical lesions) the neck. The normal function of the cranial sympathetic trunk may also be affected by lacerations at the base of the neck (or higher) or space occupying lesions in the thoracic inlet, such as mediastinal and thymic lymphosarcoma (*see* **320**) and multiple/extensive, thoracic melanoma or carcinoma. The consequences of loss of sympathetic tone include cutaneous vasodilatation with localised hyperthermia and consequent sweating. Thus, damage to the trunk in the lower or mid-cervical region, results in sweating over the side of the neck (**694**) and, in **Horners Syndrome** on the ipsilateral side (**695**). The characteristic feature of this clinical sign is the sharp cut-off of the sweating down the midline of the face (**696**). Where the lesion responsible for the damage is situated in the guttural pouch and damage to the trunk is beyond the cranial sympathetic ganglion, the area of sweating is usually limited to a small area just under the ear (**697**). Loss of sympathetic control of the upper eyelid and pupillary diameter results in a **ptosis** (**697**), **miosis** (which may not be very obvious) and **enophthalmos** (**698a/b**) on the affected side. The nictitating membrane (third eyelid) may be prominent (**698b**) as a secondary consequence of enophthalmos. Damage to the

sympathetic fibres within the spinal cord results in sweating down the whole side of the horse, as well as Horner's Syndrome, which may then be bilateral. **Equine protozoal myeloencephalitis** (*see* **736**) is one of the few generalised disorders which may produce signs of central-origin Horner's Syndrome and the condition may be attributed, in these cases, to extensive brain stem disruption and specific damage within the tectotegmental tract of the spinal cord.

   Traumatic disruption of peripheral somatic nerves having motor functions, exhibits well defined clinical signs which are entirely predictable, and which depend upon the extent and duration of the damage. Damage to nerves having sensory functions alone are more difficult to assess accurately in the horse, although, where surgical denervation has been carried out the distribution of the analgesia would also be entirely predictable. Peripheral surgical neurectomy for the relief of intractable pain is commonly performed, and, while the consequences in respect of the pain relief may be satisfactory, complications including ischemia, gangrene and the development of neuroma at the site of neurectomy (*see* **744**) are uncommon sequelae.

   Damage to individual peripheral motor nerves of visible muscles results in a very obvious and rapidly developing atrophy. The extent of the atrophy depends largely on the location of nerve disruption. Lesions occurring at or near the origins of the nerves or at

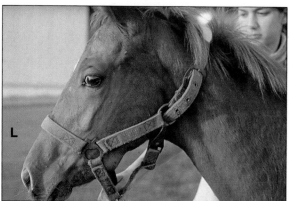

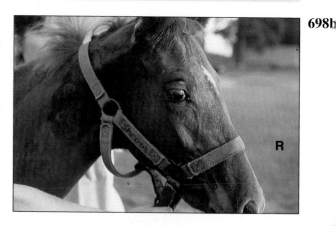

698 Horner's syndrome.
Note: Ptosis (drooping of upper eyelid), miosis (pupillary constriction) and enophthalmos (sunken eye) are visible in the right eye (**698b**) (when compared to simultaneous photograph of normal left eye (**698a**)). Right facial sweating is obvious. Condition arose following perivascular injection of irritant into right jugular groove.

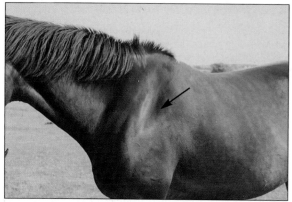

699 Denervation atrophy (infraspinatus nerve).
Note: Atrophy limited to infraspinatus muscle (arrow).
Differential Diagnosis:
i)   Equine protozoal myeloencephalitis
ii) Localised myopathy with fibrous metaplasia

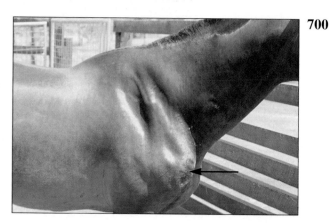

700 Suprascapular paralysis ('Sweeney') (long standing lesion).
Note: Marked atrophy of supraspinatus and infraspinatus muscles. Prominent scapular spine. Site of injury over point of shoulder (arrow).

plexuses result in widespread loss of muscular function, while damage to distal relatively minor branches of nerves results in a more localised atrophy (**699**). Specific atrophy of individual muscles is also an important clinical sign of **equine protozoal myeloencephalitis** (*see* **736**) and the **cauda equine syndrome** (*Polyneuritis equi*) (*see* **711**). It is often difficult to to establish the etiology in some cases of single muscle atrophy but denervation atrophy is usually rapid and particularly well-defined when compared to secondary atrophy following physical muscle damage or interference with blood supply.

   Fractures of the neck of the scapula, the scapular tuberosity, or blows to the shoulder, or extremes of movement (particularly caudal extension of the shoulder) may result in clinically significant damage to the **suprascapular nerve**. The resultant damage may cause a mild neurapraxia (temporarily impaired nerve function) or more severe damage, which may be permanent (neurotmesis). The path of the suprascapular nerve around the neck of the scapula makes it liable to stretching and bruising trauma, even in the absence of any obvious fractures. Damage to this nerve is often complicated by concurrent damage in the brachial plexus, and results in an acute onset of paralysis of the supraspinatus and infraspinatus muscles ('**Sweeney**'). Consequent loss of lateral support for the shoulder normally maintained by these muscles results, initially, in a sudden lateral 'popping' of the shoulder joint during movement which is usually visible. The sudden outward excursion of the shoulder joint itself may be responsible for continued stretching (and, therefore, dysfunction of

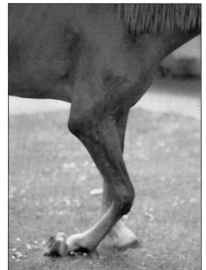

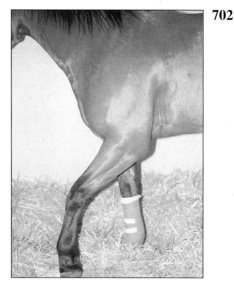

701 Brachial paralysis.
Note: Shoulder and elbow obviously dropped. Foot dragging, leg looks too long for the horse. No weight bearing possible even when the limb was placed in a normal position.

702 Radial paralysis.
Note: Dropped elbow with shoulder normal. Weight bearing possible if limb placed in normal position but forward motion was performed by lifting the whole shoulder and throwing the leg forward. An area of hypalgesia was present on the front of the antebrachium.

the nerve), even in the event that the damage is slight initially. Atrophy of the infraspinatus and supraspinatus muscles results in the scapular spine becoming very prominent (**700**).

The **radial nerve** is the largest outflow from the brachial plexus and innervates the extensors of the elbow, carpus and digit. It also has a sensory component to the front of the antebrachium (forearm). Trauma involving **brachial plexus disruption**, from simultaneous over extension and adduction of the shoulder causing overstretching of the plexus, or damage to the shaft or overlying muscles of the humerus, may affect the function of the radial nerve. The clinical signs depend upon the severity and location of the damage. True **radial paralysis** is not common; usually some brachial plexus involvement occurs simultaneously. However, recognition of the differences is important with respect to prognosis and the nursing requirements.

Brachial plexus damage involves both extensors and flexors of the forelimb and the limb is completely unable to bear weight even when placed in its natural position. The limb has a flaccid appearance with a dropped shoulder, in addition to the signs of more distal radial nerve paralysis (**701**). The limb appears to be too long for the horse. Brachial plexus disruption is also accompanied in most cases by suprascapular paralysis (*see* **700**).

Damage to the radial nerve distal to the brachial plexus results only in loss of elbow extension and limited skin hypoalgesia. Damage involving only the radial nerve is not common but is encountered both from relatively minor trauma and is associated with humeral shaft fractures. Characteristically the limb cannot be voluntarily extended and, unless placed in its natural position by an attendant, is unable to bear weight. However, once the limb is placed appropriately, the horse may bear weight relatively normally, until a step is required. In most cases the branch of the nerve to the triceps muscle is most severely involved and the elbow therefore has a dropped appearance while the distal limb is flexed (**702**). The limb typically rests with the dorsum of the pastern on the ground and voluntary movement is undertaken by thrusting the limb forward from the shoulder. Mild, partial damage to the radial nerve may only produce a tendency to stumble when the affected foot encounters a slight obstacle. Long-standing damage results in atrophy of the muscles innervated by the nerve including, most obviously, the *triceps brachialis* (**703**), *extensor carpi radialis*, *ulnaris lateralis* and the *digital extensor* muscles. The loss of triceps function does not always result in a severe handicap with some horses adapting very well (*see* **703**).

The **femoral nerve**, which innervates the *quadriceps femoris* group of muscles on the dorsal and lateral

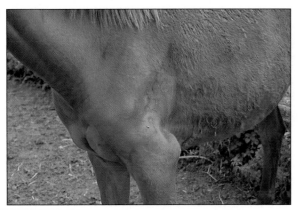

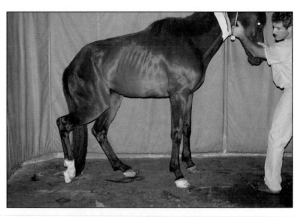

703 Radial paralysis (denervation atrophy) (long-standing lesion).
Note: Marked atrophy of the extensor muscles of the elbow and particularly the *triceps brachii* muscle. Olecranon and caudal angle of the shoulder very obvious.
Differential Diagnosis:
i) Equine protozoal myeloencephalitis
ii) Post myopathy atrophy
iii) Fibrous metaplasia following trauma.

704 Femoral (crural) paralysis.
Note: No weight bearing ability, complete lack of stifle extension. All the joints of the limb are flexed. Where the nerve is irreparably damaged, marked *quadriceps femoris* atrophy will develop.

aspects of the thigh, is prone to damage from direct trauma or from over-stretching as a result of over extension of the limb. Affected horses are unable to bear weight, with all the joints of the limb flexed (**704**). Hypoalgesia of the medial thigh may be detectable. Ultimately, atrophy of the *quadriceps femoris* and *vastus* muscle masses (*see* **736**) results in the formation of dense fibrous metaplasia, which may feel like tendons rather than muscle masses.

Damage to the **sciatic nerve** either from direct trauma, often associated with coxo-femoral luxations or fractures of the acetabulum, or from pelvic fractures and sacral/pelvic osteomyelitis, or more often, perhaps, from misdirected injections of irritant drugs in the caudal buttock, results in loss of both tibial and peroneal nerve function. While the loss of sensory functions results in hypoalgesia of the distal limb (from the stifle down), the loss of motor function results in poor limb flexion with the stifle and hock extended (i.e. virtually straight) and the fetlock flexed; possibly even standing on the dorsum of the pastern (**705**). Weight can be born on the limb if it is placed into its normal position, but if the animal moves the weight is supported by the dorsum of the hoof.

Femoral and/or sciatic nerve neurapraxia sometimes occurs in newborn foals after assisted deliveries, particularly where there has been considerable force applied as the hips are delivered through the pelvic canal in either anterior or posterior presentations.

Damage to the **obturator nerve** occurs much less frequently in the horse than in the bovine, but fetal oversize and dystocia may nevertheless cause obturator neurapraxia. The loss of adductor ability affecting the muscles of the medial upper thigh is characteristic (**706**). The affected limb may not support weight effectively, particularly when sudden movement or turning is attempted. There is a persistent danger in these cases of serious adductor muscle rupture or coxo-femoral dislocations and femoral, pelvic or sacral fractures.

Stringhalt is an involuntary hyperflexion of one or both hind limbs during movement. In most parts of the world it occurs as an isolated disorder in individual horses, but in Australasia it sometimes occurs in epidemics associated with the ingestion of Flatweed (*Hypochaeris radicata*) (**Plate 9k**, page 355), Dandelion (*Taraxacum officinale*) (**Plate 9f**, page 355) or Sweet Pea (*Lathyrus* spp.) plants. The disorder is also known as **lathyrism** when it is associated with the ingestion of *Lathyrus sativus* and the Singletary Pea (*Lathyrus hirsutis*) (**Plate 9b**, page 354). The clinical features of both forms of the disorder are similar with respect to the appearance of the involuntary flexion, but in the Australian form both hind limbs are usually affected and, occasionally, the forelimbs and neck may also be involved. The two conditions differ clinically only in degree, with the sporadic form usually being milder, sometimes unilateral and invariably permanent. Individual horses

705

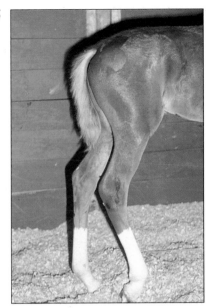

706

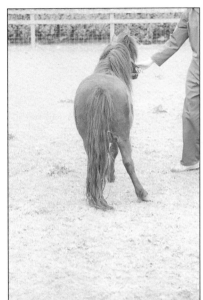

705 Sciatic paralysis.
Note: Due to *Salmonella* spp. osteomyelitis involving pelvis and adjacent soft tissues. Weight bearing adequate but metatarsophalangeal joint remains flexed. The flexor reflex was absent in the right hind limb, area of hypalgesia just below the hock.

706 Obturator paralysis.
Note: Assisted parturition 6 hours previously. Loss of adductor ability in both hind limbs with the right worse affected.

affected by the sporadic form show a sudden jerking of the hind leg during walking (**707**) of variable severity, which may be occasional or occur with every step. Less severe cases may show only a slight spasm of the leg without marked lifting of the foot. In more severe cases, however, the dorsal aspect of the fetlock may even hit the abdominal wall with considerable force and this will obviously have a marked effect upon gait. It can often be made more obvious by turning or backing the horse. The clinical syndrome presents as if the tibial nerve has been cut. Progression is sometimes ungainly, but the animal appears unconcerned, and any pace faster than a walk is usually normal or nearly normal. Although the etiology of the sporadic form is uncertain, it is considered to be a neurogenic disorder. It is often reported to be worse in cold weather, and many affected horses are of a nervous disposition.

In **Australian Stringhalt**, both hind limbs are generally, equally and severely affected (**708**), and the signs may be severe enough to prevent forward movement, with extreme spasms of both flexor and extensor muscle groups resulting in a state of tetanus. The extensor and flexor muscles of the hind limbs below the stifle, in severe cases, frequently become atrophied giving a 'peg-leg' appearance. Affected horses often develop concurrent laryngeal paralysis (usually

restricted to the left side (**Plate 5u**, page 115), but occasionally right-sided or bilateral). While the sporadic form may only be resolved by surgical interference, some cases of Australian Stringhalt may resolve spontaneously over weeks or months, provided that no further ingestion of the offending plants is allowed. In some cases, however, obvious neurological deficits including laryngeal paralysis remain.

Horses of all ages and types are occasionally affected by a granulomatous polyneuritis known as the **cauda equina neuritis syndrome** (*Polyneuritis equi*). A history of preceding immunological challenge, such as vaccination or viral infections, is often reported. While the clinical signs of the disorder are classically associated with neurological deficits within the cauda equina, the disorder has a number of alternative features. In the earliest stages the horse may be seen to rub its tail head as if irritated. Later cases have urinary and fecal incontinence, with anal flaccidity (**709**), accompanied by a well-defined area of hypalgesia or analgesia in the perineal area (**710**). Bladder sphincter atony results in urine dribbling from a flaccidly distended bladder; squirts of urine appearing during vocalisation or when the horse moves or, particularly, when it rises from recumbency. Tail paralysis is a common finding. The clinical syndrome which can usually be found closely

707

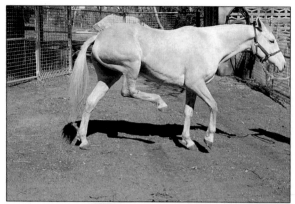

707 Stringhalt (sporadic form).
Note: Both hind legs affected for many years without any apparent progression. No visible effect when trotting or cantering. Worst in cold weather.

708

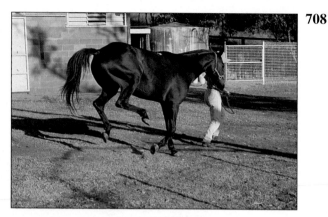

708 Stringhalt (Australian form).
Note: Both hind legs abnormal. Horse unable to make progress during movement. Urinary incontinence present.

709

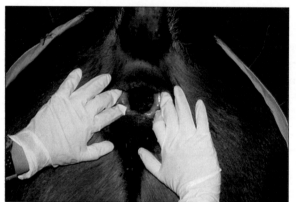

709 Cauda equina neuritis (*polyneuritis equi*).
Note: Flaccid anal ring and terminal rectum ballooned.
Differential Diagnosis:
i) Equine herpes virus (neurological) syndrome
ii) Sacral fracture
iii) Epidural anaesthesia
iv) Spinal neoplasia

710

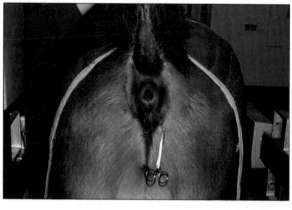

710 Cauda equina neuritis (*polyneuritis equi*).
Note: Analgesia of perineum. Tail was flaccid.

resembles the appearance of posterior epidural anesthesia. The loss of rectal, anal and bladder reflexes and perineal sensation, results in a dramatic accumulation of progressively drier food material and progressively more bladder distension often to the point where the horse develops colic symptoms associated with primary impaction of the small colon and/or chronic cystitis. Involvement of nerve roots other than those in the cauda equina including cranial nerves and individual spinal nerves may be present. In some cases subtle alterations in hind limb gait are noticeable and, in these, or occasionally independently of this sign, there may be profound unilateral muscle atrophy of the gluteal muscles, in particular (**711**). Subtle or sometimes obvious cranial nerve deficits including facial paralysis (*see* **689**), trigeminal deficits (*see* **687**), and vestibular disturbances may be present at the same time or, indeed, without concurrent cauda equina symptoms. The **cranial nerve syndromes** are often subtle and may easily be overshadowed by the more dramatic perineal and pelvic deficits or may be missed completely when, as may rarely occur, they exist on their own. Their distribution may be very localised, even to the point of affecting only one branch of the facial nerve (*see* **690**). The rate of progression of this untreatable disease may be very variable with some cases deteriorating rapidly while others appear to maintain a static state for months or years. The detection of circulating antibodies to myelin

711

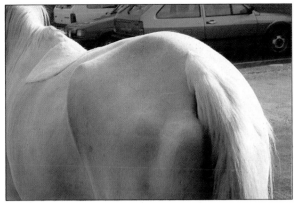

711 Cauda equina neuritis (*polyneuritis equi*).
Note: Unilateral gluteal atrophy. Tail paralysed.
Differential Diagnosis:
i)   Equine protozoal myeloencephalitis
ii) Pelvic injury / Disuse atrophy
iii) Denervation atrophy (sacral fracture/pelvic injury)
iv) Post-myopathy atrophy

712

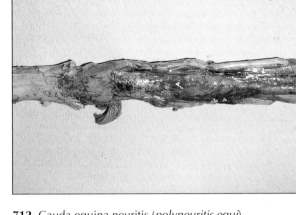

712 Cauda equina neuritis (*polyneuritis equi*).
Note: Hemorrhage and necrosis of cauda equina.

sheath (P2) proteins is a useful means of confirming the diagnosis. The prognosis is, at best, poor but the progression may be slow or almost inapparent. At post mortem examination a moderate to severe granulomatous polyneuritis with discoloration and hemorrhage of the cauda equina (**712**) can usually be found. In some cases, however, there may be little obvious pathology and histopathological examination may be required. Cases involving cranial nerves, or specific spinal nerves without cauda equina involvement, may show only histological evidence of the progressive neuropathy characteristic of the disorder.

Nutritional and metabolic derangements may exert powerful and profound effects upon nerve function. While few of these diseases present illustratable clinical features, they are of importance with respect to differential diagnosis. Thus, **reduction in circulating calcium** concentrations occurring commonly in endurance or exhausted horses, may induce a hypersensitivity in the phrenic nerve. The consequence of this is a synchronous diaphragmatic flutter occurring with each heart beat and showing a typical hiccough at the flank with each cardiac contraction.

Deficiency of thiamine either in absolute dietary terms (which is very unusual) or through the repeated ingestion of thiaminase enzymes also has significant effects upon neurological function. Most often, this disorder is seen in animals ingesting large amounts of bracken fern (*Pteridium aquilinum*) (**Plate 9c**, page 354) over prolonged periods.

Many plants from all areas of the world are known to have serious toxic effects characterised by neurological signs. In some cases the clinical signs may appear to be related to the nervous system although the plant toxins actually have their major effects upon the liver (in particular) or other organs. The neurological deficits in these cases relate to the failure of detoxification of alkaloids and/or the accumulation of abnormal concentrations of natural substances which are normally excreted or altered in such a way as to become non-toxic. **Hepatic failure due to plant poisoning** results in significantly elevated blood ammonia and organic acid concentrations which induce the signs typical of hepatoencephalopathy including dementia, mania, convulsions, head pressing (*see* **159**), circling and compulsive walking (*see* **160**). High plasma concentrations of bilirubin are also known to cause marked and often prolonged depression although the mechanism for this is not well defined. Some plants, however, are known to have marked direct toxic effects upon the central nervous system. In most cases they cause a diffuse encephalopathy with a wide range of signs including blindness, depression, dementia, seizures and in some cases subtle behavioural changes. *Astragalus* spp. (**Plate 9e**, page 354), *Oxytropis* spp. (**Plate 9h**, page 355) and crotalaria spp. (**Plate 9i**, page 355) plants, known as 'Locoweeds' in North America, and *Swainsonia* spp. (**Plate 9h**, page 355) in Australia, contain the alkaloid locoine, and are perhaps the best identified plants producing notable clinical signs including aggression, dementia, ataxia (**713**), posterior paralysis and weight loss. The same group of plants accumulate selenium and repeated ingestion over a long period may produce clinical signs typical of selenium poisoning, including laminitis (*see* **499**) and hair loss (*see* **359, 360**).

A small proportion of horses ingesting large amounts

Plate 9

a
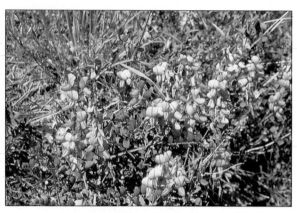
b

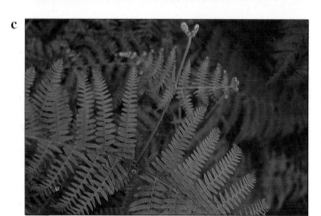
c

d
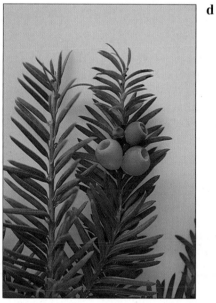

e
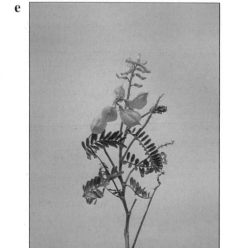

a *Sorghum* spp. grass.

b *Lathyrus hirsutis* (Singletary Pea).

c *Pteridium aquilinum* (Bracken Fern).

d *Taxus baccata* (English Yew).

e *Astragalus* spp.

Plate 9

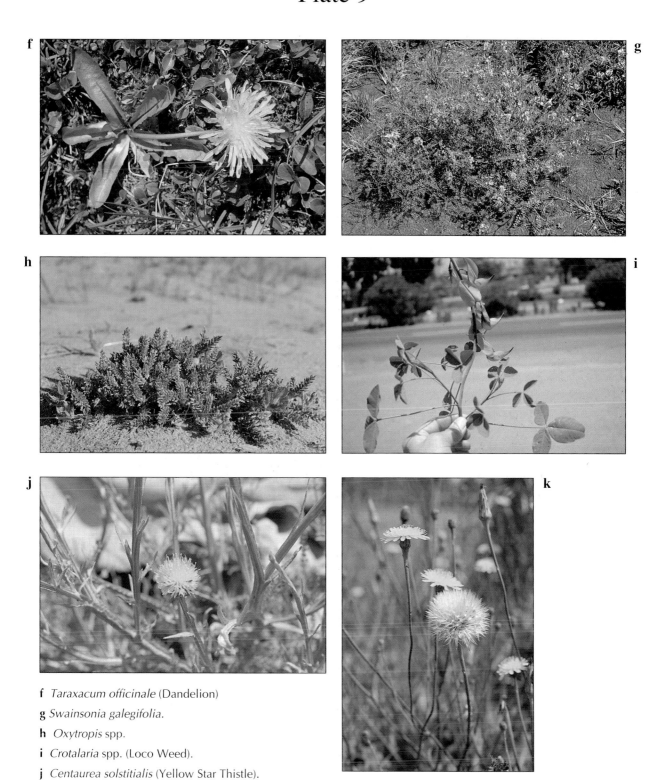

f *Taraxacum officinale* (Dandelion)

g *Swainsonia galegifolia.*

h *Oxytropis* spp.

i *Crotalaria* spp. (Loco Weed).

j *Centaurea solstitialis* (Yellow Star Thistle).

k *Hypochaeris radicata* (Flatweed).

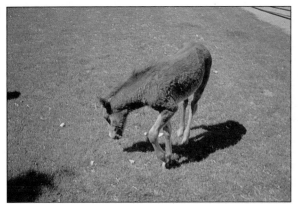

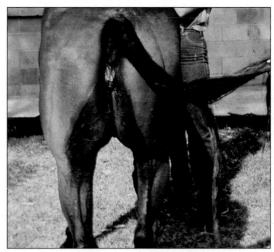

713 Selenium (*Astragalus* or *Oxytropis* spp.) poisoning. **Note:** Spatial disturbances and aggression were present. Wild behavior with repeated falling over backwards onto haunches was shown.

714 Sorghum poisoning (incontinence). **Note:** Urine scalding and hair staining of perineum. **Differential Diagnosis:**
i)   Cauda equina neuritis (*polyneuritis equi*)
ii) Epidural anaesthesia
iii) Equine herpes-1 virus infection (neurological syndrome)
iv) Sacro-coccygeal fracture/luxation
v)   Cord neoplasia (melanoma, squamous cell carcinoma, lymphosarcoma)

of *Sorghum* spp. grasses (including Sudan and Milo grass) **(Plate 9a**, page 354), over prolonged periods may develop a paralysis of the bladder with persistent urine dribbling **(714)** and, often, some degree of hind-limb ataxia. In some cases the condition may be indistinguishable from the cauda equina neuritis syndrome (*see* **709** *et seq.*) except that hind-quarter ataxia and paralysis are more prominent features of sorghum toxicity. It is possible that the syndrome is a result of repeated, subclinical cyanide poisoning derived from the cyanogenetic glycosides in these plants.

Sustained ingestion of significant amounts of the Yellow Star Thistle (*Centaurea solstitialis*) **(Plate 9j**, page 355) (and other members of this species known as Yellow Burr and Russian Knapweed), over some weeks, causes a specific equine neurological disorder characterised by difficulty with prehension, mastication and swallowing. The plant is found widely in the Western United States of America and in Australia and affected animals may obtain the plant directly from pastures or, more commonly, in preserved feeds. While the plant is not usually palatable to horses some appear to become addicted to it and this represents the most dangerous situation. The disorder is associated with a progressive and profound malacic degeneration of the *substantia nigra* and the *globus pallidus* and is known as **nigropallidal encephalomalacia**. There is a sudden onset of an obvious masticatory difficulty and affected horses are seen to prehend and then make ineffective chewing movements. Hay may be seen protruding from the mouth for prolonged

periods **(715)**, during which futile chewing movements continue. Mastication and swallowing are patently not effective and food material and water are apparently unable to be moved into the caudal parts of the oral cavity. The tongue is often drawn into a longitudinal trough **(716)** and saliva is sometimes whipped into a foamy mass which dribbles from the mouth. The tongue may be seen to move back and forth from the mouth. Attempts to drink are often frustrated, with head dipping (often up to the eyes), and some horses resort to tipping the head back to allow water to run passively into the pharynx. Persistent unrewarding feeding attempts may result in a severe edema of the muzzle and nose. Wandering, ataxia and fasciculation of the masticatory muscles, and dramatic weight-loss occur in almost all cases. More generalised central nervous signs such as head pressing, semi-conclusive seizures and incoordination are sometimes present but may reflect other aspects of the metabolic consequences of starvation and water deprivation. The condition has a very high mortality once clinical signs are present. The donkey and mule are much less susceptible to the poisoning and, in spite of ingesting large amounts over long periods, seldom show any clinical effects. At post mortem examination a pathognomonic liquefactive necrosis of the nigropallidal regions of the brain which may be extensive and obvious or subtle, with only microscopic evidence of the problem, are identified.

The **bracken fern** (*Pteridium aquilinum*) **(Plate 9c**, page 354) is very poisonous to horses when ingested

715

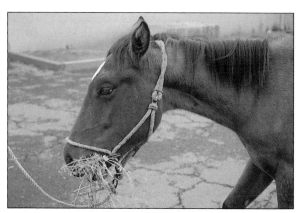

716

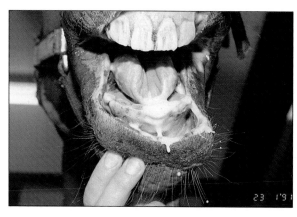

715 Nigropallidal encephalomalacia (*Centaurea solstitialis* / yellow star thistle poisoning).
Note: Dysphagia, weight loss. Food was held in mouth and ineffective chewing movements made. Excessive jaw muscle tone (dystonia).

716 Nigropallidal encephalomalacia (*Centaurea solstitialis* / yellow star thistle poisoning).
Note: Tongue drawn into typical longitudinal trough, foamy salivation as a result of mouth movements without swallowing.

717

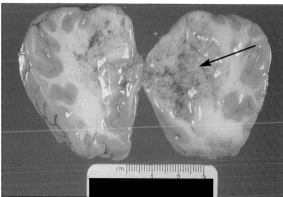

717 Leukoencephalomalacia (Mouldy corn poisoning, Fusarium Toxicosis).
Note: Frontal region of the brain of a miniature horse that died suddenly. Liquefactive necrosis can be seen best on the left side of the right-hand brain section and involves both grey and white matter (arrow).

over periods of 30 – 60 days or more, but is not usually palatable unless food is scarce. The entire plant contains a thiaminase which is not destroyed by drying and which results in a clinical thiamine deficiency syndrome. Nervous tissue is the first to suffer the effects of thiamine deficiency and the earliest signs affect the peripheral motor nerves. Gradual myelin degeneration in peripheral nerves causes a progressive weakness and incoordination (bracken staggers). Muscle weakness is initially only apparent during exercise, but progresses to recumbency and opisthotonus. Arching of the back, a base-wide, hind-limb stance and crossing of the front legs, followed by advancing weakness and recumbency are typical. Cardiac tachydysrhythmias and hemolytic crises are also encountered. The affected horse is dull and weak and there is often a concurrent pharyngeal paralysis (**Plate 6r**, page 123). A curative response to thiamine therapy is diagnostic in horses with an appropriate contact history. Poisoning with *Equisetum arvense* (Marestail) is clinically and physiologically identical.

Central nervous signs are also a feature of **mycotoxicosis** and the best defined form of this group of disorders is due to toxins produced by moulds such as *Fusarium moniliforme* in corn. Sustained ingestion of the toxin over 4 weeks or more induces a progressive liquefactive necrosis of the cerebral cortex. Characteristically this causes sudden and unexpected death in one or more animal s under the same managemental regime. Dementia, blindness, convulsions and ataxia may be seen prior to death. Death is virtually certain within 24 hours of the development of any of the clinical signs, although some horses suspected of being affected, have survived with long-standing/permanent neurological (cerebral) deficits. Cranial nerve signs include dysphagia and laryngeal paralysis, and facial and trigeminal disorders occur in some cases. Post mortem examination usually shows definite areas of liquefactive necrosis of the sub-cortical white matter in the cerebral hemispheres (**717**). In some cases hepatic pathology is also present and may produce obvious icterus, hemorrhagic diatheses and signs of hepatoencephalopathy.

Ingestion of leaves and berries of the ornamental yew tree (*Taxus baccata* and *Taxus caspicata*) (**Plate 9d**, page 354) results in sudden death related to the alkaloid, taxine. The horse is one of the most sensitive species to the effects of the alkaloid and a single mouthful may be lethal. The leaves remain poisonous in a dry state. Death is abrupt and post mortem examination shows no pathognomonic features. Fortunately the needles are distinctive and masticated pieces of them can usually be found in the mouth or stomach of affected horses. However, the small amounts required may make their detection very difficult.

One of the most puzzling disorders of the horse relating to neurological degeneration is **Grass Sickness** (*see* **129 et seq.**). The disorder is possibly connected to the ingestion of toxins (possibly mycotoxins) which result in a specific autonomic disturbance particularly relating to the loss of alimentary tract motility and coordination. The disease is confirmed by miscroscopic evidence of autonomic degeneration in ganglia and in the intrinsic myenteric plexus of the ileum in particular. The clinical effects are well defined (*see* **129 et seq.**) and the outcome of acute cases is currently regarded as always fatal.

Amongst the other neurological disorders of the horse for which there is no present explanation there are a number which occur more or less frequently and which are easily recognised. **Narcolepsy** is a rare incurable disorder of sleep which is commonest in the miniature breeds of horse including the Shetland and Welsh Ponies. Thoroughbred, Appaloosa and Standardbred horses, amongst others, have also been affected. Sleep attacks, accompanied by a dramatic loss of muscle tone, develop without warning and often in totally inappropriate places. The affected horse buckles at the knees and gently collapses without significant preparation for recumbency, and then falls into an apparently very deep sleep, during which the normal components of sleep (including rapid-eye-movements and absence of spinal reflexes) are present. The affected foal can often be aroused easily, and will then immediately regain its feet and behave normally.

Motor neurone disease is a rare disease encountered in horses of any breed or sex, associated with an apparent over activity of the neuromuscular junction. Affected horses show little or no ability to control and regulate the movement of their limbs and rapidly become exhausted. They characteristically have a hyper-alert, worried facial expression and extensive muscle fasciculations, which are most apparent in the muscles of the head and the upper limbs. Weight shifting from one leg to another, a boarded abdomen and diffuse sweating are encountered and are associated with the increased muscular effort associated with maintaining a standing posture. The animal usually takes every available opportunity to rest and lies down with difficulty, resting the head either by propping itself up by the muzzle or by profound relaxation in full lateral recumbency. The clinical features of the disease are not easily demonstrated by still pictures but the disorder may be confused with colic, tetanus, organophosphate poisoning and laminitis. However, the typical signs of these conditions are not consistently present and diagnosis of motor neurone disease in horses may depend upon careful assessment of electrical activity in muscles and their nerves and a definitive diagnosis can, at present, only be made at post mortem examination.

Neuroses (vices) are a common problem in horses, particularly those which are under-exercised and stabled. There is good evidence that these habits are quickly learned from other horses. The most common vices are **crib-biting** and **wind-sucking**. Many animals are afflicted by both vices at the same time. **Crib-biting** is the unpleasant habit of forceable grabbing of a fixed object between the incisor teeth and biting hard. Those which simultaneously wind-suck, then arch their necks and suck in air. The bolus of air is then swallowed and may create secondary disorders of gastro-intestinal function including colic and weight loss. The appearance of the cribbing behaviour is characteristic (**718**) and the wear pattern created on the incisor teeth as a result of the persistent misuse, results in a typical appearance of wear on the buccal margin of the upper incisors which may, in early or mild cases be subtle (*see* **29**) or may be very obvious (*see* **30**). Horses which simultaneously wind-suck can be seen to gulp and swallow boluses of air into the stomach. The consequences of these vices include weight loss, poor appetite and inveterate wind-suckers may suffer from colic as a result of gaseous distension of the stomach and large colon. Some cases may wind-suck without crib-biting, and while most of these have a characteristic arching of the neck, others may extend the neck. Some may show no neck-muscle involvement but still make obvious swallowing movements. The accompanying noise made by this swallowing is very similar to hiccoughs and is characteristic. In almost all cases there is a concurrent hypertrophy of the muscles of the ventral neck and the sternocephalicus in particular (*see* **718**). Horses which are treated for this condition by the application of a cribbing strap or metal cribbing bar almost always have an area of hair-loss and thickened skin over the throat on either side of the neck. The condition is virtually

718

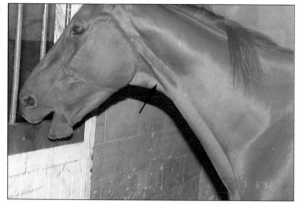

718 Crib-biting vice.
Note: Hypertrophy of sternocephalicus muscle (arrow).

719

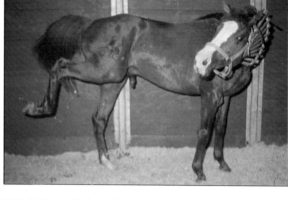

719 Self-mutilation vice.
Note: Stallion which under variable circumstances chewed at its right stifle and also spent prolonged periods kicking out with the right leg.

720

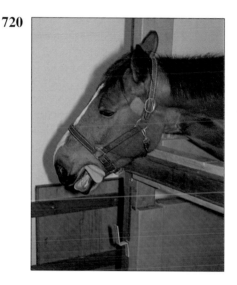

720 Tongue-sucking vice.

impossible to treat effectively without recourse to surgical myectomy and neurectomy but even this has a high rate of failure.

Mature lightweight stallions, in particular, are prone to the **self-mutilation syndrome**. Horses with a nervous disposition whose circumstances change dramatically may develop the disorder. Dramatic self-mutilation, with biting and chewing at particular sites on the body, is evident. Most cases show a variety of associated nervous signs including squealing and spinning round, and seem to pick on a particular site, usually one stifle or shoulder, biting and chewing at it incessantly (**719**). The odour of seminal fluid seems to act as a particular trigger for the behaviour which may result in alopecia, leukotrichia and localised scarring. As it occurs in horses which are bored and which have recently changed environment, it may be that the condition is a neurosis. Most cases can be temporarily and easily distracted.

Occasional foals and a few adult horses appear to have a **flaccid tongue** which is seen hanging out of the mouth. In foals it is often a temporary weakness and the tongue is palpably weak and fails to resist traction. No dysphagia or other defect is usually present and the foals develop normally. A number of adult horses show the same signs but the condition persists without any untoward effect. Some however, develop an unpleasant habit of playing with, or sucking, the tongue (**720**) and this is often a permanent vice. Saliva is sometimes whipped into a foam by the action giving the animal a foamy mouth. Usually no organic defect can be found although occasionally the tongue may be somewhat weak.

A seasonal apparently nervous disorder in which horses of all ages and types develop a severe, and often dangerous, tendency to shake or nod the head occurs in many parts of the world. The generally seasonal nature of **'head shaking'** suggests that it is due to inhaled pollen grains or dust or some other material which creates nasal irritation. An excessive nasal sensitivity, possibly due to irritant or physical factors is sometimes blamed. Many cases are, however, not seasonal, and in most there is no detectable evidence of any inflammatory process. Some cases have been ascribed to visual, oral or auditory factors or to behavioural or management problems with the rider or tack/harness. Affected horses are often unrideable, although, at rest, they may show no apparent abnormality. The head movements are often violent and may even throw the horse off balance, but are often intermittently better or worse without any apparent predisposing factors or predictability. Most cases in which a cause can be established at all, are cases of nasal hypersensitivity, possibly related to allergic rhinitis, but the condition appears to develop into a neurosis. Rubbing of the muzzle against the forelimbs or along the ground or violent twitching of the nose are some of the commoner symptoms.

Infectious Disorders

Virus Diseases: One of the most important viral disorders affecting the nervous system is **Rabies**. Although the horse is possibly less sensitive to the virus than many other species and is therefore less often affected, the disorder presents with particular but often vague clinical signs. The recognition of the syndrome is obviously of major importance. Rabies occurs in almost all parts of the world, with, at present, the exception of the United Kingdom, Australasia and a few other isolated places. After a prolonged incubation period during which the animal is normal in behaviour and appearance, Rabies may take either the furious (cerebral) form, or, more usually, the dumb (spinal) form. The furious form is characterised by vocalisation, aggression, mania, dementia, seizures and salivation. In the dumb form, depression, dementia, straining and progressive hind-quarter ataxia are common features. Cases of both types often show pharyngeal paralysis, with saliva drooling from the mouth and food and saliva at the nose **(721)**, although, in some cases, there may be little or no apparent oral involvement. A 7–10 day history of progressive self-mutilation **(722)** and persistent licking at the site of an old wound, which often has no known etiology, and which is often situated on the limbs, may be seen. A progressive ascending hind-quarter ataxia over a 7–10 day course, culminating in a distressing and complete paralysis **(723)** and coma, is strongly indicative of Rabies in endemic areas. All such cases should be treated as suspicious, until a definite alternative diagnosis can be established. The course of the disease is inexorable, with progressive dysphagia, convulsions resulting in self-inflicted trauma to the face and body and hydrophobia. Ultimately the affected horse, no matter which form of the disease has been manifest, becomes recumbent and comatose. Death is certain. A diagnosis may be confirmed post mortem, by the demonstration of pathognomonic changes in the cord and brain stem. Lesions may not be present in the brain if animals are destroyed early in the course.

721

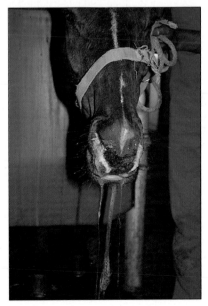

721 Rabies (dumb/spinal form).
Note: Dysphagia, salivation.
Differential Diagnosis:
i)   Choke
ii) Pharyngeal paralysis (African horse sickness, togaviral encephalitis, lead poisoning)
iii) Pharyngeal foreign body
iv) Oral foreign body

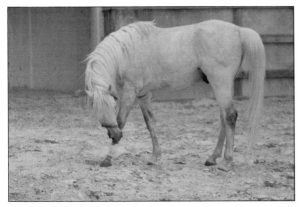

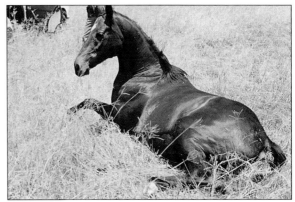

722 Rabies.
Note: Self-mutilation (persistent licking and chewing at site of injury which occurred 7 weeks previously, without any known etiology).
Differential Diagnosis:
i)   Self mutilation vice

723 Rabies (dumb/spinal form).
Note: Posterior paralysis, tail flaccidity.
Differential Diagnosis:
i)   Trauma
ii) Equine herpes-1 virus infection (neurological syndrome)
iii) Spinal lesion (parasite)

Several **arthropod-borne viruses** of the family, *Togaviridae*, have been associated with **encephalitis** in the horse. The specific viruses include Eastern, Western, Venezuelan, Japanese B and a number of other related viruses. The features of the clinical disorders which these cause are broadly similar but they differ in some aspects of their epizootic features with some being more virulent and others being less easily transmitted, while some have longer or shorter incubation periods. Apart from their often life-threatening nature in horses, many of these are of zoonotic importance. As the viruses are transmitted by arthropod vectors they are generally seasonal disorders which are geographically limited by the distribution of the vectors themselves and the seasonal fluctuations which control their prevalence. The viruses are responsible for a syndrome which is attributable to diffuse cerebral disease or, occasionally, to diffuse spinal cord disease. Initially, the diseases are characterised by a vague and non-specific, febrile malaise, with somnolence and an apparent stupidity (**724**), but more severe neurological signs develop rapidly thereafter. Behavioral changes including teeth grinding, salivation (**725**), vacant staring (**725**), blindness, circling (**726**), sweating (**726**), convulsions (**727**), hyperesthesia, photophobia, compulsive walking and recumbency with leg paddling (*see* **727**) are commonly present. Progressive ataxia, loss of conscious proprioception and postural peculiarities (*see* **726**) as well as static or progressive cranial nerve signs, such as nystagmus and facial paralysis (*see* **691**) may be found. Dysphagia (*see* **721**) as a result of pharyngeal and esophageal paralysis develops in most cases. Signs progress more rapidly when brain herniation occurs and death within 48–72 hours is then usual. Horses which survive usually have residual central neurological deficits which result in permanent, behavioural or physical disabilities. These cases are referred to as 'dummies' and often appear to spend long periods in deep sleep. Individual horses receiving low challenges of mild strains of these viruses may be unaffected and others may regain almost normal function after relatively severe clinical disease. A specific diagnosis is based on serology and on virus isolation. The cerebrospinal fluid may show xanthochromia (*see* **729**) and an elevated protein content but seldom many inflammatory cells.

Posterior paralysis resulting from an **immune-mediated ischemic vasculitis** is a rare complication of infection with **equine herpes virus-1**. Cases often have a history of previous challenge by the virus or vaccination, with recent or intercurrent coughing and/or abortion. The clinical signs associated with equine herpes virus-1 myeloencephalopathy usually have an insidious onset with mild, progressive gait deficits (ataxia). In some cases an acute onset of recumbency with posterior paralysis is present (**728**). Bladder and anal paralysis with flaccid relaxation of the vulva or penis and an area of perineal hypalgesia, very similar in distribution to that shown in cauda equina neuritis (*see* **710**) are often found. Amongst the other vague clinical signs, affected horses may show xanthochromia of the cerebrospinal fluid (**729**).

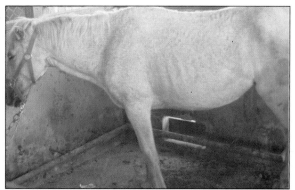

724 Venezuelan equine encephalitis (early case).
Note: Drooping of ears and somnolence.

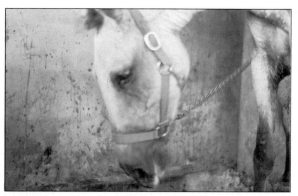

725 Venezuelan equine encephalitis (early case).
Note: Salivation secondary to dysphagia (pharyngeal and esophageal paralysis).

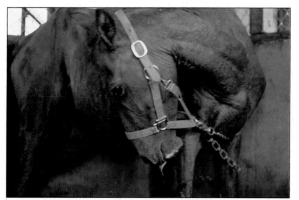

726 Venezuelan equine encephalomeyelitis.
Note: Profuse, whole body sweating, obvious right side turn of the neck (tendency to circle to the right if not tethered). Frothing from the mouth and nares attributed to dysphagia.

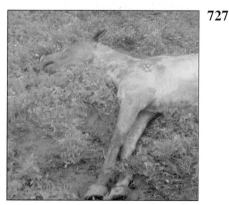

727 Venezuelan equine encephalitis (early case).
Note: Seizure appearance. Extensor rigidity. Scuff marks from paddling and head thrashing.

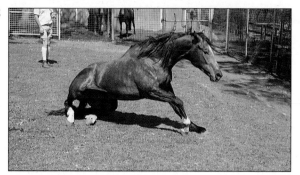

728 Equine herpes-1 virus (neurological syndrome).
Note: Posterior paralysis.
Differential Diagnosis:
i)   Rabies
ii) Traumatic/space-occupying lesion in cord
iii) Equine degenerative myeloencephalopathy
iv) Equine protozoal myeloencephalitis
v)   Vertebral osteomyelitis (e.g. tuberculosis)
vi) Secondary neoplasia (e.g. squamous cell carcinoma)
vii) Bracken fern (*Pteridium aquilinum*) poisoning
viii) Bilateral/generalised myopathy

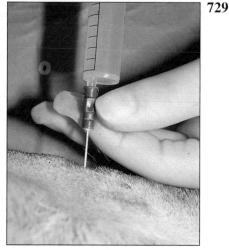

729 Equine herpes-1 virus (neurological syndrome) (xanthochromic cerebrospinal fluid).
Note: Few cells present but elevated protein.

Bacterial Diseases: Bacterial infections of the central nervous system are usually secondary effects of septicemic and bacteremic conditions. Any bacterial involvement in the brain, cord or meninges is potentially devastating in terms of the neurological consequences. Most of the clinical signs are non-specific, however. As there is a much higher prevalence of septicemia and bacteremia in foals and as the normal protective mechanisms for the central nervous system are poorly developed in neonatal foals, this is the class of horse which is most commonly affected by bacterial meningitis and encephalitis. The underlying primary bacterial condition may attract more immediate attention, but unless the earliest signs of central nervous system involvement are detected, the prognosis for the animal becomes rapidly worse. In the older horse bacterial meningitis is usually a result of direct extension of localised infective sites such as tail docking abscesses or infected epidural injections, but equally, may be the result of streptococcal septicemia in Strangles cases (*see* **226** *et seq.*), or from other septic foci. Affected horses are febrile and there is a wide variety of clinical possibilities, depending upon the site and extent of the inflammatory lesion. Blindness, seizures and coma represent the terminal stages but limited ataxia, often with spasticity and mild paresis may be seen in one or more limbs. Abscesses developing within the substance of the brain are usually more severe in one locality, in spite of being multiple or, sometimes a single lesion is responsible. Under such circumstances, the clinical signs would be expected to reflect the unilateral, space-occupying and destructive, nature of the disorder. Circling to one side, head tilt, a unilateral central blindness and ataxia would suggest this state. Definitive diagnosis in the live animal is heavily dependent upon the examination of cerebrospinal fluid which contains inflammatory cells and has a high protein content. Post mortem examination of horses with brain abscesses reveals characteristic pyogranulomatous lesions with overlying pressure necrosis (**730**). Compression of adjacent areas of the brain or brain stem cause herniation or displacement of considerable portions of the softer cerebral cortex (*see* **730**). Blood vessel disruption may result in the presence of large (often significant) hematomas, particularly in the more caudal parts of the brain (*see* **730**).

730 Bacterial pyogranuloma.
Note: Sections from a pony showing waxing and waning signs referable to the left cerebrum. There was a prominent neutrophilic pleocytosis in the cerebrospinal fluid. Severe, multifocal pyogranulo-matous meningitis (generalised ependymitis), suppurative optic neuritis (**See 643**) and choroiditis. Marked brain swelling and compression (in the top two sections) and obvious compression of the grey matter of the cerebral cortex (surface of the brain in the lower right section). The middle lower section shows herniation of the ventral portions of the occipital lobes under the *tentorium cerebelli* which compressed the mid-brain from dorsal and lateral aspects. A large hematoma is present in the bottom left section which is from the caudal cerebellum and arose from blood vessel disruption.

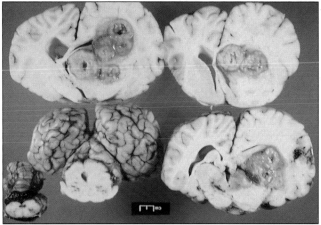

730

Abscesses in the spinal cord, either developing primarily at this site or those developing from contiguous lesions in the vertebral bodies or meninges may present a similarly variable range of symptoms. These will depend on the site, extent and rate of expansion of the septic focus. **Diffuse bacterial meningitis**, involving the meninges of both the cord and the brain, is a catastrophic disorder with a multitude of clinical signs ranging from severe depression to quadriplegia and convulsions.

Clostridium tetani in wounds produces, under suitable local anerobic conditions, a group of potent neurotoxins. While it is these toxins which are responsible for the development of the clinical signs associated with **tetanus**, the condition is best regarded as a primary bacterial infection. The horse has a much higher sensitivity to the toxin than most other domestic animals, and this, along with its considerable propensity for skin injuries and penetrating wounds, make it a prime candidate for the disease. Foals may become infected through the umbilicus. Initially, affected horses show a marked hyperesthesia with a tendency to over-respond to external stimuli. Tetanic spasm of the masseter muscles and, later, the muscles of the neck, trunk and limbs, develops with increasing severity. An apparently hyper-alert, somewhat enquiring expression and salivation are often present (**731**). Prolapse of the third eyelid (nictitating membrane) (**732**) is a characteristic feature, particularly after mild external

731

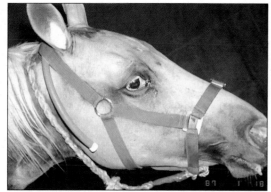

731 Tetanus.
Note: Fixed, alert facial expression, erect ears (swabs placed to avoid consequences of noise from camera), prolapsed third eyelid, nostrils drawn open and tense mouth.

732

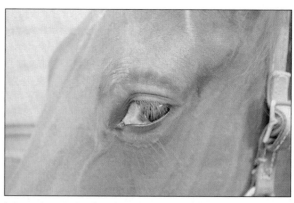

732 Tetanus.
Note: Prolapsed third eyelid and enophthalmos in response to sudden noise (and when face is tapped with a finger).

733

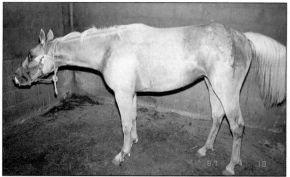

733 Tetanus.
Note: (Same horse as **731**) Tail-head elevation. Horse showed stiff, stilted gait.

734

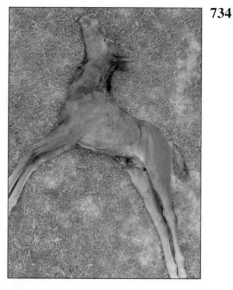

734 Tetanus.
Note: Opisthotonus and extensor rigidity of the neck, limbs, trunk and tail (hypertonia and tetanic spasm). Recumbency with these signs carries an extremely poor prognosis.

stimuli, such as a light tap below the eye or under the jaw. Progressive involvement of the body muscles results in a stiff gait and elevation of the tail head (**733**). Once a horse with tetanus becomes recumbent and exhibits opisthotonus with continuous severe generalised muscle spasms (**734**) they usually die from respiratory paralysis and exhaustion. Confirmation of the diagnosis is often difficult but the clinical appearance is usually sufficient. The finding of a penetrating injury is helpful but in many cases the wound is not apparent and indeed, some cases develop from foot infections or from other sites which are not overtly infected.

Botulism is caused by the neurotoxin produced by *Clostridium botulinum*. The toxin is extremely potent and the ingestion of even minute amounts may result in severe, and often fatal, neurological disease. Horses may become affected through direct ingestion of the toxin in food (forage poisoning), or from the production of the toxin within the gut as the organism multiplies therein, or from contamination of open wounds with the bacteria and local absorption of the toxin. Silage and poorly preserved brewer's grains have been identified as a relatively common source of the toxin. Foals are more liable to the toxico-infectious form in which the organism multiplies in the gut and the toxin is absorbed continuously. Under these circumstances it produces the **'Shaker Foal Syndrome'** in which a progressive symmetrical motor paralysis with dysphagia, a stiff gait

735 Botulism.
Note: Tongue withdrawal absent.

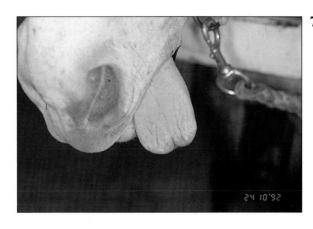

and extensive muscular tremors, are prominent signs. The tongue has a dramatic loss of tone and can easily be withdrawn from the mouth and then fails to be drawn back (**735**). Death is usually due to aspiration pneumonia. In the adult horse the clinical signs are somewhat different and are most often due to forage poisoning when the toxin is ingested from contaminated food. In these the signs are often associated with a progressive and serious paresis, recumbency and respiratory distress. Dysphagia (**Plate 6r**, page 123) with a flaccid tongue (*see* **735**), is a common early sign. Affected horses are often found 'playing' with water in a bucket; in fact, they are thirsty but are unable to prehend or swallow the water. Swallowing movements may appear to be made but are ineffectual. More extensive loss of tone in skeletal muscles results in the loss of tail tone, ptosis (drooping of the upper eyelid), and a stiff, stilted and stumbling gait. Loss of bowel and bladder tone are indicated by constipation and dribbling of urine respectively. There is a typical complete absence of normal bowel sounds. Death from respiratory paralysis is usually very quiet and peaceful although in some cases distressing agonal convulsions and struggling arises as a result of progressive anoxia. A diagnosis of botulism can be confirmed by the finding of the toxin in intestinal contents by ELISA methods. The presence of the organism or the toxin in the food or the environment of the horse is a strong supportive finding.

Protozoal Diseases: One of the more serious neurological conditions occurring in North America and parts of South America, is **protozoal myeloencephalitis**. The disease which is caused by organisms of the *Sarcocystis* genus, is characterised by a wide range of neurological dysfunction involving multifocal lesions in either brain or cord, or both. Lesions in the spinal cord appear to be more frequent than those in the brain and therefore the commonest presenting signs are those attributable to cord damage. These include progressive ataxia and occasionally long-standing, ill-defined lameness. As the condition causes degeneration of both grey and white matter, both weakness and muscle atrophy are prominent features of the spinal form of the disorder. Atrophy of individual muscle masses such as the quadriceps (**736**) and the gluteals (*see* **711**) is common. The multifocal nature of the condition means that the clinical effects are asymmetric and unpredictable. Where lesions occur in the brain the consequences are again variable and depend largely upon the site and extent of the changes. Thus, individual cranial nerves may become non-functional and result in well defined disabilities. Unilateral lesions involving the motor functions of the trigeminal nerve, resulting in dramatic atrophy of the masseter, digastricus and temporalis muscles (**737**), is a relatively common effect. This severe, apparently sharply defined atrophy is pathognomonic of the disease in endemic areas. Sensory nerves, including the sensory components of the trigeminal nerve, are maintained. Cases of equine protozoal myeloencephalitis in which both cord and brain are affected show combinations of these symptoms. Abrupt onset of asymmetric tetraparesis, ataxia, head tilt, leaning to one side, depression and generalised weakness, in limited areas of the body represent typical signs (**738**). Examination of cerebrospinal fluid is often unrewarding although in some cases there may be xanthochromia and a mononuclear pleocytosis. At post mortem examination significant lesions are confined to the central nervous system. Dark red, hemorrhagic, soft (malacic) foci ranging in size and location are to be found in either white or grey matter of brain or cord (**739**) (or both).

736

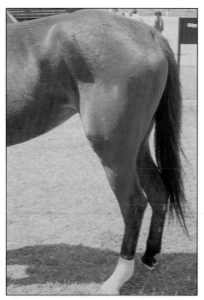

736 Equine protozoal myeloencephalitis (spinal cord form - lumbar lesion).
Note: Selective atrophy of *Quadriceps femoris* muscle only in this case.
Differential Diagnosis:
i) Peripheral nerve (femoral) degeneration or trauma.
ii) Cauda equina neuritis

737

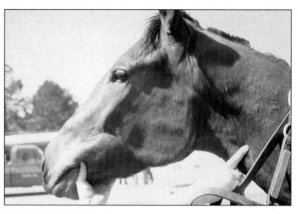

737 Equine protozoal myeloencephalitis (central [cranial nerve] form - brain stem lesion).
Note: Selective severe atrophy of masseter and temporalis muscles only.
Differential Diagnosis:
i) Peripheral nerve degeneration or trauma
ii) Cauda equina neuritis
iii) Heavy metal poisoning
iv) Masseter myopathy
v) White muscle disease

738

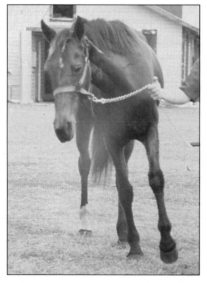

738 Equine protozoal myeloencephalitis (mixed central [cranial nerve] and spinal form).
Note: Asymmetric ataxia, hypometria (involvement of cervical spinal cord), leaning and circling.
Differential Diagnosis:
i) Cervical vertebral instability (Wobbler) syndrome
ii) Equine viral encephalomyelitis
iii) Central/cervical trauma
iv) Verminous migrations
v) Equine degenerative myeloencephalopathy
vi) Sorghum poisoning, lathyrism
vii) Heavy metal poisoning

739

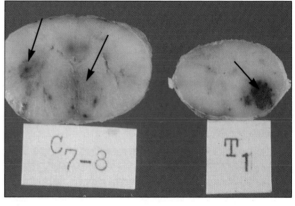

739 Equine protozoal myeloencephalitis (spinal form - cord sections from cervical and thoracic cord).
Note: Multifocal, asymmetric, necrotising, granulomatous myelitis (arrows). This case demonstrated an abrupt onset of progressive asymmetric tetraparesis and ataxia which was worse on the left side and in the right thoracic limb.

Parasitic Diseases: A number of parasites are known to cause central nervous signs when their migration involves accidental deposition in nervous tissue of cord or brain. *Strongylus vulgaris* and *Hypoderma* spp. are most often implicated. Direct migration into nervous tissue or indirect vascular occlusion or rupture, represent the mechanisms of damage which can, potentially, be afflicted by any of these parasites. Affected horses are not necessarily heavily parasitised. Most cases of **verminous myelitis** have a peracute onset of rapidly progressive asymmetric gait deficits, associated in most cases by focal infarctions caused by *Strongylus vulgaris* larvae, in the forebrain or cord. In some cases periods of remission and progression may follow longer courses. However, neurological deficits invariably persist to some extent in spite of long convalescence and prompt treatment to remove the active larvae from the body. A wide variety of clinical signs may be found including gait deficits and Horner's Syndrome (*see* **694** *et seq.*).

Neoplastic Disorders

Although **epileptiform convulsions** are often reported in the horse there are few well defined clinical syndromes related to the central nervous system which are associated with it. Most cases of convulsions have an organic origin relating to cerebral, cerebellar, or meningeal inflammation or are the result of neurotoxins or other poisonous substances, including lead, in the circulation. **Benign epilepsy of foals** has a characteristic onset in very young foals and in these cases the form of the convulsions is more or less constant with prodromal signs and post-ictic depression. **Brain tumours** responsible for central nervous disorders are particularly unusual, and are the preserve of the mature or older horse. In these cases the form of convulsion is variable from case to case, but may be similar with gradual progression in the event that there is a space-occupying lesion in the brain substance itself (**740**). Ante-mortem diagnosis is notoriously difficult unless the lesion is very large and is detectable radiographically or by scintigraphy or computer assisted tomography. Abnormal electrical activity may be detectable but a diagnosis of intracranial neoplasia often relies on secondary effects such as loss of thermoregulation, visual deficits and the presence of convulsions.

Tumours of the pituitary gland (*see* **365**) may have central effects through compression of the adjacent thalamic and brain stem tissues but in most cases the obvious clinical signs relate to the endocrine system. In many of these cases loss of thermoregulation is responsible for persistent sweating.

Tumours involving structures adjacent to the brain such as those in the paranasal sinuses and nasal cavity (**741**) may affect the cranium. Generally these do not extend into the meninges or brain itself and their significance is in their space-occupying nature (**742**). Space-occupying lesions within the cranium exert a wide variety of effects but where they are slow growing and impinge on the cerebrum there may be no detectable effect but conversely there may be a range of neurological abnormalities including epileptiform convulsions, blindness and defects of gait and posture.

Secondary tumours in the spinal cord are more common than those in the brain itself, and most arise from direct, contiguous spread from adjacent tissues such as the bone of the vertebral body or from invasion of the epidural space. **Melanomas** are the commonest form of metastasis into the cord. Hematogenous spread into central nervous tissue is extremely rare.

A common incidental post mortem finding in the lateral ventricles and choroid plexus of older horses is clusters of **cholesterol granulomata (743)**. They are probably not of any clinical significance even when they attain a considerable size.

Neuromas forming at the site of surgical neurectomy or other traumatic damage to peripheral nerves (**744**) may have serious secondary effects including persistent pain at the site and local occlusion of adjacent blood vessels, with correspondingly serious results. The commonest site for their development is at the site of posterior digital neurectomy. A few cases subjected to this form of permanent pain relief suffer from recurring, local hyperesthesia and sometimes persistent, serious pain. The masses may be small and have few other effects but occasionally they become extensive and invasion of adjacent blood vessels results in occlusive ischemia of the digit and sloughing of the foot.

740

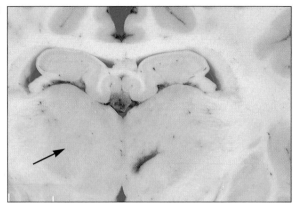

740 Undifferentiated glioma (arrow).
Note: Obvious asymmetry of brain stem. Horse suffered from epileptiform convulsions of progressively deteriorating nature over 3 months. Marked pro-dromal 'star gazing' was present and the timing of the fits could be accurately predicted. Severe post-ictic depression followed each episode.

741

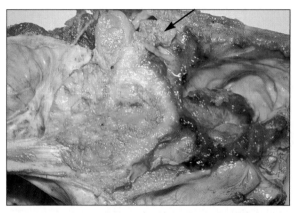

741 Cerebral compression.
Note: Horse blind in left eye and occasional seizures. Neoplastic lesion in ethmoid region of nasal cavity (arrow).

742

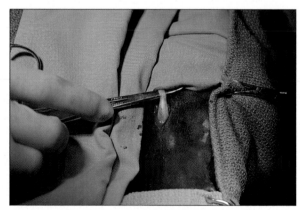

742 Cerebral compression (same horse as **741**).
Note: Loss of frontal pole sulci on left side (arrow) due to compression by neoplastic lesion in nasal cavity and extending through calvarium.

743

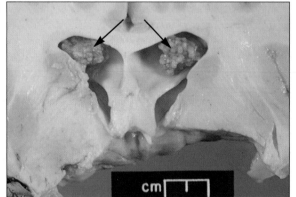

743 Cholesterol granulomata (in ventricles) (arrows).
Note: A common incidental finding in old horses.

744

744 Neuroma.
Note: Occurred at site of digital neurectomy and was associated with persistent pain and local hyperalgesia.

Tumours of peripheral nerves (Schwannoma or neurofibroma) are relatively common in the eyelids and periorbital skin. The masses may reach considerable size **(745)** and closely resemble sarcoids in this site. On occasion the more aggressive neurofibrosarcoma may be found in a similar site **(660)** and these are locally more aggressive and invasive, often spreading into the orbit and periorbital bone. Even these, however, commonly have a dermal component (possibly the origin) in the eyelid.

745

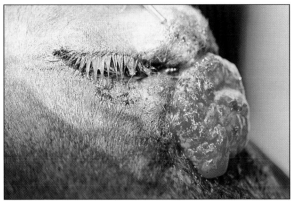

745 Neurofibroma.
Note: Tumour has eroded the skin and appears as a rapidly expanding granulomatous mass.

Further reading

Large Animal Neurology. A Handbook for Veterinary Clinicians
I.G.Mayhew (1989) Lea & Febiger, Philadelphia, USA

Current Therapy in Equine Medicine 2
Ed. N.E.Robinson (1987) Pub. W.B.Saunders, Philadelphia, USA

Current Therapy in Equine Medicine 3
Ed. N.E.Robinson (1992) Pub. W.B.Saunders, Philadelphia, USA

Manual of Equine Practice
Rose and Hodgson (1993) W B Saunders, Philadelphia, USA

Equine Clinical Neonatology
Koterba, A.M., Drummond, W.H., and Kosch, P.C. (1990) Lea & Febiger

Equine Stud Farm Medicine
Rossdale, P.D. and Ricketts, S.W. (1980) Baillière Tindall, London, UK

11. Reproductive disorders

Part 1: The Mare

Clinical examination of the mare

Adequate restraint, preferably the use of an examination stock or crush, is advisable so that undivided attention can be more safely given to the examination. It may be necessary to tranquillize some mares but a quiet, unhurried approach will often allow the initial examination to be made. Initially, the external genitalia should be assessed, the perineum cleaned and the urinogenital tract examined. This should first be observed by speculum and then by manual and digital palpation of the cervix and vaginal vault. Manual palpation per rectum of the uterine body, horns, ovaries and cervix should follow. Most reproductive examinations now require ultrasonographic examination of the ovaries and tubular tract to complete the basic examination. Specialist examination includes endometrial biopsy, the taking of uterine and clitoral swabs for cultural examination and finally, the use of endoscopy of the vagina, cervix and uterus.

A thorough history of the mare's breeding life is necessary to complete the examination. Should abnormalities be detected in the process of the examination, more detailed examination of particular areas is then warranted.

Normal ovarian development and function

The proper functioning of the reproductive system in the mare is a complex interaction of hormone release, which is governed by the length of photoperiod, nutrition and other management factors. Functional anatomy and the maintenance of a controllable disease-free status, are important factors which have a significant role in the fertility of the mare.

The ovary (and testes) undergo remarkable enlargement in the fetus between the third and ninth month, due to hyperplasia and hypertrophy of the interstitial cells, and reaches maximum size at about 200 days. Regression of interstitial cells occurs from this point with diminution of size occurring. The fetal ovary reaches its maximum size at 7 – 8 months gestation and is a reddish brown ovoid structure with a thin grey cap covering two thirds of the free border (**746**), and weighs approximately 25 – 50 grams. During the embryological development of the ovary from mesonephric ducts and tubules, defects may occur which remain in adults as cystic structures. Cranial portions of these structures, when present, form the epoöphoron which in some mares is present as a cystic structure in close proximity to the ovary (**747**), and if the caudal mesonephric tubules become dilated from the duct the paroöphoron is formed, although it rarely becomes cystic. Other remnants of the mesonephric duct may persist at various levels of uterine tubes, uterus, cervix and vagina, to the level of the vaginal vestibule and if they do occur, they may appear as cystic structures.

The paramesonephric or müllerian ducts develop and fuse to form the uterine body, cervix and vagina. The caudal end of the vaginal passage may fail to open or be only partly open, resulting in a persistent hymen. When fully closed, this may trap uterine secretion anteriorly, and also cause failure of intromission when mated. This occurs more frequently in the Arabian breed than in the Thoroughbreds and Standardbred. It is the most common major congenital defect in the tubal system of the mare. Clinically, it may be complete or partial. Where it is complete, it is often not observed until the first breeding when it is either found incidentally or, more frequently, subsequent to an unsuccessful mating. Examination shows a completely walled off posterior vagina just cranial to the urethral opening. Surgical relief often releases a milky fluid which was previously trapped in the anterior vagina and uterus. Partial hymen are common in maiden mares and are usually found when investigating post-service hemorrhage. These tears heal without serious consequences. Normal fertility can be expected after initial correction occurs.

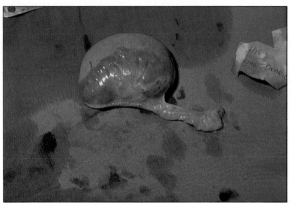

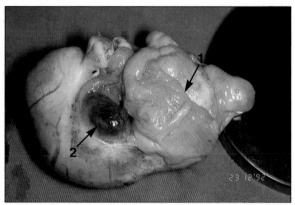

746 Fetal ovary (7–8 months gestation).
Note: Presence of thin grey cap covering most of the ovary.

747 Ovary with epoöphoron cyst (arrow 1) (12 year old mare).
Note: Four day old corpus hemorrhagicum protruding into ovulation fossa (arrow 2).

The equine ovary differs markedly from other species in that it undergoes rapid change during fetal development. It is beyond the scope of this work to discuss the complexities of this development; however, some of the more common abnormalities which persist into adult life are described later.

The Breeding Cycle

The estrus cycle in the mare may be regarded as the period between the ovulation of a mature follicle through to the ovulation of the next mature follicle. This is usually a period of approximately 21 days in Thoroughbred mares and up to 25 days in pony mares. The period between ovulations may be conveniently divided into separate identifiable periods which reflect changes in behaviour and in ovarian function. Estrus display and acceptance of the stallion begins before ovulation and normally lasts for 24–48 hours post ovulation. Thereafter the mare loses receptivity.

The luteal phase commences with the formation, first of the corpus hemorrhagicum which develops into the corpus luteum. The corpus luteum is responsible for progesterone production which peaks at approximately the ninth day after ovulation. Luteal regression, which then follows, is under the control of prostaglandins (PGF2). Following the regression of the corpus luteum the pattern of follicular development, which may be followed accurately with the aid of ultrasonography, changes in late diestrus and early estrus when the number of small follicles present, which had decreased in number with the approach of estrus, now increases. The number of medium size follicles remains relatively constant in the inter-ovulatory period due to recruitment from the smaller follicles. These medium-size follicles then continue to grow into larger follicles or alternatively become atretic. Those which continue to enlarge from mid to late diestrus, are probably stimulated by follicle stimulating hormone. This group of larger follicles (16–20mm diameter) reach their maximum size 5–7 days prior to ovulation, and then as either one or two ovulatory follicles undergo final maturation, the remainder of the group regresses. This peak of follicular activity is reached at the commencement of luteinizing hormone release and the onset of estrus.

The dimensions of mare ovaries, on average, are 50mm x 28m x 33mm, and the average weight is 120 grams. Pony mares have smaller ovaries with an average weight of only 43 grams. Equine ovaries have distinctive differences from other species. There is a relatively small ovulation fossa **(748)** with the ovarian stroma having a very fibrous appearance. Large areas of the surface are usually devoid of follicles **(749)**. Mature follicles may be as large as 70 – 80mm **(750)** and may be numerous. They may also persist for long periods without causing interference to a pre-ovulatory follicle proceeding to final maturation. A palpably large follicle (>70mm) should be carefully evaluated as this may, especially in Thoroughbreds, be due to the presence of more than one mature follicle. Up to 40% of Thoroughbred mares may have a double ovulation. Once ovulation occurs, a large corpus hemorrhagicum,

748

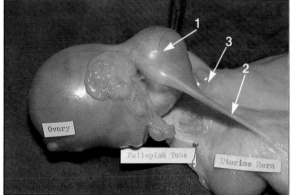

748 Normal ovary (showing follicle, infundibulum covering ovulation fossa (arrow 1), isthmus of uterine tuba (arrow 2), round ligament of uterus (arrow 3)).

749

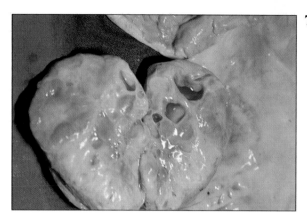

749 Ovary of 10-month pregnant mare.
Note: A small fibrous ovary showing some luteal tissue, a few atretic follicles and very few small follicles.

750

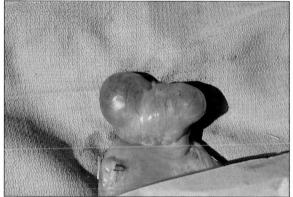

750 Normal ovary (showing mature, pre-ovulatory follicle - round but approaching pear shape of full maturity).

751

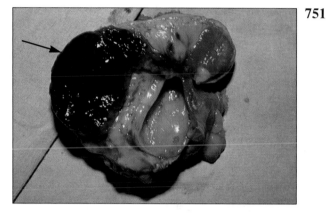

751 Normal ovary (showing corpus hemorrhagicum (arrow), 24 hours after ovulation).

approximately 70% of the size of the preovulatory follicle, develops (**751**). This may often be difficult to differentiate manually as it becomes smaller and is progressively luteinized. The primary corpus luteum, which on section has a yellowish hue (**752**), develops at the site.

The development of a dominant preovulatory follicle occurs with rapid enlargement to 45mm or more, and may be identified up to 6 days prior to ovulation. Based on ultrasonographic findings, this follicle undergoes shape changes as ovulation approaches, maturing from spherical shape to a pear-shape (*see* **750**). Ovulation occurs as a result of rising levels of luteinizing hormone, which reaches its peak concentration 1 – 2 days after ovulation, and culminates in the collapse of the preovulatory follicle and release of the oocyte. Service by a fertile stallion either results in pregnancy and the termination of the estrus cycle, or in the absence of conception, the recommencement of the next estrus cycle.

Variations from this cycle of events include ovulation in the luteal phase in approximately 9% of mares, and this can be responsible for a prolonged luteal phase (diestrus). Estrus, service and pregnancy can, rarely, occur in this period, but more often, the mare remains unreceptive.

Small atretic follicles occur in the mare (**753**) and are a phase in the maturation process when preovulatory-follicle growth is about 30mm; regression and atresia of the remaining follicles occurs. It is a gradual process, the initiating factors being unknown.

Follicular cystic degeneration which occurs in other domestic species does not occur in mares. It is frequently diagnosed clinically but cannot be substantiated on gross or histological examination. Mares may exhibit a long transitional phase from winter anoestrus to spring estrus, with estrus cycles up to 40 days being recorded. Typical ovaries show numerous slow growing follicles to be present, leading to the

752

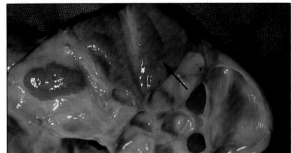

752 Normal ovary (showing mature corpus luteum (brownish/yellow tissue) (arrow), smaller corpus luteum and atretic follicles).
Note: Thickened walls of atretic follicles.

753

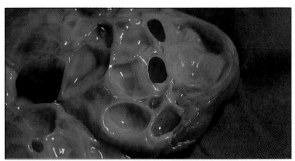

753 Normal ovary (transitional, pre-seasonal, 'spring estrus' ovary).
Note: Numerous small atretic follicles with a few medium follicles developing.

754

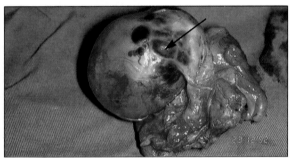

754 Normal ovary - aged mare.
Note: Marked varicosity of veins (arrow).

755

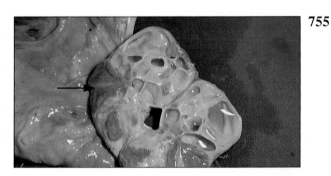

755 Normal ovary - Day 45 pregnancy.
Note: Primary corpus luteum (arrow) with numerous small secondary corpora lutea.

756

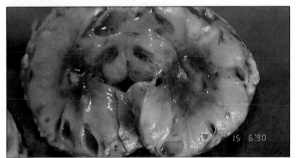

756 Normal ovary - pregnant mare.
Note: Fibrotic appearance with absence of normal breeding season cyclical structures (compare with **752**).

757

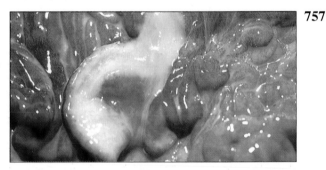

757 Normal uterus showing endometrial cups (50 days pregnant).

erroneous belief that this represents a cystic condition.

Prominent vessels are often present on the surface of the ovary and in some normal aged mares, may display even more marked varicosity (**754**).

Following conception, and at about Day 40 of pregnancy, secondary corpora lutea are formed (**755**). There is wide variation in their number between different mares. Both the primary and secondary corpus luteum begin to regress and are usually completely atrophic by about 210 – 220 days. From this stage forward, the ovaries of pregnant mares show little follicular activity (**756**).

The uterine horn and uterus receive the developing embryo 6 – 7 days post conception. At or around Day 36, a process of implantation of the girdle cells of the trophoblast into the uterine mucosa occurs. This is responsible for the creation of the endometrial cups (**757**) which are present from about Day 37 to Day 150.

One: The Ovary

Developmental Disorders

Embryological abnormalities of the reproductive organs include **intersexes**, **cystic aberrations of the genital tract**, **teratoma of the gonads** and **malformations of the tubular portions** of the system. Foetal and placental abnormalities are complicated by lack of sufficient knowledge of their embryological development.

Normal sexual development proceeds providing the embryo carries the normal karyotype which is expressed by the chromosome pattern 64.XX and the male as 64.XY; the sex chromosomes XX or XY being the principal determinant of the eventual physical and reproductive capacities of the individual horse. Chromosomal sex (either XX or XY) is determined at the time of fertilisation. **Defects of individual chromosome structure** and of chromosomal numbers may be of a very minute character but almost always have extremely serious consequences on future reproductive ability, leading in most instances, to partial if not complete **infertility**.

The use of karyotyping to determine individual abnormalities is a biological means of determining the gene status of that individual. Aseptic peripheral blood lymphocytes are cultured for 64 – 72 hours and then processed to eventually allow electron microscopic examination and comparison of 31 paired chromosomes plus 1 pair of sex chromosomes; differences are determined and so allow the identification of chromosomal abnormalities.

Mares presenting with chronic and primary **infertility**, having small ovaries, a flaccid uterus and cervix and hypoplastic endometrium, which fail to cycle regularly (or at all), are prime suspects for some type of chromosomal abnormality.

Of these abnormalities, **63.X gonadal dysgenesis (or 63.X0)** is the most common. Mares with this condition are often slightly undersize, and while they may have complete genital systems, they often have vestigial ovarian tissue which is difficult to palpate rectally **(758)**.

Abnormalities of the gonads where intersexuality occurs, may be classified according to their morphology. **True hermaphrodites** have one or both gonads containing both ovarian and testicular tissue **(759)**, or may have one male and one female gonad. **Pseudo-hermaphrodites** have the gonads of one sex and the accessory genitalia of the other. A female hermaphrodite has ovaries and male accessory reproductive organs (and the male hermaphrodite the reverse). Ovarian tissue may be extremely small or even absent. Predominant external features of equine hermaphrodites are ventral displacement of the vulva with an enlarged clitoris **(760)** or a short, backward-projecting penis **(761)**. Testes may be present with mammary tissue and teats. Testes, epididymis and vesicular glands are usually present abdominally as well as a poorly developed uterus. The genetic nature of this abnormality is uncertain but recorded cases indicate that individual stallions may sire intersex foals from different mares.

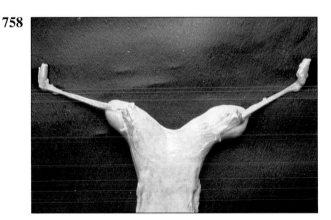

758 Chromosomal abnormality (**63.X0**) genital tract. **Note:** Very small ovaries and under-developed uterine horns and body.

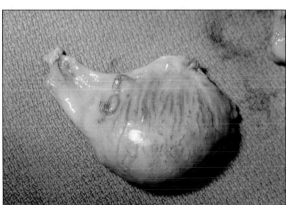

759 Intersex ova-testis (a gonad being an intersex mix of ovarian and testicular tissue cells)

760

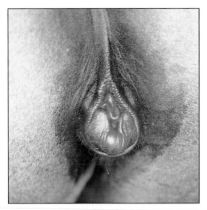

760 Female hermaphrodite.
Note: Vestigial opening of vulval lips, enlarged clitoral body.

761

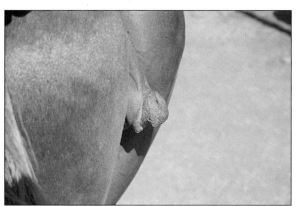

761 Pseudo-hermaphrodite (male horse with vestigial vulva and penis).
Note: Effectively used as a teaser.

Non-Infectious Disorders

A cystic condition of the ovaries has been reported following the feeding of melengestrol acetate (MGA), the cystic follicles so produced, remaining for a prolonged time through the winter until spring.

Luteinization is a normal process following ovulation; however, where apparent ovulatory failure occurs in late autumn, the maturation of the pre-ovulatory follicle would appear to be slow and it may either not fully develop, or it may fail to ovulate. It is possible for the **follicle to fill with blood (762)** which may persist for long periods. Ultrasonography is an essential aid in the diagnosis of this condition. Occasionally, surgical removal has erroneously been used as a treatment of these persistent hemorrhagic ovaries but when affected mares are examined after a winter anestrus they show full regression of this problem. Very occasionally, **granulosa cell tumours** can contain a large blood filled cavity (*see* **768**) and when this occurs, the diagnostic protocol should include both blood hormone levels and ultrasonography.

Persistent *corpora lutea* occur in the mare with and without a previous stallion cover. Mares exhibit anestrus and resent the teaser. These may occur at any stage in the breeding year but are most frequently associated with a prolonged interval without a return to estrus in a non-pregnant mare.

Epithelial inclusion cysts are multiple and occur in close proximity to the ovulation fossa increasing both in size and number with advancing age and these may interfere with ovulation. The other ovary usually continues to function normally and pregnancy may also occur.

Other structures occurring near the ovary include cysts of the mesonephric tubules; **epoöphoron cysts** (*see* **747**) and **paroöphoron cysts**. These slowly enlarge with time and consequently are more frequently found in aged mares. Epoöphoron cysts can reach up to 7 cm diameter and, on manual palpation, may be mistaken for part of the actual ovary. Paroöphoron cysts are smaller and less common.

762

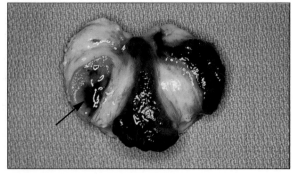

762 Autumn ovary.
Note: Follicle showing two corpora hemorrhagica and a blood filled follicle (arrow). Normal non-pathological finding.

Neoplastic Disorders

Epithelial cell tumours are rare and reports are confined to **cyst adenoma**. Clinically these may be identifiable per rectum as large cystic masses; fertility of the other ovary appears to remain normal and pregnancy may be uninterrupted following the surgical removal of the tumour. Affected ovaries are large (**763**) and enclose multiple, large cysts containing clear, yellow fluid (**764**); these masses probably originate from the epithelial cells of the ovulation fossa.

Papillary adenocarcinoma have also been described but are very rare. The affected ovary has a coarse nodular surface and the tumour may metastasize to other organs.

Germ cell tumours are also very rare but **dysgerminomas** may be associated with hypertrophic osteopathy of the lower limbs (*see* **416**), loss of condition and stiffness when walking. They are reported to vary in size but appear to metastasize early to the regional lymph nodes.

Teratomas have also been reported in equine ovaries which are enlarged and the mass contains fluid and an amorphous material with hair-like structures.

By far the most common ovarian neoplasm is the **granulosa cell tumour**. These are usually unilateral and vary considerably in size, but may reach 5 kg or more in weight. The tumours have a characteristic, multi-cystic appearance, and are seldom invasive. Affected mares show gross disturbances of hormone production, frequently showing altered behaviour patterns, including stallion-like behaviour (**765**), teasing, herding and mounting other mares and attacking geldings. Almost all have disturbances of the estrus cycle. Usually, one very small inactive ovary is found in conjunction with a grossly enlarged smooth (but occasionally nodular) mass in the other. Tumours vary in size from 6 – 40 cm diameter (**766**). Pregnancy may not be affected by the development of the tumours after conception but mares do not conceive if the tumour is established prior to mating. The majority of mares return to near-normal fertility after surgical removal of the affected ovary. Tumour bearing ovaries are often grossly enlarged with a smooth thickened capsule but sometimes give an impression of follicular structures being present (*see* **766**). On section, early tumours show multiple cysts with a thin stroma (**767**); older tumours show marked thickening of the stroma and may on occasion be filled with blood (**768**). The clinical diagnosis may be confirmed by the presence of increased plasma concentrations of testosterone and/or inhibin. The ultrasonographic appearance is also very typical (**769**), although this, on its own, may be confused with a number of the other cystic-like ovarian disorders such as the rarer dysgerminoma.

Other **mesenchymal tumours** such as hemangiomas, leiomyoma, fibroma and lymphoma (**770**), have been described but appear to be extremely uncommon.

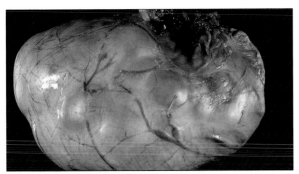

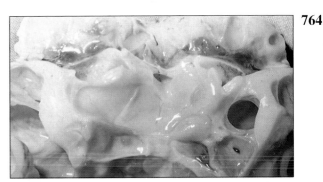

763 Ovarian cyst adenoma.
Note: Multiple follicle like cysts throughout ovary.

764 Ovarian cyst adenoma.
Note: Yellow tissue in stroma of ovary.

765 Granulosa cell tumour (mare showing stallion-like behaviour).

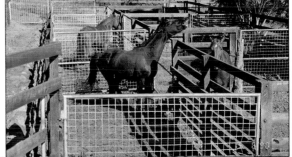

766

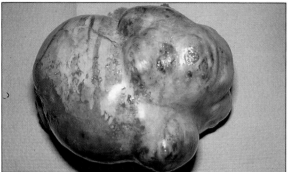

767

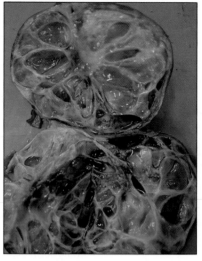

768

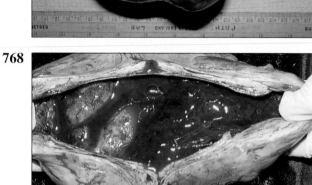

766 Granulosa cell tumour.
Note: Very large mass with a smooth surface having 'follicle-like' protuberances.

767 Granulosa cell tumour.
Note: Early tumour with thin fibrous tissue around multiple loculated cysts.

768 Granulosa cell tumour.
Note: Long-standing lesion showing hemorrhagic cyst within grossly enlarged ovary. Responsible for abdominal bleeding and persistent mild colic.

769

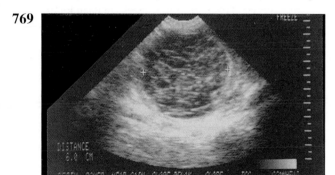

770

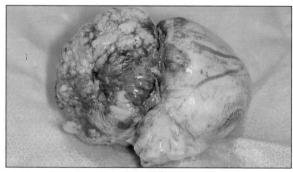

769 Granulosa cell tumour (ultrasound image).
Note: Older lesion with some loss of loculated appearance.

770 Ovarian lymphosarcoma.
Note: Ovary from 10 – year old mare with generalised lymphosarcoma involving the heart, diaphragm and colon. Complete loss of normal ovarian structure inside capsule; mare was found to be 5 months pregnant.

Two: The Fallopian Tubes and Uterus

The uterus comprises the two uterine horns, uterine body, and cervix.

Developmental Disorders

Congenital abnormalities of the uterus are rare in the mare but the finding of a bifid placenta without avillous areas (**See 888**) suggests that bifid uterus may occur, although this has not so far been described.

Non-Infectious Disorders

Accidental injury to the uterus or uterine wall occurs principally at parturition. The most common accident is the result of a foal's foot piercing the wall of a uterine horn (**771**). Mares with uterine tears of this type often appear to be clinically normal for some time after foaling, but after 1 – 8 days, become febrile and develop signs of peritonitis and progressive parietal pain. Many such cases die because of the insidious nature of the injury; the condition often is not recognised until the clinical situation is irretrievable.

The cervix is subject to **physical trauma** principally during parturition. This may show as slight to severe bruising, or more serious injury where full thickness tears can occur. These tears cause infertility if the integrity of the canal has been breached (**772**). Diagnosis can be difficult and requires methodical manual palpation of the entire perimeter of the cervical canal and possibly endoscopic examination. It may be necessary to examine the cervix during both diestrus and estrus to make a definitive diagnosis. Rough handling as a result of dystocia or medication may result in a reddened, inflamed cervix covered with a muco-purulent exudate (**773**). This may be complicated by an intercurrent endometritis. Adhesions between opposite

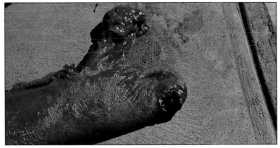

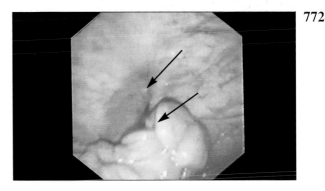

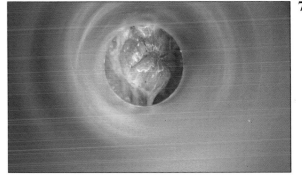

771 Uterine tear (caused by foal's foot).
Note: Mare died 8 days after foaling, lesion partly healed but severe peritonitis ensued. Note reddened serosa of uterus (See **890** for placental changes of this case).

772 Cervical and vaginal tear (endoscopic view of healed lesion).
Note: Tear in cervix and vagina in upper right quadrant (arrows). Found during investigation of infertility.

773 Cervicitis (speculum examination).
Note: External os inflamed and purulent exudate over surface.

774

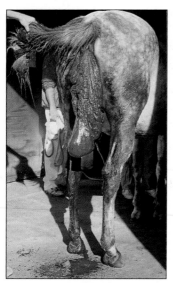

775

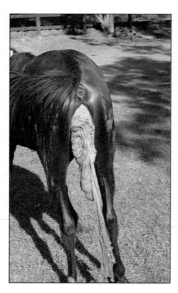

774 Prolapsed Uterus (followed prolonged dystocia)

775 Partial Uterine Prolapse (with retained fetal membranes still attached)

sides of the cervix may cause complete closure and lead to a closed pyometra and complete sterility (*see* **787**).

Prolapse of the uterus is a particularly serious event in the mare and if left unattended, a complete eversion rapidly ensues (**774**). The complications of this accident include rupture of the ovarian artery(ies) with consequent massive internal hemorrhage and/or shock from edema and trauma to the exposed uterus (*see* **774**) The condition carries a high mortality unless treated early and correctly. Prolapse of the uterus can occur after prolonged dystocia (*see* **774**), from the effect of abortion and undue abdominal straining due to irritation caused by retained fetal membranes (placental retention) (**775**).

Another condition which is part accident, part vascular lesion, occurs when **rupture of the middle uterine artery** (and less commonly utero-ovarian or iliac arteries) occurs, with hemorrhage into the broad ligament (**776**). It may occur in late pregnancy, following galloping over inclines, ditches, or immediately prior to, or during, parturition. Copper deficiency has been suggested as a contributory cause. Mares exhibit signs of restlessness, sweating, extreme pallor (**Plate 8e**, page 179), trembling and low-grade abdominal pain. Older mares, in which the condition is more common, may be found dead at, or immediately following, foaling. The findings at rectal examination vary according to whether the bleeding is contained in the broad ligament or whether blood escapes into the peritoneal cavity. In the former a tense fluid filled (often very large) mass can be identified in one broad ligament (*see* **776**) and there is usually no free blood in the peritoneal cavity. In these cases the mare may survive. Where bleeding is not contained there may be no significant rectal findings but the abdomen will contain

a large quantity of free (often clotted) blood, which can be identified by paracentesis. Surviving mares show a relatively high incidence of recurrence, with further rupture of the vessels in any subsequent pregnancy. Post mortem examinations suggest that the site of previous hemorrhages of this type becomes fibrosed and adhesions occur between the site and other abdominal organs. The reduction in natural, local elasticity may be sufficient to increase the likelihood of tearing during a subsequent pregnancy or parturition.

Hemorrhage may also occur **within the wall of the uterus** and should the consequent hematoma rupture into the lumen or into the abdominal cavity, the mare will probably have a fatal hemorrhage. Post mortem examination shows rupture of major intramural blood vessels, forming either large hematomas within the uterine wall (*see* **776**) or evidence of rapid exsanguination with profound anemia (**Plate 8e**, page 179) and large volumes of blood in the abdominal cavity or within the uterus.

Cystic conditions of the uterine wall occur and these can be small multiple cysts or one or more large 5–50 mm sub-mucosal cysts. Ultrasonography has considerably aided in their location and detection; many become thick-walled and remain as permanent features, appearing on ultrasonograms as relatively thick-walled, fluid-filled structures (**778**). Up to 6% of mares show mild (**779**) to severe uterine cysts, but the majority appear to have little effect on the mare's fertility. Indeed, the blastocyst may attach at the site of these cysts without any apparent deleterious effect upon the course of the pregancy (*see* **778**).

Retained fetal membranes (placental retention, retained afterbirth) is not an uncommon occurrence in

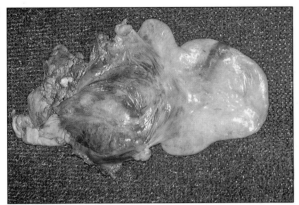

776 Broad Ligament Hematoma (post partum).
Note: Mare died from ruptured middle uterine artery. Large swelling (hematoma) visible in broad ligament, which was palpable per rectum before death.

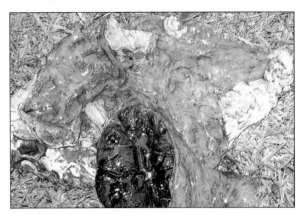

777 Uterine Wall Hematoma.
Note: Swelling incised to show large intramural hematoma with hemorrhage into uterus; pressure in uterine wall caused colic; loss of blood caused shock and death.

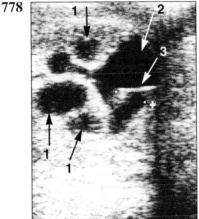

778 Uterine/Endometrial Cyst (Ultrasonographic appearance).
Note: Three small endometrial cysts (arrows 1) under a normal 28 day blastocyst (arrow 2) in which the embryo is visible (arrow 3). Sequential examinations showed normal advancing pregnancy which terminated normally at full term. There was no apparent change in size or structure of the cysts which were detected prior to the next breeding season.

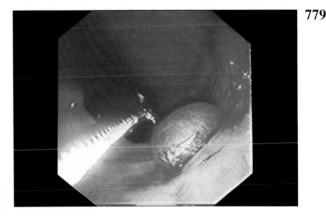

779 Endometrial Cyst (Endoscopic appearance).
Note: Small cyst identified during routine ultrasonographic examination.

the mare. The definition of retained fetal membranes varies according to the accepted duration of the third stage of labour. Individual veterinarians consider that membranes are retained if stage three of labour (placental delivery) is not completed within 4 hours, while others accept a normal of up to 12 hours or sometimes even more. In colder climates (or in winter), it may not be unreasonable to suggest 12 – 24 hours to be normal, but in stressed mares after abortion, difficult dystocia, or where ambient environmental temperatures are high, prolonged retention leads to severe and often fatal endometritis. There is a relatively high incidence of uterine prolapse amongst mares having retained fetal membranes (*see* **775**). Clinically, the fetal membranes may be either visible and partly expelled, or they may be totally contained in the uterus and therefore, unfortunately, unaccountable. Commonly, the mare becomes clinically ill before this is detected and rectified. One of the most common types of retention of fetal membranes is where the chorio-allantois attached within the non-pregnant horn is broken off and retained in the uterus. Unless all placentas are carefully examined immediately they are passed, it may not be discovered until the mare becomes dangerously ill. Small fragments of placenta attached to the endometrium (**780**) are, possibly, an even more dangerous problem as the fragment may not be missed on a cursory examination of the placenta. The onset of endometritis may be even more insidious but is, ultimately, no less dangerous. In either case the mare usually becomes ill 2 – 3 days after

780

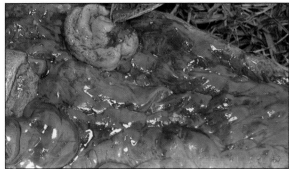

781

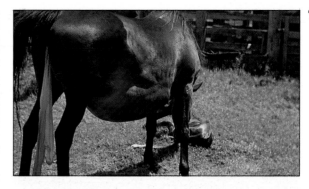

782

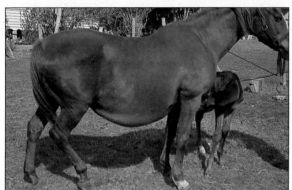

780 Retained fetal membranes (portion).
Note: Remnant of necrotic placenta still attached to uterine wall in mare dying of endotoxic shock, laminitis and septicemia 6 days after foaling. Dark brown, fetid, soupy exudate in uterus.

781 Rupture of prepubic tendon (Abdominal Wall).
Note: Massive edema and collapse—ventral abdominal wall level with hocks developed 6 weeks before foaling. Assisted parturition produced a normal foal. Swelling remained after foaling. No further breeding.

782 Abdominal wall edema.
Note: Subcutaneous edema only; had been present for over 7 weeks prior to foaling; swelling regressed by 10 days post partum.

foaling due to endometrial infection and consequent toxemia. Laminitis (*see* **409**) and endotoxic shock are commonly encountered in mares with retained fetal membranes of all types. Furthermore the rate of progression of the laminitis is usually particularly rapid and the prognosis for these cases is particularly poor.

Other physical conditions which can affect the uterus are related to **ventral or lateral abdominal herniation of the uterus** and/or rupture of the prepubic tendon which occurs in older mares. The latter condition often arises spontaneously without obvious previous excessive exercise or injury. A lowered ventral abdominal wall is usually obvious—usually level with the hocks or lower (**781**). Where ventral hernias are also present, careful monitoring of parturition is essential as foals can be deformed by mal-positioning due to entrapment within the hernia or, alternatively, the mare may have difficulty in delivering the foal and/or the placental membranes. This condition must be carefully differentiated from the commoner, benign, subcutaneous edema of the ventral abdominal wall which is due to circulatory changes caused by the weight of the foal (**782**).

Uterine torsion occurs in late pregnancy, but not usually in the last month; mares show discomfort and signs of low-grade, or sometimes more severe, colic. Diagnosis is usually possible by rectal palpation but mares may require sedation for this. Vaginal palpation is not always a reliable indicator of mild or early cases but where torsion is extensive it is usually a useful aid to the diagnosis.

Infectious Disorders

Salpingitis occurs more frequently than fertility results would suggest, and although little is known about the disorder it is possibly due, in some cases, to infection. Many cases however, have no identifiable pathogenic (or other) organism and these are assumed to be due to other types of tubal obstruction and may then be classified as hydrosalpinx. In all cases the narrowing and possible complete occlusion of the fallopian tube results in the accumulation of fluid (**783**) and partial or total infertility. The latter arises most often when infection is responsible and both fallopian tubes are involved, either equally or to different degrees. Concurrent uterine infection would further reduce fertility. Unilateral adhesions are also more common than might be expected - the cause of both the inflammatory changes and the adhesions is not clear.

783

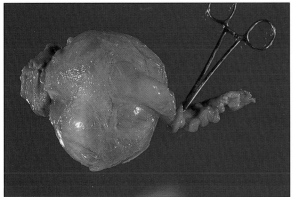

783 Salpingitis (hydrosalpinx).
Note: Found on autopsy; normal fertile mare with no history of infertility. No other abnormalities present.

784

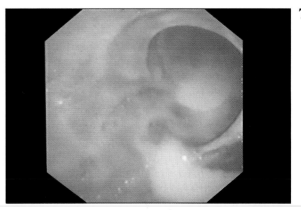

784 Endometritis (chronic) (endoscopic appearance).
Note: Purulent exudate in horns and body of uterus. Surface detail of blood vessels etc. obliterated by exudate, and inflammation and edema of mucosa.

785

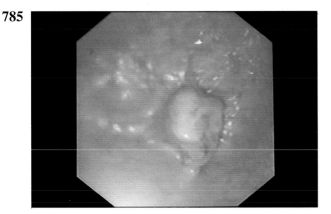

785 Endometritis (chronic) (endoscopic appearance of cervix).
Note: Cervical and vaginal discharge can be identified by direct observation using a speculum.

786 Pyometra/endometritis/vaginitis.
Note: Typical vaginal discharge associated with endometritis or purulent vaginitis; aged mare 3 days post service. Infertile.

786

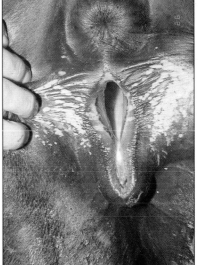

Infectious conditions of the uterus include **fungal and bacterial disease** causing **acute, chronic and low-grade endometritis**. Common uterine bacterial pathogens include *Streptococcus* spp., *Klebsiella* spp, *Pseudomonas* spp., *Escherichia coli* and *Proteus* spp.. Other bacteria are often isolated but most are contaminants and are frequently related to vaginal 'wind-sucking' (pneumovaginum) (*see* **796**) or poor perineal conformation (*see* **800**).

Acute endometritis (inflammation of the uterine mucosa) is usually associated with infectious processes immediately after parturition. Retention of the fetal membranes is one of the commonest causes of this serious disorder. Affected horses are seriously ill and show pyrexia, progressive endotoxemia, septicemia and laminitis. The mortality amongst these mares is high. A diagnosis can usually be reached from the presenting clinical features and vaginal and uterine examinations, during which an obvious, fetid uterine discharge is detected.

Chronic endometritis is a relatively common occurrence in older mares; clinically, cases show a mild uterine discharge which may be visible both inside the uterus, when viewed endoscopically (**784**) and at the cervix, when examined with the help of a speculum (**785**). Externally there is almost always an obvious vaginal discharge (**786**). Where uterine defence mechanisms are fully functional, some degree of endometritis is a frequent (and possibly, normal) transient stage following mating or foaling, but where local (or general) immunity is compromised, the condition may deteriorate to result in a persistent inflammation and a chronic discharge. Sustained infection results in overt metritis (deeper inflammation of the uterine wall and endometrium). The presence of a dark-tan, tarry, mucoid exudate is a normal finding 2 – 3 days post-partum and should not be confused with the potentially disasterous forms of metritis; the number and character of polymorphonuclear leucocytes can be used to assess the extent and severity of the condition and the benefit of therapeutic measures.

Post-partum pyometra, is a disease of older mares, or mares which undergo trauma and subsequent infection at parturition. The uterus becomes distended **(787)** with a purulent exudate which may be watery **(788)** or more creamy in consistency. There is usually little or no evidence of systemic disease and bacteria may, or may not, be isolated from the uterine contents. The commonest organisms identified include *Streptococcus zooepidemicus*, *Escherichia coli*, *Pasteurella* spp., *Pseudomonas* spp. and *Actinomyces* spp. The accumulation of purulent material is usually most severe in the body of the uterus and is often accompanied by concurrent severe endometritis with loss of endometrial integrity. The cervical canal often develops adhesions and may be completely sealed in 'closed' pyometra. While there is, in these cases, no vaginal evidence of an abnormality, the uterus is often particularly distended and easily recognised per rectum. The diagnosis of pyometra may also be confirmed by ultrasound and endoscopic examination and biopsy of uterine mucosa. The fertility of these mares is reduced to very low levels and usually they are best regarded as completely infertile.

Contagious equine metritis (CEM) is a highly contagious venereal disease of horses. The disease may be spread by fomites, instruments and gloves in addition to coitus and is caused by *Taylorella equigenitalis*. Clinically mares show a muco-purulent white discharge between 2 and 10 days post service (*see* **786**). The discharge may persist for up to 3 weeks and shortening of the estrus cycle is a common finding in affected animals. Experimentally infected mares showed mild, bilateral salpingitis. The inflammation is most severe at approximately 14 days after infection. There have, however, been no recorded erosions or hyperplasia of any of the glandular portions of the uterus. Diagnosis is confirmed by microaerophilic incubation of uterine, cervical and clitoral swabs on special media (chocolate or Amies agar). The disease is important because of its venereal nature and its deleterious effect on fertility.

Other bacteria, including some strains of *Klebsiella* spp. or *Pseudomonas* spp. can also be regarded as contagious and are usually the result of poor hygiene, allowing their establishment within the genital tract. In the case of *Pseudomonas* spp. the use of antiseptics prior to service as a control measure for other venereal infections, may allow, and even encourage, its proliferation and spread. Mares infected after service by stallions contaminated with *Pseudomonas* spp. may show ulceration and erosion of the clitoris and vagina.

Most mares affected by any of these opportunist pathogens, show early return to service, mucopurulent discharges after coitus with inflammation of the cervix, and a cervico-uterine discharge; isolation of organisms from uterine swabs must always be related to active clinical infection. Routine isolation of potentially pathogenic organisms from clinically normal mares must be interpreted carefully before prolonged antibiotic treatment is commenced to avoid possible harmful alteration of the normal bacterial flora in the uterus.

787

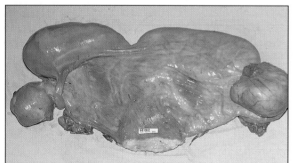

787 Pyometra.
Note: Easily recognised per rectum and by ultrasonography. Specimen showing entire uterine body with ovaries, grossly enlarged uterine horns. Infertile.

788

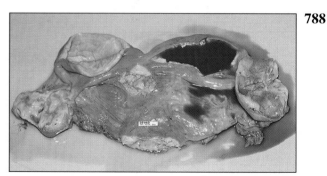

788 Pyometra.
Note: Uterus-autopsy specimen (same mare as **787**) showing red/brown purulent contents. Histopathological examination showed complete loss of normal uterine structures with severe fibrosis.

Neoplastic Disorders

Neoplasms of the uterus of the mare are most uncommon. Adenocarcinoma, fibroma, lymphosarcoma, rhabdomyosarcoma have been reported emanating from the uterine wall. A large **leiomyosarcoma (789)** may sometimes be misdiagnosed as a pregnancy but the solid pendulant nature of the mass is typical of the tumour. Metastatic secondary tumours in the wall of the uterus do not occur with any frequency.

789

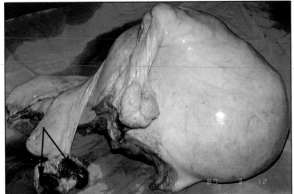

789 Leiomyosarcoma.
Note: Found in uterine cavity attached to ventral wall; mare had been anestrus for 4 months of breeding season and had been presumed in foal despite previous history of infertility. Note large hemorrhagic areas resembling corpora hemorrhagica in ovary (arrows).

Three: The Vagina, Vestibule and Vulva

Developmental Disorders

Very few developmental defects occur in this region in the horse. True hermaphrodites often have rudimentary anatomical features and some mares have a complete hymen which results in failure of intromission, complete infertility and, often, gross accumulation of uterine and vaginal secretions behind the membrane.

Non-Infectious Disorders

Varicose veins occur most commonly on the anterior, dorsal segment of the vagina **(790)**, but are found in other locations in the vaginal wall and vestibule **(791)**. The majority of severely affected mares are over 12 years of age, and show intermittent vaginal bleeding which is not necessarily (or even usually) related to mating or parturition. Most incidents, however, occur during the last month of pregnancy and may be mistaken for impending abortion or parturition. It is rare for more than 50 – 100 ml of blood to be lost but an occasional case may develop a fatal blood loss. Not all cases show prominent large veins and a definite diagnosis can often only be made immediately after, or during, a bleeding episode, when the hemorrhagic site can be directly visualised. By far the majority of cases are recognised sometime after the hemorrhage and the lesions have usually healed by the time they are examined. A reddish tinge may be detectable along the vulval margins in these cases.

Immunological conditions affecting the vulva rarely occur. **Bullous pemphigoid**, a vesico-bullous ulcerative disease which occurs at muco-cutaneous junctions, may affect the vulval-skin junction where ulceration with epidermal collarette formation may be seen.

Depigmented vulval and perineal skin (**vitiligo**) occurs following traumatic damage from service and foaling injuries or from viral and bacterial infections.

790

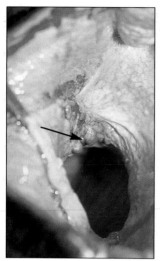

791

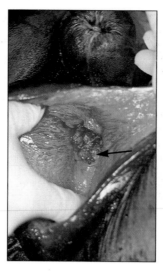

790 Vaginal varicosity (anterior).
Note: Varicose veins in anterior vault of vagina. Veins bleeding with clots of blood overlying veins (arrow); mare died 12 months later from a fatal hemorrhage, 1 month before foaling.

791 Vaginal varicosity (posterior).
Note: Small hemorrhagic 'grape-like' varicose veins in the posterior vagina (arrow). Bled frequently after service and occasionally following urination. Owner reported blood staining of vulval lips.

Mating and Foaling accidents

The mare is notoriously unpredictable with respect to foaling dates and times. Some mares run milk for several days (or sometimes weeks) prior to foaling, others have a normal udder or even no mammary gland development up to delivery, yet foal normally without any premonitory signs. Normally, parturition passes through the three stages of labour, often with minimal need for either interference or assistance. However the second stage of labour in the mare is particularly rapid, and usually so short that the equine obstetrician has little time for delay

792

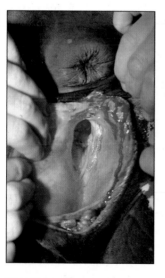

793

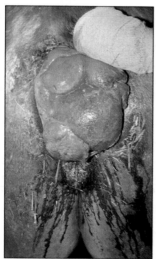

794

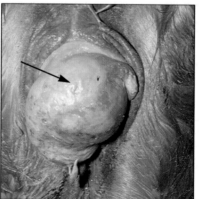

792 Vaginal scarring.
Note: This unusual, post-foaling complication followed severe, prolonged dystocia. Adhesions obliterated the vagina and cervix completely and the picture shows complete adherence of the urethral opening around perimeter of vagino-vulval junction. The opening shown is the urethral opening.

793 False cover (rectal prolapse following anal penetration by stallion).
Note: Severe edema of exposed rectal mucosa; care must be exercised not to further traumatize area during examination.

794 Vaginal prolapse (maiden mare).
Note: Prolapse of posterior vagina caused by irritation due to injury and vaginitis from stallion service. Note healing scar from trauma to vaginal wall caused by stallion (arrow).

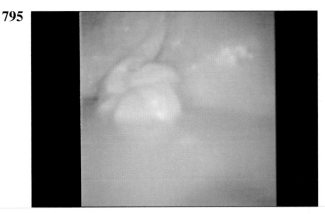

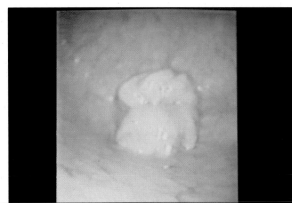

795 Urovagina (urine pooling) (endoscopic view).

796 Pneumovagina (vaginal wind-sucking).
Note: Dilated vagina with pale mucosa. Caused by poor vaginal conformation (vulval angle of 80°—see **800**).

if a live foal is to be delivered. Correction of malpresentation should be done as soon as it is evident. Failure to do so may lead to death of the foal and/or perineal lacerations or uterine tears. Other severe post partum injuries concerning other body systems include prolapse and eversion of bladder, or small intestine through the vaginal wall, vaginal and uterine tears (*see* **771**) or rupture of the mesocolon and/or small colon wall or small colon prolapse through the rectum.

Trauma to the vagina may occur at foaling, during service or as a result of examination or surgery. Mares are frequently bruised during foaling but this resolves quickly. Where trauma is more extensive, adhesions and fibrosis of the vaginal wall may occur leading to vaginal scarring and loss of elasticity. Some degree of urine pooling in the anterior vagina (with or without pneumovagina) is relatively common (*see* **795**). Subsequent fertility may be reduced in all these cases. Extensive vaginal tearing may occasionally result in extensive vaginal adhesions which may even occlude the vagina (**792**).

The vagina may also be traumatised during service, resulting in bruising of the cervix and vaginal vault in mild cases, actual rupture of the dorsal vaginal wall, above or adjacent to the cervix (*see* **772**). Affected mares strain vigorously and persistently after service and may show a blood stained discharge. Where contamination of the peritoneal cavity occurs as a result of both bacterial contamination and seminal fluid, low grade peritonitis results. Most cases respond to medical treatment and, only when the injury and peritonitis are associated with traumatised bowel, do mares commonly die following this injury. The complications arising from

herniation of bowel through the vaginal tear can be avoided in most cases by preventing the mare from lying down.

'False cover', a term used to indicate that a stallion has served the mare rectally and not vaginally, may result in severe straining and (temporary) **rectal mucosal prolapse (793)**. Some stallions become particularly adept at this and the stallion handler of such horses must be alert to prevent its continuing occurrence. Only rarely do mares show severe inflammatory damage and it is rarely fatal unless full thickness rectal tears have occurred. Great care must be taken as the mucosa is frequently bruised or torn and the defect may develop into a full thickness tear if rough manual examination follows the injury.

Vaginal prolapse occurs infrequently in the mare and is generally the result of persistent irritation or inflammation of the vaginal walls, bladder problems or impending abortion. A reddish mass of mucosa usually protrudes from the vulval lips (**794**) and careful clinical assessment must be undertaken to differentiate this from a prolapsed bladder (*see* **338**) or a bladder eversion (*see* **337**).

Urinary pooling, the accumulation of varying quantities of urine in the anterior vagina, which often covers the cervix, commonly occurs following difficult parturition, but may also be associated with nerve injuries, dropped abdomen (where the pelvic contents are dragged forwards and downwards), pneumovaginum, or from anterior displacement of the urethral opening for any reason. Clinical examination by speculum shows the accumulation of fluid in the anterior vagina (**795**). Where this is associated with estrus and

797

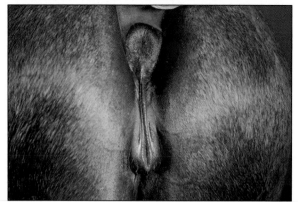

798

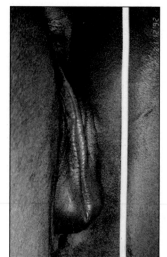

799

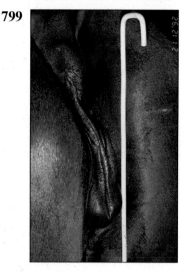

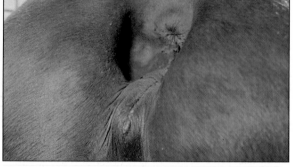

800

797 Normal Vulval (Perineal) Conformation.

798 Vulval angulation (10°).
Note: Common (near-normal) conformational shape; requires vulvoplasty (Caslick's operation) for best fertility results.

799 Vulval angulation (40°).
Note: Very poor conformation; always needs vulvoplasty (Caslick's operation). Surgery possible. Fertility often reduced significantly.

800 Vulval angulation (80°).
Note: No prospect of conception without combined perineal reconstruction (Pouret's Operation) and vulvoplasty (Caslick's Operation).

an open cervix, urine may run into the uterus, causing chronic infertility.

Pneumovaginum, a condition which is closely related to poor perineal conformation, is characterised by the ballooning of the entire vaginal vault with air, a blanched mucosa (**796**) and, in severe cases, the presence of fecal, and other particulate matter in the vagina. Where the condition is chronic, the vaginal walls and cervix may be inflamed. Affected mares often make flatulent noises when trotting. Racing fillies which have this condition are often poor-performers on the track, showing intermittent, low-grade, colic-like signs, 'cramps', straddling and frequent attempts to urinate after exercise.

Normal mares with good perineal conformation (**797**)

rarely exhibit pneumovaginum. However where the abdominal organs sink, due to a stretched or aged abdomen, they draw the rectum and anal sphincter cranially and, in so doing, progressively change the angle of declination of the vulva (**798**). Mares with vulval angles of less than 30°–40° (**799**) are most amenable to surgical treatment with Caslick's operation (vulvoplasty) (*see* **813**). Extremely poor conformation associated with vulval angles of over 70° (**800**) are very difficult to repair and while being assisted by surgery, these mares are never fully corrected and so they have a permanently reduced fertility. Surgical correction (Caslick's operation (vulvoplasty) or Pouret's operation for perineal reconstruction) are the only satisfactory solutions for most mares. Following Caslick's operation

801

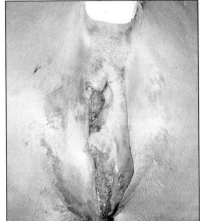

802

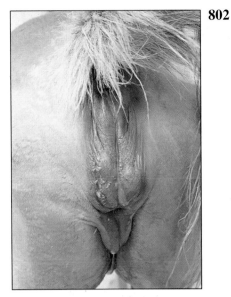

801 Vulval laceration (mare previously subjected to Caslick's operation).
Note: Severe lacerations following failure to carry out surgical episiotomy prior to parturition.

802 Vulval bruising.
Note: Unassisted foaling.

804

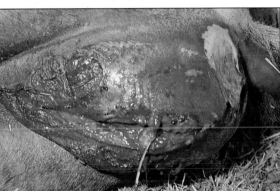

803

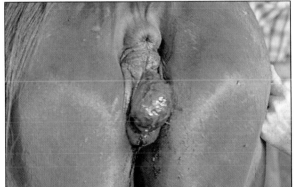

803 Vulval hematoma.
Note: Unassisted foaling.

804 Vulval bruising and laceration.
Note: Extreme bruising from foaling unattended for over 12 hours. Mare had showed complete foaling paralysis, never regained her feet and was killed.

805

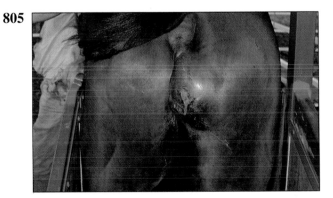

806

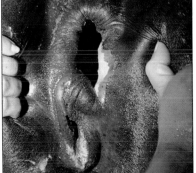

805 Vulval hematoma.
Note: Due to kick from another horse. Note marked, localised bruising over buttock -different in appearance to that shown in **803** which is entirely within the vulval tissue.

806 Recto-vaginal fistula.
Note: Perineal skin largely intact but fistula extended between dorsal vaginal wall and rectum. Resulted in gross fecal contamination of vagina and total infertility.

807

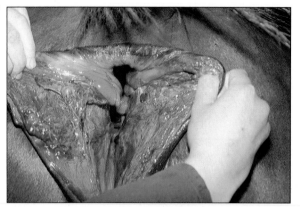

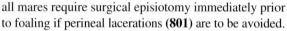

807 Third degree perineal laceration (fresh).

808 Third degree perineal laceration (Healed).
Note: Same mare as **807**, after 6 weeks; granulated
sufficiently for preparation for surgical repair.

808

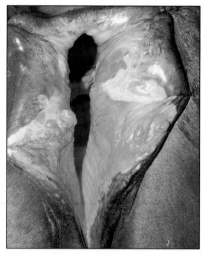

all mares require surgical episiotomy immediately prior
to foaling if perineal lacerations **(801)** are to be avoided.

Physical injury to the vulva occurs principally at
parturition and may result in bruising of the vulval lips
(802). With difficult foaling, vulval tearing and
hematoma formation occurs **(803)**, while more severe
and prolonged dystocia or grossly oversized foals may
cause very deep bruising and contusions to the vulva
(804). The most severe cases are occasionally
complicated by posterior paralysis which may not
recover and they then have to be killed. Trauma as a
result of kicking by other horses can also cause
hematoma and swelling of the vulva and perineum but
this has a different appearance **(805)**.

Fetal malpresentation in which one (or more) foot,
and even the head in some cases, may be forced to
penetrate and rupture the vagina and the rectum causes a
recto-vaginal fistula (806). When the trauma is more
severe and the foaling unattended, the foal may rupture

all the structures of the perineum between the rectum and
the vagina, resulting in a third degree perineal laceration
(807), in which an effective cloaca is created, with a
common anal and vulval external opening. The cranial
extent of the resulting cloaca depends upon the original
site of penetration. This may be within the anterior
vagina or at any point more caudal to this. Direct fecal
contamination of the vagina causes, in almost all cases,
a consequent moderate or severe endometritis and
complete infertility. Penetrations which occur anterior to
the pelvic reflection of the peritoneum result in opening
of the abdomen and possible prolase of intestine and, or
moderate, severe or extreme peritonitis. Repair of
perineal lacerations at the time of foaling is frequently
unsuccessful unless bruising is minimal and repair is
undertaken within 4 hours of the injury; otherwise it is
more appropriately carried out about 6 weeks later, once
second intention healing has occurred **(808)**.

Infectious Disorders

Infectious processes in the vagina are usually related to
events already described such as concurrent metritis or
endometritis or infected, traumatised mucosa from service
or parturition. Most such infections are bacterial or fungal
in origin. While **infectious vulvo-vaginitis** has been
reported in mares, specific causal organisms have not
been consistently demonstrated. Gross contamination of
the vagina with fecal material (where either rectovaginal
fistula or third degree perineal lacerations are present) or
urine (where poor vulval, vestibular, vaginal or perineal

conformation results in urovagina) inevitably results in
bacterial infection of the vagina (and in most cases of the
uterus). The organisms involved in these cases are usually
mixed contaminants and are seldom specific pathogens.

Infectious diseases affecting the vulva are principally
of viral and bacterial origin.

Viral Diseases: Viral disease such as **coital
exanthema** which is caused by equine herpes virus-3,
manifests short-lived vesicles which rapidly progress to
yellow-pigmented papules and, within 5 days, to crusty

erosions of the perineal skin (**809**). The disease is usually venereally transmitted but can be spread by fomites, gloves and gynecological instruments. Usually spread of this virus requires the vulval or vaginal mucosa to be abraded. Affected mares should not be served in the active stages of the infection; however no residual infertility has been found in mares recovering from the disease.

Bacterial Diseases: The clitoral sinuses which fill with smegma (**810**) are excellent repositories for **contagious equine metritis** (*Taylorella equigenitalis*). *Klebsiella* spp, *Pseudomonas* spp in carrier mares and other diseases due to *Streptococci* can also accidentally be located in these sinuses to readily contaminate or infect the stallion during service. Swabs taken for routine or clinical reasons, are obtained from the clitoris, clitoral sinuses, smegma pea, if present, and the urethral opening.

Bacterial diseases of the vulva are usually related to contamination from service or examination during breeding procedures. Organisms such as *Pseudomonas* spp. and *Streptococcus* spp. have been isolated. Generalised diseases such as **Bastard Strangles** (*see* **230, 231**) occasionally cause abscesses in and around the vulva. Such infections are frequently responsible for leukoderma and leukotrichia around the vulval lips.

Protozoal Diseases: Dourine, a venereal disease of equidae, caused by *Trypanosoma equiperdum* is spread by sexual contact. The disease has been known and recorded since 400AD and it is thought to have originated in North Africa and spread to other parts of Africa, Asia, Europe, USSR, Indonesia and the Americas. Currently it has been eradicated from parts of Africa, USA and Western Europe. Edematous vulval swelling occurs 8-14 days post contact with a variable dirty mucopurulent discharge from the vulva, but these signs are not pathognomonic and the organism responsible is often difficult to detect. Irritation of the vulvovaginal mucosa leads to frequent attempts to urinate with the mare showing discomfort by leg stamping, tail twitching and rapid blinking of the vulval lips and clitoris. Severe swelling of the vulva and perineum can occur with a cloudy red vaginal discharge. Chronic lesions appear after the acute phase with raised circular to oblong urticarial plaques 'Dollar plaques' in the vulva and adjacent skin. These may disappear and be replaced by others within hours or days. Later, the same area may show areas of depigmentation of skin and clitoris. Characteristically with this disease, weakness and ataxia of the hindquarters occurs with stumbling and knuckling of the lower limb joints. Terminal stages of the disease show anemia, cachexia, intermittent irregular fevers, severe nervous signs such as posterior paralysis, hyperesthesia and hyperalgesia. Signs of disease may persist for up to 2–4 years, although most cases progress over 1–2 months; few horses recover from the disease either being destroyed or die. The disease may be diagnosed by complement fixation tests and identification of the organism from vaginal discharges. Abortion may occur in pregnant mares.

809

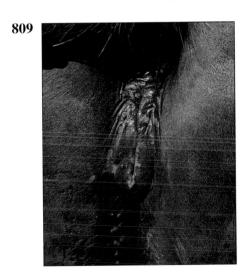

810

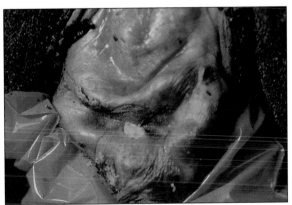

810 Clitoral sinus smegma accumulation (arrow).
Note: This often harbours pathogenic bacteria as well as commensal organisms.

809 Equine herpes virus-3 infection (coital exanthema).
Note: Lesions approximately 10 – 11 days after infected service.

Neoplastic Disorders

Neoplasms occur on the wall of the vagina and may even protrude from the vulval lips. **Hemangiomas (811)** are occasionally found on the vaginal wall but have little particular significance.

Pale skinned horses, with white or non-pigmented skin around the vulva are liable to develop **squamous cell carcinoma** at this site **(812)**. This may extend into the walls of the vagina. The tumour is most common in areas where high levels of ultraviolet light are present, such as the tropics.

Perineal melanotic masses frequently occur in grey mares **(813)** and often offer a mechanical obstruction to service or foaling. Traumatic damage of these masses during foaling or service can lead to discharge of black, glutinous, amorphous material. Occasionally, **melano sarcoma** is involved in this area and surgical removal appears to stimulate metastases to the spinal cord, leading to posterior paralysis.

811

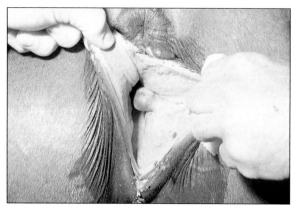

811 Cavernous hemangioma (on vaginal wall).

812 Squamous cell carcinoma.
Note: Involvement of vulva and adjacent vaginal mucosa. Cream colored horse with non-pigmented perineal skin.

812

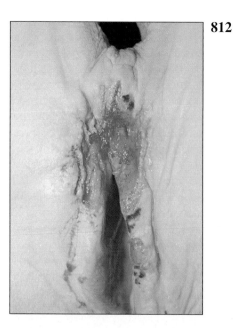

813

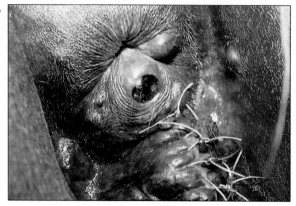

813 Melanoma (vulval).
Note: Grey horse. Numerous nodular melanoma lesions in perineum involving anus and vulval lips; slowly enlarging over 4 years; mare killed 4 seasons later. Note vulvoplasty (Caslick's operation) performed - sutures still *in situ*.

Four: Mammary Gland

Developmental Disorders

Congenital abnormalities are uncommon; most mares have at least two ducts in each teat, but may not produce equal quantities of milk through each duct. The mare has a lactiferous sinus which is less likely to blockage than are cow's teats. There is a marked variation in size of teats, both in length and diameter. Maiden mares may have relatively short teats set close on the mammary gland, making it difficult for foals to suck, particularly if the foal is weak; equally, some mares have excessively large teats which can also be difficult for weak foals to suckle.

Non-Infectious Disorders

Although proximity to foaling is often indicated by the presence of wax 'candles' adherent to the teat orifice (**814**) some mares may run milk for up to six weeks prior to foaling, and others may show no waxing and no mammary development prior to foaling. The running of milk prior to foaling may be related to placentitis, death of one twin foal, impending abortion, but may be a normal physiological event in multiparous mares with large udders. This is often manifest as milk stain on the back legs (**815**) and, when this occurs, it should be a warning of impending problems with the foal, or that the foal will be deprived of colostrum.

Because of the protected anatomical location of the mare's mammary gland it is much less commonly affected by trauma than in the cow or goat. Occasionally gross edema and even serum exudation occurs during allergic reactions to drugs or other allergens and it is also occasionally involved in urticarial, allergic reactions. Swelling and pain in the udder area results in a painful stiff gait and obvious discomfort. Most cases presenting with these signs are, however, due to infectious mastitis.

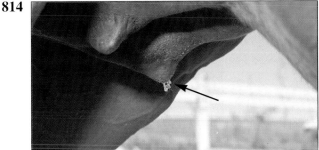

814

814 Pregnant mare mammary gland (12 hours pre-foaling).
Note: Normal 'wax candles' on end of teat (arrow).

Infectious Disorders

Infectious diseases are restricted to **acute, chronic and indurative mastitis**. The most common organisms involved are *Streptococcus* spp. and *Staphylococcus* spp. Acute cases are febrile, stiff in the hind quarters and the glandular edema may extend into the perineum (**816**) caudally and anteriorly with obvious enlargement of the transthoracic veins (**817**). Where the gland remains hard after weaning, and does not return to its normal contracted state, a chronic fibrotic induration (**818**) may have occurred. This may be due to inflammation of the gland tissue related to overfeeding of the mare during weaning and may resolve in time, or it may be related to persistent fibrosis from chronic, low-grade mastitis.

815

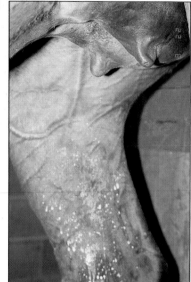

816

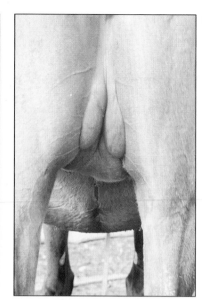

815 Pregnant mare mammary gland (milk running).
Note: Stained hind leg - pre-parturient milk 'run'. Loss of colostrum prepartum. Foal would require colostral supplementation or serum transfusion.

816 Mastitis.
Note: Gland was hot, painful, and had stringy milk without clots. Edema above gland.

817

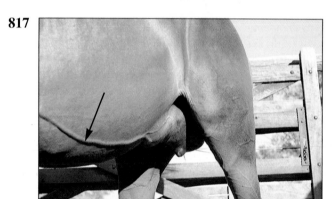

818

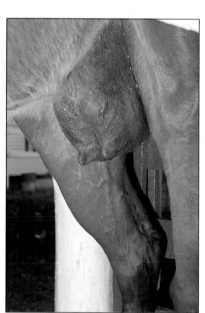

817 Mastitis.
Note: Enlarged gland, mare lame; foal refused to suckle this side of the udder. Obvious engorgement of transthoracic vein (arrow).

818 Mastitis (chronic).
Note: Weaned mare showing enlarged gland. No milk present and all enlargement related to fibrous induration; foal poorly grown due to reduced milk supply.

Neoplastic Disorders

Mammary tumours are not common, but verrucose, fibroblastic and nodular sarcoids are found on the skin overlying the gland (*see* **525**).

Very rarely, **primary adenocarcinoma (819)** affects the glandular tissue and the size, progression and high propensity to metastasis make the clinical syndrome more dramatic than most other swellings of the gland. Early gross enlargement of the iliac lymph nodes may be detected per rectum.

Secondary melanoma and **melanosarcoma (820)** occur occasionally in aged grey mares and are associated with mammary enlargement.

819
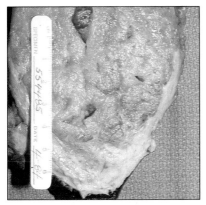

820
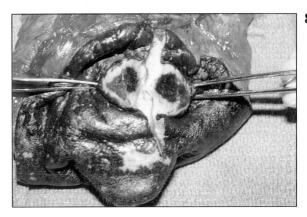

819 Mammary adenocarcinoma.
Note: Cross section of gland after surgical removal showing loss of lactiferous sinus. Metastases developed over following 3 months and the mare was killed.

820 Mammary melanoma.
Note: Grey mare. Melanosarcoma and melanin deposits in mammary tissue above lactiferous sinus.

Part 2: The Stallion and Gelding

Clinical examination of the stallion (or gelding)

Any previous breeding or other history pertinent to the genital tract examination should be collected and assessed.

Examination of the male horse should include thorough observations of the horse in a totally relaxed state to observe the natural state of prepuce, scrotum and the number, relative size and shape of the testes. Without undue excitement, the stallion should be allowed to approach mares, again if possible, to allow natural tumescence of the penis, rather than full erection, to occur. This permits examination for defects, skin abnormalities, or infective processes to be quietly observed before any manual examination of the genital tract is carried out.

A detailed palpation of the external genitalia, and particularly the scrotum and both inguinal canals, should be made, preferably without recourse to sedation. Great care must be taken and the use of stocks is recommended for thorough examination of the internal accessory glands per rectum. If suitable ultrasonography equipment is available, scanning of the accessory glands and bladder should be performed.

The next step in the examination is the actual process of mating; assessment of mating behaviour, libido and demeanour towards the mare and the handlers.

For a full and complete examination, a collection of semen (using an artificial vagina) should be made.

Wherever changes or abnormalities are encountered, these should be further explored as necessary for the completion of the examination.

The male equine reproductive system includes the testes and spermatic cord, penis, prepuce and accessory sex organs. The testes descend just prior to, or at birth in normal horses. Anatomically each testis is comprised of the gonad and the attached spermatic cord and epididymis. When the normal testis is transected, the cut surface bulges (**821**), and where this does not occur, severe degenerative changes of the seminiferous tubules have occurred. The normal colour of the cut testis varies, tending to be darker in older horses (**822**).

The appendix testis (**823**), which is the homologue of the infundibulum of the uterine tube, is a common normal structure to be seen on the surface of the testis. It always occurrs on the surface of the stallion's testis adjacent to the head of the epididymis (*see* **823**). It may be flat or rounded and is usually only a few millimetres across. The appendix epididymis is a vestigial remnant of the mesonephric duct origin and is occasionally found as a cystic structure located between the head of the epididymis and the body of the testis, or just adjacent to this area.

Aggressive behaviour in the stallion often occurs from many causes such as bad handling, poor or insufficient exercise, over-feeding, poor management (including persistent use as a teaser without subsequent

821

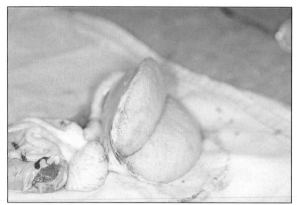

822

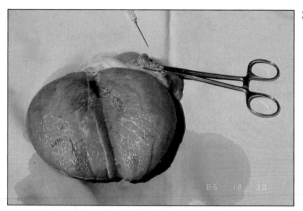

823

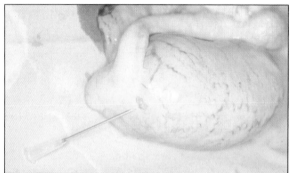

821 Normal testis (2-year-old colt) (sagittal section).
Note: Marked normal 'bulging' of tissue above level of tunic edge. Testes which are abnormal, fibrotic or have severe degenerative changes, do not 'bulge' in this manner.

822 Normal testis (aged stallion).
Note : Very dark colour compared with testis of 2 year old colt shown in **821**.

823 Normal testis (appendix testis visible at end of needle).
Note: Appendix testis is a normal structure found on the majority of testes. This is the vestigial remnant, similar to the infundibulum of the uterine tube in the mare.

service). It may also be a characteristic behaviour in some blood lines but may be related to either overwork or underwork in stud duties. Clinically, it may take the form of aggression towards the handler, the mare, or other horses in general. Among the more common causes are over-use in 2, 3, and 4 year old stallions in their first season, and it is for this reason, if no other, that 2 year old colts are better not mated at all, and 3 and 4 year old horses are worked sparingly and extremely carefully. Any serious disturbances to normal mating habits which occur in these young horses may affect mating behaviour for the rest of their breeding life. Ejaculatory failure is more commonly a problem of the young stallion in contrast to intermittent ejaculation which occurs in the older stallion.

Developmental Disorders

Normal anatomical features of the penis and prepuce of the stallion include the urethral process, head (glans penis), body of the penis and the prepuce. Congenital abnormalities have rarely been recorded but deviations of the penis in stallions **(824)** may have a familial relationship. Such stallions have obvious difficulty

824

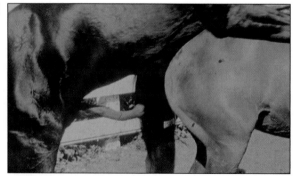

824 Penile deviation.
Note: Spiral and lateral deviation of penis; required hand guidance. This stallions father had been similarly affected but showed more lateral deviation.

825

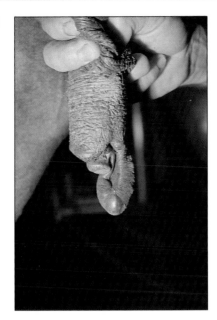

826

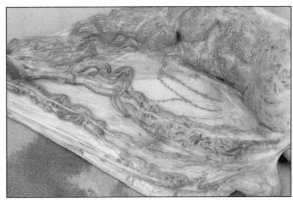

825 Developmental deformity of *caput glandis*.
Note: Horse unable to get corona enlargement. He was gelded.

826 Varicose testicle (developmental vascular abnormality of spermatic cord).
Note: Testis from 18 month old colt with unilateral scrotal enlargement; structural changes included a secondary venous system, by-passing the pampiniform plexus; testis was smaller and firmer than normal; scrotal swelling was due to secondary vasculature.

serving mares without assistance. Congenital abnormalities of the glans penis include penile hypoplasia and deformities of the corona (**825**) but are rarely recognised.

Vascular malformations of the spermatic cord are uncommon but **varicosity** has been observed in the spermatic vein and the pampiniform plexus (**826**). As the plexus plays a very important role in the thermoregulation of arterial temperature to the testis, any abnormality such as this might easily result in reduced fertility or, sometimes even in complete infertility.

Congenital absence of one testis is extremely rare and extra testes are even rarer (and probably do not occur). A suspected polyorchid horse is almost always found to be either an incomplete abdominal cryptorchid, or has cystic structures on the cord which have been mistaken for an extra testis. Fusion of the left testis and spleen has been reported in cryptorchids and ectopic adrenocortical tissue has been found in the lower segments of the spermatic cord, adjacent to the head of the epididymis, and in the mediastinum testes.

Congenital absence of the cremaster muscle may be found in horses having no ability to lift the testicle. The scrotum of affected horses may have a pendulous nature but it is more usually found incidentally (**827**).

Rotation of the testis is not uncommon in racing horses (**828**) Opinions are divided as to the pathological significance of this state, but it may be a normal variation. In other cases surgical correction has been performed. The condition can be recognised by the abnormal (anterior) positioning of the tail of the epididymis (*see* **828**); attempts to re-locate are successful only as long as the testis is restrained in the normal position; release leads to an immediate return to the original dislocated position. More severe rotation leads to **torsion of the spermatic cord (829)**, which leads to dramatic vascular compromise, abdominal pain, and edema of the scrotum with an enlarged, very firm and extremely painful testis.

Probably the most common abnormality relating to the testes is the **cryptorchid testis** when one (or both) testes fail to descend completely into the scrotum. A temporary, usually unilateral (the right-side testis is most commonly involved), **inguinal retention** is relatively common amongst ponies with small testicles. **Permanent inguinal retention** occurs in all types of horse, and is recognised when the testis is lodged within the inguinal canal. The affected testis (usually unilateral but either can be involved) may be palpable and may be misshapen. **Abdominally retained testicles** may be freely mobile within the abdomen and may, furthermore, be found in a wide variety of locations. Usually, however, they are to be found deep to the internal inguinal ring. The abdominally retained testicle is commonly very much smaller than the descended one although in some cases, and particularly those in which teratomatous changes are present, they may be considerably larger than the normal one and are then often 'flabby' in consistency. Incomplete abdominal retention occurs when the tail of the epididymis is in the

827

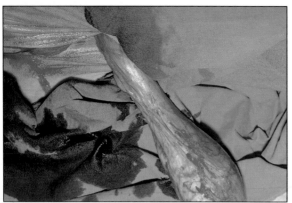

827 Developmental Absence of Cremaster Muscle.

828

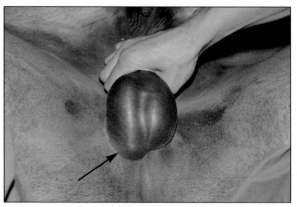

828 Rotation of (left) testis.
Note: Tail of rotated (left) testicle lying cranially and not obvious to view. Normal (right testis) epididymis lying caudally in correct position and visually obvious (arrow).

829

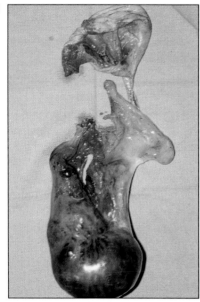

830

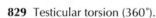

829 Testicular torsion (360°).
Note: Rotation of testis resulted in vascular compromise, swelling of the scrotum, severe pain and lameness in a 3-year-old Quarterhorse.

830 Cryptorchid testis.
Note: Small testicle located in abdominal cavity following removal of tail and body of epididymis via scrotum some time previously. This is a common error by novice surgeons who mistakenly identify the tail of the epididymis for a 'small' testicle.

831

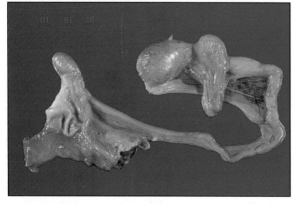

831 Cryptorchid testis.
Note: Excessive length of body of epididymis (> 25 cm)

inguinal canal while the body of the testicle lies at or above the internal inguinal ring. The gross appearance of a cryptorchid testicle is often abnormally dark and where there has been a previous attempt to castrate the animal the epididymis may be removed in the mistaken belief that it is the testicle (**830**). The anatomical structure and relationship between the tail and body of the epididymis of the cryptorchid testis to the rest of the testis is often changed with elongated epididymal bodies up to 30cm long being present (**831**) which often leads to inexperienced surgeons removing these portions, leaving the testis and the balance of the epididymis in the abdominal cavity. A simple confirmatory test to avoid this error is to cut the tail of the epididymis or body transversally and examine for the coiled tubes of vas deferens rather than testicular tissues.

Other developmental abnormalities of the inguinal canal include **herniation of the small intestine** which appears to have a slightly higher incidence in Standardbred and Quarter horses than in other breeds. Inguinal and scrotal hernias are frequently present at birth (*see* **88**), causing gross enlargement of the scrotum. This most often resolves within a few days and does not require intervention. The defect is sometimes large enough to warrant manual reduction over the first few days after birth. Acquired hernias with accompanying swelling (*see* **106**), pain on palpation and reluctance to move, occur as a result of accidents due to kicks, or falls when horses become caught over rails. In older horses, herniation can be encountered at castration (*see* **837**) if a large inguinal canal remains patent.

One: The Testis, Scrotum and Spermatic Cord

Non-Infectious Disorders

Where stallions are unable to exercise due to painful hind leg conditions such as fractures, there can be excessive weight bearing on the other normal leg, leading to edema of the scrotum (**832**) only, and unless this quickly resolves, it may cause future infertility. A similar appearance is often presented by stallions in which there is gross accumulation of peritoneal fluid (ascites) with consequent hydrocele in the *tunica vaginalis*.

Physical trauma to the scrotum of the horse occurs from kicks and injuries acquired by hanging over rails, but may also occur where horses are ridden or driven through spiky, awned grasses, thistles or shrubs. Thistle spikes may penetrate the skin of the legs, lower abdomen and scrotum causing exudate of serum, crusting and gross edema of the scrotal skin (**833**). The scrotum should be examined carefully in all cases where there is swelling in order to establish the cause. Some such conditions are very serious while others are less so in the short term but all may result in temporary (or sometimes permanent) infertility as a result of temperature changes, adhesions or vascular compromises of one (or both) testicle(s).

Orchitis or inflammation of the testis may be initiated by either trauma or infection. Clinically, the accompanying edema causes enlargement of the affected testis and, almost always, the scrotum. Occasionally, it occurs as a result of racing and may be due to a more-pendulous-than-normal scrotum, leading to physical injury. In other cases it may be a result of infection, particularly from *Streptococcus* spp.. Clinically, in acute cases, the affected testis is enlarged, hot and often very painful, and unless the condition is quickly relieved, irreversible damage occurs, leading to a testicular atrophy and fibrosis (**834**). Examination of the scrotum and its contents with the help of ultrasonography can be most useful in establishing the true nature of scrotal swellings and an accurate diagnosis dramatically improves the chances of returning the animal to normal reproductive function.

Testicular degeneration (which may or may not be accompanied by an obvious reduction in testicular size and weight) has many causes, the most common being thermal injury. Normal spermatogenesis occurs at a slightly lower temperature than the general body temperature and any condition which results in an elevation of the scrotal temperature will necessarily impair the normal fertility and result in testicular atrophy. Vascular changes as a result of impaired heat-exchange mechanisms in the vessels of the spermatic cord and pampiniform plexus and fluid (blood, serous or peritoneal fluid) accumulations within the *tunica vaginalis*, as well as any condition which causes edema and inflammation of the scrotum have harmful effects upon spermatogenesis. Systemic infections or even prolonged exposure to high ambient temperatures have also been associated with testicular atrophy and

832

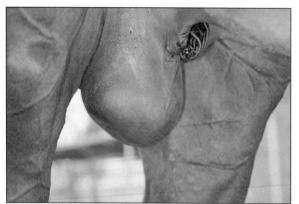

832 Scrotal edema.
Note: Severe edema due to inactivity (horse pivoted in circle on normal hind leg) caused by pain associated with pastern fracture.
Differential Diagnosis:
i)   Hydrocele
ii) Inguinal/scrotal hernia
iii) Testicular torsion
iv) Orchitis (traumatic or infective)
v)   Ascites
vi) Uroperitoneum
vii) Hemoperitoneum
viii) Varicose testicle
ix) Testicular neoplasia
x)   Plant (thistle etc) or trauma induced edema

833

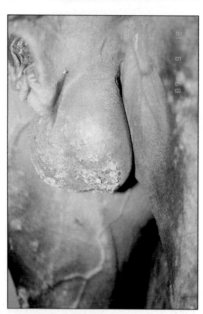

833 Scrotal edema.
Note: Edema, scabs and scurf caused by imbedded plant (thistle) awns.
Differential Diagnosis:
i)   Hydrocele
ii) Inguinal/scrotal hernia
iii) Testicular torsion
iv) Orchitis (traumatic or infective)
v)   Ascites
vi) Uroperitoneum
vii) Hemoperitoneum
viii) Varicose testicle
ix) Testicular neoplasia
x)   Horse pox

834

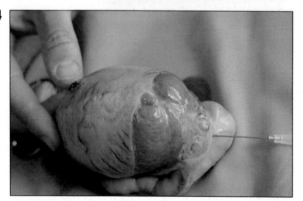

834 Orchitis.
Note: Enlarged painful scrotum. The horse was febrile and lame; responded to antibiotics but testicle was left shrunken and on removal, showed marked degenerative changes.

consequent infertility. **Equine viral arteritis** (*see* **298, 299**) has been specifically implicated as a cause of testicular atrophy. Furthermore, testes which have reduced blood supply as a result of cord torsion, scrotal and inguinal hernia and varicocele of the spermatic vein (*see* **826**) may be affected similarly. The effects of malnutrition, ingestion of toxic plants and physical obstruction to the epididymis can all cause degenerative changes. Diagnosis must depend on clinical assessment by manual palpation, examination of semen and ultimately, test mating.

   Testicular atrophy may be encountered after 10 – 12

years of age in some specific genetic lines. The onset can be very sudden with an abrupt onset of complete infertility. No satisfactory explanation has been found to date, although degenerative vascular lesions have been seen in some testes. Testicular biopsy is a technique for sampling but its use can be hazardous and may cause further degenerative changes to occur.

Hypertrophy may occur in one testis due to injury and atrophy of the other and is commonly encountered where one testis has been previously removed.

In the case of cryptorchids used as stallions, increase in size of the undescended testicle may occur. Frequently, where an undescended testicle has been left in situ for a long period, hypertrophy can be found on removal.

Epididymitis is a rare condition in stallions and is poorly documented. Infection with *Salmonella abortus equi* and *Streptococcus zooepidemicus* have been recorded as being initially related to trauma, orchitis or infections of the accessory sex glands. Clinically there is both pain and swelling of the scrotal area which, if associated with orchitis, quickly becomes edematous and tight, causing difficulty in palpation of structures within the scrotum. Ultrasonographic examination can be used very effectively to establish the nature of this (and many other) scrotal problem.

Complication arising from castration

Many different surgical procedures are used for castration including the use of open and closed methods. The closed methods are usually performed on a recumbent horse under general anesthesia and under these circumstances it is possible to pay particular attention to hemostasis and primary wound healing of the scrotal incision is usual. Open castration (in which the *tunica vaginalis* is incised) is frequently performed in the sedated (and sometimes unsedated) standing horse under local anesthesia. The resulting scrotal wound is usually left open to allow drainage and second intention healing. Where no (or minimal) infection or post-surgical hemorrhage occurs, there is usually only minor swelling and a slight amount of serous fluid. Occasionally however, significant scrotal swelling, with edema of the prepuce and ventral abdomen, develops

835

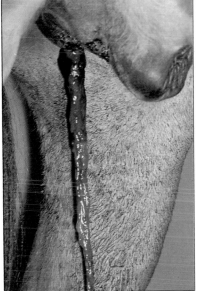

836

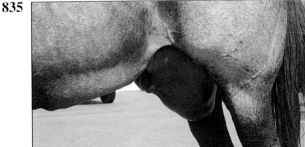
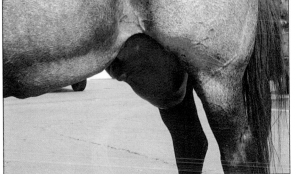

837

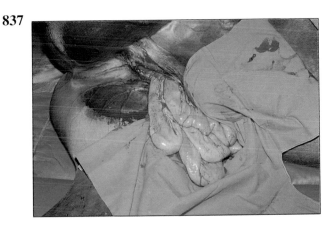

835 Post castration swelling.
Note: Massive swelling of scrotum and abdominal wall occurred 5 days post castration; scrotum contained several large blood clots.

836 Omental hernia (prolapse).
Note: Mass appeared 24 hours after castration.

837 Post-castration eventration.

401

over the first few days after surgery. This is generally due to the presence of variably-sized blood clots retained in the scrotum (**835**) or to fluid accumulation and gravitation. It may be related to poor hemostasis, poor drainage (possibly as a result of an inadequate scrotal incision), or lack of appropriate post-operative exercise.

Occasionally, following castration, a 'tail' of red-coloured tissue may be seen to hang from the scrotum (**836**). This is almost always omentum and very occasionally, may precede herniation of small intestine. Fortunately, the latter complication is particularly unusual. **Herniation of small or longer lengths of small intestine** is an unfortunate and extremely serious complication of castration (**837**). Open castration in horses having wide or patent inguinal canals and those with inguinal or scrotal hernias seems particularly likely to predispose to this disorder. Closed castration may also be complicated by herniation of small intestine into the scrotal sac, resulting in severe and intractable colic associated with strangulating small intestinal obstruction. Standing, open castration of a horse with an inguinal or scrotal hernia is almost bound to lead to dangerous herniation of intestine.

Accumulation of lymph or serum around the remnants of the spermatic cord leads to the formation of a sterile **seroma** (**838**). These are often non-painful, warm swellings which develop over the first few days post operatively. The seroma is made up of a multi-loculated mass of clotted blood and fibrin strands (**839**). Improved drainage of the operative site or surgical excision of the mass is usually followed by a rapid and full recovery.

An infected operative site following castration causes hot painful swelling and the persistent discharge of sero-sanguineous or purulent material from the affected side(s) (**840**). Affected horses are often systemically ill, being febrile and innappetant. Serious infection usually develops after 5–10 days and may be particularly difficult to control. In some cases little or no apparent discharge will be encountered for up to 6 weeks, but it will be noticed that the wound fails to heal and slight or moderate local swelling persists (**841**). Infected castration sites may persist for years, particularly when the site is infected by *Staphylococcus* spp. bacteria. This chronic infective process is called **scirrhous cord**. Where castration is accompanied by cord ligation there is an added opportunity for local reaction and persistent infection. The use of non-absorbable suture material, string or non-surgical wire has been commonly associated with persistent infection and draining sinuses from castration sites. Evidence for all of these unpleasant and debilitating complications of castration may be very difficult to obtain as some cases have little local swelling and the surgery may have been performed years previously. Usually, however, the clinical signs include gross swellings of the scrotum, prepuce and abdominal wall, pain on movement, loss of appetite, elevated temperature and the presence of a draining serosanguineous to purulent discharge (*see* **841**). Surgical drainage, antibiotics and exercise usually remedy the early post-castration problems. However, where infection slowly becomes established, the scrotal incisions may heal and swelling regress temporarily for short to long periods. Lesions of dense fibrous tissue and chronic, multiloculated or focal abscess of the cord remnants are found during surgical exploration (**842**), which is the only effective way of diagnosing the extent of the problem.

838

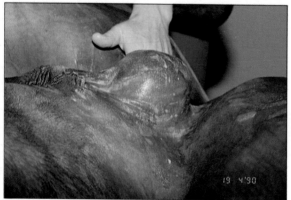

838 Scrotal seroma.
Note: Enlarged indurated scrotal area 3 years after castration. No pain or discharge.

839

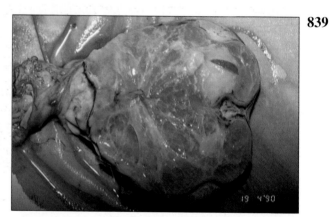

839 Scrotal seroma.
Note: Incised scrotal area showing seroma on distal cord-end, 3 years after castration (same horse as **839**).

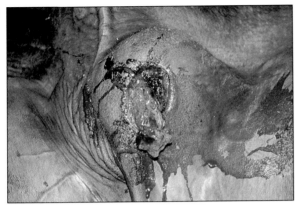

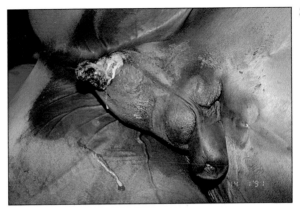

840 Infected castration site.
Note: Scrotum 30 days after 'lay' castration. Abdominal wall edema and swollen prepuce and scrotal area. Serosanguineous discharge from site developed at induction of anesthesia.

841 Scirrhous cord.
Note: Discharging sinus of bloody purulent exudate 6 months after castration.

Infectious Disorders

The testicle is seldom directly involved with infectious processes but many systemic virus and bacterial infections exert considerable harmful effects upon spermatogenesis through their febrile nature and the consequent thermal inhibition (and possibly hypoplasia) of the testicular tissue. **Equine viral arteritis, African Horse Sickness** and some other virus infections may cause orchitis. **Orchitis (see 834)**, as a result of direct sequestration of bacteria (particularly, *Staphylococcus* spp., *Streptococcus* spp. and *Brucella* spp.), is rare in the horse but may cause severe painful swelling of one (or both) testis(es). The condition is indistinguishable from traumatic orchitis. The long term effects upon fertility are considerable with many affected horses becoming infertile following even relatively minor episodes of infective or traumatic orchitis. A diagnosis may be supported, in the acute stages, by examination of the scrotum and its contents using ultrasonography. Testicular biopsy is an effective, if somewhat risky, technique for definitive diagnosis. It is usually reserved for the advanced case because of the risk of aggravating an already reduced fertility.

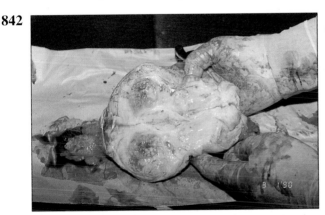

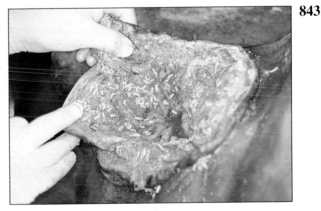

842 Scirrhous cord (Botryomycosis, *Staphylococcus aureus*).
Note: Abscess, presence of pus and marked fibrous tissue reaction at end of cord with milliary, interlinked abscesses and tracts.

843 Myiasis.
Note: Castration wound 24 hours after castration showed heavy infestation with Blowfly (*Lucilia* spp) maggots. Scrotum smelt unpleasant but not necrotic; compare to screw worm (*Callitroga* spp.) infestation, when severe malodour is present due to necrosis.

Botryomycosis of the spermatic cord is due to infection from *Staphylococcus aureus* and clinically shows as a chronic granulating thickening of the cord stump (*see* **842**). The lesion shows miliary small or minute abscess foci and, similar to other scirrhous cords, may show a persistent discharging sinus (*see* **841**).

Occasionally in warm weather, even in temperate climates, scrotal wounds can become 'fly-struck' (**myiasis**). This can be due to *Lucilia* spp. flies (**843**). In tropical areas where the screw worm fly (*Callitroga* spp.) occurs. Navel cords and scrotal wounds are frequently affected.

Neoplastic Disorders

Tumours of the testes are not common; however two types do occur more frequently than others. Retained testes quite frequently show **benign teratomatous changes** (**844**). These may be found to contain cartilage, bone, fibrous tissue and cysts which may contain hair, glandular tissue and other amorphous material. Testicular teratomas occur predominantly in young cryptorchid stallions and may well be congenital neoplasms.

Seminomas occur in older stallions and these slow growing tumours may reach considerable size. Seminomas become clinically apparent when the affected gonad increases markedly and rapidly in size (**845**). Usually, only one testis is involved. The tumour mass has an obvious, nodular appearance and while some are single and large, others are multiple and smaller (**846**). Metastases into the spermatic cord, inguinal and lumbar lymph nodes, are not uncommon in this condition. **Interstitial cell tumours** are commonly recorded in old stallions and may be easily overlooked as they have very little effect on the size of the gonad. Other types of neoplasms have been recorded in stallions but are of very low incidence. This may only reflect the fact that the majority of male horses are castrated at a young age.

844

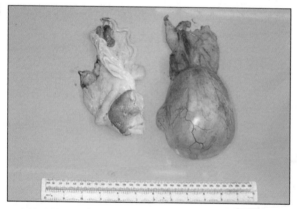

844 Testicular teratoma (two types).
Note: LEFT: Teratoma containing cartilage and bone
RIGHT: Large fluid-filled, cystic teratoma.

845

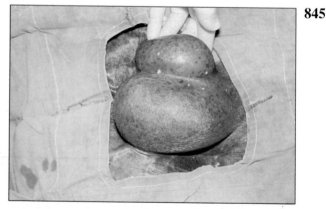

845 Seminoma.
Note: Grossly enlarged testicle compared to the normal one.

846

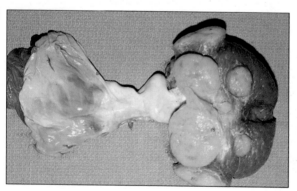

846 Seminoma.
Note: 15 year old Quarter horse. Normal (dark) testicular tissue with several areas of pale neoplastic tissue.

Two: The Penis and Prepuce

Non-Infectious Disorders

The penis of the neonatal foal may be seen to hang from the prepuce for the first day or two of life but this normal occurrence usually resolves within the first two weeks as increasing retractor strength develops. In some foals the opposite occurs when the penis is not relaxed during urination and urine scalding of the sheath and hind legs is a further temporary complication. In the adult horse urination is accompanied by appropriate posture and penile relaxation.

Traumatic damage to the penis is a serious condition in the horse. Physical injury may arise from kicks, accidents caused by falls on rails, fences or even by tail hairs of mares during service. **Damage to the urethral process (847)** occurs most commonly when natural (paddock) mating occurs and the sharp hairs of the mares tail are pulled across the erect *glans penis*. Minor bleeding from the area may be noted immediately after service and, while a single such episode is unlikely to cause any long-term ill-effect, repeated trauma may result in localised fibrosis and urethral infection. Accidental tears to the urethral process and *corona glandis* may lead to hemorrhage following service. Where this occurs, there is usually a lowered fertility or even infertility until hemorrhage ceases, or is controlled and healed. Clinically, semen samples show pink discoloration **(848)** due to the presence of blood (hemospermia).

Direct kicks to the erect penis of stallions are particularly serious conditions which commonly result in **hematoma formation (849)**. Usually these injuries result in hemorrhage from the rich plexus of veins outside the *tunica albuginea*; rupture of this, such as occasionally occurs in bulls, probably does not occur in the horse. The penis may become very heavy with blood and edema and its dependent nature serves only to aggravate the condition. A kick to the prepuce and non-erect penis may cause severe local swelling **(850)** but seldom affects the penis directly. Gross preputial swelling of this type has more effect upon urination and commonly shows particular difficulty in resolving naturally. Most of these injuries will resolve if urgently and correctly treated but long term injury may result unless appropriate emergency medical attention is provided.

Contusions to the penis with swelling due to hemorrhage and edema of the injured tissues, or inability to pass small cystic calculi may cause occlusion of the urethra (*see* **336**) cause urinary retention which if untreated, leads to colic and, even, rupture of the bladder. Poorly fitted stallion rings may also cause occlusion, and in severe cases, lead to sloughing of the glans penis. Urethral injury may result from kicks, laceration to the glans or urethral process during coitus from tail hairs of the mare (*see* **847**), or acute or chronic *Habronema* spp. infestation (*see* **862**).

847

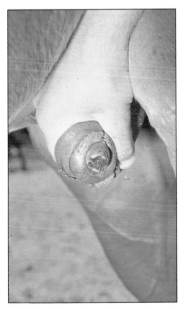

848

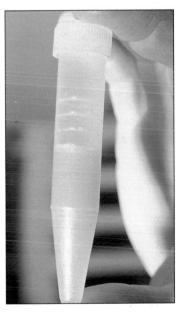

847 Urethral process damage (by mare's tail hairs during service).
Note: Natural (paddock) service; this is a natural hazard when mares tails are not bandaged prior to service.

848 Hemospermia.
Note: Semen sample taken from stallion with injury to urethra process which bled during service, contaminating semen. Reduced fertility occurs with presence of blood in semen.
Differential Diagnosis:
i)   Penile trauma
ii) Urethral infection (ulcerative)
iii) Bladder hemorrhage (cystitis, calculi neoplasia)
iv) Accessory gland inflammation
v)   Hemorrhagic diatheses

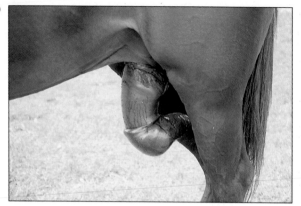

849 Penile hematoma/bruising.
Note: Injury to erect penis during actual service. Swollen, enlarged penis which cannot be retracted.

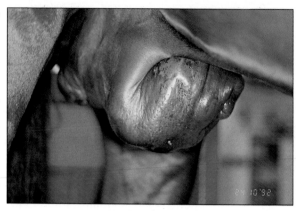

850 Preputial bruising.
Note: Injury to prepuce only; kick by mare during service but penis not erect and not injured.

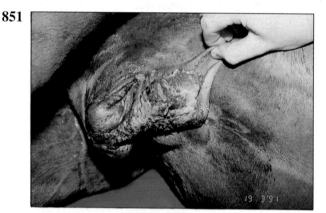

851 Preputial scalding.
Note: Scalding and smegma inside prepuce caused by intra-prepucial urination.

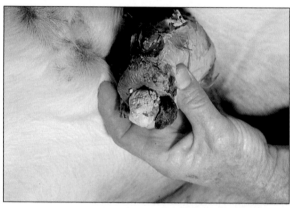

852 Smegma accumulation (in the diverticulum of penis/urethral fossa).
Note: Contamination of this area with such organisms as *Taylorella equi genitalis*, *Klebsiella* spp. and/or *Pseudomonas* spp. is associated with a high risk of genital transfer of disease.

In the adult male horse, where urination occurs without penile relaxation, or where phimosis (narrowing of the opening of the prepuce) occurs following injury, infection due to *Habronema* or neoplasia (such as squamous cell carcinoma or melanoma), urination within the prepuce frequently leads to **scalding (851)** and increased smegma formation within the sheath. In white skinned or coloured horses, this often leads to pre-cancerous skin changes occurring on both prepuce and penis (*see* **863**). Accumulation of dried smegma occurs particularly in the urethral fossa (**852**), in old geldings and may lead to occasional low grade inflammatory changes such as frequent urination or straining to pass urine.

Defects in the vascular, nervous control and musculature of the penis lead to serious and sometimes permanent changes to the use and carriage of the penis. **Priapism** (persistent abnormal erection of the penis) may occur either as a fully or semi-erect condition. Occasionally, full erection occurs in states of sexual excitement in racing horses, and may be very difficult to treat. A semi-erect condition (**853**), occurs in conjunction with a variety of other diseases including injuries and inflammation of the spinal cord, purpura hemorrhagica, complication of castration and the use of some phenothiazine tranquilizers, (either alone or in combination with other drugs). This condition often fails to respond to any treatment.

Paraphimosis (painful constriction of the glans penis by a phimotic preputial ring) or the inability to withdraw the penis into the preputial cavity, occurs from a variety of causes. Trauma from kicks (**854**), debility, or following

853

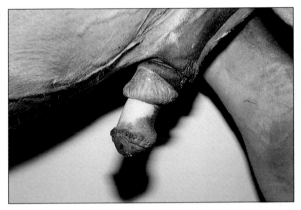

854

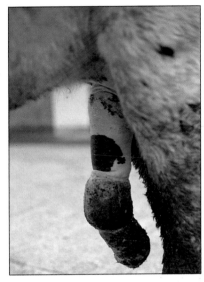

853 Priapism (continuous tumescence of the penis).
Note: Gelding which failed to respond to any treatment.

854 Paraphimosis.
Note: Shire stallion kicked during service; became severely swollen and was untreated; failed to retract penis and condition is now permanent.

penile paralysis related to the use of some types of tranquilizers are possible causes. **Paraphimosis** has also occurred as a result of surgical error during castration where the root of the penis is incised instead of a testicle (**855**).

Penile prolapse is also a possible secondary complication of disease conditions in other organs including malabsorption, lymphosarcoma and debility. Paralysis of the penis may also be of neurological origin with spinal cord or sacral, or cauda equina disease resulting in a loss of retractor ability. Clinically, the acute swelling associated with these conditions and with accident-related paraphimosis should be treated as an emergency. The penis should be catheterized, pressure bandaged and supported under the horse's abdomen (**856**) to prevent progressive edema and undue tension on the retractor muscles. A number of these cases are incurable, failing to respond to any treatment and amputation may be the only recourse and as it occurs almost exclusively in stallions the potential consequences of failure to resolve are considerable.

Untreated **hematoma of the penis** may lead to fibrosis of the site and the development of permanent paraphimosis (**857**). Some affected stallions, while able to mount mares, cannot attain a full erection, but providing sensory innervation is still present, may be able to ejaculate into an artificial vagina.

Vascular defects in the genital tract result in **hemospermia** (*see* **848**) which may occur as a result of bleeding from sites in the accessory sex glands, bladder, urethra and glans penis. Consequently, it may be difficult to positively identify the exact point of hemorrhage. Clinically the ejaculate may be pink, due to small amounts of blood (*see* **848**), or may contain obvious blood clots, or may be overtly hemorrhagic with several hundred millilitres of blood being discharged on dismount after service. Most stallions become sub-fertile until the condition is remedied. Diagnosis is by careful evaluation of the external genitalia, and ultrasonographic and fiberoptic examination of the urethra, bladder and openings of the accessory glands.

855

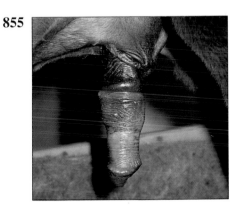

855 Paraphimosis.
Note: 'Lay' castration led to severance of base of penis; correction by amputation.

856

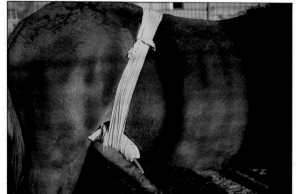

857

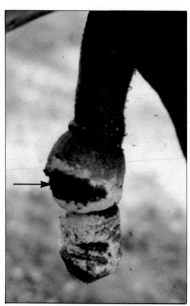

856 Paraphimosis.
Note: Injury induced paraphimosis treated by catheterisation of urethra, pressure bandaging and slinging until swelling had regressed and retraction of penis returned to normal.

857 Paraphimosis (permanent).
Note: Following a kick, a hematoma of the penis developed which was neglected. A penile-shaft fibrous (scarred/organised) hematoma is present (arrow).

Infectious Disorders

Viral Diseases: Clinically important viral infection of the penis and prepuce, is restricted to **Equine herpes virus-3 (Coital exanthema)** which in maiden stallions, occurs after contact with a clinically affected or carrier mare. The disease initially appears as blisters over the penis and preputial mucosa, which rapidly rupture, leaving a yellowish necrotic area (**858**) which exudes serum, forming small encrusted sores on the preputial reflection. This site corresponds with the longest duration point of contact with the vulval region of carrier mares (*see* **809**). The condition is often transient provided that the stallion is rested until the condition has healed completely. Diagnosis is by viral isolation from early lesions and paired sera using both complement fixation and serum neutralization tests.

Bacterial Diseases: Bacterial urethritis occurs in the stallion, usually from extension of infection from the urethral process (**859**) and may cause erosion of the mucosa at any point along the urethra. Endoscopic examination shows superficial and sometimes deep erosions of the mucosa (**860**) which may be hemorrhagic and lead to hemospermia and infertility. *Pseudomonas* spp. is the organism most commonly isolated from such infections.

The bacterial fauna of the prepuce is usually fairly diverse and involves a number of species which when in normal numbers are regarded as normal commensal organisms. Over zealous hygiene measures taken in stallions (particularly the use of strong disinfectants and antiseptics) may result in a difficult and persistent inflammation of the penis and preputial lining with over-production of smegma.

Bacterial infections of the penis and prepuce may occur subsequent to trauma, Dourine, coital exanthema and habronema, and may be caused by *Pseudomonas* spp., *Klebsiella* spp. or *Taylorella equi genitalis* (CEM). Frequently, the stallion remains free of clinical signs of infection, but may continue to transmit infection to mated mares. Serial samples for bacterial culture should be taken from the prepuce, diverticulum, urethral fossa (*fossa glandis*) and free portion of the penis. Culture of smegma from the *fossa glandis* may yield a pure culture of pathogenic organisms.

Protozoal Diseases: Dourine is a protozoal venereal infection due to *Trypanosoma equiperdum* and probably originated in North Africa, spreading to other parts of Africa, Asia, Europe, Indonesia and the Americas. The disease has been eradicated from North Africa, Western Europe and North America. Early clinical signs in the stallion include edema of penis, prepuce and testes, followed by raised plaques on the penis and prepuce, leading to so called 'Dollar plaques'; so named because the lesions are hardened disc-like masses under the skin the size of a dollar coin. These characteristically appear and disappear over variable intervals of a few hours to a few days, only to be replaced by others. Paraphimosis and penile edema with edema and swelling of the

858

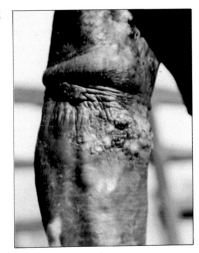

859

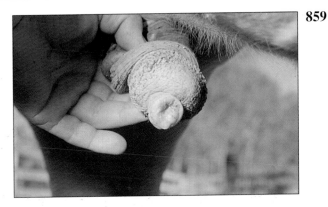

858 Equine coital exanthema (equine herpes virus-3).
Note: Lesions developed 10 days after infected service. Note the position of the lesions at the preputial reflection (the point of most prolonged contact with the vulva of the infected mare).

859 Bacterial urethritis (*Pseudomonas* spp.).
Note: Enlarged urethra, mildly painful and caused occasional inhibition of service.

860

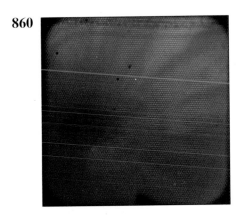

861

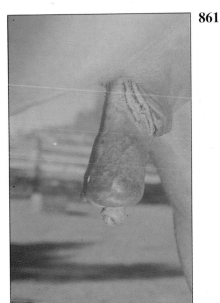

860 Urethritis (endoscopic view).
Note: Erosion of mucosa (approximately 40cm from the prepucial opening). Caused mild intermittent hemospermia.

861 Dourine (*Trypanosoma equiperdum*).
Note: Edema of urethral process, prepuce, penis and surrounding skin.

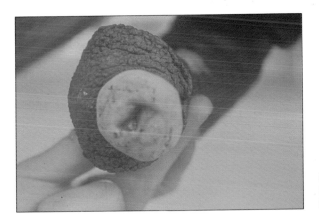

862 Habronemiasis (Urethral) (Chronic).
Note: Enlarged urethral process due to chronic infection from Habronema larvae.

urethral process are commonly present **(861)**. Depigmentation of the mucosa of the genital tract may occur; paralysis of the hind quarters and cachexia develop and death ensues. The disease is transmitted by coitus and trypanosomes may be present in seminal fluid, or mucus exudate from the penis.

Parasite infestation of both the prepuce and urethral processes occur; commonly due to *Draschia megastoma*, *Habronema musca* or *Habronema microstoma*. Larval worms may be deposited into cuts,

tears or other areas of broken mucosa or skin where they can induce a granulomatous reaction. The lesions are small at first and lead to ulceration of the external surface of the urethral process. Progressively there is enlargement of the urethral process **(862)** and variable ulceration. It may occur in both geldings and stallions; in the stallion, bleeding occurs during and following mating and may lead to both temporary inhibition due to pain and irritation, and to reduced fertility due to the presence of blood intermixed with ejaculate.

Neoplastic Disorders

Neoplasia of the external genitalia is particularly rare in stallions but relatively common in geldings. Smegma has been incriminated as having carcinogenetic properties and this especially applies in horses with poorly pigmented skin such as Appaloosa, and coloured horses such as Cremello, Palamino, Pinto and Overo.

Squamous cell carcinomas are found on the prepuce of geldings of any age, often showing as small

granulomatous tumours. The earliest stage of the development of squamous cell carcinoma in geldings is a well-recognised 'pre-cancerous', plaque-like inflammatory change which is most obvious at the preputial reflection **(863)** but which may affect larger areas of the preputial lining **(864)** with adjacent lesions on the penis. These pre-cancerous plaques frequently respond to regular washing to prevent smegma

863

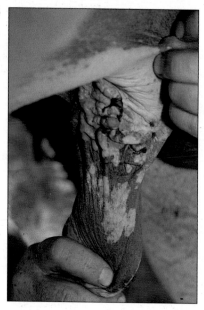

864

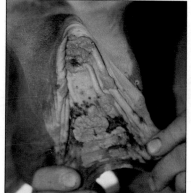

865

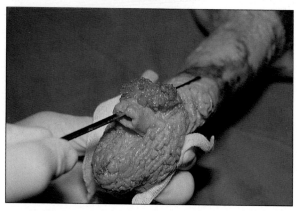

863 Squamous Cell Carcinoma (Precancerous Stage).
Note: Multiple ulcerative lesions distributed particularly at preputial reflection.

864 Squamous cell carcinoma (precancerous stage).
Note: Multiple ulcerative lesions distributed particularly at preputial ring, associated with smegma accumulations.

865 Squamous cell carcinoma (penile shaft) (early cauliflower-like lesion).
Note: Erosion of penile shaft to urethra.

accumulation and then may not develop overt squamous cell carcinoma. The extent of the true neoplastic lesions which develop quickly from the pre-cancerous stage is variable with some lesions being relatively localised and cauliflower-like (**865**). These, like the others may be locally invasive and result in defects of local anatomy including erosion and perforation of the urethra some way back from the urethral process (*see* **865**) or may occur at the preputial reflection (**866**). In some cases massive proliferative neoplastic lesions develop and may even result in an inability to withdraw the penis into the prepuce (pseudo-paraphimosis) (**867**). In most cases, and particularly when the condition develops in old horses, the tumour is not highly malignant, growing rather more slowly than might be expected from its nature. Spread to local lymph nodes and other remote structures such as the vertebral bodies and lungs does however occur. When it develops in younger horses the outlook is much poorer. The more invasive type of penile squamous cell carcinoma which occurs in younger horses is often less proliferative in appearance (**868**) but palpation of the penis will often identify an irregular firmness occupying a variable length of the free length. Metastasis to inguinal and iliac lymph nodes is relatively common in these and their life expectancy, even following radicle surgery, is much reduced.

Melanomas occur relatively commonly in grey horses and occasionally are found affecting the preputial ring where they may cause phimosis.

Nodular and fibroblastic sarcoids commonly occur on the preputial skin (**869**). Multiple lesions are commonly encountered although single (or few) nodular lesions are also common. Only very rarely do these masses occur on the preputial skin and they are only rarely found on the free part of the penis.

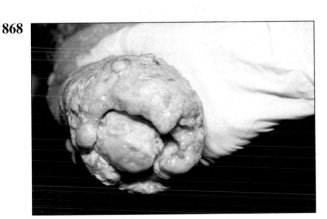

866 Squamous cell carcinoma (penile base) (late cauliflower-like lesion).
Note: Extensive ulcerative and proliferative nature.

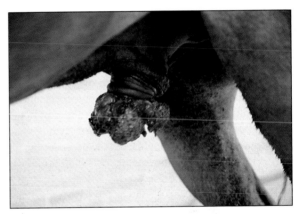

867 Squamous cell carcinoma (penile shaft) (late cauliflower-like lesion).
Note: Pseudo-paraphimosis resulted from an inability to withdraw the mass into the prepuce.

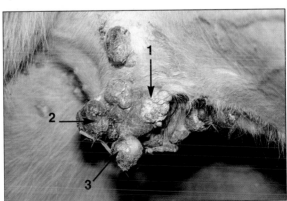

868 Squamous cell carcinoma (penile shaft) (malignant form).
Note: Young horse with extensive thickened feel to shaft of penis and gross enlargement of both inguinal and iliac lymph nodes.

869 Preputial sarcoid.
Note: Verrucose (arrow 1), fibroblastic (arrow 2) and nodular (arrow 3) lesions are present.

411

Part 3: The Placenta

The placenta is the physiological unit made up entirely of fetal tissues which lies in contact with the endometrium of the mare and is responsible for the exchange of nutrients and waste matter between the foal and the dam. Any factor or condition which alters this relationship has the potential to cause changes to the foal which may lead to death, resorption, abortion, deformity or infection of the neonate. Such a wide ranging set of conditions can be encountered that it behoves the reproductive clinician to undertake a careful study of every placenta at parturition. A great deal of useful information can be gleaned, concerning, not only itself, but also the endometrium, to which it was attached during the pregnancy. Indeed it is possible that, in many cases of abortion, more may be learnt from the placenta than from the aborted fetus itself. A careful examination of the placenta may furthermore provide useful information regarding future pregnancies.

Abortion represents a traumatic event for the mare and the fetus (and indeed the mare owner), and few events occur which cause more anguish, recriminations, deceit and poor relationships between owners of mares and stallions. It is a time for particular tact on the part of the veterinarian who should exert the greatest possible effort to reach a conclusive diagnosis, and hopefully establish a definitive etiology.

The fetus and placenta should be thoroughly examined both externally and internally in a situation where the risks of cross-contamination of other mares and the surroundings is minimal. A full examination is performed, specimens taken, and the fetus and placenta properly disposed. Measurement of the foals crown-rump length should be made and it should be examined for the presence (or otherwise) of hair on the mane, muzzle, eyelids and coronet. These will provide a reasonable estimate of the gestational age and this may be compared with the computed gestational age derived from accurate service dates. A full range of samples, including liver, lung, kidney, thymus, lymph node and adrenal gland, should be taken and preserved in 10% formal saline and stomach contents placed in a sterile, iced, sealed bottle. Fresh specimens of all the above organs should also be taken on ice and despatched to the laboratory immediately for virus, bacterial and fungal isolations. Where delay in transit may occur, viral samples may be frozen until suitable transport can be arranged.

Portions of placenta (allanto-chorion) should be taken, for both microbiological examination and histopathology, from the region of the cervical star and any other areas where discoloration or thickening is detected. Samples from the allanto-amnion for bacterial and fungal culture complete the range of specimens needed for a full investigation.

Visual examination of the placenta will also, often, provide indicators as to the future fertility of the mare and potential septic problems which may develop in the neonatal foal. In order to gain familiarity with this important organ, it is necessary to have a good knowledge of the anatomy, function and normal variations of the placenta.

It is beyond the scope of this book to describe the early embryonic changes which occur in the fetus and placenta, apart from some aspects of endometrial cup-formation and their recognition as part of the embryological development of the structure found in the mature placenta. Embryologically, the chorionic girdle cells of the conceptus invade the maternal endometrium to cause implantation after about 35 days. This leads to the formation of distinctive irregular plaques of tissue, the endometrial cups (*see* **757**) which form a disconnected ring of tissue at the point of implantation, which usually occurs at the mesometrial side of the uterus at the caudal end of one horn.

Due to the developmental relationship of the girdle cells to the allantoic stalk, the umbilical cord is always located at the centre of the ring of cups. Physiologically the endometrial cups consist of trophoblast cells derived from the girdle cells, and are responsible for the production of (equine) chorionic gonadotropin. While the endometrial cups occupy much of the endometrial stroma in the area of implantation, they do not destroy the underlying endometrial glands and indeed, may in some cases even implant on structures such as endometrial cysts (**870**) without any other detectable abnormalities or deficiencies. The endometrial cups gradually become less recognisable as they regress, usually from about Day 130. Their regression however does leave remnants and scars in the placenta (**871**) and in some cases the resultant sloughed endometrial surface forms the core of allantoic pouches which frequently project into the allantoic cavity (**872**). Examination of the placenta in the area of attachment characteristically shows a ring of cup remnants surrounding a central avillous area (caused by the remains of the yolk sac) (**873**).

Embryologically, the placental circulation gradually takes over the function of the yolk sac circulation from about Day 60. The allantois, which becomes visible from about Day 20, grows rapidly to assume the major blood supply to the chorion at about Day 30. The fused

870

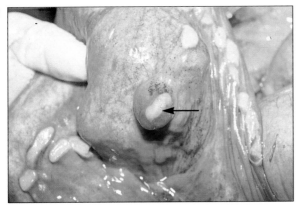

870 Endometrial cups (day 70).
Note: Normal interrupted ring of cups on the uterine wall. Endometrial cup implanted on uterine cyst (arrow).

871

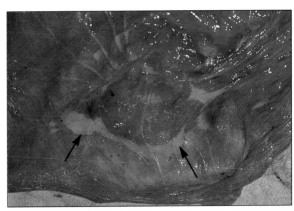

871 Endometrial cups (scars).
Note: Full term placenta showing endometrial cup remnants (scars)(arrows).

872

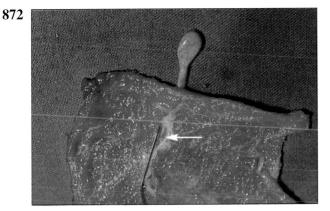

872 Chorionic (endometrial) pouch.
Note: Segment of placenta showing remnant of endometrial scar on chorionic surface (arrow) and formation of endometrial pouch and stalk (on allantoic side).

873

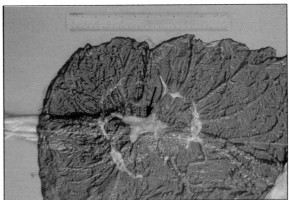

873 Endometrial cups (scars) and central avillous area.
Note: Full term placenta showing interrupted circle of endometrial cup remnants around a central avillous area (arrow). Allantoic blood vessels arise on allantoic surface opposite this area.

chorion and allantois (the allanto-chorion) then attaches to the endometrium to form the placenta.

The gross anatomical features of the placenta may be visualised best by placing the easily identified cord and the two uterine horns in the form of an 'E' configuration on an open flat surface (**874**). Normal structures which can then be observed from the inverted allanto-chorion (*see* **874**) are the thickened (edematous) pregnant horn, the much thinner, smaller, non-pregnant horn, the body, the umbilical cord, and the attached allanto-amnion.

The placement of the umbilical cord may be close to the non-pregnant horn (*see* **874**) or the pregnant horn (**875**) or may be located at some place intermediate between these two locations (**876**). The variation in this location is related to the trans-uterine migration of the fetus which occurs in some mares after implantation occurs. There is no migration of the point of implantation over the surface of the endometrium.

Examination of the chorionic surface of the normal placenta shows normal avillous structures such as the placental star (**877**). This scarred area is the site of rupture during normal parturition, and represents the point of contact between the avillous cervix and the chorionic surface of the placenta. The avillous imprint of the opening of the oviduct is usually also obvious (**878**). Also, folds in the chorion appear as avillous areas of varying size and location. A particular and very important situation occurs with twinning, where one developing chorion abuts against the other, resulting in the development of a relatively large avillous area (**879**). This deficit can usually be identified no matter what stage of pregnancy has been reached before absorption, abortion or full time delivery occurs and its recognition is of paramount importance to the equine obstetrician.

874

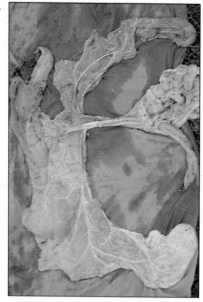

875

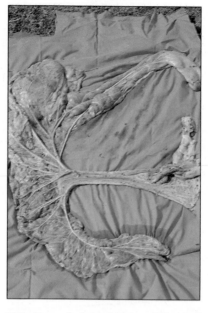

874 Normal placenta (viewed from allantoic side).
Note: Attachment of umbilical cord close to smaller, non-pregnant horn.

875 Normal placenta (viewed from allantoic side).
Note: Attachment of umbilical cord in larger, pregnant horn.

876

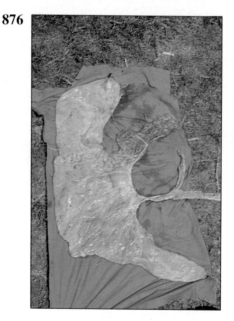

877

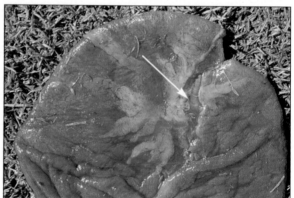

876 Normal placenta (viewed from allantoic side).
Note: Attachment of cord centrally between the uterine horns.

877 Normal placenta (showing placental star).
Note: Normal foaling, showing delivery tear in star region (arrow).

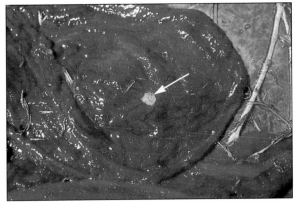

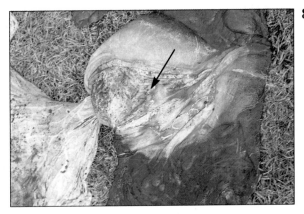

878 Normal placenta (avillous area of oviduct opening) (arrow) in pregnant horn.
Note: Thickened, more edematous appearance of the tip of the pregnant horn.

879 Twin pregnancy placenta.
Note: Heavily fibrous area (arrow) where opposing surfaces of twin placentas abut. Normal villous placental surface visible above and below avillous area.

Non-Infectious Disorders

Twinning

Twinning in horses is widely feared amongst breeders and a variety of permutations can be encountered. One apparently normal twin and the placental remnant of the second fetus (**880**), or abortion of a resorbing twin with a dead premature foal (**881**) may be detected. Alternatively, there may be a full term delivery of twins, either both alive, one alive or both dead. (Triplets are exceptionally rare and are not viable).

The placentas of all types of twinning are very characteristic and show marked fibrosis at the common site of contact (**882**). Care should always be taken to examine both sides of the placenta as viewing of a twin placenta from the allantoic side only, could be misleading if only one placenta and foal had been found (**883**). It is certainly true that almost all twin foals which are born alive (either at full term or before term) are handicapped by having a poor placental surface area. Most experienced equine obstetricians consider that all twins are dysmature regardless of their gestational age.

Placental defects

The presence of specks of material known as '**amnionic pustules**' (**884**) are frequent findings on the umbilical cord and amnion. There is no evidence to suggest that these are in fact pustules or have any inflammatory origin and are probably normal depositions of urinary salts.

Serious, and sometimes even minor, defects in the development of the placenta (and/or its individual components), almost always results in abortion but some embryological structures may remain and become calcified, such as a **yolk sac remnant** found in the infundibulum (**885**). Deposition of calcium salts in plaques in various locations on the urachus and amnion

may become twisted and further calcified, leading to quite large calcified structures (**886**). These are often mistaken for fetal remnants. Dilatations of the urachal vessel to the allanto-amnion can give rise to urachal cysts (**887**).

A bifid, non-pregnant horn (**888**) is an unusual developmental defect of the placenta. Both segments of the apparently divided horn are fully villous, with no avillous areas present, such as would be seen with abutting twin placentas. This situation suggests that there might be a bifid uterine horn in these mares but such an anatomical abnormality has not been described.

880

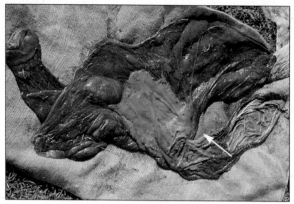

880 Twin pregnancy (remnants of resorbed twin fetus) (arrow).
Note: Live twin was normal but somewhat small for breed and showed a prolonged adaptive period.

881

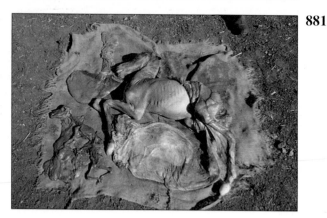

881 Twin pregnancy (resorption and abortion).
Note: Abortion at 7 months; poorly conditioned larger fetus and resorbed mummified, very small fetus.

882

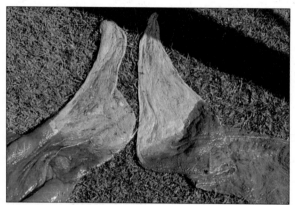

882 Twin pregnancy placenta (viewed from chorionic side) (large avillous fibrous area of apposition of placentas from twins).
Note: Both foals born alive but small and both showed slow adaptation.

883

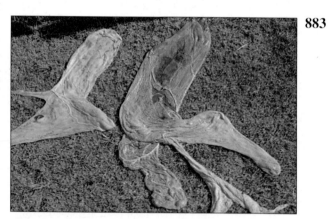

883 Twin pregnancy placenta (viewed from allantoic side).
Note: Same placentas as **882** viewed from allantoic side.

884

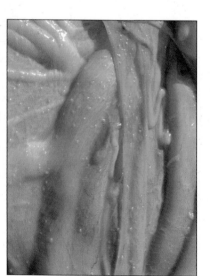

885

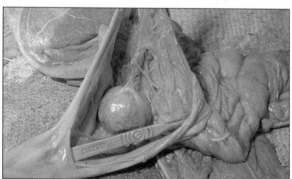

884 Amnionic 'pustules'.
Note: Probably normal deposits of urinary salts in amnion.

885 Calcified yolk sac remnant (contained in infundibulum).

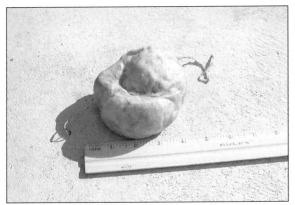

886 Calcified plaque (remnant of calcified area of urachal vessel).

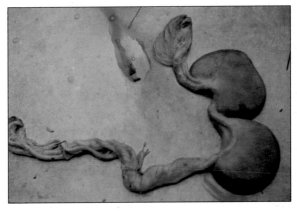

887 Urachal cysts.
Note: Compression and twisting of urachus may lead to sacculation - the so-called urachal cysts.

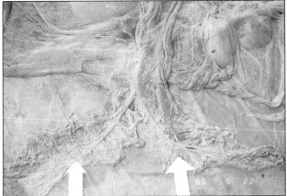

888 Bifid non-pregnant horn abnormality (viewed from amnionic side).
Note: Showing distribution of blood vessels in the divided chorio-allantois (arrows).

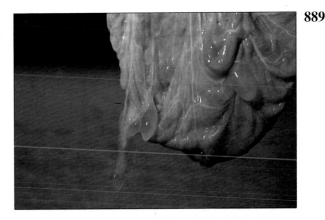

889 Chorionic cysts / edema (resembling cysts) of allantoic surface of chorion.
Note: Placenta from premature foal. Also seen in specimens taken from normal, near-term mares.

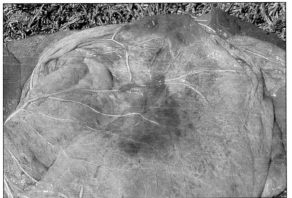

890 Intramural hemorrhage.
Note: Caused by foal kick, resulted in perforation of mare's uterus (see **771**).

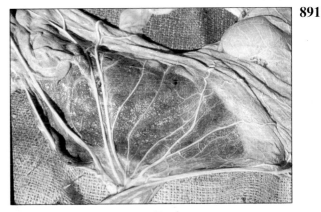

891 Placental hemorrhage (moderate).
Note: Foal lethargic, slow to rise, slow to suckle; normal after 3 days.

Physical disorders of the placenta

A wide variety of physical changes may be detected in the placenta. Edema of the inside surface of the chorion (with cyst-like formation) (**889**) is most frequently seen in placentas from premature deliveries or in apparently normal, pre-term placentas from mares which are examined after death for other reasons. The significance of the 'defect' is equivocal but it would seem likely that circulatory and inflammatory factors may be involved in some cases while in others it may be an entirely incidental (normal) occurrence.

Severe foal struggling or abnormal pressure within the uterine wall-allanto-chorionic interface due to uterine contractions, causes **hemorrhage into the allanto-chorion**. This may be mild (**890**), more extensive (**891**) or severe and life-threatening to the foal (**892**). Large **hematomas** may develop at the site of such hemorrhage (**893**). Other indications of fetal stress related to malpositioning include tears through the body of the allanto-chorion other than at the cervical star, and the presence of meconium staining of both the foal (**894**) and the placental contents. In all these circumstances the placental (or fetal) findings are indicators of excessive fetal movement which is possibly due to fetal stress. Any of these may be found associated with abortion or sometimes with normal delivery of foals which are slow to adapt and may be affected by the neonatal maladjustment syndrome (*see* **676**). Careful placental examinations may provide some effective indicators of impending problems and provide the clinician with an opportunity to take appropriate preventive measures.

The umbilical cord is normally twisted on its length. Up to 6 – 9 twists may be observed in normal foals *in utero* and it is unlikely that these are of any significance with respect to umbilical efficiency. These normal twists are usually evenly distributed and the cord lacks obvious constrictions in its length (**895**).

The length of the umbilical cord is variable. In the Thoroughbred it is approximately 85 cm long at term, and is related to the attachment area on the allanto-chorion. Longer cords may have a greater tendency to become more twisted than shorter cords; a normal number of 6 to 9 twists can be found on most, but where this number is grossly exceeded, compromise to the fetal circulation may well occur, leading to abortion. Pathologically significant twisted umbilical cords show irregular twists and areas of passive congestion in the umbilical vessels (**896**). Foals with shorter cords appear to be more liable to fetal stress syndromes immediately prior to, and during, delivery and it is easy to imagine that these might be more affected by fewer twists. This may lead to earlier vascular occlusion during delivery. In these cases fetal distress or even death may ensue. While rotation of the fetus on the cord is normal, it does always require total rotations of the fetus. Where a portion of the fetus (such as the head and neck, or one limb) is prevented from attaining a normal position during these twists, circulatory compromise may occur in the fetus. Usually such compromise results in rapid fetal death and subsequent abortion (**897**).

Other physical events which may terminate pregnancy are travel, galloping by heavily pregnant mares, fetal death/resorption, and forced service in pregnant mares (**898**). A detailed history and examination of the foal and the placenta usually establishes the relevant unusual features of management or behaviour.

892

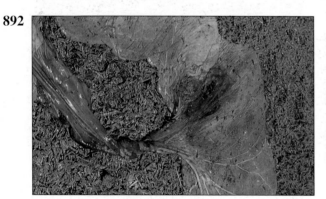

892 Placental hemorrhage (severe).
Note: Foal anemic and weak, and required supportive therapy for 5 – 6 days post partum.

893

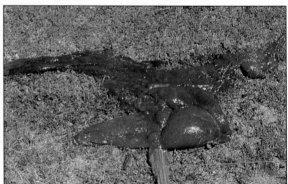

893 Placental hemorrhage (severe).
Note: Same placenta as **892**, viewed from chorionic surface, showing considerable blood clot lodged in placental wall.

894

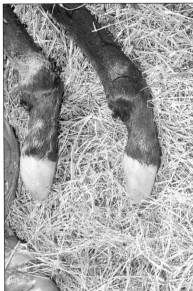

895

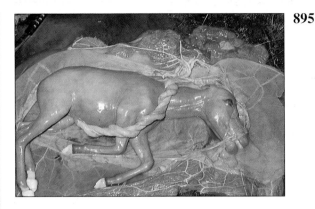

894 Meconium staining.
Note: Placenta also stained; indicative of fetal distress prior to or during parturition. This foal was born dead.

895 Umbilical cord twisting (normal 8 month fetus *in situ*).
Note: Mare killed for other reasons. Normal, regular twisting of cord.

896

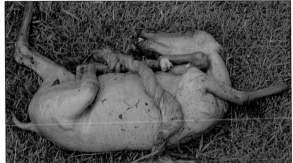

897

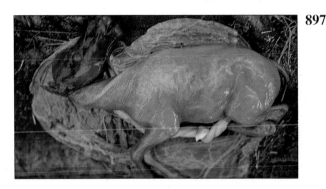

896 Umbilical cord twisting (excessive) (Approximately 8 month fetus).
Note: Foal aborted. Note anoxia (blue skin), excessive irregular twists and distortion of umbilical cord.

897 Malposition of foal's head leads to asphyxia (8 to 8½ month fetus).
Note: Severe cyanosis of head from mal-positioning in uterus, leading to asphyxia; cord, itself normal.

898

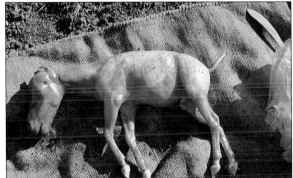

899

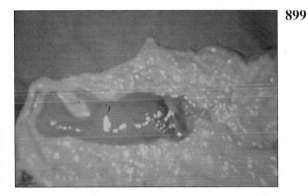

898 Fetal trauma.
Note: Mare approximately 6 months pregnant showed strong estrus behaviour, including willingness to be covered. Aborted foal 30 minutes later. Severe subcutaneous hemorrhage (bruising) of foal's skin; mare had retained fetal membranes for 4 days.

899 Fetal resorption (80 days).
Note: Aborted membranes with autolysed fetus enclosed.

Fetal resorption

Fetal resorption is a frustrating and expensive problem encountered in many mares, which may be related to a host of conditions associated with the immediate uterine environment and the health status of the mare, as well as the genetic, physical and nutritional development of the foal. Uterine infections, uterine fibrosis and glandular abnormalities, poor nutritional status of the mare, hormonal imbalances, twinning (and many other reasons for the development of a hostile uterine environment), are possible factors. Fetal resorption may occur as early as 15 days. In the case of twins embryonic reduction of (one or both) embryo(s) occurs naturally through to 70 – 80 days. The resorbing remnants of foals (**899**) may be only clinically observed in those mares which abort, and only luck dictates that the very small amount of aborted membranes and the foal are actually found. Ultrasonographic monitoring of pregnancies may provide definitive proof of resorption in some mares, and particularly in those which resorb early, when monitoring is usually performed. Later stage fetal resorption or mummification may pass unnoticed until the expected pregnancy fails to result in delivery on the expected date. It is more likely that twinning is responsible for later fetal resorption and this may be seen at any stage from 70 days to full term, either as increased areas of brown necrotic mucoid material on a normal placenta or one (or two) larger, more mummified fetus(es) (**900**).

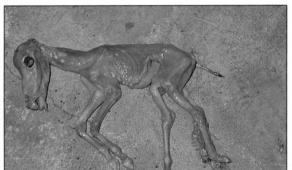

900 Fetal resorption (twin foal).
Note: Advanced autolysis resulting in abortion at 7½ months, along with otherwise normally developed but non-viable foal.

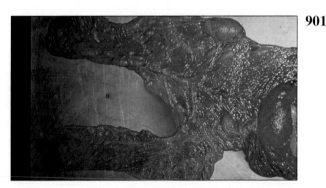

901 Body pregnancy (fetal abortion).
Note: Chorionic side of placenta displaying two equal size and density horns of a type typical of a non-pregnant horn.

Body pregnancy

Body pregnancy (fetal development within the uterine body instead of either of the uterine horns) almost always has marked effects upon the development of the fetus. These terminate either in abortion, or a premature foal (gestational age of less than 320 days) or a dysmature foal (a foal born after a normal gestational period but with characteristics of prematurity). The placentas of these cases characteristically show placental horns of equal size and density (**901**) and the allantoic surface frequently shows edema and cystic formations (**902**).

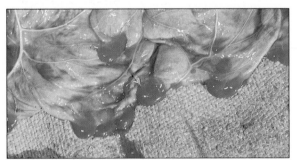

902 Body pregnancy (full-term) (allantoic pouches).
Note: Foal was alive but undersized, undernourished and underweight and died in a few hours. Edema and cystic condition of allantoic lining.

Premature placental separation

Premature placental separation is a very serious complication of parturition. It may cause death of a full term fetus as a result of serious hypoxia if delivery is delayed at all. As the term implies, separation of the placenta occurs before normal delivery of the foal, thereby depriving the foal of adequate gaseous-exchanges. It is, furthermore, uncommon for the placenta to separate over limited areas only. More usually the entire placenta separates within a short period of time, making delivery all the more urgent. The condition can be recognised by the appearance of the placental star at the vulva and the enclosed legs of the fetus, the so called 'red-bag' delivery (**903**). In normal placental separation, the placenta ruptures at the cervical star and this remains within the vagina following delivery of the foal, but with premature separation, the placenta continues to be expelled with, eventually, either complete or incomplete tearing of the placenta in the mid-body, with delivery of the foal. All foals which are delivered under these conditions are compromised to some extent and many are born dead. It is imperative that this particular problem of parturition is recognised and acted upon as an extreme emergency.

903

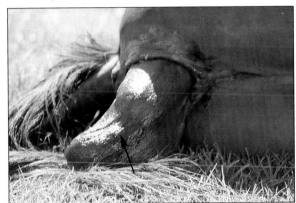

903 Premature placental separation ('red-bag' delivery). **Note:** Supervised parturition. Placental star (arrow), presence of chorionic surface of placenta extruded more than normal; foal only slightly depressed at birth. Full recovery.

Infectious diseases

Viral Diseases: Infection with **equine herpes virus-1** is capable of causing respiratory disease (*see* **211**), posterior paralysis (*see* **728**) and is a particularly common cause of abortion (*see* **212**). Foals which are infected *in utero* are usually born dead or very weak, succumbing early to a progressive pneumonia (and other organ failure). Abortion may occur at any time between 7 months and full term, and usually occurs without any sign of illness in the mare. The disease is spread by ingestion of the virus from contaminated food or water, or from contact with an infected placenta, fetus or uterine discharges from an aborted mare. The nasal discharges from infected horses are particularly liable to transmit the condition, which is highly contagious. Abortion may occur singly or as a 'storm', involving several (or more) mares under the same management and severe losses have been reported, even in vaccinated mares. When abortion occurs, there is rapid separation of the placenta within the uterus. The fetus is often delivered within the placenta, with the chorionic side of the placenta still on the outside - the so called '**red-bag**' **abortion**. Some pregnancies may continue to full-term, but the foals are usually weak and most die from intractable virus pneumonia (*see* **212**) and/or hepatic and adrenal collapse within 10 days. The fetus may show any number of gross lesions such as subcutaneous edema, jaundice, increased body fluids, and an enlarged liver with varying numbers of 1 mm diameter, whitish-yellow, necrotic foci. The placenta is either normal in appearance and consistency, or the chorion has a much-thickened, edematous, red appearance. It is either delivered immediately with the foal, or shortly afterwards. Retention of fetal membranes under these conditions is particularly unusual.

Abortion is a very common clinical sign associated with **equine viral arteritis** and usually occurs within a few days of the onset of clinical signs. Mares may be infected via the respiratory tract or venereally. There are no remarkable lesions of either placentas or aborted foals in case reports of this disease. Experimental infections have suggested that abortion is due to fetal anoxia caused by myometrial vessel compression which is in turn due to edema in the uterine walls.

Bacterial Diseases: Although placental histo-pathology and bacterial cultures are frequently unrewarding, no opportunity should be missed to extend our knowledge of these conditions. Diligent and meticulous sampling does occasionally reward the clinician with possible pathogens in some cases.

Bacterial infection of the placenta (**bacterial placentitis**) may be as a result of residual infection of the endometrial crypts and/or glands prior to conception. It may also occur from a patent cervix or from hema-togenous infection. The most common placental findings are usually related to the placental star area (*see* **877**), which becomes thickened, edematous and inflamed (**904**). There is usually an accompanying, obviously muco-purulent discharge from the mare (**905**). In some cases these areas can be more generalised, or, where chronic endometrial gland infection has occurred, there may be more generalised placental changes (**906**). The colour changes from the normal, rich red/brown to yellow-brown in the area associated with infection and necrosis (**907**). More severe inflammation in the uterine mucosa will result in an increased production of mucoid material from the chorio-allantoic - uterine junction, and this leads to

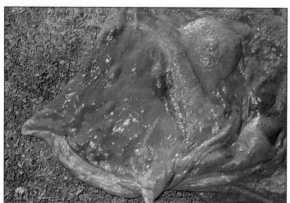

904 Placentitis (placental star region) (full-term placenta).
Note: Weak, sickly, septicemic foal, died after 24 hours. Thickened, inflamed placental star with purulent exudate over surface.

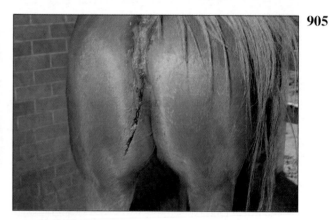

905 Placentitis (vulval discharge).
Note: Four weeks pre-partum. The mare had been running milk, and delivered a live but weak and small foal which survived; a large area of the placenta showed a yellow, necrotic area of villous degeneration.

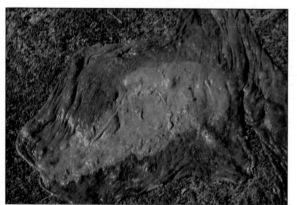

906 Placentitis (bacterial).
Note: Mare foaled premature, weak, septicemic foal which died after 24 hours. Large areas of placenta show mucoid, 'putty'-like degenerative changes. *Escherichia coli* isolated from placenta and foal.

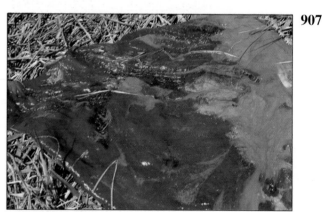

907 Placentitis.
Note: Mare delivered full-term, normal foal which developed neonatal maladjustment syndrome within 24 hours; placenta showed marked degenerative (yellow area) changes over approximately ⅓ of placental surface; more than 3 sites involved; no organisms cultured but bacterial bacilli seen in sections of affected area.

large aggregations of a putty-like material (**908**). This should be carefully examined, as it may contain remnants of resorbed foals. Placentas affected in this way are often associated with premature running of milk and the premature delivery of weak septicemic foals.

Bacterial infection causing inflammatory changes to the blood vessels has been found in some mares. The appearance of the placenta in these infections is variable and related largely to the species of organism involved and the duration and route of infection. Infections associated with *Klebsiella* spp. produce a characteristic

diffuse and often severe, inflammatory change along the placental blood vessels (**909**) while that due to *Streptococcus* spp. tends to be less severe but more extensive (**910**), involving blood vessels over almost the entire placental surface. **Bacterial infection of the embryonic yolk sac** also occurs and is usually found as a result of an abortion investigation (**911**). Bacterial infection causing abortion may also present a normal yolk sac area with green coloration of the entire allantois, probably as a result of concurrent placental hemorrhage and consequent hemoglobin breakdown (**912**).

908

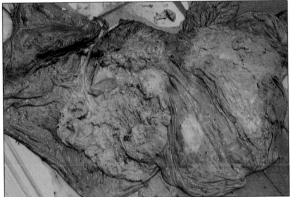

908 Placentitis.
Note: Mare aborted foal near full-term; placenta showed aggregation of thick 'putty'-like, mucoid material in more than 3 locations in the body of the uterus. Cultures were negative.

909

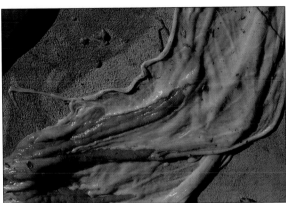

909 Placentitis (*Klebsiella pneumoniae*).
Note: Bacterial infection extending from yolk sac area along blood vessels. Foal born dead.

910

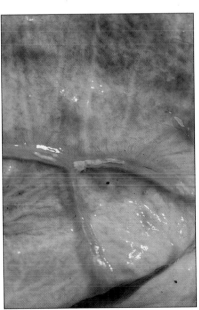

910 Placentitis (ß-hemolytic *Streptococcus*).
Note: Premature foal survived. ß-hemolytic *Streptococcus* isolated from placenta and foal.

911

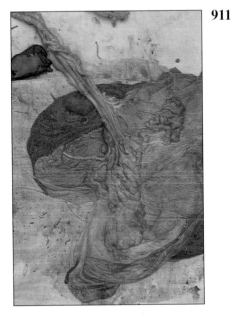

911 Yolk sac infection.
Note: Aborted fetus (7 months). No organisms isolated, foal dead for some period of time before delivery; autolysis present.

912

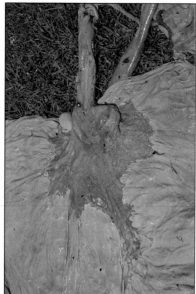

913

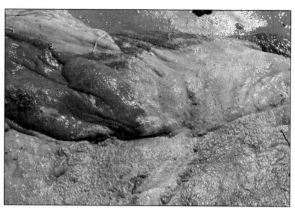

912 Discoloured placenta (aborted 9 months).
Note: Normal coloration of endometrial cup and yolk sac areas with obvious green discoloration of allantoic surface; possibly related to hemorrhage between uterus and placenta with pigment staining of placenta (possibly associated with blood pigments).

913 Fungal placentitis (diffuse form).
Note: Placental star area shows grey-brown, infected, leathery placenta. Premature foal, born dead. *Aspergillus* spp. fungus isolated.

Fungal Diseases: Fungal placentitis is not common but occurs under similar circumstances and in similar locations as the bacterial infections. While it is more commonly located in the region of the placental star (**913**), suggesting that the likely route of infection is via the cervix, it may occur in other locations, such as body and horn extremities (**914**). Clinically the lesions appear as thickened, leather-like areas around the placental star or edematous avillous areas, with a tenacious exudate of brownish mucus in other areas of the placenta. These areas of avillous necrosis often lead to poor intra-uterine nutrition for the foal and commonly lead to abortion, with a severely malnourished foal (**915**); lesions may also be present in the foal, and therefore, stomach contents should always be taken for a microbiological study. **Aspergillus** spp are the commonest isolates both from placenta and fetus.

914

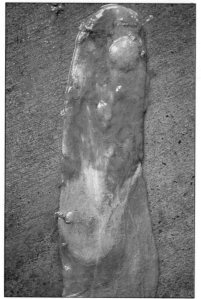

915

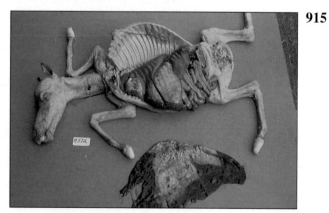

914 Fungal placentitis (focal or horn form).
Note: Lesion restricted to pregnant horn; premature dead foal. *Aspergillus* spp isolated.

915 Fungal placentitis (chronic form).
Note: Aborted foal shows marked malnutrition.

Further reading

Current Therapy in Equine Medicine (2) Ed. Robinson, N.E. (1987) W B Saunders, Philadelphia USA

Current Therapy in Equine Medicine (2) Ed. Robinson, N.E. (1987) W B Saunders, Philadelphia USA

Equine Stud Farm Medicine Rossdale, P.D. and Ricketts, S.W. (1980) Ballière Tindall, London, UK

Surgery of the Reproductive Tract Cox, J.E. (1987) Liverpool University Press, Liverpool, UK

Fertility and Obstetrics in the Horse Allen, W.E. (1988) Blackwell Scientific Publications, Oxford, UK

Pathology of Domestic Animals (3rd Edition) Jubb, K.V.F., Kennedy, P.C. and Palmer, N. (1985) Academic Press, Philadelphia, USA

Manual of Equine Practice Rose and Hodgson W B Saunders

Equine Reproduction McKinnon A.O. and Voss, J.L. (1992) Lea & Febiger

Fertility and Obstetrics in the Horse; Allen, W.E. (1988) Blackwell Scientific Publications;

Diseases and Management of Breeding Stallions D.D. Varner, J. Schumacher, T.L. Blanchard, L. Johnson (1991), American Veterinary Publications

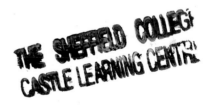

Index